Ocular Manifestations of Systemic Disease

OCULAR MANIFESTATIONS OF SYSTEMIC DISEASE

Edited by

Bernard H. Blaustein, O.D.

Associate Professor
Department of Clinical Sciences
The Eye Institute
Pennsylvania College of Optometry
Philadelphia, Pennsylvania
Chief
Optometry Services
Veterans Affairs Medical Center
Coatesville, Pennsylvania

Churchill Livingstone
New York, Edinburgh, London, Madrid, Melbourne, Milan, Tokyo

Library of Congress Cataloging-in-Publication Data

Ocular manifestations of systemic disease / edited by Bernard H.
　Blaustein.
　　　　p.　　cm.
　　Includes bibliographical references and index.
　　ISBN 0-443-08883-7
　　1. Ocular manifestations of general diseases.　I. Blaustein,
Bernard H.
　　[DNLM: 1. Eye Manifestations.　WW 475 021 1994]
　RE65.026　1994
　617.7—dc20
　DNLM/DLC
　for Library of Congress　　　　　　　　　94-22058
　　　　　　　　　　　　　　　　　　　　CIP

Distributed in the United Kingdom by Churchill Livingstone, Robert Stevenson House, 1–3 Baxter's Place, Leith Walk, Edinburgh EH1 3AF, and by associated companies, branches, and representatives throughout the world.

Accurate indications, adverse reactions, and dosage schedules for drugs are provided in this book, but it is possible that they may change. The reader is urged to review the package information data of the manufacturers of the medications mentioned.

The Publishers have made every effort to trace the copyright holders for borrowed material. If they have inadvertently overlooked any, they will be pleased to make the necessary arrangements at the first opportunity.

Acquisitions Editor: *Carol Bader*
Copy Editor: *Elizabeth Bowman-Schulman*
Production Supervisor: *Sharon Tuder*
Cover Design: *Jeanette Jacobs*

Printed in the United States of America

First published in 1994　　　7　6　5　4　3　2　1

Contributors

John L. Baker, O.D.
Associate Professor and Director of Clinical Residencies, Illinois College of Optometry, Chicago, Illinois

G. Richard Bennett, M.S., O.D.
Associate Professor, Department of Clinical Sciences, The Eye Institute, Pennsylvania College of Optometry; Adjunct Associate Professor, Department of Ophthalmology, Hahnemann University School of Medicine, Philadelphia, Pennsylvania

Bernard H. Blaustein, O.D.
Associate Professor, Department of Clinical Sciences, The Eye Institute, Pennsylvania College of Optometry, Philadelphia, Pennsylvania; Chief, Optometry Services, Veterans Affairs Medical Center, Coatesville, Pennsylvania

Chris J. Cakanac, O.D.
Clinical Instructor, Department of Ophthalmology, The Eye and Ear Institute, University of Pittsburgh School of Medicine, Pittsburgh, Pennsylvania; Adjunct Faculty, Pennsylvania College of Optometry, Philadelphia, Pennsylvania

Connie L. Chronister, O.D.
Associate Professor, Department of Clinical Sciences, The Eye Institute, Pennsylvania College of Optometry; Consultant, Department of Optometry, Sidney Hillman Medical Center, Philadelphia, Pennsylvania

John E. Conto, O.D.
Associate Professor, Department of Clinical Education, Illinois Eye Institute, Illinois College of Optometry, Chicago, Illinois

Sarah L. Foster, O.D.
Clinical Instructor, Department of Clinical Sciences, The Eye Institute, Pennsylvania College of Optometry, Philadelphia, Pennsylvania; Consultant, The Nemours Health Clinic, Wilmington, Delaware

Andrew S. Gurwood, O.D.
Assistant Professor, Department of Clinical Sciences, The Eye Institute, Pennsylvania College of Optometry, Philadelphia, Pennsylvania

Nicky R. Holdeman, O.D., M.D.
Associate Professor, University of Houston College of Optometry; Chief of Medical Services and Director, University Eye Institute, Houston, Texas

Helene M. Kaiser, O.D.
Assistant Professor, Department of Clinical Sciences, The Eye Institute, Pennsylvania College of Optometry, Philadelphia, Pennsylvania

Brian P. Mahoney, O.D.

Associate Professor, State University of New York College of Optometry, New York, New York; Associate Professor, Pennsylvania College of Optometry, Philadelphia, Pennsylvania; Chief, Optometry Services, Department of Veterans Affairs Medical and Regional Office Center, Wilmington, Delaware

Susan E. Marren, O.D.

Assistant Professor, Department of Clinical Sciences, The Eye Institute, Pennsylvania College of Optometry, Philadelphia, Pennsylvania

Jean Marie Pagani, O.D.

Instructor, Department of Physiology and Clinical Medicine, Pennsylvania College of Optometry; Clinical Instructor, Department of Clinical Sciences, The Eye Institute, Pennsylvania College of Optometry, Philadelphia, Pennsylvania; Consultant, The Nemours Health Clinic, Wilmington, Delaware

Anastas F. Pass, M.S., O.D.

Assistant Professor, University of Houston College of Optometry; Director, Emergency Care, University Eye Institute, Houston, Texas

Marcus G. Piccolo, O.D.

Associate Professor, University of Houston College of Optometry; Attending Optometrist, Medical Clinic, University Eye Institute, Houston, Texas

Mark Sawamura, O.D.

Clinical Instructor, Southern California College of Optometry, Fullerton, California

Mark A. Shust, O.D.

Clinical Consultant, Department of Optometry, Sidney Hillman Medical Center, Philadelphia, Pennsylvania

George E. White, O.D.

Associate Professor, Department of Clinical Sciences, The Eye Institute, Pennsylvania College of Optometry; Director of Eye Services, Department of Ophthalmology, John F. Kennedy Memorial Hospital, Philadelphia, Pennsylvania

Preface

To the poet, the eyes are the windows to the soul. To the optometrist, the eyes are the windows to the general state of the patient's health. Indeed, many systemic diseases manifest initially in the eyes or ocular adnexa.

Ocular Manifestations of Systemic Disease discusses a broad range of diseases and conditions in a manner relevant for the practicing optometrist. The book includes many topics not typically reviewed in the optometric literature: the ocular manifestations of substance abuse, pregnancy, connective tissue disease, metabolic disease, oncologic disease, hematologic disease, and the phakomatoses.

To ensure clinical relevance, each chapter revolves around a prototypical case presentation. Emphasis is placed on the pertinent tests and procedures that the clinician should perform to establish a differential diagnosis. Chapters on laboratory testing and neuroimaging techniques are included to assist the clinician in interpreting enigmatic clinical data. The pathophysiology of the disease process is also emphasized so that the reader may gain a conceptual understanding of the ocular manifestations. Finally, the specific management of the ocular manifestations of the disease are addressed as well as ways the optometrist can participate in the total care of the patient.

The authors were carefully selected for their skill as optometric clinicians and educators with a particular expertise in the area covered. All have worked hard to bring this book to fruition. I am in their debt for their contributions. Also, special thanks are due to Ms. Jane Stein of The Eye Institute of the Pennsylvania College of Optometry for the many excellent photographs.

Finally, I must acknowledge the help of Ms. Carol Bader and Ms. Elizabeth Bowman of Churchill Livingstone who never flagged in their support and assistance. During the many moments that the editor doubted that this project would ever be completed, Ms. Bader and Ms. Bowman were ever reassuring.

Bernard H. Blaustein, O.D.

Contents

Color plates appear following page 214.

1 Laboratory Tests

JEAN MARIE PAGANI

INTRODUCTION

The optometrist, as the primary eye care practitioner, must be familiar with basic laboratory diagnostic testing. The optometrist can use laboratory blood analysis as a screening device for disease, to format a working differential diagnosis, or to confirm a clinical impression. Laboratory blood testing can also give baseline information to monitor a patient's condition and demonstrate the effectiveness of therapeutic treatment.[1] Information gained from appropriate laboratory blood testing can be invaluable to the optometrist to ensure the correct diagnosis and management of the patient.

This chapter focuses on common laboratory blood tests of hematology, serum blood chemistry analysis, serology/immunology studies, serologic analysis of infectious disease, and laboratory analysis of disorders of the endocrine system.

HEMATOLOGY

The laboratory hematologic work-up of a patient suspected of having a systemic disease with ocular manifestations includes the complete blood cell count (CBC) with red blood cell (RBC) indices and white blood cell (WBC) differential (Table 1-1).

The CBC is ordered from the hematology laboratory to evaluate the body's reaction to inflammation or infection. It also indicates the presence of anemias, leukemias, polycythemias, and other disease processes.[2] The CBC permits individual assessment of RBCs, WBCs, and platelets. Each of these is reviewed.

The RBC transports oxygen to the tissues and maintains hemoglobin function. Additionally, the RBC helps to rid the tissue of carbon dioxide and acts as an acid–base buffer of the blood.[3] RBCs must maneuver through the small capillaries in the microcirculation. Diseases of RBCs include disorders of RBC formation, anemias caused by excessive RBC loss, and disorders of hemoglobin synthesis.[4] The RBC count is a measure of erythrocytes per cubic millimeter of peripheral blood. The RBC parameters, listed in Table 1-2, help to differentiate between the various types and causes of RBC disease, such as iron-deficiency anemia, thalassemia, vitamin B_6 and B_{12} deficiency, and pernicious anemia.[5]

The WBC functions as the mobile element of the body's protective system. It is formed in the bone marrow and in the lymph tissue and then transported in the blood to those parts of the body where it acts against infectious agents.[3] The WBC count, or leukocyte count, is a measure of WBCs per cubic millimeter of whole blood. The differential WBC count determines the qualitative and quantitative variations in the WBC numbers[6] (Table 1-3).

Table 1-1. The Complete Blood Count With Indices and Differential

Red blood cell
    Red blood cell count
    Red blood cell morphology
    Red blood cell indices
        Mean cell volume
        Mean cell hemoglobin
        Mean cell hemoglobin concentration
    Red cell distribution width
    Hematocrit
    Hemoglobin
White blood cell
    White blood cell count
    White blood cell differential
        Granular basophils, eosinophils, neutrophils
        Agranular lymphocytes, monocytes
Platelet count

Table 1-2. Red Blood Cell Tests and Definition

Red Blood Cell Tests	Definition
Red blood cell count	Red blood cells per cubic millimeter of peripheral blood
Red blood cell morphology	Manual review of red blood cells
Red blood cell indices	
Mean cell volume	Size of average red blood cell
Mean cell hemoglobin	Weight of hemoglobin/cell
Mean cell hemoglobin concentration	Amount of hemoglobin in average red blood cell as compared to its size (%)
Red cell distribution width	Index of size variation of red blood cells
Hematocrit	Packed red blood cell volume (%)
Hemoglobin	Index of oxygen-carrying capacity of blood

Table 1-3. White Blood Cell Differential

Types of Leukocyte	Increase or Decrease in Differential Count	Example
Neutrophils	↑ Infection Inflammation Hematologic disorders Physical/emotional stimulation ↓ Infections Hematologic disorders Miscellaneous	Bacterial/viral Rheumatoid arthritis Leukemia, anemia Viral Iron deficiency anemia Shock, cirrhosis
Eosinophils	↑ Allergic disorders Skin disease Hematologic disorders Malignant neoplasms Miscellaneous	Asthma Eczema Pernicious anemia Rheumatoid arthritis, sarcoid, tuberculosis
Basophils	↑ Myeloproliferative disorders Miscellaneous ↓ Endocrine disorders	Chronic myeloid leukemia Hypersensitivity reaction Hyperthyroidism
Lymphocytes	↑ Infection Hematologic disorders ↓ Acute infections	Cytomegalovirus, tuberculosis, syphilis Systemic lupus erythematosus
Monocytes	↑ Infections Granulomotous disease Hematologic disorders Collagen vascular disease ↓ Bone marrow injury	Viral Tuberculosis, syphilis, sarcoid Leukemia Systemic lupus erythematosus, rheumatoid arthritis

↑, increase in differential count; ↓, decrease in differential count. (Adapted from Tietz,[6] with permission.)

Platelets function in clot formation and may serve as a substrate for the coagulation factors in the blood.[2] The platelet count determines the number of platelets per cubic millimeter of whole blood. This number is important for evaluation of bleeding disorders and hemorrhagic diseases.[7]

The CBC gives helpful information for the standard inflammatory work-up, such as in a patient with recurrent uveitis. Also, it is beneficial when evaluating unexplained hemorrhages in the retina and suspected systemic disorders such as anemia and when monitoring the hematologic composition of a patient undergoing drug therapy.

HEMATOLOGIC DISEASE AND GIANT CELL ARTERITIS

Tests used for assessment of hematologic disease and giant cell arteritis are listed in Table 1-4.

Anemia

Anemia by definition is a reduction in RBC mass, measured by a decrease in the concentration of RBCs or hemoglobin, or both in the peripheral blood. The patient with anemia generally has a low hematocrit or hemoglobin concentration. The RBC indices may show abnormalities in the size of the RBCs (mean corpuscular volume) and the color of the RBCs (mean corpuscular hemoglobin concentration). The RBC morphology, performed by microscopic examination of a peripheral blood smear, permits manual evalua-

tion of the RBC changes that may occur in anemia. The reticulocyte count, which is an evaluation of erythropoietic activity, is increased in hemolytic anemias and in acute and chronic hemorrhage.

General Hemoglobinopathies

A pattern of suspicion, characteristic features, and familial studies is extremely important in ascertaining the nature and type of hemoglobinopathy suspected in a patient. A CBC with erythrocyte indices and examination of the erythrocytes of the blood smear, both routine procedures, provide a good starting point to yield information on the presence and degree of hemolytic anemia associated with most of the hemoglobinopathies. The examination of RBC morphology by a peripheral blood smear provides clues in character-

Table 1-4. Hematologic Tests for Hematologic Disease and Giant Cell Arteritis

Anemia	Thalassemia
Complete blood cell count	Complete blood cell
Blood indices	count
Hematocrit	Fetal hemoglobin
Hemoglobin	Hemoglobin
Red blood cell morphology	electrophoresis
Reticulocyte count	Giant Cell Arteritis
General hemoglobinopathies	Complete blood
Complete blood count	count
Blood indices	Histopathology of
Differential count	temporal artery
Fetal hemoglobin	Erythrocyte
Red blood cell morphology	sedimentation rate
Sickle cell preparation	C-reactive protein
Hemoglobin electrophoresis	(quantitative)
Sickle cell anemia	Alkaline phosphatase
Complete blood count	
Sickle cell screening test	
Red blood cell morphology	
Hemoglobin electrophoresis	

izing the hemoglobinopathy. In the normal patient, RBCs are normochromic and normocytic. In the thalassemia syndromes, however, the RBCs are hypochromic and microcytic. In cases of sickle cell anemia, the hematocrit is usually 20 to 30 percent, the peripheral blood smear demonstrates irreversibly sickled RBCs, and the WBC count may be elevated to 12,000 to 15,000/MM^3.[1] If a hemoglobinopathy associated with hemoglobin S is suspected, a sickle cell screening test, such as a sickle cell preparation or the Sickledex is a quick and easy next step. Last, hemoglobin electrophoresis identifies the most common hemoglobinopathies and allows for genetic and clinical classification.

Sickle Cell Anemia

Sickle Cell Screening Tests

Sickle cell screening tests may not be used in the assessment of infants younger than 6 months old.

Sickle Cell Preparation (Slide Test)

Sickle cell preparation is performed by placing a sample of blood on a blood smear and covering it with a clover slip. It is then examined by microscopy for sickle forms after exposure to a reducing agent, such as sodium metabisulfite. Sodium metabisulfite is responsible for oxygen depletion on the slide, which causes erythrocytes that contain hemoglobin S, to

form their characteristic sickle shape. The degree of abnormal sickling is a function of the amount of hemoglobin S per cell. Even in the sickle cell trait, however, where hemoglobin S is approximately 50 percent or less, enough hemoglobin S is present to cause sickling. Sickle cells are formed after about 30 minutes of incubation. This test is positive in hemoglobin SS, SA, SC or S-thalassemia combinations. Thus, it is a screening method, and positive results must be followed by hemoglobin electrophoresis.

Sickle Cell Solubility Testing

Sickle cell solubility testing is available commercially as Sickledex hemoglobin high-salt-solubility test. This is a rapid, simple screening test for the presence of hemoglobin S. A sample of blood is exposed in a test tube to a reagent. Unstable hemoglobins, then precipitate after exposure, producing a turbid solution. This screening method does not differentiate between sickle anemia, trait, and other hemoglobin S genetic variants.[8] Thus, positive results must be followed by hemoglobin electrophoresis.

Hemoglobin Electrophoresis

Hemoglobin electrophoresis is indicated if a positive sickle screening test has been obtained. Many forms of electrophoretic techniques, including alterations in the pH of buffers, ionic strength, and supportive medium, are used in the identification of hemoglobins.[9] The easiest and most common hemoglobin electrophoresis occurs on cellulose acetate or starch gel at a pH of 8.6. Hemoglobin separated by this method can then be quantified by spectrophotographic analysis or densitometry scanning. This technique is useful for detecting hemoglobins A, S, C, E, and D. It does not discriminate between hemoglobin A and F. The characteristic electrophoretic patterns distinguish the normal patient from the patient with sickle cell trait, sickle cell disease, sickle C disease, sickle-thalassemia, thalassemia major, and thalassemia minor. In rare variants, additional testing may be needed from a research laboratory.

Giant Cell Arteritis

Histopathology of the Temporal Artery

A histologic evaluation of the temporal artery is a definitive surgical method to confirm the diagnosis of cranial, giant cell arteritis. A 3.0-cm or larger section of the artery is removed, then examined in serial sections by microscopy.

Erythrocyte Sedimentation Rate

The erythrocyte sedimentation rate (ESR) is a hematology test that determines the rate at which RBCs settle to the bottom of a vertical tube of anticoagulated blood within a specific period. Three laboratory techniques are used: zeta sedimentation rate, Wintrobe method, and Westergren method.[10] The Westergren method is recommended as the standard because of its simplicity and reproducibility.[4] It uses a 200-mm column of anticoagulated blood, diluted 20 percent with saline or sodium citrate solution, which is then allowed to settle for 1 hour. Measurement of the distance from the top of the column of settled RBCs to the top of the fluid level determines the ESR. In normal values, relatively little settling occurs. Normal values for men younger than age 50 are 0 to 15 mm/h; for men older than age 50, 0 to 20 mm/h; for women younger than age 50, 0 to 25 mm/h; and for women older than age 50, 0 to 30 mm/h.[11] Because reference levels may vary, it is imperative to check with the laboratory from which the test was ordered.

The ESR aids in detecting nonspecific activity of infections, inflammatory states, autoimmune disorders, neoplastic conditions, and plasma cell dyscrasias. Additionally, the ESR has value in following disease activity and in monitoring therapy regimens. It is relatively nonspecific for any single disease entity. Yet, it is a moderately sensitive test that is widely used. Finally, a normal ESR does not rule out organic disease. Most acute and chronic inflammatory and neoplastic conditions, however, result in an increase in the ESR.

For the eye care practitioner, the ESR is especially useful in the diagnosis of temporal (cranial or giant cell) arteritis. Generally, the ESR is very high, 60 mm/h or more, when measured in patients with giant cell arteritis. Interpretation, however, should be correlated with the clinical findings of giant cell arteritis, because "normal" levels of 40 mm/h have been documented in some elderly patients, and patients with biopsy-proven giant cell arteritis have had ESR levels of less than 30 mm/h.[12]

C-Reactive Protein Test

The C-reactive protein test (acute-phase reactant), like the ESR, is a nonspecific index of infectious diseases, inflammatory states, and tissue injuries.[2] The C-reactive protein test is used when the ESR is equivocal, because it is more sensitive and responds more rapidly than the ESR. C-reactive protein is a plasma protein, not normally found in blood or body fluids, that rises in response to acute disease and trauma. It rapidly decreases once the process has dissipated. It is measured by a hematologic test that is quantitated by immunologic laboratory methods.

The results of the C-reactive protein test in patients with giant cell arteritis invariably show a rise in C-reactive protein in their blood serum.

Alkaline Phosphatase

Alkaline phosphatase levels may be elevated in the blood of those patients with giant cell arteritis (see the section *Blood Chemistry Analysis*).

Complete Blood Cell Count

Normocytic normochromic anemia, leukocytosis of less than 20,000/mm^3, and a thrombocytosis of less than 1,000,000/mm^3 can be found in patients with giant cell arteritis.[13] (See this section **Hematology.**)

BLOOD CHEMISTRY ANALYSIS

Different chemical substances within the blood can be measured and analyzed. These constituents are related to a particular organ or organ system and can reflect metabolic and physiologic process. Alterations in the chemistry levels of a patient's blood are evaluated when determining a diagnosis of systemic illness and for the planning and monitoring of drug therapy.

Blood chemistries can be ordered as a single test (i.e., serum cholesterol) or in specific groupings referred to as profiles, or panels. Specifically, chemical analysis of the blood and serum is conducted to examine enzymes that are released from cells as a result of cell damage, abnormal cell permeability, or abnormal cellular proliferation. Also included are studies of liver and kidney metabolite waste products being cleared from the blood such as uric acid and blood urea nitrogen. Substances that normally function in the blood such as blood glucose and blood lipid levels are also evaluated.[14] The sequential multiple analysis (SMA-6, SMA-12, Chem 20) are common blood chemistry panels. Table 1-5 is a listing of those constituents included in one of the panels testing for 12 blood chemistries. Panel testing can be less expensive and often is quicker than individually ordered tests. Profiles and

Table 1-5. Chemistry Panel

	Function	Diagnostic Information
Alkaline phosphatase	Enzyme that mediates bone, lung, and liver function	Orbital/bone fracture, Paget's disease, Liver disease, renal disease
Lactate dehydrogenase	Enzyme that participates in glycolytic pathway	Anemias, neoplastic states, hepatitis, liver disease, myocardial infarction (MI)
Aspartate aminotransferase	Enzyme useful to evaluate the liver, heart, and skeletal muscle	Hepatitis, alcoholism, liver disease, myocardial infarction trauma and striated muscle disease
Creatinine kinase	Enzyme indicative of brain, heart, and smooth muscle function	Malignant cancer, MI, myocarditis, skeletal muscle damage
Calcium	Bone formation, neuromuscular excitability, blood coagulation, integrity of membranes, messenger for hormone action	↑ Primary hyperparathyroidism, malignant cancer, granulomatous disease, sarcoidosis, ↓ hypoparathyroidism, vitamin D deficiency
Phosphorus	Inorganic compound involved in structural and metabolic function	Endocrine disease, renal function, bone disease
Cholesterol (total)	Ingested and synthesized in liver; used in skin and hormone function	Atherosclerosis, coronary artery disease
Glucose	Main carbohydrate in production of cellular energy	Diabetes mellitus, endocrine disorders, severe liver disease
Total protein/albumin	Cotransporters and buffers of the blood	Malnutrition, acute chronic inflammation
Bilirubin	Liver and kidney metabolites	Hepatocellular damage
Blood urea nitrogen (BUN)	Liver and kidney metabolites	Chronic renal disease, hypertension
Uric acid	End product of purine metabolism	Renal disease, gout, endocrine disorders

(Adapted from Tietz,[6] with permission.)

panels are considered screening devices. Abnormal results may then be followed by specific blood chemistry level testing.[4]

CARDIOVASCULAR AND CEREBROVASCULAR DISEASE

The diagnostic work-up of the patient with suspected cardiovascular disease or cerebrovascular disease includes a few simple laboratory blood tests (Table 1-6). The purposes of the CBC blood chemistry panel, and urinalysis are to look for a curable cause of hypertension; to look for organ damage, especially the existence of myocardial dysfunction; and to determine whether other common conditions co-exist with cardiovascular disease and/or cerebrovascular disease. Furthermore, these laboratory tests should be run to determine a baseline before drug therapy is initiated.

Lipid Profile

A lipid profile is often helpful in patients suspected of coronary and other arterial disease and in those patients with a family history of atherosclerosis or hy-perlipidemia. The lipid profile commonly includes the measurement of triglycerides, total cholesterol, high-density lipoprotein (HDL) cholesterol, and low-density lipoprotein (LDL) cholesterol. The test is performed after the patient has fasted for at least 12 hours. High levels of HDL are a protective factor against atherosclerosis. Elevated levels of other blood lipid coupled with specific risk factors pose a major health threat leading to coronary artery disease (CAD). Clinically, patients who deliberately lower their cholesterol through diet and decrease risk factors such as smoking and hypertension have effectively lessened their risk of CAD. The National Cholesterol Education program sponsored by the National Heart, Lung and Blood Institute established guidelines for testing persons older than 20 years of age, with the initial classification based on total cholesterol. Patients with serum cholesterol levels of less than 200 mg/dl should be tested every 5 years. Borderline results are those between 200 and 239 mg/dl. Levels greater than 240 mg/dl are considered high risk for CAD. For patients who are at high risk or borderline with two other risk factors, LDL and HDL levels

Table 1-6. Laboratory Tests for Suspected Cardiovascular Disease and Cerebrovascular Disease

	Laboratory Tests	Nonlaboratory Tests

Cardiovascular disease	Complete blood count
	Blood chemistry panel
	Complete urinalysis
	Lipid profile, including
	    Triglyceride
	    Total cholesterol
	    HDL cholesterol
	    LDL cholesterol
		Blood pressure measurement
		Electrocardiogram
		Chest radiograph

Cerebrovascular disease
Carotid artery disease
	Complete blood count
	Blood chemistry panel
	Complete urinalysis
	Lipid profile, including
	    Triglyceride
	    Total Cholesterol
	    HDL Cholesterol
	    LDL Cholesterol
		Blood pressure measurement
		Duplex scanning
		Carotid artery auscultation (carotid bruit)
		Magnetic resonance imaging
		Digital intravenous subtraction angiography
		Arterial angiography

Abbreviations: HDL, high-density lipoprotein; LDL, low-density lipoprotein.

should be assessed. Normal triglyceride levels are less than 165 mg/dl.

High LDL cholesterol and low HDL cholesterol are risk factors for atherosclerotic disease, whereas high HDL cholesterol and low LDL cholesterol lower the risk of atherosclerotic disease or CAD. According to the general guidelines for LDL, values of less than 130 mg/dl are low risk, 130 to 159 mg/dl are borderline, and greater than 160 mg/dl are high risk. Because reference levels may vary, it is imperative to check with the laboratory that performed the blood work.

Blood Pressure

High blood pressure, or hypertension, is an important preventable cause of cardiovascular disease. It occurs in over 60 million adults in the United States. Left

Table 1-7. Blood Pressure Classification

Diastolic Blood Presure (mmHG)	
Normal	<85
High normal	85–89
Mild hypertension	90–104
Moderate hypertension	105–114
Severe hypertension	≥115
Systolic Blood Pressure (mmHG)	
Normal (when DBP <90 mmHg)	<140
Borderline systolic hypertension	140–159
Isolated systolic hypertension	≥160

Abbreviation: DBP, diastolic blood pressur.
(Data from the Joint National Committee.[15])

untreated, hypertension increases the incidence of cardiac failure, CAD, myocardial infarction, stroke, and renal failure.

Generally, the diagnosis of hypertension in adults is established when the average of two or more diastolic measurements on at least two consecutive visits is 90 mmHg or higher or when the average of multiple systolic measurements on two or more consecutive visits is greater than 140 mmHg (Table 1-7).

More specifically, the classification of borderline isolated or isolated systemic hypertension is more critical than a classification of high normal blood pressure. However, a diastolic blood pressure within the high normal range is more critical than a systolic blood pressure within the borderline range.[15]

Blood pressure measurements are taken with a stethoscope and a standard-size cuff. Large-size adult and pediatric-size cuffs should be available to obtain accurate readings in the obese and in children. The patient should be seated comfortably for approximately 10 minutes before the initial blood pressure determination. At any given visit, the average of two or more measurements taken at least 2 minutes apart will aid in avoiding aberrant measurements. Systolic and diastolic pressures, right or left arm, lying or sitting position, and time of day should be recorded in the patient's file.

Table 1-8. Serology/Immunology Studies for Collagen Vascular Disease and Connective Tissue Disease

Laboratory tests
  Antinuclear antibody
  Anti-DNA
  Extractable nuclear antigen
  Rheumatoid factor
  Human leukocyte antigen typing, HLA-B27
  C-reactive protein
  Erythrocyte sedimentation rate
  Histopathology
  Complete blood count
  Urinalysis
Nonlaboratory tests
  Radiograph studies
  Synovial fluid studies

SEROLOGIC AND AUTOIMMUNE DISEASE

Antinuclear Antibody

The blood test for antinuclear antibody (ANA) is an immunologic screening test performed by indirect immunofluorescence for autoimmune diseases, systemic lupus erythematosus and chronic active hepatitis (Tables 1-8 and 1-9).

Results are reported as either negative or positive. A negative test result is strong evidence against the diagnosis of systemic lupus erythematosus. On obtaining a positive test result, the laboratory will usually run a titer, which reflects the concentration of the antibody and reports a pattern of microscopic fluorescent staining distribution. Fluorescent patterns reflect specificity for various autoimmune diseases. Nuclear peripheral (rim) or homogeneous (diffuse) staining bears correlation to systemic lupus erythematosus, mixed connective tissue disease, rheumatoid arthritis, progressive systemic sclerosis, or Sjögren syndrome. A speckled appearance correlates to systemic lupus erythematosus, mixed connective tissue disease, Sjögren syndrome, progressive systemic sclerosis, or rheumatoid arthritis. A nucleolar pattern is seen in patients with progressive systemic sclerosis and Sjögren syndrome. The centromere staining pattern indicates the syndrome of calcinosis, Raynaud's phenomenon, sclerodactyly, and telangiectasia. Last, cytoplasmic staining indicates biliary cirrhosis and chronic active hepatitis. A positive specimen should be screened for anti-DNA.

Finally, the test ANA cannot be regarded as a fool-

Table 1-9. Serology and Immunology Studies

	ANTI-DNA	ANA	RF	HLA	ESR
AS	(−)	(−)	(−) 1–6% (+)	90–99% HLA-B27	85% Elevated
Behcęt's disease				HLA-B5	Often elevated
JRA		50% (+)	(−)	HLA-DW5 HLA-DPW2 75% (+) HLA-B27	Often elevated
Psoriatic arthritis	(−)	(−)	(−) 1–15% (+)	HLA-B17 50% (+) HLA B27	Usually elevated
Reiter syndrome	(−)	(−)	3–6% (+)	63–99% HLA-B27	Normal/elevated
Rheumatoid arthritis	(−)	Low titers 15–50% (+)	70–90% (+)	HLA-B27 10% HLA-DR4	85% Elevated
Inflammatory bowel disease			(−)	10–20% HLA-B27	Often elevated
Sjögren syndrome	Rare	(+)	(+)	HLA-DR3	Often elevated
SLE	80–90% (+)	90–100% (+)	20–40% (+)	HLA-B27 6–10% (+) HLA-DR2 HLA-DR3	Usually elevated
MCTD	Rare	(+)			Often elevated
Scleroderma	Rare	(+)	Titer 20% (+)		Often elevated
Osteoarthritis	(−)	(−)	(−)	6–8% HLA-B27	Usually normal

Abbreviations: ANA, antinuclear antibody; AS, ankylosing spondylitis; ESR, erythrocyte sedimentation rate; HLA, human leukocyte antigen; RF, rheumatoid factor; JRA, juvenile rheumatoid arthritis; SLE, systemic lupus erythematosus; MCTD, mixed connective tissue disease.

proof screening method for systemic lupus erythematosus or other disorders. One percent of the "normal population" demonstrates serum ANA, while various medications produce a lupus-like condition and positive ANA titers. Additionally, the elderly have also demonstrated positive low ANA titers without significant systemic disease.[16]

Anti-DNA

The test for anti-DNA is an indirect immunofluorescent technique that assays blood for the presence of antibodies to DNA. Antibodies to single- or double-stranded DNA are found in 80 to 90 percent of patients with active systemic lupus erythematosus (Table 1-9). They are less commonly seen in patients with other rheumatic disorders. This test therefore, confirms a diagnosis of systemic lupus erythematosus. It is also useful for monitoring the course of systemic lupus erythematosus and determining therapeutic efficacy.

Extractable Nuclear Antigen

The tests for extractable nuclear antigen (ENA) and ANA are typically the most commonly used screening tests for patients suspected of having autoimmune disease. The test for ENA works similarly to that for ANA; it identifies autoantibodies directed against antigens present in many cells of the body.[4] The ENA blood test is specifically useful in the differential diagnosis of systemic lupus erythematosus, mixed connective tissue disease, and ANA-negative lupus. It is performed by immunodiffusion on a patient's blood serum.

Rheumatoid Factor

The test for rheumatoid factor is performed by slide latex test, latex agglutination, and various other methods. It aids in the differential diagnosis and monitoring of rheumatoid arthritis (Table 1-9). Rheumatoid factors are antibodies, immunoglobulin M antigammaglobulins directed against immunoglobulin G, that react with other immunoglobulins to form immune complexes. Rheumatoid factor is detected in the blood serum of rheumatoid arthritis patients approximately 75 percent of the time. A positive result for rheumatoid factor may occur, however, in other rheumatic conditions—syphilis, tuberculosis, hepatitis, sarcoidosis, and aging, to name a few.

Human Leukocyte Antigen B27

Human Leukocyte Antigen Typing

The human leukocyte antigens (HLAs) make up a complex system of antigens present in the blood. They are used in clinical medicine for organ transplantation, transfusions, disease associations, and paternity testing. Specific genetic material located on the short arm of chromosome 6 is inherited from each parent and is expressed as an HLA haplotype. At least five different series of antigens, A, B, C, D, and DR belong to the HLA system. In each series, a number of distinct antigens exist. For laboratory testing purposes, the best association between disease and the HLA involves the rheumatologic diseases and the antigen HLA-B27 (Table 1-9). HLA-B27 is strongly associated with ankylosing spondylitis and less strongly associated with Reiter syndrome, juvenile rheumatoid arthritis, psoriatic arthritis, and other arthritides. In fact, a patient who is HLA-B27 positive with significant clinical and radiographic findings of ankylosing spondylitis is 100 times more likely to develop the disease than someone who is HLA-B27 negative. Approximately 90 percent of patients with ankylosing spondylitis are HLA-B27 positive. Associations between B and D loci and other diseases such as sjögren syndrome, myasthenia gravis, Addison's disease and insulin-dependent diabetes also exist. Generally, the diagnosis of rheumatoid disease is made by radiographic evidence and clinical and laboratory findings. HLA typing should not be considered as a screening procedure for ankylosing spondylitis or other disorders of this nature.

Erythrocyte Sedimentation Rate

The ESR (Table 1-9) and C-reactive protein test are a general index to the presence and quantitative amount of the inflammatory process present in the body. These two tests are not diagnostic of a specific connective tissue or collagen vascular disease, but may be considered diagnostic screening tests.

INFECTIOUS DISEASE

Sexually Transmitted Diseases

Syphilis

Dark-Field Microscopy

The diagnosis of syphilis can be made by dark-field examination of live *Treponema pallidum*, the spirochete that causes syphilis. Dark-field microscopy confirms the diagnosis of syphilis before seroconversion occurs, 10 to 20 days after contact.[17] Fresh serous transudate material from the chancre of primary disease or the condyloma latum of secondary disease is collected from the patient. A drop mixed with saline is then placed on a microscope slide, cover-slipped, and examined with a microscope equipped with a dark-field condenser. Spirochetes that appear motile tightly coiled, and that flex and rotate along their longitudinal axes are considered positive specimens.[4]

Serologic Tests

Serologic tests for syphilis are the primary method of diagnosis in the absence of lesions for dark-field microscopic examination (Table 1-10). Syphilis serology is based on detection of either nontreponemal antibodies or reagin directed against lipid-containing antigens from damages host cells or treponemal antibodies directed against surface antigens of *T. pallidum*.

Table 1-10. Serologic Analysis of Infectious Diseases

Sexually Transmitted Diseases
  Syphilis
    Nontreponemal tests
      Dark-field microscopy
      Venereal disease research laboratory test, (VDRL)
      Rapid plasma reagin (RPR)
      Toluidine red unheated serum test (TRUST)
    Treponemal Tests
      Fluorescent treponemal antibody absorption test (FTA-ABS)
      Hemagglutination treponemal test for syphilis (HATTS)
      Treponemal pallidum hemagglutination assay (TPHA-TP)
      Microhemagglutination *T. pallidum* test (MHA-TP)
  Acquired Immunodeficiency Syndrome
    Antibody to human immunodeficiency virus (ELISA/enzyme immunoassay)
    Western blot
Bacterial diseases
  Tuberculosis
    Purified protein derivative (PPD)
    Mantoux test
    Mycobacteria culture and acid-fast smear
    Nonlaboratory tests
    Chest radiograph
  Lyme disease
    Lyme ELISA for IgG and IgM
    Lyme indirect fluorescent antibody assay for IgG and IgM
    Western blot

Abbreviations: ELISA, enzyme-linked immunosorbent assay; IgG, immunoglobulin G.

Nontreponemal Tests. The tests for nontreponemal antibodies are used to screen patients for syphilis and to provide a gauge to measure the response of the patient to drug therapy.[18] Therefore, nontreponemal tests are best suited when signs and symptoms of disease are minimal. When the likelihood of syphilis is high, for example, in a case of suspected ocular syphilis, latent syphilis, or uveitis with a clinically significant history, a treponemal test should be ordered.[19] The nontreponemal test is associated with frequent false-positive reactions which may be due to intercurrent infections, pregnancy, drug addiction, collagen-vascular disease, and related treponemal infections.[20] Reactive-positive tests must be confirmed by performing a treponemal test.

Treponemal Tests. Treponemal tests confirm positive nontreponemal antibody test results. These serology tests have a higher predictive value because treponemal tests are at least as sensitive and are more specific than nontreponemal tests.[21] Unlike the nontreponemal test, a positive treponemal test remains positive after treatment and is a permanent marker of present or past syphilis.[22] The microhemagglutination *T. pallidum* test (MHA-TP) and *T. pallidum* hemagglutination assay (TPHA-TP) may be falsely negative in early primary syphilis. False-positive results for the treponemal tests may occur in systemic lupus erythematosus, infectious mononucleosis, leprosy, and treponemal infections other than syphilis.

The Centers for Disease Control (CDC) suggest that lumbar puncture and cerebrospinal fluid (CSF) studies should be performed in patients with ocular syphilis for the diagnosis of neurosyphilis.[23] No test is ideal for the diagnosis of neurosyphilis. The CDC recommends the use of the CSF in Venereal Disease Research Laboratory (VDRL) test. Although controversial, a CSF fluorescent treponemal antibody absorption test is more sensitive but less specific than the nontreponemal CSF-VDRL. Additionally a CSF leukocytosis and elevated CSF protein concentration in a patient at any stage of syphilis, with neurologic symptoms for longer than 1-year duration is consistent with the diagnosis of neurosyphilis.[21]

Last, there is a strong association both historically and serologically between infection with *T. pallidum* and the increased risk of infection with the human immunodeficiency virus (HIV).[24,25] Therefore, if a patient tests positive for syphilis, a test for HIV type 1 (HIV-1) should be administered and vice versa.[26]

Acquired Immunodeficiency Syndrome

HIV-1 is the causative pathogen for the acquired immunodeficiency syndrome (AIDS). Serology for this fatal disease detects the HIV-1 antibodies produced by the host or patient. The most widely used serologic test, the enzyme-linked immunosorbent assay (ELISA), is used in conjunction with the confirmatory test, the Western blot, for HIV-1 antibody.[27]

A person is considered HIV-1 seropositive after three tests are positive: two successive ELISAs and one confirmatory Western blot.[28]

Antibody to HIV by Enzyme-Linked Immunosorbent Assay

Several screening serologic tests for HIV antibody measure immunoglobulin G or total antibody. The ELISA is the most commonly used. Enzyme immunoassays (EIAs) have become popular in recent years because they lend themselves well to automation and instrumentation. Along with the radioimmunoassays, the EIAs are the most sensitive of the assays performed in general laboratories.[4] ELISA technology uses known disrupted HIV as the source of p24 antigen, which is the most antigenic gene product of HIV.[29] It detects the antibody, produced by the patient, by specific immune binding to the antigen. A color change in proportion to the amount of antibody fixed to antigen is then read. Sensitivity of this these tests varies, but generally ranges between 90 and 99 percent.

The ELISA has a high false-positive rate and therefore must test positively two times in succession before the Western blot technique is used for confirmation.

Western Blot

The Western blot is a complex procedure, requiring technical expertise and informed interpretation.[16] It is performed by a reference laboratory.

This procedure enables separation by electrophoresis of individual viral proteins, such as viral core and envelope proteins, into well-defined bands for use as HIV-1 antigen standards. The separated bands are transferred to nitrocellulose membrane that is cut into strips and exposed to the serum sample. Serum antibodies to the antigen standard are detected and characterized as discrete colored bands. These diagnostic pattern bands are more specific than ELISA for viral antibodies.

Technologic advances in HIV-testing include polymerase chain reaction and in situ hybridization testing for HIV nucleic acid sequences.[28,30]

Tuberculosis

Purified Protein Derivative

The purified protein derivative (PPD) test (Tinetest) is a routine screening method that tests for a delayed hypersensitivity reaction of the skin for *Mycobacterium tuberculosis*. It uses PPD of tuberculin coated on four prongs, which puncture the volar surface of the arm, 2 to 4 inches below the bend of the elbow. The test is read after 48 to 72 hours by outlining the diameter of induration in millimeters at the largest of the four puncture points. Erythema frequently occurs, but the reaction should be discounted. A test is considered positive when induration is 10 mm or greater. When results of 5- to 10-mm induration are obtained, the test should be repeated.[31] A positive reaction indicates previous exposure to *M. tuberculosis,* not necessarily an active infection. Immunocompromised patients and cases of advanced tuberculosis (TB) may be anergic. Anergic patients may give false-negative skin test results in the presence of active TB. Therefore, a negative skin test should not be the sole criteria used for excluding the diagnosis of TB.

Mantoux Test

The Mantoux test is an intradermal injection of 0.1 ml of diluent containing the desired amount of PPD of tuberculin. The doses of tuberculin PPD can be varied. The PPD can be applied at first strength (I tuberculin unit [ITU], intermediate (STU), and secondary strength (250TU). This test is ordered when the PPD reacts positively or as a first-choice test method.

All HIV-infected patients suspected of developing TB should be tested with an intermediate-strength Mantoux test, because many of these patients may be anergic. Only one-third to one-half of AIDS patients with TB will test positive to PPD, and 50 to 80 percent of HIV-seropositive patients (without AIDS) and TB will react to PPD.[32]

Anergy Panel

The anergy panel is a delayed hypersensitivity skin test that uses a common battery of antigens such as tetanus, diphtheria, streptococcus, old tuberculin, *Candida, Trichophyton,* and *Proteus* spp.

Mycobacteria Culture and Acid-Fast Smear

A definitive diagnosis of active TB can be made by acid-fast stain and culture of sputum, urine, skin, gastric fluid, bone marrow, and/or CSF. The noninvasive sputum mycobacteria culture and acid-fast stain by microscopy are performed on an early morning specimen of at least 5 ml of thick mucus accumulated when the patient coughs deeply. The specimen may be collected over a 1- to 2-hour period. Additionally, the medical laboratory may require first morning specimens submitted on 3 consecutive days. Cultures are more sensitive than smears; therefore, the smear may be negative when the culture is positive.

Lyme Disease

The diagnosis of Lyme disease, caused by *Borrelia burgdorferi*, is by serologic confirmation of the patient's history, clinical appearance, and symptomatology.[33] Culturing and direct examination of a lesion from the skin or serum for *B. burgdorferi* may yield a definitive diagnosis of Lyme disease, but both these methods are notoriously difficult.[34]

The serological tests most commonly ordered are the Lyme enzyme immunoassay (EIA/ELISA) for immunoglobulins G and M and the Lyme immunofluorescent assay for immunoglobulins G and M. These methods have been developed to specifically detect *B. burgdorferi* antibodies. Many of the available assays, however, cross-react with other spirochetal antibodies, such as *T. pallidum*, which may yield false-positive tests results.[33,36] *T. pallidum* is the causative agent for syphilis. Additionally, specific serum antibodies produced vary with the stage of infection. Thus, the results may be false-negative in the very early stages or in the late or chronic stages of the disease. Frequently, clinicians propose that a serum sample be tested by multiple laboratories if there is a strong suspicion of Lyme disease. Lyme disease testing results, however, vary considerably. Lyme disease test kits need greater sensitivity and specificity, and laboratories performing the tests must improve quality controls.[37] Therefore, Lyme disease blood analysis is of questionable value without appropriate clinical appearance and symptomology. The most sensitive and specific confirmatory test for Lyme disease is the Western blot.[1]

Lyme ELISA/EIA for Immunoglobulins G and M

ELISA/EIA is used to detect immunoglobulins G and M antibodies to *B. burgdorferi* (see the section *Antibody to HIV by Enzyme-Linked Immunosorbent Assay*).

Lyme Indirect Fluorescent Antibody for Immunoglobulins G and M

The indirect fluorescent antibody (IFA) assay is an immunofluorescence technique that assays for antibodies to infectious agents. It requires the use of a microscope that provides ultraviolet illumination or an instrument capable of producing and detecting ultraviolet light-induced fluorescence. IFAs generally require less than 4 hours to complete, with most of the time being the incubation periods.

Western Blot

The test of current choice for the confirmation of the diagnosis of Lyme disease appears to be the Western blot, in which antibodies to a group of *B. burgdorferi* antigens are detected individually. The results may be negative in the first few weeks of the infection but are almost 100 percent positive in stage II and stage III of the disease[34] (see the section *Acquired Immunodeficiency Syndrome, Western Blot*).

ENDOCRINE DISEASE

Thyroid Function Testing

The active hormones produced by the thyroid gland are triiodothyronine (T_3) and thyroxine (T_4). Although 99.97 percent of T_4 and 99.7 percent of T_3 circulate bound to serum proteins, physiologic activity results from the unbound form of the hormones. The effect of the thyroid hormones on physiologic activity includes control of oxygen consumption, carbohydrate and protein metabolism, the mobilization of electrolytes, the conversion of carotene to vitamin A, and the development of the central nervous system.[4] The pituitary gland releases a hormone known as the thyroid-stimulating hormone (TSH), which controls the secretion of T_3 and T_4. Pituitary production of TSH is regulated by the hypothalamus through the secretion of thyrotropin-releasing hormone, which responds to active levels of free T_3 and T_4 in blood.

Included in this discussion is a brief but practical overview of thyroid function tests (Tables 1-11 and 1-12). Clinical interpretation of signs and symptoms, in addition to test interpretation, has primary significance in the analysis of thyroid disease. Many nonthyroidal factors influence T_3 and T_4 levels. In vivo tests, such as radioiodine uptake and radioactive scans, to evaluate thyroid function are of less importance with the advent of radioimmunoassays but are still used. Histo-

Table 1-11. Laboratory Analysis of Disorders of the Endocrine System

Thyroid profile
    Serum T_4
    T_3 Uptake
    Free T_3 index
    Thyroid-stimulating hormone

Hyperthyroidism
    Serum T_4
    T_3 Uptake
    Free T_4 index
    Thyroid antibody

Hypothyroidism
    Serum T_4
    T_3 Uptake
    Free T_4 index
    Thyroid antibody
    Thyroid-stimulating hormone
    Lipid profile

Other thyroid tests
    T_3 by radioimmunoassay
    Free T_3 and free T_4

Parathyroid disorder
    Serum calcium
    Phosphorus
    Parathyrin

Diabetes mellitus
    Fasting blood glucose
    2-Hour postprandial glucose
    Glucose tolerance test
    Glycosylated hemoglobin
    Routine urinalysis

Abbreviations: T3, triiodothyronin; T_4, thyroxine.

logic analysis by biopsy of the thyroid gland may also be necessary. Ultrasound, computed tomography, and magnetic resonance imaging are adjunct procedures used to distinguish the exophthalmos of Graves disease, from nonendocrine causes of exophthalmos. Finally, normal ranges for thyroid function test results are method dependent; interpretation depends on the individual laboratory where the tests were performed. No normal values are given.

Thyroxine

The serum T_4 concentration is the most important single test for thyroid function.[38] It is an accurate, widely used measurement of the total concentration of serum T_4. This laboratory blood chemistry test is performed by EIA or RIA.

Triiodothyronine Uptake

T_3 uptake (T_3U) test is performed, with the serum T_4 concentration, as part of the thyroid profile. It indirectly measures thyroid-binding globulin and does not directly measure serum T_3 levels. It is used for the diagnosis of hypothyroidism or hyperthyroidism when used in conjunction with the T_4 (RIA/EIA) results and provides a mathematical approximation of free T_4 concentration in the blood. It is called the estimated free T_4 index (FT_4I).[39] This laboratory blood chemistry test uses radioactive T_3 and is performed as a resin sponge uptake or related method.

Table 1-12. Thyroid Profile

	Hyperthyroidism	Hypothyroidism (Thyroid Gland Failure)	Graves' Disease
T_4	Increased	Decreased	Increased
T_3 Uptake	High	Low	High
Free T_4 index	Increased	Decreased	Increased
Thyroid-stimulating hormone	<0.1 m μ/L	Quite increased (>6.0 m μ/L)	Decreased
Thyroid antibodies Antimicrosomal Antithyroglobulin Antithyroglobulin			Positive
Thyrotropin-receptor antibody			Positive
T_3 by radioimmunoassay	Increased	Decreased	Increased
Free T_4	Very high	Decreased	Increased
Free T_3	Increased	Decreased	Increased

Abbreviations; T_3, triiodothyronine; T_4 thyroxine.

Free Thyroxine Index

The estimated FT$_4$I is a calculation from results of the serum T$_4$ level and the T$_3$ uptake test (FT$_4$I = T$_3$U × T$_4$/100). It is an estimate of the concentration of unbound T$_4$ in the blood serum that allows meaningful interpretation of the T$_4$ and T$_3$U by excluding most nonthyroidal factors or protein-binding problems.

Thyroid-Stimulating Hormone

The most recently developed immunoassays for the detection of TSH are extremely sensitive and specific. Assays for TSH include immunochemiluminometric assays, sandwich immunoradiometric assays, and fluorometric enzyme assays with the use of monoclonal antibodies. They may be considered screening tests for thyroid disease.[40]

Thyroid Antibodies

Most thyroid diseases can result in the release of thyroglobulin or microsomal antigen of thyroid epithelial cells. The patient responds by producing circulating antibodies to these materials, usually retained in the thyroid gland. Immunologic measurement of thyroid antibodies can be performed by passive hemagglutination, indirect immunofluorescence, or EIAs. Thyroid antimicrosomal antibody is used in the differential diagnosis of hypothyroidism and thyroiditis. Thyroid antithyroglobulin antibody is useful in the diagnosis of autoimmunothyroiditis and Hashimoto's thyroiditis. Both are usually ordered together because of their cross-reactivity with other antigens.

Long-Acting Thyroid Stimulator

The thyrotropin-receptor antibody test, or thyroid-stimulating autoantibody or immunoglobulin test, is not commonly ordered in the thyroid profile but gives additional information about Graves disease. The serum of patients with Graves disease contains an immunoglobulin G antibody that is thought to stimulate the thyroid gland. This antibody is measured by bioassay or radioreceptor assay and helps to detect and confirm hyperthyroidism and Graves disease. It is found in 90 percent of patients with Graves disease, 50 percent of patients with euthyroid Graves disease, and in hyperthyroid patients.

Triiodothyronine by Radioimmunoassay

RIA to detect T$_3$ is a thyroid function test that measures total serum T$_3$. It is useful in patients with clinical evidence of hyperthyroidism with a normal or border-line thyroid profile. It is needed in the diagnosis of T$_3$ thyrotoxicosis in which T$_3$ is increased and T$_4$ is normal. This condition is occasionally found in Graves disease.

Free T$_4$ and Free T$_3$

Free T$_4$ and free T$_3$ make up a very small fraction of total T$_4$ and T$_3$. These unbound hormones can be measured directly by the reference method, equilibrium dialysis, which is both difficult and expensive. This test is useful when the thyroid profile is inconsistent with the clinical findings.[41]

Parathyroid Function Testing

The evaluation of the parathyroid glands includes the measurement of serum calcium, phosphorus, and parathyrin, the secretory product of the parathyroid glands. Testing often includes and evaluation of the alimentary tract, renal function, and acid–base relationship.[1]

Diabetes Mellitus

The blood glucose level test for the diagnosis of diabetes mellitus is one of the most common chemistry tests individually ordered. It usually tests a fasting blood glucose level or a 2-hour postprandial glucose level.

Fasting Blood Glucose Test

The fasting blood glucose test is performed after the patient fasts for at least 8 hours. A venous blood specimen is drawn. Serum or plasma glucose is then determined by enzyme-based assays, glucose oxidase, or hexokinase. The normal range of blood glucose varies with age, but generally for the average, nonpregnant adult, 60 to 115 mg/dl is expected. Results of 115 to 140 mg/dl bear reexamination, but, if consistent, imply impairment of glucose tolerance. Fasting levels of over 140 mg/dl on at least two occasions are considered definitive for the diagnosis of diabetes mellitus.[40]

Two-Hour Postprandial Glucose Test

The 2-hour postprandial glucose test is performed 2 hours after the patient has eaten a meal or has consumed a premeasured glucose load. The patient must be instructed to eat an adequate meal (breakfast or lunch) and complete the meal in 15 to 20 minutes. A venous blood specimen is drawn 2 hours from the beginning of the meal. The preferred method is to have the patient consume a 75-g glucose solution in 5 minutes, then collect a blood sample in 2 hours. For the average nonpregnant adult patient, a 2-hour postprandial blood glucose is normal when measured as less than 140 mg/dl. A result of 140 to 200 mg/dl is classified as impaired glucose tolerance. A 2-hour test result greater than 200 mg/dl on at least two occasions supports a diagnosis of diabetes mellitus.[40,43]

Glucose Tolerance Test

The fasting and 2-hour postprandial glucose tests are used to establish the diagnosis of diabetes mellitus. The glucose tolerance test is used when the fasting or postprandial blood levels are equivocal.[44] When the glucose tolerance test is performed, the patient should have been fasting for 12 hours and should not have smoked or consumed any liquids other than water. A fasting venous blood specimen is drawn. The patient then drinks a standard dose of glucose solution. This usually is 75 g of glucose, or the glucose load may be tailored to the individual body size. Blood samples are then collected at various times, most frequently 30, 60, 90, and 120 minutes for the duration of the test. Interpretation is variable. Generally, for the non-pregnant adult, fasting levels should be 60 to 115 mg/ dl; 1-hour levels should be 184 mg/dl or less; and 2-hour levels should be 138 mg/dl or less.[43]

The glucose tolerance test is used to establish the presence of glucose intolerance. Most commonly, it supports or rules out the diagnosis of diabetes mellitus in patients with borderline results from the fasting and postprandial glucose tests. It is contraindicated in patients with the presence of obvious diabetes mellitus.

Glycosylated Hemoglobin Test

The diagnosis of diabetes mellitus is established by the fasting blood glucose test and the 2-hour post-prandial glucose test. Glycosylated hemoglobin values are recommended for monitoring diabetes control. The percentage of glycosylated hemoglobin depends on the average level of glucose to which the RBCs have been exposed during their life span or preceding 100 to 200 days. The exact percentage depends on the method of measurement used, such as elution from resin columns, affinity chromatography, electrophoresis, and isoelectric focusing affinity. In general, in patients who demonstrate good diabetic control, 4 to 7 percent of their hemoglobin is in the glycosylated form. In uncontrolled diabetics, this range may in-

crease threefold to fourfold.[45] Most interesting to the eye care practitioner is the correlation noted between the glycosylated hemoglobin value and the incidence and progression of diabetic retinopathy.[46]

REFERENCES

1. Rosenbaum J, Wernick R: Selection and interpretation of laboratory tests for patients with uveitis. Int Ophthalmol Clin 30: 238, 1990
2. Covington S, May D, Karcioglu Z: Hematologic tests. In Karcioglu Z (ed): Laboratory Diagnosis in Ophthalmology. Macmillan, New York, 1987
3. Guyton A: Textbook of Medical Physiology. WB Saunders, Philadelphia, 1981
4. Sacher R, McPherson R: Widmann's Clinical Interpretation of Laboratory Tests. FA Davis, Philadelphia, 1991
5. Dayhaw-Barker P: Hematological testing. p. 41. In Classe J (ed): Optometry Clinics. Vol. 2, No. 1. Clinical Laboratory Testing. Appleton & Lange, Norwalk, CT, 1992
6. Tietz NW (ed): Clinical Guide to Laboratory Tests. WB Saunders, Philadelphia, 1983
7. Dayhaw-Barker P: Medical laboratory tests. p. 566. In Ebkridgetal J (eds.): Clinical Procedures in Optometry, J.B. Lippincott, Philadelphia, 1991
8. Wallach J: Interpretation of Diagnostic Tests. Little, Brown, Boston, 1992
9. Hall A: Disorders of synthesis, structure and function of hemoglobin. p. 482. In Halsted, Halsted (eds): The Laboratory in Clinical Medicine. WB Saunders, Philadelphia, 1981
10. Wall M: Laboratory tests in neurophthalmology. In Karcioglu Z (ed): Laboratory Diagnosis in Ophthalmology. Macmillan, New York, 1987
11. Tilzer L, Demott WR: Hematology. p. 457. In Jacobs DS (ed): Laboratory Test Handbook. Lexi-Comp, Hudson, Ohio, 1990
12. Kanski JJ, Thomas DJ: The Eye in Systemic Disease. Butterworth-Heinemann, London, 1990
13. HO G, Kammer GM: Musculoskeletal and connective tissue disease. p. 634. In Ancheoli T, Carpenter C, Plum F, Smith L (eds): Cecil Essentials of Medicine. WB Saunders, Philadelphia 1990
14. Matthews D, Smalley D: Blood chemistries, serology and immunology. p. 53. In Classe J (ed): Optometry Clinics. Vol. 2, No. 1. Clinical Laboratory Testing. Appleton & Lange, E. Norwalk, CT, 1992
15. Joint National Committee: The 1988 report of the Joint National Committee on detection, evaluation and treatment of high blood pressure. Arch Intern Med 148:1023, 1988
16. Wolfson WL: Immunology and serology. p. 554. In Jacobs D (ed): Laboratory Test Handbook. Lexi-Comp, Hudson, Ohio 1990
17. Sommers HM: Sexually transmitted diseases. p. 447. In Youmans GP, Paterson PY, Sommers HM (eds): The Biology and Clinical Basis of Infectious Disease. WB Saunders, Philadelphia, 1985
18. Romanowski B, Sutherland R, Fick G et al: Serologic response to treatment of infectious syphilis. Ann Intern Med 114:1005, 1991.
19. Descheres J, Seamone CD, Baines MG: Acquired ocular syphilis: diagnosis and treatment. Ann Ophthalmol 24:134, 1992
20. Department of Pathology: Episcopal Hospital Lab User's Guide. Lexi-Comp, Hudson, 1990
21. Hitchinson CM, Hook EW III: Syphilis in adults. Med Clin North Am 74:1389, 1990
22. Margo C, Hamed L: Ocular syphilis. Surv Ophthalmol 37:203, 1992

23. Centers for Disease Control: Sexually transmitted disease treatment guidelines. MMWR, 38:5, 1989
24. Schultz S, Araneta MRG, Joseph SC: Neurosyphilis and HIV infection (letter). N Engl J Med 317:1464, 1987
25. Stamm WE, Sandsfield HH, Rompalo AM et al: The association between genital ulcer disease and acquisition of HIV infection in homosexual men. JAMA 260:1429, 1988
26. Rufli T: Syphilis and HIV infection. Dermatologica 179:113, 1989
27. Schuman J, Orellana J, Friedman A, Teich S: Acquired immunodeficiency syndrome (AIDS). Surv Ophthalmol 31:384, 1987
28. Sloand E, Pitt E, Chiarello R, Nemo G: HIV Testing. JAMA 266:2861, 1991
29. Yoser S, Forster D, Rao N: Systemic viral infections and their retinal and choroidal manifestations. Surv Ophthalmol 37:5, 1993
30. Knowles JG: DNA amplication in the detection of viral genes (HIV-1). Am Clin Prod Rev 7:42, 1988
31. ATS Committee on Diagnostic Skin Testing: The Tuberculin Skin Test, Supplement to Diagnostic Standards and Classification of Tuberculosis and Other Mycobacterial Disease. American Lung Association, New York, 1974
32. Chaisson RE, Sluticin G: Tuberculosis and HIV infection. J Infect Dis 159:96, 1989
33. Florakis GJ, Vrabec MP, Krachmer JH, et al: Lyme disease. p. 229. In Gold DH, Weingeist TA (eds): The Eye in Systemic Disease. JB Lippincott, Philadelphia, 1990
34. Banyas G: Difficulties with Lyme serology. J Am Optom Assoc 63:135, 1992
35. Park M: Ocular manifestations of Lyme disease. J Am Optom Assoc 60:284, 1989
36. Magnarelli L, Anderson J, Johnson R: Cross reactivity in serological tests for Lyme disease and other Spirochete infections. J Infect Dis 156:183, 1987
37. Bakken L, Case K, Callister S et al: Performance of 45 laboratories participating in a proficiency testing program for Lyme disease serology. JAMA, 268:891, 1992
38. Van Middleesworth L: Function and diseases of the thyroid. p. 649. In Halstead, Halstead (eds): The Laboratory in Clinical Medicine, Interpretation and Application. WB Saunders, Philadelphia, 1981
39. Surks M, Chopra I, Mariash C et al: American Thyroid Association guidelines for use of laboratory tests in thyroid disorders. JAMA 263:1529, 1990
40. Jacobs DS, Demott W, Strobel S, Fodry E: Chemistry. p. 58. In Jacobs DS (ed): Laboratory Test Handbook. Lexi-Comp, Hudson, Ohio 1990
41. Chattorai SC, Watts NB: Endocrinology. p. 533. In Tietz NW (ed): Fundamentals of Clinical Chemistry. 3rd Ed. WB Saunders, Philadelphia, 1987
42. National Diabetes Data Group: Classification and diagnosis of diabetes mellitus and other categories of glucose intolerance. Diabetes 28:1039, 1979
43. Moltich M: Diabetes mellitus: pathophysiology and current trends in management. J Am Optom Assoc 59:842, 1988
44. Solomon SS, Duckworth WC, Kitabchi A: Disorders of carbohydrate metabolism: obesity, diabetes mellitus and hypoglycemia. p. 697. In Halsted, Halsted (eds): The Laboratory in Clinical Medicine. WB Saunders, Philadelphia, 1981
45. Klein R, Klein BEK, Moss SE et al: Glycosylated hemoglobin predicts the incidence and progression of diabetic retinopathy. JAMA 260:2864, 1988

2 Diagnostic Imaging Techniques

CHRIS J. CAKANAC

INTRODUCTION

With the increasing scope of primary care, optometrists can often use radiologic tests to aid in the diagnosis of many ocular disorders.

This chapter reviews plain film radiography, computed tomography (CT), and magnetic resonance imaging (MRI). Included in the discussion are how these tests work, when to use them, and how to order them. Although the ordering of radiologic test is a component of every medical specialty, their interpretation is the duty of the radiologist. It is the optometrist's responsibility to recognize an anomaly, provide pertinent clinical information, and work in conjunction with a radiologist to achieve an accurate diagnosis.

CASE REPORT

A 28-year-old white man was struck in the left eye with a tennis ball while charging the net. He presented with a black eye and the complaint of numbness of the left cheek. He reported no double vision. His past systemic and ocular history was unremarkable. He currently took no medications and had seasonal allergies.

Uncorrected visual acuity was OD 20/20 and OS 20/25 at distance. Pupillary responses were normal, no afferent pupillary defect was noted, and extraocular muscle motility was without restriction. Ecchymosis of the inferior orbital area was prominent. External slit lamp examination was unremarkable, and intraocular pressures via Goldmann was OD 18 mmHg and OS 17 mmHg. A slight enophthalmos was noted in the left eye, and Hertel exophthalmometry showed a 5-mm difference.

Dilated fundus examination revealed a small area of retinae commotio of the inferior temporal retina, which later resolved. The peripheral retina was intact bilaterally. The optic nerve heads exhibited minimal cupping, normal coloration, and clear margins in both eyes.

An orbital series of radiographs with Caldwell's and Waters projections was ordered (Fig. 2-1). A left inferior blow-out fracture was found. No muscle entrapment was observed. The patient was referred for oculoplastic consultation and later underwent surgical repair.

Discussion: This case demonstrates the need to know and use radiologic tests. Despite the minimal ocular findings of only a black eye, a potentially disfiguring fracture was present. In this case, no extraocular muscle entrapment was noted and no diplopia was elicited, which usually identifies a blow-out fracture. The fracture, however, caused an expansion of the orbital space and enophthalmos. Surgery was indicated because the criteria for repair of a blow-out fracture is either compromised binocular function or altered cosmesis.

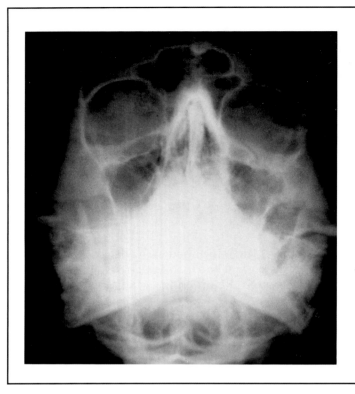

Fig. 2-1. Plain film of the patient in the Case Report exhibiting a left inferior orbital fracture without muscle entrapment. Waters projection.

PLAIN FILM X-RAY

Basic Principles

The x-ray has been used for medical applications since the early 1900s.

X-rays are produced whenever fast-moving electrons with enough energy slam into an object. Usually, most of the electron's energy is converted to heat on collision. If the electron is moving fast enough, a small amount of the electron's energy is converted to x-rays at impact. The original x-ray tube used a heated filament to produce a steady stream of electrons. A large electrical force then propelled these electrons against a target. Most of the energy from the collision was transferred as heat to a copper bar on which the target rested. A small amount of energy, however (less than 1 percent), was reflected from the target and out a window in the tube in the form of x-rays.[1]

X-rays closely resemble other rays of light. Their wavelength, however, is much shorter than visible or even ultraviolet light. Because of their high energy and short wavelength, x-rays can pass through a surface, rather than being reflected, as typical light waves are. This penetrability gives x-rays their medical significance. In the plain film study, a controlled amount of x-rays are directed at a film cassette. A part of the body is placed in the path of the x-ray between the point of emission and the film (its final destination). Because the body tissues (muscle, fat, bone) impede the x-ray's passage at different rates, various densities or shadows are produced on the film.[2]

In radiologic terms, *increased density* means less penetrance of the x-ray and therefore decreased radiolucency, with a resulting whiter image on the film. Conversely, decreased density and increased radiolucency appear as dark shadows on film.

To obtain useful information and establish a diagnosis based on ophthalmic x-ray films, the investigator should have a thorough understanding of the structures of the skull and their relationships.

Techniques of Orbital Radiology

Most of the bones of the skeleton can be projected separately on x-ray film without interference from other structures. Projections of the orbit, however, are somewhat more difficult. The skull comprises 22 relatively small bones, and their proximities make it impossible to isolate a single bone by means of x-rays. Interpretation of the radiograph is complicated by the superimposed shadows of nearby bones as well as by movement of the head during exposure, which blurs the shadows.

The general rule of radiology is that two views of an anatomic part are taken 90 degrees from one another. A routine orbital series usually consists of one or two posteroanterior projections and a lateral view of the affected side. Occasionally, additional views such as oblique or submentovertical may be needed to make the diagnosis.

Projections

One of the most important factors in obtaining a clear picture of a particular body part is appropriately positioning the patient and the x-ray unit.

In studying the skull, the posteroanterior projection is one of the primary positions used. In this projection, the patient's face is placed parallel against the film, and the x-ray is aimed directly perpendicular to the film. Although this projection will exhibit many cranial features, it is of little use in evaluating the orbit. With this position, the petrous portions of temporal bones fall in direct line with the orbits, thereby obscuring any clear view of the orbits on the film.

Caldwell's Projection

Caldwell's projection uses the same position of the patient's head against the film as described for the posteroanterior projection. The x-ray, however, is angled toward the feet, approximately 15 degrees from perpendicular[3] (Fig. 2-2). An exaggerated (the x-ray is tilted 30 degrees) Caldwell's projection is occasionally used. With this view, the petrous portions of temporal bones are projected below the orbits, leaving a much clearer visualization of orbits as compared to the straight posteroanterior projection.[4] Caldwell's projection is especially helpful in evaluating the orbital roof, ethmoid air cells, and nasal cavity.[5]

Waters Projection

Instead of using a tilted x-ray, in the Water's projection, the head is tilted upward approximately 30 degrees from the film toward the feet (Fig. 2-3). The x-ray is projected directly vertically, like the straight

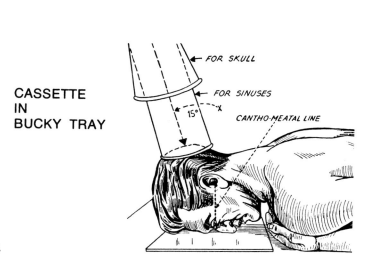

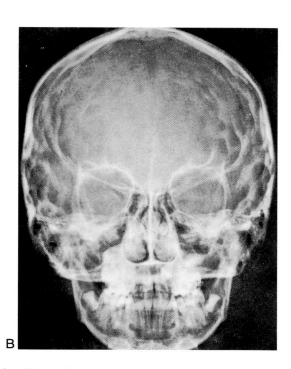

A

B

Fig. 2-2. (A & B) Appropriate positioning and resulting image for Caldwell's projection. (From Meschan,[3] with permission.)

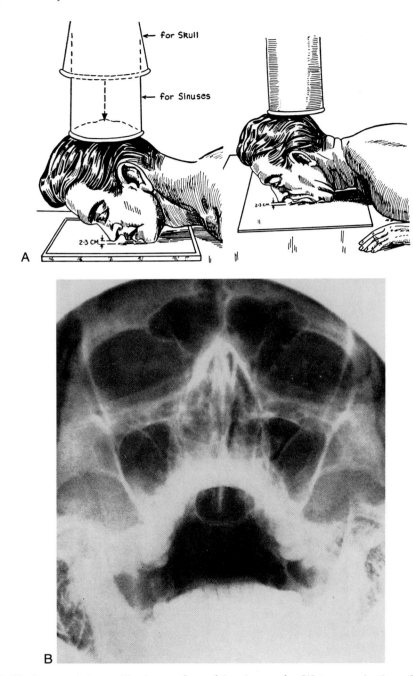

Fig. 2-3. (A & B) Appropriate positioning and resulting image for Waters projection. (From Meschan,[3] with permission.)

posteroanterior view.[5] This technique also allows an extremely clear view of the orbits by projecting the temporal bones out of this area. The Waters projection is especially helpful in evaluating the floor of the orbit and the maxillary and ethmoidal sinuses.

Submentovertical Projection

To examine the lateral walls and zygomatic arches, the submentovertical projection may be employed. With this position, the film is placed against the top

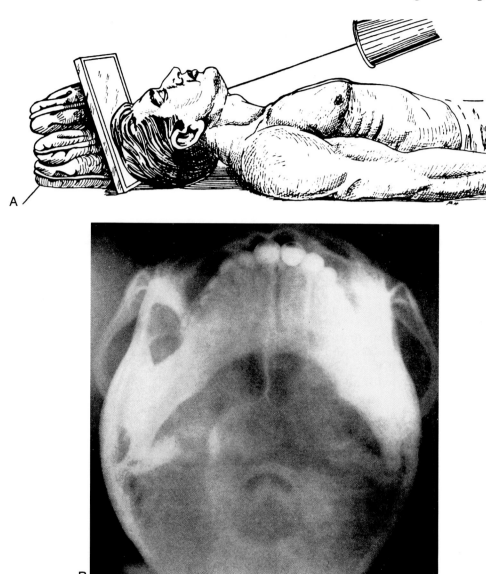

Fig. 2-4. (A & B) Appropriate positioning and resulting image for submentovertical projection. (From Meschan,[3] with permission.)

of the patient's head, and the x-ray aimed under the patient's chin[5] (Figs. 2-3B and 2-4). The result is a clear view of the zygomatic arches, which otherwise can be difficult to evaluate.

Lateral Projection

The lateral projection is useful in visualizing the lateral orbit as well as the sinuses and the sella tursica. In this projection, the film is placed on the side of the face parallel with the sagittal plane, and the x-ray is directed between the ear and the outer canthus of the eye.

Indications and Contraindications

At its inception, the plain film was used to evaluate all pathology, including trauma, tumors, and foreign bodies. With the advent of the CT scan and MRI, the plain film is now used mainly for ruling out orbital fractures. Some experts believe that even this use should be left to CT. Plain films, however, are extremely economical and are highly accurate for most simple fractures.

Foreign bodies in the globe or orbit can also be detected with plain film radiographs. In fact, increasingly, the plain film is used to rule out metallic objects in the orbit in patients with a foreign body history before MRI is performed.

The single contraindication to plain film radiographs is pregnancy. Because plain films use ionizing radiation, which is toxic to the fetus, they should not be used on patients who are at any stage of pregnancy or if pregnancy is suspected.

COMPUTED TOMOGRAPHY

Although plain films are helpful in assessing simple trauma, CT is far superior to plain film radiography for most other conditions. CT is useful for diagnosing complicated fractures, stroke, visual loss, and certain tumors. The great advantage of CT is that soft structures can be seen simultaneously with bone in cross section.

Basic Principles

In contrast to plain film radiography, during which a broad x-ray beam is aimed at the object of interest, CT uses an x-ray tube and collimators to narrow the x-ray beam to penetrate a thin slice of tissue. Sodium iodide detectors, rather than film, absorb the x-ray as it leaves the body. The x-ray tube and detectors are used to take pictures at 1-degree increments of a 180-degree arc. The information of each picture at each degree is computer analyzed, which mathematically creates a cross-sectional image.[6]

Images can be obtained in an axial, coronal, or sagittal plane. Axial (transverse images) are the most common for viewing the head. These are horizontal sections of the head taken from top to bottom[7] (Fig. 2-5). The usual scan of the head will use 5-mm slices. For the orbit, thinner slices of 1.5 mm are recommended for greater anatomic detail.[6] The axial scan is the primary section for beginning to analyze the orbit and visual pathways.

Coronal sections are vertical sections taken front to back (Fig. 2-6). This section is useful in determining

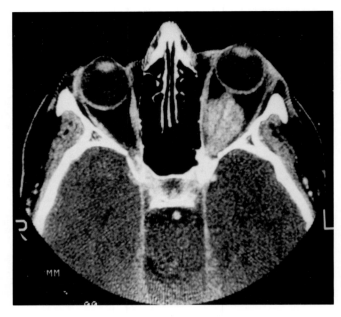

Fig. 2-5. Axial CT scan exhibiting a meningioma of the left optic nerve.

extraocular muscle enlargement and masses of the optic nerve and in localizing foreign bodies.[6]

Sagittal scans are lateral vertical sections between the ears. Sagittal sections are optimal for viewing the optic chiasm.[7] They are also used to assess changes in the floor and roof of the orbit.

Sagittal and coronal scans can be obtained from direct scanning of the head or can be reformatted from axial scans via computerized image re-creation. Reformatting affords the advantages of exposing the patient to less radiation, shorter scan times, and less repositioning of the head. Some resolution, however, is lost after the reformatting, which is why direct scanning is employed.[8]

CT scans can be obtained with or without contrast-enhancing agents. Contrast enhancement increases the images of the blood–brain barriers. The orbit images quite well without enhancing agents, because orbital fat provides a natural contrast background; thus, contrast administration is not required for all intraorbital pathology.[9] Enhancing agents should be used when extracranial extension is suspected or when evaluating the optic chiasm. Enhancing agents will image vascular lesions quite well, such as angiomas, meningiomas, and gliomas. Enhancement is

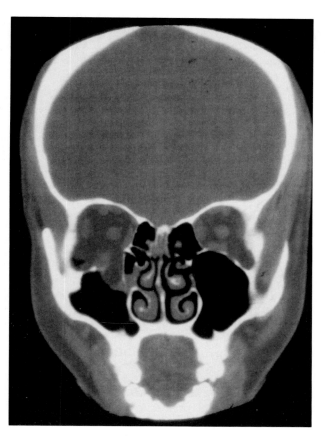

Fig. 2-6. Coronal CT scan exhibiting a blow-out fracture of the right orbit with muscle entrapment noted.

not required in instances of trauma or foreign body localization.

Indications and Contraindications

CT is recommended for complicated fractures, localizing foreign bodies for removal, and much soft tissue pathology.

Orbital fractures with suspected muscle entrapment or fractures involving many bones are better left to CT than plain films.

CT will aid in localizing a foreign body for removal within the posterior two-thirds of globe or orbit, especially if the surrounding media is opaque (as in vitreous hemorrhage). Plain films suffice for merely ruling out a foreign body, but CT provides much more information if removal must be made. Metals as small as .05 mm in diameter can be visualized.[10] Materials such as wood or glass may need to be somewhat larger to be visualized. Usually, axial and coronal sections are ordered with 1- to 2-mm cuts to evaluate intraocular or intraorbital foreign bodies.[11]

With its inception in the early 1970s, CT rapidly became the standard for evaluating soft tissue pathology. Since then, MRI has supplanted CT for most soft tissue lesions. However, CT remains useful in many instances.

Because the orbit has moderately thin bones and a good contrast background, orbital tumors image quite well on CT. Tumors of the posterior fossa are imaged better with MRI because these bones are much thicker and produce artifacts with CT.

Tissue pathology with calcifications image well with CT because calcium will absorb more of the x-rays than surrounding normal areas.[6] Therefore, optic nerve head drusen and tumors with calcification such as meningiomas and retinoblastomas image as well or better on CT than on MRI.[12]

MAGNETIC RESONANCE IMAGING

Basic Principles

MRI is the most recent advancement in diagnostic imaging and has been available since the 1980s. The instrumentation of MRI is not based on ionizing radiation but on radio and magnetic waves. The image obtained is not the result of how much x-radiation the tissue absorbs but, rather, the chemical and physical properties of the tissue. This makes MRI very sensitive in the detection of subtle biochemical changes such as degeneration or demyelination, which often precede anatomic alterations.[13] By contrast, CT images by one parameter (x-ray attenuation) and is relatively insensitive to early disease.

The concept of MRI is based on the hydrogen atom, which is found extensively throughout the body. Hydrogen possesses an odd number of protons and neutrons, which gives it a small magnetic field. Mathematically, a vector, which has a specific direction and magnitude, can be assigned to this small magnetic field. In the body, these vectors are in random disarray and tend to cancel each other out. If a strong external magnetic field is applied to the body, however, these vectors realign with the external field, and a net magnetic vector is achieved.

An MRI unit places the patient in the bore of a large magnet, which causes the hydrogen nuclei to align. Next, a radio frequency is quickly applied along the axis perpendicular to the patient, to temporarily knock the atoms out of alignment. As the nuclei realign, various parameters are measured by an antenna surrounding the body. These parameters are fed to a computer, which generates the image by complicated analysis.

Two of the parameters usually analyzed are T_1 and T_2. T_1 represents the time it takes for the atoms to realign in the magnetic field after being perturbed by the radio frequency pulse. The chemical state of the tissue dictates how quickly the protons regain their orientation. T_1 is also termed the "spin-lattice" function.

In addition to the vectors of hydrogen nuclei aligning in a strong magnetic field, the vectors precess, or spin, independently along the transverse plane. With application of the radio frequency pulse, the vectors precess exactly the same for a brief instant. This is termed *phase coherence*. As soon as the radio frequency pulse is removed, the phase coherence decays to random spinning again. T_2 represents the time it takes for phase coherence to decay. It is a much shorter time than T_1. T_2 is also termed the "spin-spin" function and depends largely on the physical state of tissue.[13]

Obviously, the images generated by MRI depend highly on the hydrogen content of the tissue. Cortical bone and air have very little hydrogen and therefore do not image well with MRI. The different water content of white and gray matter allows them to image separately with MRI.[13]

The image brightness of various tissues will depend on whether the image is T_1 or T_2 weighted. For the eye and orbit, T_1 will exhibit a bright orbital fat background and a dark vitreous, optic nerve, and extraocular muscles. The brightness of the these structures tends to reverse with T_2 weighting (Fig. 2-7). A general rule is that T_1 is best for viewing normal anatomy and T_2 highlights pathology.

With MRI, coronal and sagittal sections can be obtained without repositioning the patient. However, reformatting these images from axial sections is currently not available, although it is with CT.

Indications and Contraindications

MRI is rapidly becoming the test of choice for most soft tissue pathology. MRI is particularly useful for scanning the cranial posterior fossa. With CT, the thick petrous bones in the posterior fossa produce many artifacts, making this area difficult to view. MRI does not image bone, so tissues in the posterior fossa

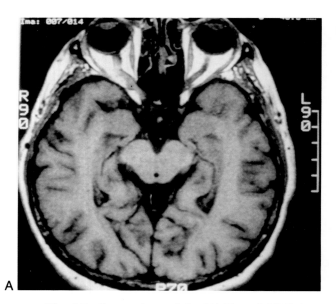
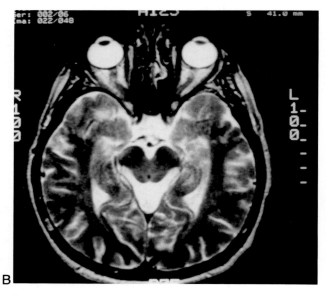

Fig. 2-7. Comparison of the **(A)** T_1 and **(B)** T_2 images with magnetic resonance imaging.

are easily visualized. Thus, pathology such as cranial neuropathies, gaze palsies, nystagmus, and papilledema are indications for MRI.[12]

MRI is also superior to CT for detecting demyelination and therefore has become the test of choice to support the often elusive diagnosis of multiple sclerosis.

Because no x-rays are involved in MRI, radiation exposure is not a concern. The National Institutes of Health, however, suggests avoiding MRI during the first trimester of pregnancy.[7] Because of the strong magnetic field applied to the body, metallic foreign bodies of any type contraindicate use of MRI. A history of ocular foreign body requires investigation before an MRI scan is performed. The presence of metallic aneurysm clips is an absolute contraindication. The strong magnetic field can also interfere with the electronics of pacemakers, causing them to malfunction.[13] Finally, life support systems and respirators may have metallic components, which prevents patients from being placed into the magnetic bore while sustained on them.[7]

Patients who are claustrophobic may need sedation before being placed in the narrow confines of an MRI unit, and some obese patients may not fit into certain MRI scanner models.

PATHOLOGY

Types of Fractures

The orbit consists of a roof, a floor, and two side walls, all of which converge posteriorly to form an apex. A fracture can involve any wall or the apex. Each fracture location produces a characteristic clinical appearance.

Floor Fractures

Blow-out fractures of the orbital floor occur when the force of a blunt object contacts the orbital area, causing the orbital contents to compress. The increased hydraulic pressure within the orbit causes a blow-out at the weakest portion of the orbit, the floor.[14] This mechanism is considered a safety valve that acts to decompress the orbital cavity and protect the globe from injury.[15] The object responsible is usually larger than the orbital opening, such a a fist or baseball. Smaller objects (e.g., a golf ball) can pass through the orbital opening and directly contact the globe, result-

ing in more serious intraocular damage but not usually a blow-out fracture.

An alternative theory suggests that trauma to the inferior rim causes a buckling force, which creates a hole in the thinner, more posterior orbital floor.[16]

Regardless of which theory the reader ascribes to, a pure blow-out fracture is considered to have no associated rim fracture.[15] An impure or complicated blow-out implies fracture of the rim as well as the floor.

The classic findings in blow-out fracture are ecchymosis of the infraorbital area, enophthalmos, and diplopia on upgaze. Occasionally, the patient may also complain of anesthesia of the skin under the orbit as a result of injury to the infraorbital nerve.

The enophthalmos results from enlargement of the orbital space by a hole in the floor.[17] In rare cases, the entire globe can herniate into the maxillary sinus.

Diplopia may or may not be present in blow-out fractures, depending on whether entrapment of orbital tissues occurs at the blow-out site. Orbital fat, the inferior rectus, or inferior oblique can prolapse into the maxillary sinus. When this occurs, superior gaze (and to a lesser degree, inferior gaze) of the involved eye is restricted.[14] Motility restriction can occur from orbital edema and hemorrhage, which will usually resolve with time. Diplopia from muscle entrapment, however, usually improves minimally without intervention.[14]

Roof Fractures

Fractures to the roof of the orbit are uncommon because of the thickness of the bone.[18] They are usually caused by severe trauma to the frontal area. Isolated roof fractures occur more commonly in children, presumably because their softer bones have a tendency to buckle when subjected to blunt force.[19] Unlike floor and wall fractures, roof fractures usually are associated with exophthalmos rather than enophthalmos.

Patients with fractures generally have superior ecchymosis and possibly ptosis from damage to the levator. Because of the direct communication of the orbit with the cranial vault created by the fracture, cerebrospinal fluid can leak into the orbit, giving the appearance of epiphora. Cerebrospinal fluid can also leak into the nasal cavity, causing rhinorrhea.

The severity of injury necessary to create roof fractures often results in intracranial damage and can cause life-threatening complications.

Medial Wall Fractures

The medial wall of the orbit is composed of the paper-thin lamina paprycea reinforced by the pillars of the ethmoidal cells.[17] Fractures of this area occur in a hydraulic nature similar to the blow-out mechanism or from a direct blow to the mid-face.[18,20]

The classic symptom of an ethmoid fracture is orbital emphysema and crepitus. When the ethmoidal area is fractured, a direct communication exists with the orbit and nasal area, allowing air to enter the orbit. Small air pockets around the orbit can occasionally be palpated. Additionally, if the patient sneezes or blows the nose, the periorbital skin can temporarily inflate.

Because of its close proximity, nasolacrimal damage and obstruction can occur. Finally, a fracture that extends to the cribiform plate can allow rhinorrhea to occur.[20]

Lateral Wall Fractures

The lateral orbit is composed of zygomatic bone, which is the thickest but also the most exposed part of the orbit.[18] It is the most common site of orbital fracture.[17]

The body of the zygomatic arch is so strong that it rarely fractures. More commonly, fracture lines occur where the zygomatic meets other bones. This occurs superiorly with the frontal bone, medially with the maxillary bone, and laterally with the temporal bone. This three-point fracture is called a *tripod fracture*. A free-floating zygomatic bone is created with this mechanism.

A patient with a tripod fracture may have enophthalmos and loss of the malar eminence (loss of a prominent cheekbone).[17] Anesthesia of the lateral cheek can occur from damage to the zygomatic nerve. Finally, patients with tripod fractures may report problems opening the mouth.[14]

Apex Fractures

Fractures of the most posterior portion of the orbit, the apex, are rare and serious. They are seldom isolated and are usually extensions of facial or skull base fractures.[21]

The principal finding with orbital apex fractures is optic nerve injury. The damage can range from reduced visual acuity to immediate blindness.

Superior orbital fissure syndrome can also occur. This damages structures passing through the superior orbital fissure (cranial nerves III, IV, V, and VI). It manifests as ophthalmoplegia, ptosis, proptosis, and a fixed dilated pupil. Orbital apex syndrome consists of optic nerve damage plus superior orbital fissure syndrome.[21]

Foreign Bodies

Foreign bodies can be detected by radiograph or CT scan. Radiographs permit determination of the presence of a foreign body; however, CT is the method of choice for precisely localizing a foreign body, especially if removal is required. Radiologic techniques are helpful, especially for imaging a foreign body that cannot be directly visualized, such as in vitreous hemorrhage.

Mass Lesions

Retinoblastoma

Retinoblastoma is the most common intraocular tumor of childhood. The vast majority of patients present before the age of 3 years.[22] The most common accompanying sign is a pupil that appears white. Occasionally, strabismus is present, and a previous family history can be elicited.

Retinoblastomas have intraocular calcification, which is readily detectable with CT.[22] CT is also useful in demonstrating extraocular spread to the optic nerve, orbit, or brain.

Meningioma

Meningiomas of the orbit nerve sheath occur predominately in middle-aged women. These tumors have an insidious onset with slow progressive visual loss. Disc edema, optic atrophy, proptosis, and afferent pupillary defects can be variably present.[22]

With imaging, meningiomas exhibit a diffuse enlargement of the optic nerve and sheath. Differences in density between the tumor and the optic nerve can give a characteristic tram-track appearance. Calcification is also very common and may provide a coarse or punctate character to the lesion, especially on CT.[22]

Glioma

Optic gliomas usually occur in the first decade of life, with the peak incidence between 2 and 6 years of age. The typical case presentation is a preschool-age child with visual loss and optic atrophy or less commonly, proptosis. Compared to meningioma, glioma has a younger age of onset, early and more severe visual loss, and visual disturbance that precedes proptosis.[23]

In early stages, gliomas are imaged as homogenous enlargements of the optic nerve. When large or medium in size, they have a greater tendency to appear lobulated.[23]

Ocular Metastases

Metastatic disease to the eye most commonly involves the uveal tract. Carcinoma of the breast and lung are the most common primary malignancies, although metastasis can occur from other areas. With imaging, these lesions are generally small, multiple, flat areas of increased density.[22]

Uveal Melanoma

Uveal melanoma is the most common primary intraocular malignancy in adults. Its peak incidence is in the fifth and sixth decades. Most lesions arise from choroid with less likely occurrence in the ciliary body and iris.[22]

A melanoma will usually image as a soft tissue mass next to the outer layer of the globe, which bulges toward the vitreous. If the mass breaks through Bruch's membrane, a characteristic mushroom appearance may be found.[22]

Pituitary Adenoma

Pituitary adenoma occurs most commonly in the 25- to 55-year age group. The lesion causes headaches, endocrine dysfunction, and visual field loss. As the tumor grows in an upward direction, it compresses the optic chiasm, creating a bitemporal field defect, which is denser above the midline.[24]

The adenoma will image as rounded lobulated ares of equal or slightly greater density than surrounding

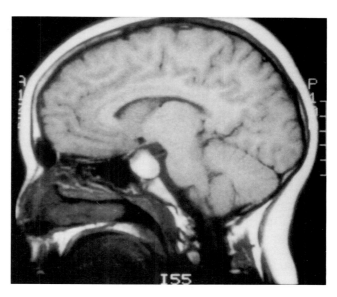

Fig. 2-8. Sagittal magnetic resonance image illustrating a pituitary adenoma that appears as a hyperintense mass.

tissue (Fig. 2-8). MRI is now considered the imaging modality of choice for investigating pituitary tumors.[24]

Other Pathology

Thyroid Ophthalmopathy

Thyroid disease is the most common cause of exophthalmos in the adult. Other accompanying ocular signs of thyroid disease include dry eyes, lid lag, scleral show, and diplopia from extraocular muscle involvement.[22]

The characteristic radiologic finding in thyroid disease is enlargement of extraocular muscles. The belly of the muscle is expanded, but the tendon insertion to the globe is spared. The exophthalmos from thyroid disease can be mistaken for orbital pseudotumor; however, the CT appearance of pseudotumor will not show tendon sparing.

Demyelinating Disease

Plaques of demyelinated neural tissue can be dramatically demonstrated by MRI as compared to CT.[23] Thus, MRI is the imaging technique of choice for evaluating optic neuritis and isolating demyelinating areas elsewhere in the brain (as in multiple sclerosis).[10]

TEST ORDERING

To request any of these tests, an order can be written on a prescription pad. It should contain the following information:

Line 1: List the test requested and the area to be scanned.
Example: X-ray left orbit.
Example: CT scan right orbit.

Line 2: Give a tentative diagnosis or instructions to rule out certain conditions. This will help the radiologist to obtain the best possible scan.
Example: Tentative diagnosis: blow-out fracture.
Example: Rule out foreign body.

Line 3: List any specific views or section definitely required.
Example: Include submentovertical view.
Example: Include coronal sections.

CONCLUSION

Like many other optometric procedures, radiologic tests are tremendous diagnostic tools. Just as these tests are a tool of the primary care physician, they should become part of the armamentarium of primary eye care as well.

REFERENCES

1. Meschan I: An Atlas of Anatomy Basic to Radiology. WB Saunders, Philadelphia, 1975
2. Semat H, Baumel P: Fundamentals of Physics. Holt, Rinehart & Winston, New York, 1974
3. Meschan I: Synopsis of Radiologic Anatomy. WB Saunders, Philadelphia, 1980
4. Gombos GM: Handbook of Ophthalmologic Emergencies. 2nd Ed. Medical Exam Publishing, New York, 1977
5. Meschan I: Radiographic Positioning and Related Anatomy. 2nd Ed. WB Saunders, Philadelphia, 1967
6. Meschan I, Farrer-Meschan R: Orbital roentgen signs in diagnostic imaging. WB Saunders, Philadelphia, 1985
7. Tower H, Oshinskie L: An introduction to computed tomography and magnetic resonance imaging of the head and visual pathways. J Am Optom Assoc 60:619, 1989
8. Peyster R: Computed Tomography in Orbital Disease and Neuro-ophthalmology. Yearbook Medical Publishers, Chicago, 1984
9. Hammerschlag S, Hesselink J, Weber A: Computed Tomography of the Eye and Orbit. Appelton-Century-Crofts, East Norwalk, CT, 1983
10. Haik B: Advanced imaging techniques in ophthalmology. Int Ophthalmol Clin 26:79, 1986
11. Deutsch T, Feller D: Management of Ocular Injuries. WB Saunders, Philadelphia, 1985
12. Slamovits T, Gardner R: Neuro imaging in neuro-ophthalmology. Ophthalmology 96:555, 1989
13. Elster A: Cranial Magnetic Resonance Imaging. Churchill Livingstone, New York, 1988
14. Deutsch TA, Feller DB: Fractures of the orbit. p. 37. In: Management of Ocular Injuries. WB Saunders, Philadelphia, 1985
15. Ohare TH: Blow-out fractures: a review. Emerg Med Rev 9:253, 1991
16. Kersten RC: Blow-Out fracture of the orbital floor with entrapment caused by isolated trauma to the orbital rim. Am J Ophthalmol 103:215, 1987
17. Vermeersch H, Heintz F, Matton G: The management of orbital roof fractures. Acta Chirurg Belg 91:277, 1991
18. Terry JE: Ophthalmic radiology. p. 563. In: Ocular Disease: Detection, Diagnosis and Treatment. Charles C Thomas, Springfield, IL, 1984
19. Penfold CN, Lang D, Evans B: The management of orbital roof fractures. Br Orbital Maxillofac Surg 30:97, 1992
20. Gruss GS: Naso-ethmoid-orbital fractures: classification and role of primary bone grafting. Plast Reconstruct Surg 75:303, 1985
21. Unger JM: Orbital apex fractures: the contribution of computed tomography. Radiology 150:713, 1984
22. Newton TH, Bilaniuk LT: Radiology of the Eye and Orbit. Raven Press, New York, 1990
23. Jacobs L, Weisberg L, Kinkel W: Computerized Tomography of the Orbit and Sella Tursica. Raven Press, New York, 1980
24. Gonzalez CF, Becker MH, Flanagan JC: Diagnostic Imaging in Ophthalmology. Springer-Verlag, New York, 1986

3 Cardiovascular Disease

JOHN E. CONTO

INTRODUCTION

Whether directly or indirectly, the vast majority of Americans are affected by cardiovascular disease, which accounts for over half of all deaths in the United States. Cardiovascular disease spans all age, racial, and socioeconomic groups. The cost to our society, both emotionally and economically, is enormous, and extensive research has been devoted to prevent these conditions and to treat affected patients. Because cardiovascular disease is common, the level of public awareness and education in general is high; unfortunately, significant misinformation persists.

Because the signs and symptoms of cardiovascular disease are often not specific, the medical examination of patients with cardiovascular disease must be performed carefully and thoughtfully.[1,2] A complete review of symptoms and medical history should begin any entry physical examination. The electrocardiogram has become an important tool to investigate a patient suspected to have a cardiovascular disorder. Chest radiograph and echocardiography are other useful noninvasive tests that may uncover important diagnostic findings. Cardiac catheterization and angiocardiography are invaluable but invasive tests.

The ocular manifestations of cardiovascular disease are well known, with hypertension and arteriosclerosis representing the most common causes of vascular damage to the eye. Unfortunately, routine ophthalmic evaluation of patients with vascular disease is still not standard, and most patients tend to present for examination when the vision has already been adversely affected. The ocular effects of cardiovascular disease are easily discovered on routine eye examination, often before notable systemic symptoms arise. Awareness of significant ocular signs can lead to early diagnosis and treatment, which is a key factor in reducing the degree of morbidity and mortality associated with the complications from cardiovascular disorders.

HYPERTENSION

Systemic hypertension is one of the most prevalent health conditions in the United States, affecting 50 to 75 million Americans, or about 20 to 30 percent of the adult population.[3–6] It is a leading risk factor for the development of coronary heart, cerebral vascular, and renal vascular disease, which are responsible for about one-half of the deaths in the United States.[7] Hypertension represents the most common cause of vascular damage to the eyes. Before the onset of menopause, hypertension is less common in women than in men but thereafter is equally distributed between the sexes.[8,9] Blacks are afflicted with hypertension two times as frequently as whites in the United States and suffer higher morbidity from hypertension than other racial groups.[5,10] The Framingham study demonstrated that the risk of developing coronary disease in both middle-age and elderly patients is directly correlated with increasing systolic and diastolic pressure.[11] In women and men older than 45 years of age, systolic elevation is a stronger risk factor for the development of coronary heart disease than diastolic elevation or mean blood pressure.[11,12] Isolated systolic hypertension is rare before the age of 55 years and is a risk factor for cardiovascular morbidity and mortality, especially stroke.[13]

Because blood pressure is a continuous variable, systemic hypertension is generally defined when diastolic blood pressure is greater than 90 mmHg or systolic blood pressure is greater than 160 mmHg on subsequent readings.[13] In 80 percent of newly diagnosed hypertensive patients, the blood pressure is mildly elevated, with diastolic pressures between 90 and 104 mmHg.[7] Borderline hypertension is considered when the blood pressure is 140 to 160 mmHg systolic or 90 to 95 mmHg diastolic. About 20 percent of the population have a blood pressure higher than 160/95 mmHg, while 45 percent have a blood pressure higher than 140/95 mmHg.[14]

From 90 to 95 percent of systemic hypertension is classified as essential hypertension, which is usually apparent by the age of 40.[15–17] The cause of essential hypertension remains unknown. Both genetic and environmental factors are thought to have a role in increasing the peripheral vascular resistance, one of the basic processes involved in hypertension. Other secondary causes of hypertension include primary aldosteronism, pheochromocytoma, Cushing's disease, toxemia of pregnancy, coarctation of the aorta, anemia, and hyperthyroidism.[7]

The lowering of blood pressure appears to reduce the morbidity and mortality even in severe cases. Hypertension may be controlled with diet or with various antihypertensive agents. In general, the higher the blood pressure elevation, the greater the chance of developing complications, which include stroke, congestive heart failure, myocardial infarction, dissection of the aorta, and kidney failure.[7,18]

Structural damage to the retinal and choroidal vascular supply from untreated hypertension manifests as hypertensive angiopathy, retinopathy, choroidopathy, and ischemic optic neuropathy. The effects are most pronounced with acute or severe elevations in blood pressure, but permanent vision loss can occur even in moderate cases. The major complications include retinal vascular occlusions that result either from the direct effects of hypertension on the vessels or from the acceleration of arteriosclerotic disease.

CASE REPORT #1

A 46-year-old black man presented with the chief complaint of a sudden onset of a floater in the right eye of 3 weeks' duration, which was also accompanied by a decrease in vision. The vision loss had not progressed since onset and appeared to be improved when he indirectly looked at objects. The floater was located centrally, and the position did not change with eye movement. He also reported photopsia in the right eye that began 1 week after the development of the floater. No other significant ocular symptoms were elicited. Ocular history was unremarkable for pathology or surgery. General medical history was remarkable for hypertension, diagnosed 10 years earlier, which was not under medical care. He denied any symptoms related to his hypertension. He was not currently using any medications and did not have any known allergies.

Best corrected visual acuities at distance were OD 20/80 and OS 20/20. Pupils were reactive to both light and near targets, with no relative afferent defect noted. Extraocular muscles demonstrated full range of motion in all positions of gaze. Confrontation fields were full to finger counting in each eye, but Amsler grid testing demonstrated an inferior nasal area of metamorphopsia in the right eye. Color vision was decreased in the right, with a 30 percent desaturation to a red target.

Evaluation of the anterior segment demonstrated mild chemosis of the bulbar conjunctiva, a clear cornea, and normal iris appearance in each eye. The anterior chamber was quiet without evidence of present or previous inflammation. The anterior chamber angles appeared to be open by von-Herrick estimation in both eyes. The intraocular pressures were OU 17 mmHg. The sitting blood pressure was 190/125 mmHg of the right arm and 185/127 mmHg of the left arm. The radial pulse was strong and steady.

Dilated examination of the posterior segment showed numerous cotton-wool spots (CWS) in the posterior pole of the right eye, along with scattered intraretinal and flame hemorrhages (Fig. 3-1 and Plate 3-1). The retinal arteries appeared narrowed, and beading and dilation of the retinal veins was evident. Hard exudates were present in the right macula in a star-shaped pattern, along with obvious edema. The right optic disc appeared to be edematous in the inferior and superior poles. Choroidopathy was not apparent. The presentation of the left posterior pole was similar to that in the right eye but without complete exudative star formation in the macula (Fig. 3-2 and Plate 3-2).

The diagnosis was severe systemic hypertension with advanced hypertensive retinopathy in both eyes. The patient was referred to internal medicine for additional studies, which did not locate any specific cause for the hypertension. The blood pressure was stabilized by a combination of clonidine hydrochloride (Catapres), atenolol (Tenormin), and furosemide (Lasix) over 3 weeks. During the following 3 months, the retinal exudates and hemorrhages resolved, with best corrected distance visual acuity of OD 20/25 and OS 20/20. Automated central visual fields demonstrated no deficits in either eye. The retinal vessels showed mild arteriosclerotic changes in both eyes. The optic disc margins were distinct, with no apparent nerve fiber layer edema.

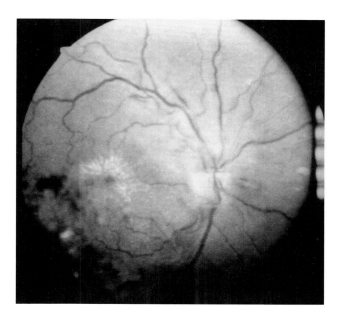

Fig. 3-1. Moderate hypertensive retinopathy in the right eye, with scattered intraretinal hemorrhages and macular star formation. The optic disc appears edematous. (Photograph courtesy of Drs. Leonard V. Messner and Stephanie S. Messner.) (See also Plate 3-1.)

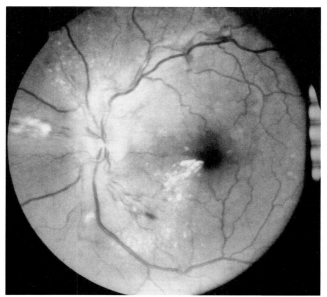

Fig. 3-2. Moderate hypertensive retinopathy in the left eye, with scattered intraretinal hemorrhages, cotton-wool spots, and optic disc edema. A partial macular star is present. (Photograph courtesy of Drs. Leonard V. Messner and Stephanie S. Messner.) (See also Plate 3-2.)

Clinical Considerations

Mild essential hypertension is almost always asymptomatic and may remain undiagnosed for many years. When symptoms occur, they usually are characteristically general and include morning headaches, tinnitus, dizziness, fainting, or increased nervousness. In accelerated or malignant hypertension, the signs and symptoms are related to the organ involved, such as transient ischemic attacks or stroke from cerebral effects, angina or myocardial infarction from coronary artery involvement, or uremia with kidney damage.

If essential hypertension is untreated, the blood pressure will continue to elevate over time, and progressive vascular damage to target organs, such as the heart, brain, or kidney may result. Secondary hypertension is usually discovered during the medical management of the primary condition and is usually controlled by treating the specific disorder.

Systemic essential hypertension is thought to be multifactorial, and although the specific factors are not known, both genetic and environmental factors are believed to be involved. When there is a positive family history, the chance of developing hypertension is increased two to four times.[19] Factors that may be inherited include a transport defect of sodium across cell membranes, an intensified sympathetic stress response, and a renal defect in sodium excretion.[20,21]

Hypertension is two to three times as prevalent in obese persons, especially those with predominantly upper body obesity.[13,22,23] Other risk factors associated with the development of hypertension include sleep apnea, physical inactivity, heavy alcohol intake, cigarette smoking, diabetes mellitus, polycythemia, and gout.[1,4,5,7] The likelihood of developing cardiovascular complications from hypertension increases significantly with older age, male sex, cigarette smoking, hypercholesterolemia, and a higher entry level of systolic pressure.[24]

The most consistent sign of hypertension is elevated blood pressure, which may vary throughout the day. Hypertension may be diagnosed when the average of multiple readings over several months is greater than or equal to a diastolic blood pressure of 90 mmHg or greater than or equal to a systolic blood pressure of 140 mmHg, or both. A diastolic blood pressure between 85 and 89 mmHg is considered to be in the high normal range. The chance of developing compli-cations is high when the diastolic blood pressure exceeds 105 mmHg, and prompt treatment is indicated.

A diastolic blood pressure between 90 and 104 mmHg is classified as *mild hypertension;* between 105 and 114 mmHg, *moderate;* and greater than 115 mmHg, *severe.* If the diastolic blood pressure is less than 90 mmHg, but the systolic blood pressure is between 140 and 159 mmHg, hypertension is defined as *borderline isolated systolic hypertension;* if greater than 160 mmHg, *isolated systolic hypertension. Malignant hypertension* usually refers to a blood pressure level greater than 200/140 mmHg. *Accelerated hypertension* refers to a significant elevated blood pressure rise over previous levels.

Pathophysiology

Blood pressure depends on the degree of blood flow or cardiac output and the vascular peripheral resistance to the blood flow.[4,13,25–28] An increase in either parameter can lead to the development of hypertension. When a defect to excrete excess sodium exists, and the intake of dietary sodium is high, the total sodium level in the body becomes elevated. Chronic sodium retention promotes increased intracellular sodium levels, which in turn leads to increased intracellular calcium. This causes vascular contraction and increased arteriolar tone, with the result of increased vascular resistance and cardiac output. Subsequently, the blood pressure becomes elevated.

Vascular contraction, and the increase in peripheral resistance, may also be initiated by a pressor mechanism. The two pressor systems thought to primarily contribute are the renin–angiotensin–aldosterone system and the sympathetic nervous system.[4,7,25] Renin, with angiotensinogen, produces angiotensin I, which with angiotensin-converting enzyme (ACE) reacts to produce angiotensin II, a potent vasoconstrictor. Angiotensin II then stimulates the release of aldosterone, which causes impaired sodium excretion from the kidneys. Stimulation of the sympathetic nervous system releases epinephrine and norepinephrine, causing vasoconstriction, increased cardiac output, release of renin, and impairment of renal sodium excretion. Epinephrine, norepinephrine, and angiotensin II also promote vascular wall hypertrophy, which causes an increase in the contractility of vascular smooth muscle tissue.

Complications

Untreated systemic hypertension is known to significantly increase the risk of cardiovascular complications, either from direct hypertensive effects or from the acceleration of atherosclerosis. About 50 percent of patients with untreated hypertension die from coronary heart disease or congestive heart failure, about 33 percent from stroke, and 10 to 15 percent from renal failure.[7] An elevation in the systolic blood pressure is probably more damaging than an elevation in the diastolic blood pressure. Men have greater cardiovascular morbidity and mortality than women for any level of hypertension.[11] Renal hypertensive involvement is more prevalent and severe in blacks than in other racial groups.[29]

The early morning rise in blood pressure is thought to be responsible for the increase in acute cardiovascular incidents in the waking hours between 5 and 10 in the morning.[30] Hypertension causes left ventricular hypertrophy, promotes coronary artery arteriosclerosis, and increases the likelihood of myocardial infarction, sudden death, arrhythmias, and congestive heart failure.[11] Silent infarction is more prevalent in hypertensive patients.[31]

Ocular Manifestations

The ocular manifestations of systemic hypertension are variable in presentation and depend on the rate, degree, and duration of the blood pressure elevation. In mild-to-moderate hypertension, eye signs are usually found during a routine eye or general medical examination, often prompting further assessment of the blood pressure level. A decrease in visual acuity is most often seen with accelerated or malignant hypertension and is caused by macular exudates, choroidal ischemia, associated serous detachment, or optic neuropathy.[32,33] Other causes of decreased visual acuity related to hypertension include amaurosis fugax and retinal vascular occlusions. The effects of systemic hypertension on the anterior segment are not specific to hypertension alone, although cataracts and primary angle glaucoma occur with increased frequency in hypertensive patients.[34]

The direct effects of hypertension on the posterior segment depend on the severity of the blood pressure elevation and present as hypertensive retinopathy, choroidopathy, and optic neuropathy.[6,14,32,35] Previous classifications of the hypertensive fundus findings, such as the Keith-Wagner-Barker, Scheie, and Leishman systems, were descriptive and attempted to correlate the fundus appearance with prognosis.[36–38] Interexaminer consistency is poor with these classifications, and with the advent of effective treatment for hypertension, they offer limited predictive value.[14,32,39]

Hypertensive Retinopathy

In untreated hypertension, the autoregulatory ability of the retinal arteries eventually fails when the blood pressure rises beyond a particular level. In mild-to-moderate elevation of the arterial blood pressure, the retinal arteries initially narrow from hypertonus or spasm of the vessels.[6,32,33] These slowly progressive changes appear as generalized or focal vasoconstriction of the arterioles, which is most evident near the optic disc and second- or third-order arterioles.[6] Distal to the arteriovenous crossings, the retinal venules may become dilated and tortuous. If the blood pressure returns to normal during this stage, the arterioles can recover without permanent damage to the vascular muscle wall.[33,40] With progressive and sustained elevations in blood pressure, however, alternating focal constrictions and dilation of the retinal arterioles develop, giving a sausage string or bead string appearance to the vasculature.[32,40,41] In the areas of constriction, hyperplasia of the vessel wall is evident, whereas collagen replacement is found where vessel dilation occurs.[6] In most patients with chronic hypertension, the prolonged elevated arterial blood pressure accelerates arteriosclerotic thickening of the vessel wall. Intimal hyalinization, medial hypertrophy, and endothelial hyperplasia are characteristic vessel alterations. These compensatory arteriosclerotic changes cause a widened arteriolar light reflex, increased arterial tortuosity, and arteriovenous crossing changes, such as nicking and banking of the retinal vessels.[6,33,40]

If the blood pressure is acutely or severely elevated, as in accelerated or malignant hypertension, the vascular wall is damaged, and the smooth muscle necroses. The arteriole can no longer constrict, and the vessel becomes dilated from the increased arterial pressure.[32,33,40,42,43] Eventually, the inner blood–retinal barrier is disrupted, resulting in decompensated exudative retinopathy. This manifests clinically as CWS, retinal hemorrhages and exudates, macular edema, and optic disc edema.[6,14,32]

CWS, or inner retinal ischemic spots, are focal infarcts of the retinal nerve fiber layer.[44] They develop following the obstruction of retinal arterioles.[44,45] Loss of the retinal nerve fiber layer and formation of intraretinal microvascular abnormalities are also evident in the involved retinal tissue.[32,44] CWSs are usually located in the peripapillary region and appear as superficial white lesions with indistinct edges. They tend to appear before retinal hemorrhages.

Extravascular retinal hemorrhages are thought to arise from the border of perfused and nonperfused retinal capillaries, where the capillaries are prone to rupture.[46] The hemorrhages initially appear in the peripapillary retina but become randomly distributed throughout the retina in later stages. Most are flame-shaped in appearance and located in the nerve fiber layer; occasionally, however, punctate hemorrhages are seen in the deeper retinal layers. A subhyaloid hemorrhage may develop when the blood breaches the inner limiting membrane.

Hard exudates also result from the breakdown of the inner blood–retinal barrier, with the deposition of plasma lipoproteins in the outer plexiform layer of the retina.[6,47] The location of intraretinal exudates is usually confined to the posterior pole. When located in the macular region, the anatomy of the retinal elements often cause the exudates to form a star-shaped configuration.[48]

Unlike in mild or moderate hypertension, arteriolar narrowing apparently does not occur in the acute phase of malignant hypertension. Instead, intraretinal perimacular transudates represent the earliest retinal changes seen in malignant hypertension.[41] These round and opaque lesions of the deep retinal layer are transient and are usually found in clusters along the posterior pole arterioles or occasionally on the optic disc surface. Intraretinal perimacular transudates can be as large as one-quarter disc in diameter. They are believed to be intraretinal plasma deposits that result from focal leakage of the vessel. Fluorescein angiography demonstrates multiple punctate arteriolar leaks caused by focal dilation of precapillary retinal arterioles. They appear to resolve without permanent retinal damage.

After intraretinal perimacular transudates develop, the next sign of malignant hypertensive retinopathy to develop is macular edema, followed by optic disc edema, acute focal retinal pigment epithelial lesions, and CWS.[6,32,33] Flame retinal hemorrhages are only occasionally seen. Hard exudates and arteriosclerotic vessel changes tend to be later manifestations of chronic malignant hypertension.

Hypertensive Choroidopathy

The effect on the choroidal vasculature from chronic essential hypertension is not as apparent as the retinal vascular changes. Because of certain physiologic characteristics, the choroidal vessels are easily damaged by acute hypertensive states, and hypertensive choroidopathy is more likely to develop when accelerated, malignant, or acute secondary hypertension exists.[6]

The choroidal vasculature will vasoconstrict when blood pressure elevates. This response is controlled by the sympathetic nervous system but lacks an autoregulatory mechanism.[42] When the blood pressure rises acutely and beyond a certain level, this response can no longer compensate, and damage results to the delicate endothelium of the smooth muscle layer. Patchy nonperfusion of the choriocapillaries develops, producing acute ischemia and necrosis of the retinal pigment epithelium. This appears as outer retinal lesions known as acute Elschnig spots or Siegrist streaks.[6,42,49,50] In chronic cases, subretinal leakage from the choroidal vessels results from the decompensation of the blood–retinal barrier, producing serous retinal detachments of the posterior pole.

Elschnig spots, or acute focal retinal pigment epithelium lesions, are pale yellow or reddish outer retinal layer lesions that develop primarily in the posterior pole. They may arise as early as 24 hours after the onset of acute hypertension.[49] Fluorescein angiography demonstrates choriocapillary hypoperfusion, with late diffuse leakage produced by localized detachments of the sensory retina from the retinal pigment epithelium.[50] Siegrist streaks, similar in appearance to Elschnig spots, are linear-aligned lesions of hyperplastic retinal pigment epithelium that are located above sclerosed choroidal vessels.[50,51] With control of the elevated blood pressure, the damaged choroidal arteries and choriocapillaries are replaced by new blood vessels, and the choroidal circulation is restored. The Elschnig spots become pigmented centrally with a surrounding depigmented halo, and the subretinal fluid is absorbed. Fluorescein angiography will show window defects without leakage.

Hypertensive Optic Neuropathy

Acutely or severely elevated blood pressure may cause ischemia of the optic disc, resulting in optic nerve head edema.[6,32,52,53] The nerve head appears hyperemic, with dilation of the surface capillaries.

Flame hemorrhages can occur at the disc margin, and edema of the nerve fiber layer may be evident. If severe, this type of anterior ischemic optic neuropathy can result in loss of vision. Optic atrophy develops from chronic disc edema, with pallor of the neuroretinal rim tissue. Papilledema may develop from the increased intracranial pressure associated with hypertensive encephalopathy.

Ocular Complications

Hypertension is a risk factor for retinal or choroidal artery occlusion, retinal arterial macroaneurysm, and central retinal vein occlusion.[54–57] Neovascularization of the retina, optic disc, or iris can develop from central retinal artery or vein occlusions, and panretinal photocoagulation should be considered in these cases. Hypertension is associated with non-arteritis ischemic optic neuropathy, especially in patients younger than age 65.[58] Systemic hypertension may be a risk factor for the development of age-related macular degeneration.[54,59] Juxtafoveal choroidal neovasculization tends to response less favorably to laser therapy.[60,61] In diabetic patients younger than age 30, hypertension may hasten the development of diabetic retinopathy.[62] Hypertension may worsen the ocular effects of connective tissue disorders, such as systemic lupus erythematosus, or polyarteritis nodosa.[35] If hypertensive retinopathy is asymmetric between the eyes, then carotid occlusive disease should be considered on the side with the lesser degree of changes. The retinopathy in pregnancy-induced hypertension is similar in appearance to that seen in essential systemic hypertension; however, a serous retinal detachment is often present.

If the blood pressure is lowered to normal levels within several months, the ocular effects from hypertension usually resolve. However, the arteriosclerotic changes that can develop from hypertension are probably permanent. Exudates in the macular region may cause depigmentation following reabsorption and reduce the visual acuity. If blood pressure is normalized too rapidly, the perfusion pressure to the optic nerve may be deceased. This may cause acute infarction of the prelaminar nerve head or increase the risk of developing normotensive glaucoma.[14,34] Ocular hypertension may progress to primary open angle glaucoma, when the blood pressure levels are reduced too quickly.[34]

Therapy

The objective in the management of systemic hypertension is to reduce the likelihood of complications. General agreement suggests that the necessary blood pressure level is below 140/90 mmHg.[4,25,63] Nondrug therapy, such as weight reduction and dietary sodium restriction, or antihypertensive medications are used as single or combined treatment regimens. Hypertension usually responds to treatment; only about 5 percent of patients fail to respond.[64] Complaints and side effects from medications, such as fatigue, weakness, and postural dizziness, are minimized when several smaller 10- to 15-mmHg reductions in blood pressure are attempted instead of a single large lowering of the blood pressure.[63] Because patients are often asymptomatic before the initiation of medical therapy, treatment noncompliance increases when the medication side effects are more pronounced. The side effects of antihypertensive medications may be related to reduced cerebral blood flow, producing cerebral hypoperfusion. Between 30 and 50 percent of patients cease therapy within 1 year of the initial diagnosis.[4,63] To promote compliance, the objective of antihypertensive medical therapy is to use the medication with the fewest side effects and the least amount of daily doses.

Because even patients with mild hypertension are at increased risk of early development of cardiovascular disease, the elevated blood pressure is usually treated either by nondrug therapy or with antihypertensive medications. Treatment is also indicated for minimally elevated diastolic blood pressure in the presence of other conditions, such as coronary artery disease, cholesteremia, cigarette smoking, family history of premature heart disease, or diabetes with early evidence of glomerulosclerosis.[65] Drug therapy is mandatory when diastolic blood pressure is above 105 mmHg or systolic blood pressure exceeds 170 mmHg.

Nondrug Therapy

Nondrug therapy—which includes weight reduction, cessation of cigarette smoking, dietary sodium restriction, reduction of alcohol ingestion, isotonic exercise, and relaxation techniques—is useful alone when mild hypertension exists or as an adjunctive treatment with medication.[4,63,66–72] When possible, weight reduction to within 15 percent of ideal body weight, reduction of alcohol to less than 1 ounce daily, and limiting daily sodium intake to 2 to 4 g can be effective in reducing the diastolic blood pressure up to 10 mmHg in some patients.

Drug Therapy

In the choice of antihypertensive medications, important considerations are race, age, and concurrent conditions such as diabetes, arthritis, chronic lung disease, angina, myocardial infarction, and congestive heart failure.[73] Fifty percent of patients with mild hypertension can be managed with monotherapy, and 90 percent with the combination of two drugs.[4] Lowering of the blood pressure below 85 mmHg has not shown to provide additional benefits and may actually increase the likelihood of complications, especially coronary events.[74] A reduction in perfusion pressure to the myocardium, either from narrowed coronary vessels, or an impaired vasodilation response, is thought to be the mechanism. β-Blockers or diuretics are believed to be more likely to produce this effect.

Diuretics are considered to be an effective class of antihypertensive medications. They include the thiazides and related sulfonamide compounds, loop diuretics, and potassium-sparing agents. Diuretics reduce the blood pressure level by volume depletion and sodium diuresis, resulting in improved hemodynamics.[4,25,63] Their use has declined because of induced metabolic disturbances, including hypokalemia, hypercholesterolemia, glucose intolerance, and hyperuricemia. Diuretics should be used with caution for patients with diabetes mellitus, gout, or digitalis toxicity. Diuretics may be more effective in blacks and the elderly. Because diuretics enhance the effectiveness of other antihypertensive medications, diuretics are considered to be useful ancillary agents.

β-Adrenergic-receptor–blocking agents, both nonselective and selective, lower arterial pressure by reducing cardiac output.[4,25,63] Nonselective β-blocking agents include propanolol, pindolol, and timolol. Cardioselective agents, such as metoprolol and atenolol, are useful in patients with bronchospasm. In general, β-blocking agents can incite bronchospasm, cause fatigue or depression, and induce hypoglycemia. They are contraindicated in patients with asthma or heart block and should be administered with caution in patients with peripheral vascular disease, insulin-dependent diabetes, allergy, coronary spasm, or withdrawal angina. β-Blockers help to relieve co-existing anxiety, angina, migraine, and glaucoma.

α-Adrenergic blockers block the effects of norepinephrine at α-receptor sites, causing peripheral vasodilation and reduced peripheral resistance.[4,25,63] They do not decrease cardiac output. Prazosin, doxazosin, and terazosin are agents that selectively block the postsynaptic α-receptors, whereas phentolamine and phenoxybenzamine provide both presynaptic and postsynaptic α-blockade. Common side effects include sudden syncope, postural dizziness, fatigue, and tachycardia. They are contraindicated in patients with advanced coronary artery disease or if orthostatic hypotension is present. α-Adrenergic blockers do not affect blood lipids levels or cause sedation.

Centrally acting antiadrenergic agents reduce sympathetic outflow by stimulating the vasomotor centers of the brain, resulting in lowered arterial pressure and cardiac output.[4,25,63] The most common drugs in this class are methyldopa, clonidine, and guanabenz. Frequent side effects include sedation, dry mouth, and postural hypotension. They are contraindicated in patients with orthostatic hypotension and liver disease. They do not alter blood lipids and do not cause fluid retention.

ACE inhibitors promote peripheral vasodilation by preventing the conversion of angiotensin I into angiotensin II.[4,25,63] The most common agents in this class include captopril, enalapril, and lisinopril. They are particularly useful in controlling accelerated or malignant hypertension. Patients receiving ACE inhibitors may complain of increased coughing, taste disturbances, or nonspecific dermatitis. These agents can induce leukopenia or proteinuria. ACE inhibitors should not be used during pregnancy and should be used with caution in patients with renal insufficiency and renovascular disease. They have the advantages of not causing central nervous system effects, congestive heart failure, or coronary vasoconstriction.

Calcium antagonists cause peripheral vasodilation, reducing arterial pressure and peripheral resistance.[4,25,63] This class of antihypertensive medications includes diltiazem, verapamil, nifedipine, and nicardipine. Flushing, local edema, and constipation are possible side effects. Because they can affect atrioventricular conduction, care should be taken when these drugs are used by heart patients. Calcium antagonists are thought to be particularly effective in blacks and the elderly.

Hydralazine and minoxidil cause vasodilation by relaxing arterial smooth muscle tissue.[4,25,63] Because these drugs have significant side effects, their use is limited to severe hypertension that is resistant to other antihypertensive agents. They are contraindicated in coronary artery disease. With higher doses, hydralazine may cause a lupus-like syndrome.

ARTERIOSCLEROSIS

Arteriosclerosis is a progressive disease of the arteries in which the vessel wall becomes rigid and thickened. Arteriosclerosis is highly prevalent in the United States and is a major cause of death and morbidity.[75–77] Vascular disorders are estimated to be re-sponsible for greater than 50 percent of deaths in the United States, with 85 percent of those due to arteriosclerotic disease.[78] Myocardial infarction from coronary artery disease is the leading cause of death secondary to arteriosclerosis, followed by cerebrovascular accident.[78]

Direct ocular complications from arteriosclerosis include central and branch retinal vessel occlusions. Arteriosclerotic carotid disease may result in the ocular ischemic syndrome. The effects of arteriosclerosis on the central nervous system may cause amaurosis fugax, visual field defects, cranial nerve palsies, gaze disturbances, and nystagmus.

CASE REPORT #2

A 69-year-old white man presented with the chief complaint of a decrease in vision in his right eye of 3 months' duration. The vision loss was not progressive. He reported a similar episode 4 years previously, which resolved within 2 weeks. No other significant symptoms were elicited. Ocular history was otherwise unremarkable for pathology or surgery. General medical history was remarkable for insulin-dependent diabetes mellitus, diagnosed 15 years earlier. He did not personally monitor the blood sugar level. He had also been hypertensive for 20 years, which he reported as under moderate control. Medications included verapamil hydrochloride (Calan) and reserpine-hydrochlorothiazide (Hydropres) for the hypertension, and twice-daily insulin injections for the diabetes. He denied any known allergies.

Best corrected visual acuities at distance were OD 20/100 and OS 20/20. Pupils were reactive to both light and near targets, with no relative afferent defect noted. Extraocular muscles demonstrated full range of motion in all gaze positions. Confrontational fields were full to finger counting in both eyes. Formal visual fields demonstrated a depression of the central field in the right eye and a full central field in the left eye. Color vision was normal in both eyes.

Biomicroscopy showed normal-appearing ocular adnexa in both eyes. The anterior chamber was deep, without signs of inflammation. No rubeosis irides was noted in either eye. The cornea was clear in each eye. Intraocular pressures were OD 18 mmHg and OS 19

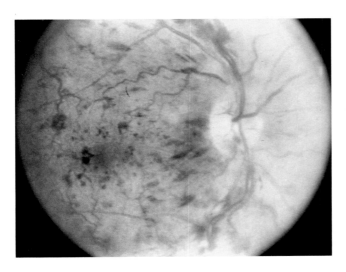

Fig. 3-3. Nonischemic central retinal vein occlusion in the right eye. Intraretinal hemorrhage, retinal edema, and retinal vein engorgement are evident. (Photograph courtesy of Dr. Leonard V. Messner.) (See also Plate 3-3.)

mmHg. Sitting blood pressure of the right arm was 168/88 mmHg.

Ophthalmoscopy of the right eye demonstrated extensive intraretinal and flame hemorrhages of the posterior pole, with substantial macular edema (Fig. 3-3 and Plate 3-3). The veins appeared to be engorged and irregular in caliber. Moderate arteriosclerosis of the retinal arteries was observed. The optic disc was slightly hyperemic, with retention of the physiologic cup. Scattered background diabetic retinopathy was evident in the posterior pole of the left eye. No flame hemorrhages or hard exudates were present. Neovascularization of the disc or elsewhere was not observed in either eye. The retinal periphery was unremarkable in each eye.

The tentative diagnosis was central retinal vein occlusion of the right eye and mild nonproliferative diabetic retinopathy of the left eye. Fluorescein angiography confirmed the diagnosis of nonischemic central retinal vein occlusion of the right eye. The patient was referred to internal medicine for additional studies, which did not reveal any medical conditions other than moderately controlled hypertension and diabetes mellitus. The central retinal vein occlusion resolved over a period of 12 weeks, with restoration of distance visual acuity of OD 20/20. The macular region showed slight pigmentary changes; however, no macular edema was present. The patient was reminded to maintain compliance of his systemic medications and was scheduled to return in 6 months for additional evaluation.

Clinical Considerations

Depending on the size and type of artery affected, arteriosclerosis may be classified as atherosclerosis, medial sclerosis, or arteriolosclerosis.[76,79] Atherosclerosis involves the intimal layer of larger arteries, such as the cerebral arteries, the carotid artery system, coronary arteries, and the abdominal aorta.[79] Atherosclerosis of the cerebral and peripheral arteries is as common as coronary artery involvement.[75] Calcification of the medial muscular layer of medium-size arteries occurs in medial sclerosis, which is also known as *focal calcific arteriosclerosis*.[79] It seldom appears before the age of 50, and appears to be equally distributed between genders. Medial sclerosis may be the result of sympathetic denervation of the smooth muscle cells, causing calcification of the vessels to become rigid.[76,79] It tends to develop in the pelvic and femoral arteries, which supply the lower extremities. Total occlusion of the affected vessel is rare, unless concurrent atherosclerosis is present. Medial sclerosis may be more severe in diabetics. Arteriolosclerosis develops in the smaller arteries and arterioles of the retinal, pancreatic, splenic, and renal vascular supply.[76,79] Proliferative and degenerative disease are the two main forms of arteriolosclerosis. The degenerative or hyaline type is an involutional process and is commonly found in the elderly population. It is characterized by the formation of lipid and collagen deposits in the intimal and medial layers of the vessel. Proliferative arteriosclerosis most often develops from acute and severe hypertension and causes smooth muscle hyperplasia and thickening of the vessel wall.

The risk of developing arteriosclerosis has been linked to several factors, including hypertension, hypercholesteremia, hyperlipidemia, hyperglycemia, cigarette smoking, and stress.[75,79–81] Obesity, aging, male gender, and genetic predisposition are also significant risk factors.[75,79–81] The Framingham study indicated that an increase in cholesterol levels is directly correlated to the degree of intimal involvement and occlusion of the vessel.[75]

Atherosclerosis of the coronary arteries has been associated with the development of ischemic heart disease, resulting in fatal arrhythmias or myocardial infarction from a decreased blood supply to the myocardium.[76] Thrombosis may also result in myocardial ischemia. When the carotid and vertebrobasilar arteries develop atherosclerosis, ischemia may result in transient ischemic attacks or stroke. Cerebral vascular disease may be detected by carotid auscultation and palpation, ultrasound, and angiography. Intermittent claudication, peripheral nonhealing ulcers, gangrene, impotence, and renal hypertension may be caused by atherosclerotic disease of the peripheral arteries.[76]

Pathophysiology

Although the exact mechanism of the arteriosclerotic process is still in debate, several theories have been proposed to explain the initiation of the fatty streak, the subsequent lipid deposition, and eventual occlusion of the artery. The endothelial injury hypothesis, or response to injury theory, proposes that endothelial cell loss occurs from the mechanical stress effects of lipids and other chemicals in the bloodstream.[75,76,]

[79,81-83] The by-products of the hydrolysis of triglyceride, chylomicrons, and very low-density lipids have damaging effects on the endothelium. An immune-related process may also contribute to endothelial injury by causing macrophages to release cytotoxic factors, along with proteolytic and lipolytic enzymes. Following endothelial cell injury and lysis, primary chemotactic and growth factors may be released. These agents help to initiate plaque formation by promoting smooth muscle cell proliferation and fibrosis.[75,76,79,82] Viruses, such as the herpesvirus and cytomegalovirus, have also been suggested as a cause of initial endothelial cell insult.[75]

Hemodynamic factors may contribute to the initiation of arteriosclerosis. Plaques tend to develop where an artery curves or bifurcates into tributaries. The hemodynamic shear pressure is relatively low at these sites, which is optimal for the accumulation of platelets or deposition of leukocytes.[75] Lesions can also develop in areas where increased lateral pressure is present, such as in hypertension, or when permeability of the endothelium is increased.[75] The endothelium may also be damaged during coronary vasospasm.

The tumor or monoclonal theory states that individual smooth muscle cells act as the initiating factor.[75,76,79] These cells promote arteriosclerotic lesion formation by serving as progenitors for subsequent cells. A failure in the feedback loop to prevent cell proliferation is thought to be the basic defect. The lysosomal theory proposes that an altered cellular enzyme function is responsible for beginning the arteriosclerotic process.[75,76,79] Lysosomal enzymes are thought to be responsible for the degradation of cellular products, and a deficit in this process would lead to an accumulation of cholesterol and lipids in the smooth muscle tissue.

The fatty streak is believed to be the first lesion to appear in atherosclerosis and the precursor to the fibrofatty plaque or atheroma.[75,76,79] Diffuse intimal thickening may also represent an early atherosclerotic change. Fatty streaks may first develop in the aorta as early as the first decade of life, and develop in the cerebral and coronary arteries, usually after the second decade. Most fatty streaks remain harmless and disappear with time. Fatty streaks appear grossly as narrow and longitudinally oriented lesions located in the intima of the vessel wall. The overlying endothelium is usually intact but may be distorted. The streaks consist of subendothelial accumulation of cholesterol esters, free cholesterol, smooth muscle cells, and macrophages or foam cells. With progression, the level of smooth muscle cells increases and becomes the dominant cell type over macrophages.

The fatty streak may develop into a fibrous plaque or atheroma, which appears as a nodular, subendothelial deposition in the intima of large and medium arteries.[75,76,79] The vessel lumen becomes narrowed, and the endothelial surface is damaged, causing disrupted blood flow and thrombosis formation. Aneurysms may develop when the intima ruptures. Atheromas form equally in the coronary and cerebral vessels. When the peripheral vasculature is involved, lower extremity claudication may occur. Renal artery atheromas cause renal vascular hypertension.

Ocular Manifestations

The ophthalmic artery and central retinal artery can develop atherosclerosis, but atheromatous plaque formation in the retinal arterioles is rare.[84] The earliest sign of arteriosclerosis is a broadening of the retinal arteriolar light reflex from increased vessel wall thickness. With continued sclerosis, the light reflex acquires a copper hue, and when the blood column becomes obscured, the arteriole will take on a silver wire cast.[85] Fluorescein angiography, however, may demonstrate normal blood flow. The arterioles may also become attenuated, with increased angulation at bifurcations, which is caused by a decreased flexibility of the vessel wall.[85,86]

The intraocular effects of arteriosclerosis often appear as changes in the venules, especially at an arteriovenous crossing, where the arteriole and the venule share a common adventitial sheath.[32] The retinal venous blood column may appear to be narrowed or tapered by a retinal artery at an arteriovenous crossing. This venous compression is referred to as *Gunn crossing sign*.[48,85] This is most likely from arteriolar wall thickening and perivascular glial cell proliferation. When the venule becomes totally obscured, the appearance is referred to as *venule nicking*.[85,87] If the sclerotic arteriolar wall causes severe blockage of venous blood flow, the venule becomes banked, and venous occlusion may occur.[85,88] Another arteriovenous crossing change, Salus sign, is a deflection of the venule in a sinusoidal pattern, or in the extreme, at right angles to the arteriole.[48,85,87]

Ocular complications from arteriosclerosis include branch retinal vein occlusion at an arteriovenous crossing, or central retinal vein occlusion at the level of the lamina cribosa. Obstruction of the branch or central retinal arteries from thrombosis or emboli from a distant site may also occur. The main source of emboli in central retinal artery occlusion is from carotid occlusive disease.[76,89,90] These emboli, known as Hollenhurst's plaques, are cholesterol particles that are yellow and glistening. They are characteristically refractile and are found usually in branch arteries, often near bifurcations. Fibrin-platelet plaques are dull gray and usually arise from the heart but can also originate from the carotid arteries. They can cause branch vessel occlusions. Calcific emboli from the heart and heart valves are white and may result in a retinal vasculitis. Fluorescein angiography should be performed in all patients with vascular occlusions, specifically to determine the degree of retinal tissue perfusion. If moderate ischemia is present, panretinal photocoagulation should be considered to discourage the development of neovascularization. Persistent cystoid macular edema from vein occlusion may require focal laser therapy. Degenerative arteriosclerosis and emboli can damage the vessel wall, promoting the development of macroaneurysms.

Ocular ischemic syndrome and resistant neovascular glaucoma may result from atherosclerotic carotid artery disease. Other cerebrovascular effects of arteriosclerosis appear as visual field defects, gaze palsies, extraocular muscle paresis, transient vision loss, and nystagmus.[76] Permanent motility disturbances may benefit from the occlusion of the affected eye or the prescribing of spectacle prism. For severe defects, low-vision devices may expand the remnant visual field.

Management

Because arteriosclerosis cannot be directly treated, management is directed at reducing the risk factors associated with the development of complications.

Hypertension, hypercholesteremia, hyperlipidemia, and glucose intolerance should be brought under control.[76] Dietary modification, weight loss, cessation of cigarette smoking, and reducing stress are important measures that may provide a beneficial effect. The Collaborative Coronary Prevention Trial of the Lipid Research Clinics demonstrated that lowering LDL by 2 mg/dl can result in a 1 percent reduction in risk of coronary artery disease.[75] Other studies have shown that aggressive cholesterol-lowering therapy may promote regression of established lesions.[79,80] Management of the complications associated with late-stage disease has improved over the last decade, with a reduction in the overall morbidity and mortality.

MITRAL VALVE PROLAPSE

Superior displacement or billowing of one or more of the mitral valve leaflets into the left atrium during systole is known as mitral valve prolapse (MVP), Barlow syndrome, or floppy valve syndrome.[91–97] MVP is considered to be one of the most common valvular disorders and is estimated to affect 3 to 10 percent of the general population.[97–101] It may occur in up to 10 percent of young women between the ages of 14 and 30.[97,99,100] Although the cause in most cases remains unknown, current research suggests that MVP may be inherited as an autosomal dominant trait.[91,96,102,103] It can present with systemic features also seen in connective tissue disorders, including thoracic deformities, spinal column disorders, and increased joint flexibility.[91,96,97] Connective tissue disorders that have been associated with MVP include Marfan syndrome, Ehlers-Danlos syndrome, pseudoxanthoma elasticum, osteogenesis imperfecta, and periarteritis nodosa.[91,96,97] Acquired heart disease, such as rheumatic heart disease, cardiomyopathy, and coronary heart disease, may also contribute to the development of MVP.[91,96,97]

CASE REPORT #3

A 36-year-old black woman presented with the chief complaint of recurrent episodes of transient vision loss of her left eye, each lasting about 1 hour, and with a full return in visual function. She reported no other symptoms related to the episode, such as scintillating phenomenon, headaches, or extremity weakness. Her mental status and speech were not affected during or after the episodes. She did not note an increase in fatigue, recent fever, or unexplained sweating. She denied incidents of syncope. Positive medication history included a congenital heart murmur. She underwent dental surgery 3 weeks previously but had received a course of prophylactic antibiotics.

Best corrected visual acuities at distance were OU 20/20. Pupils were reactive to both light and near targets, without a relative afferent defect noted. Extraocular muscles demonstrated full range of motion in all gaze positions. The eyelids were normal in position and appearance. Automated central visual fields were full in both eyes, and color vision was normal, without desaturation to red targets.

Biomicroscopy demonstrated normal-appearing anterior segment structures and ocular adnexa in each eye. No conjunctival hemorrhages were noted in either eye. The anterior chamber angles appeared to be open by von Herrick estimation in both eyes. The intraocular pressures were OU 20 mmHg. Dilated examination of the posterior segment revealed normal-appearing retinal periphery of both eyes. The maculae were healthy without any sign of edema. The retinal vascular tree in each eye was normal without any obvious emboli or vasculitis. The optic discs were healthy in appearance. Located superior temporally and adjacent to the left optic disc was an intraretinal white-centered hemorrhage (Fig. 3-4 and Plate 3-4). A second retinal hemorrhage was located in the superficial nerve fiber layer, superior to the left optic disc. No retinal hemorrhages were present in the right eye.

The sitting blood pressure was 125/80 mmHg in each arm with a strong radial pulse. Auscultation of the carotid arteries demonstrated no bruit, and the heart sounds appeared to be normal. The tentative diagnosis was noninfectious white-centered hemorrhage in the left eye, and the patient was referred to internal medicine for further studies, including a cardiac evaluation.

Echocardiography demonstrated mitral valve displacement and confirmed the diagnosis of MVP. Blood cultures were negative, and hematologic studies were normal. The patient was placed on aspirin therapy and had no further transient vision loss episodes. Subsequent examinations over a 12-week period showed resolution of the retinal hemorrhages in the left eye without permanent changes to the retinal tissue. No other hemorrhages developed, and no emboli were evident in either eye.

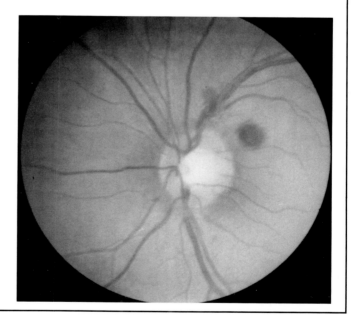

Fig. 3-4. White-centered hemorrhage in the left eye, temporal to the optic nerve disc. Additional nerve fiber hemorrhage is located directly superior to the optic disc. The patient has a history of transient vision loss and a mitral valve prolapse. (See also Plate 3-4.)

Clinical Considerations

MVP is usually detected during a routine physical examination and is characterized by the presence of one or more mid- to late systolic clicks followed by a late systolic murmur.[91,97,104] The electrocardiogram findings are usually abnormal but not specific for MVP. Confirmation is usually made by two-dimensional echocardiography demonstrating systolic displacement of the mitral valve leaflets.[54,91] Chordal rupture, mitral regurgitation, and annular dilation may also be evident. In general, the clinical course of MVP is usually benign, but some patients may develop significant regurgitation and ventricular dilation. The vast majority of patients are asymptomatic. When symptoms are present, however, they are related to either the degree of valvular prolapse, and the subsequent effects on the intracardiac hemodynamics, or arrhythmia. In severe cases, patients may complain about fatigue, difficulty breathing, fainting, atypical chest pain, and heart palpitations.

Pathogenesis

The pathogenesis of MVP is unclear but is thought to be related to a defect in collagen metabolism.[105,106] The result is a myxomatous proliferation of the mitral valve leaflet, with the resultant prolapse during systole. Gross examination of the diseased valve demonstrates an increase in the surface area of the leaflets, elongated or ruptured chordae tendinae, and enlargement of the annular diameter.[96] The combination of the diseased valvular surface and abnormal blood flow may stimulate platelet coagulant hyperactivity resulting in the development of intravascular thromboemboli.[107,108] Emboli to the brain and retina may cause transient ischemic attacks, reversible neurologic deficits, or completed stroke. Transient visual obscurations and hemifield defects have also been reported.[54,107–110] Although most cases are considered benign, complications include sudden death, acute myocardial infarction, arrhythmias, and infectious endocarditis.[91,96,97]

Ocular Manifestations

The local effects of platelet coagulant hyperactivity are thought to cause most of the ocular complications seen in MVP.[97] However, small fibrin and platelet retinal emboli have been reported.[111–114] Amaurosis fugax is reported in about one-quarter of cases.[97,113,115,116] Retinal hemorrhages may be seen in the nerve fiber layer or intraretinally. Unilateral or bilateral retinal and choroidal arteriolar occlusions can occur. Retinal venous occlusions have been associated in patients with MVP and platelet coagulant hyperactivity that are younger than 50 years of age.[97,117,118] Occlusion of the short posterior ciliary arteries may result in anterior ischemic optic neuropathy. Other less common ocular associations include atypical Eales disease, keratoconus, cataracts, high myopia, and progressive external ophthalmoplegia.[97,111,119,120]

Management of the ocular complications associated with MVP depends on the particular condition. Fluorescein angiography is indicated in all cases with associated retinal vascular occlusion. A careful history and ocular examination must be performed to exclude other conditions that may present with amaurosis fugax, such as migraine, sickle cell disease, or hypercoagulation conditions. In elderly patients, carotid occlusive disease and giant cell arteritis must be also considered.

Therapy

Treatment of MVP is usually limited to symptomatic patients or patients with arrhythmia. Antiarrhythmic agents may be used if necessary, and a β-blocker, such as propanolol, is the preferred medication to control ventricular arrhythmia. β-Blockade has also been reported to relieve the chest pain associated with MVP.[91,96,97] Oral antiplatelet therapy with aspirin or dipyridamole or anticoagulants are employed in patients suffering transient ischemic attacks. If medical therapy fails to prevent embolization, mitral valve replacement surgery should be considered. As with any valvular heart disease, patients with MVP often receive prophylactic antibiotics before dental manipulation.[91,96] This is believed to reduce the possibility of the development of bacterial endocarditis. It should be emphasized that the vast majority of patients with MVP are asymptomatic and require only periodic observation every several years, including echocardiography.

INFECTIOUS ENDOCARDITIS

Infectious endocarditis (IE) is an infection of the heart valves or the endocardium, most often caused by bacteria. Fungi, chlamydia, and rickettsia are also known to cause IE, but primary viral infection is relatively rare.[96,121,122] Endoarteritis, a microbial invasion of a large artery, can have a clinical presentation similar to that of IE.[123] If left untreated, IE is almost always fatal. IE affects all age groups and is usually related to an underlying defect in the heart tissue. IE appears to exhibit no preference in race or gender. In children, congenital heart defects, such as septal defects, stenotic valves, tetralogy of Fallot, and patent ductus arteriosus, are the most common disorders found in association with IE.[124] MVP, aortic and mitral valve degeneration, congenital heart disease, and rheumatic heart disease are the major contributing disorders in adults.[125] Other major risk factors are intravenous drug abuse and prosthetic valve replacement.

Clinical Considerations

The clinical presentation of IE may follow an acute or subacute course, which is determined by the virulence of the organism, and the general medical status of the patient. Acute IE is caused by highly virulent organisms, such as *Staphylococcus aureus*, *Streptococcus pneumoniae*, or *Neisseria gonorrhoeae*, while less virulent pathogens, such as *Streptococcus viridans*, enterococcus, anaerobic streptococcus, rickettsieae, or fungi, usually cause subacute disease.

The symptoms of IE usually present within 2 weeks of the initial infection, with common complaints of malaise, night sweats, fatigue, loss of appetite, and weight loss. These symptoms can be confused with those seen in influenza, tuberculosis, collagen vascular disease, congestive heart failure, stroke, carcinoma, lymphoma, or atrial myxoma. Most patients have an intermittent low-grade fever, with afternoon or evening peaks. Heart murmurs are evident in 95 percent of cases and often are related to valvular damage.[121] Murmurs may be absent in acute disease and in right-sided heart infection.

Acute bacterial infectious endocarditis usually followed a suppurative infection, with a fulminant and rapid presentation. A high fever with chills is common. The normal heart is more often involved in acute disease, particularly in intravenous drug abusers.[126]

Prosthetic valve endocarditis occurs in 1 to 4 percent of patients, within the first year after surgery.[127] Early infections within 2 months of surgery usually are caused by resistant strains, and a high rate of death occurs from valve dehiscence, myocardial invasion, or septic shock.[126] Delayed prosthetic valve endocarditis is typically caused by a nonsterile prosthetic

valve, or by transient bacteremia following other surgical procedures, and has a better prognosis.[126]

The physical findings in infectious endocarditis are not specific and can be quite variable among patients. Splenomegaly and clubbing of fingers or toes can develop in one-third of cases longer than 6 weeks in duration.[128,129] Damage to cutaneous blood vessels may result in widespread petechial hemorrhages. They commonly occur in the conjunctival, palate, or buccal mucosa, and in the skin above the upper trunk region. These hemorrhages are not tender and do not blanch on pressure. Linear and splinter hemorrhages may appear under the nailbeds. Osler's nodes are tender, pea-sized nodules that are red or purple and are located on the finger or toe pads.[130,131] They can last for hours to days and are thought to represent an accumulation of immune-complex substance or septic embolization. Janeway lesions are painless, reddish-blue macules on the soles and palms that more commonly occur in acute IE. They are thought to result from septic emboli.[132]

Infection of the heart valves may cause leaflet perforation, obstruction, or chordae rupture.[96,121,126] Cardiac abscesses and purulent pericardial infusions are also possible complications. Cardiac arrhythmias, interchamber fistulas, or sinus aneurysms may develop, causing fatigue, shortness of breath, chest pain, palpitations, and progressive heart failure.[133] Postinfection scarring may promote valvular stenosis or insufficiency. The most common complication from IE is congestive heart failure.[134] Myocardial infarction and myocarditis are usually the result of coronary artery emboli, myocardial abscesses, or immune complex vasculitis.

The extracardiac effects of IE are usually as a result of emboli, especially in acute disease.[96,121,126,133] Emboli to distal foci originate from the left side of the heart and may be septic or bland. The most common complications of distant embolization are organ infarction, localized abscesses, and mycotic aneurysms. Pulmonary infarction may occur if the right side of the heart is involved. Other complications from emboli can arise and include acute vascular insufficiency of the extremities, hematuria, and acute mesenteric infarction. Emboli to the kidneys may result in infarction or abscess.

Both the humoral and cell-mediated immune systems become activated in the presence of sustained infection, and circulating antigen–antibody complexes are commonly found with chronic subacute disease.[135] Arthritis, Osler's nodes, glomerulonephritis, or cutaneous vasculitis are common complications associated with immune complex deposition.[136,137]

IE can cause neurologic complications, such as strokes, brain abscesses, mycotic aneurysms, and purulent meningitis, in about one-third of the patients.[121,122,138] The most common complaint is headaches, followed by transient ischemic attacks. One-half of patients suffer cerebral vascular accidents, with infarction of the middle cerebral artery causing hemiplegia.[129] Cerebral arteritis, cranial nerve palsies, intracerebral hemorrhage, and toxic encephalopathy are also common central nervous system complications.

IE should be considered when the characteristic clinical signs are present. Blood cultures are mandatory and are positive in 95 percent of cases.[121,126] Normocytic anemia in subacute endocarditis is often found. The white blood cell count is usually normal in subacute infection, but leukocytosis is usually seen with acute disease. Thrombocytopenia may also occur, and the erythrocyte sedimentation rate is almost always elevated. Urine abnormalities include proteinuria, microscopic hematuria, and microscopic pyuria. In chronic endocarditis, the serum globulin may be elevated, and a positive rheumatoid factor is found in one-half of the cases lasting longer than 3 weeks.[139] Echocardiography may demonstrate vegetative deposits on the heart valves.

Pathophysiology

Although highly virulent microorganisms can invade normal cardiac tissue, the usual mechanism by which IE develops requires a predisposing heart defect. Deposition of fibrin and platelets at the site of the injured endothelium occurs and is known as noninfectious thrombotic endocarditis.[96,121,122,126] Circulating microorganisms can then adhere to and proliferative on the altered endothelial surface. Blood-borne foreign particles, as seen in intravenous drug abuse; systemic conditions, such as systemic lupus erythematosus; and prosthetic cardiac valves can also damage the cardiac endothelium, producing noninfectious thrombotic endocarditis.

Bacteria, the most common microorganism causing IE, typically cross into the bloodstream following trauma to the upper respiratory area during dental procedures or oropharynx surgery. The most common bacterial species are streptococci followed by staphylococci.[96,121,122,126] When transient bacteremia develops from the gastrointestinal or urogenital tract, enterococci are usually isolated. Staphylococcal, gram-negative bacilli and fungi infections are more prevalent in intravenous drug abusers and typically enter through the skin.[96,121,122,126] Prosthetic valve endocarditis is commonly caused by staphylococci.[96,121,122,126]

Ocular Manifestations

Most of the ocular complications of IE are the result of emboli to either the eye or brain, and usually resolve with successful systemic treatment of the infectious agent. Involvement of cranial nerves III, IV, and VI can produce diplopia, and damage to the facial nerve may lead to lagophthalmos or tearing abnormalities.[140] The palpebral and bulbar conjunctiva may show petechial hemorrhages.

The classically described finding is the white-centered intraretinal hemorrhage, or Roth spot, which is thought to be the result of focal retinitis caused by infectious emboli or a fibrin-platelet clot.[122,141–143] Leukocyte aggregation or focal ischemia are thought to cause the white-centered appearance.[122] Roth spots occur in less than 5 percent of patients with IE and are more commonly associated with an acute course.[121,141] Superficial retinal hemorrhages can also occur. Central retinal artery or branch artery occlusion can result from emboli, whereas occlusion of smaller retinal vessels produce CWS. Occlusion of the short posterior ciliary arteries may cause anterior ischemic optic neuropathy. In one-third of cases, papilledema may develop, with the enlargement of the blind spot.[144] If the globe is infected by highly virulent organisms, acute endophthalmitis may develop. Intraocular infection from less virulent organisms may cause choroiditis, focal retinitis, vitritis, or uveitis.[144–146]

Therapy

Therapy is geared toward the use of bactericidal agents, since the vegetations must be rendered sterile so that relapse does not occur. High doses of antibiotics are required. A variety of antibacterial agents are used, such as penicillins, cephalosporins, vancomycin, aminoglycosides, or quinolones.[121] Fungal endocarditis is very unresponsive to the standard antifungal agents currently available, with the outcome very poor and often characterized by relapses. Most patients respond to effective antibiotic therapy within 3 to 7 days. Recovery from untreated endocarditis is rare.

Surgical intervention is indicated when standard trials of antibiotic therapy fail or if secondary cardiac complications arise. Damaged valves can be replaced or resected, and surgical drainage of myocardial or valve ring abscesses may be necessary. Recurrent emboli also indicate the need for surgical intervention. Anticoagulants are of no value in the treatment of IE and do not prevent emboli or augment antibiotic therapy.[147]

The curative rate for patients with endocarditis is greater than 90 percent for streptococcal endocarditis, 75 to 90 percent for enterococcal endocarditis, and 60 to 75 percent for *S. aureus* endocarditis.[121] Death usually is from superinfection, rupture of mycotic aneurysms, emboli, heart failure, cardiac surgery complications, and renal failure.[121] Poor prognosis is associated with the elderly and very young, aortic versus mitral valve involvement, left-sided versus right-sided endocarditis, myocardial abscess, ruptured mycotic aneurysm, emboli, heart failure, renal insufficiency, and cardiac surgery.[121] The survival rate in patients with prosthetic valve endocarditis is about 50 percent in late disease and 20 percent in early infection.[121]

The optimal approach in preventing endocarditis is the correction of underlying systemic defects. Antibiotic prophylaxis is of value in patients who undergo procedures that may result in bacteremia and have a prior knowledge of a predisposing cardiac effect. Most patients, however, are not aware of underlying defects before the onset of IE.

REFERENCES

1. Braunwald E: Approach to the patient with heart disease. p. 863. In Braunwald E, Isselbacher KJ, Petersdorf RG et al (eds): Harrison's Principles of Internal Medicine. 11th Ed. McGraw-Hill, New York, 1987
2. Bates B: A Guide to Physical Examination and History Taking. 4th Ed. JB Lippincott, Philadelphia, 1987
3. Newcomb R: Epidemiology of hypertension and diabetes mellitus. Optom Clin 2:1, 1992
4. Schwartz G: Diagnosis, pathogenesis, and management of essential hypertension. Optom Clin 2:31, 1992
5. Joint National Committee on Detection, Evaluation, and Treatment of High Blood Pressure: The 1984 report of the Joint National Committee on the detection, evaluation, and treatment of high blood pressure. Arch Intern Med 144:1045, 1984
6. Lewis H: Hypertensive ocular disease. Curr Opin Ophthalmol 2:169, 1991
7. Kaplan N: Systemic hypertension: mechanisms and diagnosis. p. 852. In Braunwald E (ed): Heart Disease, A Textbook of Cardiovascular Medicine. 4th Ed. WB Saunders, Philadelphia, 1992
8. Dustan H: Racial differences in hypertension. Vas Pract 6:4, 1989
9. Rowland W, Roberts J: Blood pressure levels and hypertension in persons aged 6–74 years: United States, 1976–1980. In: Advandced Data From Vital Health Statistics. National Center for Health Statistics (Public Health Service), Hyattsville, MD, 1982
10. Otten M, Teutsch S, Williamson D et al: The effect of known risk factors on the excess mortality of black adults in the United States. JAMA 263:845, 1990
11. Levy D, Wilson P, Anderson K et al: Stratifying the patient at high risk from coronary disease: new insights from the Framingham Heart Study. Am Heart J 119:712, 1990
12. Page L, Sidd J: Medical management of primary hypertension. N Engl J Med 287:960, 1972
13. Joint National Committee on Detection, Evaluation, and Treatment of High Blood Pressure: The 1988 report of the Joint National Committee on detection, evaluation, and treatment of high blood pressure. Arch Intern Med 148:1023, 1988
14. Hayreh S: Hypertension. p. 664. In Gold D, Weingeist T (eds): The Eye in Systemic Disease. JB Lippincott, Philadelphia, 1990
15. Rudnick K, Sackett D, Hirst S et al: Hypertension in family practice. Can Med Assoc J 3:492, 1977
16. Danielson M, Dammstrom B: The prevalence of secondary and curable hypertension. J Intern Med 209:451, 1981
17. Sinclair A, Isles C, Brown I et al: Secondary hypertension in a blood pressure clinic. Arch Intern Med 147:1289, 1987
18. MacMahon S, Petp R, Cutler J et al: Blood pressure, stroke, and coronary heart disease. Part I. Prolonged differences in blood pressure: prospective observational studies corrected for the regression dilution bias. Lancet 335:765, 1990
19. Williams R, Hunt S, Hasstedt S et al: Definition of genetic factors in hypertension: a search for major genes, polygenes, and homogenous subtypes. J Cardiovasc Pharmacol, suppl. 12:S7, 1988
20. Williams R, Hunt S, Hasstedt S et al: Current knowledge regarding the genetics of human hypertension. J Hypertens, suppl. 7:S8, 1989
21. Julius S: Autonomic nervous system dysregulation in human hypertension. Am J Cardiol 67:3B, 1991
22. Stamler R, Stamler J, Riedlinger W et al: Weight and blood pressure-findings in hypertension screen of 1 million Americans. JAMA 240:1607, 1978
23. Frohlich E, Messerli F, Reisin E et al: The problem of obesity and hypertension. Hypertension, suppl. 5:S71, 1983
24. Medical Research Council Working Party: MRC Trial of treatment of mild hypertension: principle results. Br Med J 291:97, 1985
25. Williams G, Braunwald E: Hypertensive vascular disease. p. 1024. In Braunwald E, Isselbacher KJ, Petersdorf RG et al (eds): Harrison's Principles of Internal Medicine, McGraw-Hill, New York, 1987
26. Genest J, Kuchel O, Hamet P et al: Pathophysiology of experimental and human hypertension. p. 1. In Genest J, Kuchel O, Hamet P (eds): Hypertension: Physiopathology and Treatment. 2nd Ed. McGraw-Hill, New York, 1983
27. Pickering G: Hypertension: definitions, natural histories and consequences. Am J Med 52:570, 1972
28. Lund-Johansen P: Central haemodynamics in essential hypertension at rest and during exercise: a 20 year follow-up study. J Hypertens, suppl. 7:S52, 1989

29. Whelton P, Klag M: Hypertension as a risk factor for renal disease. Review of clinical and epidemiological evidence. Hypertension, suppl. 13:S1, 1989

30. Muller J, Tofler G, Stone P: Circadian variation and triggers of onset of acute cardiovascular disease. Circulation 68:733, 1989

31. Kannel W: Contribution of the Framingham Study to preventive cardiology. J Am Coll Cardiol 15:206, 1990

32. Locke L: Ocular manifestations of hypertension. Optom Clin 2:47, 1992

33. Hayreh S: Classification of hypertensive fundus changes and their order of appearance. Ophthalmologica 198:247, 1989

34. Alexander L: Diagnosis and management of primary open-angle glaucoma. Optom Clin 1:19, 1991

35. Tso M, Abrams G, Jampol L: Hypertensive retinopathy, choroidopathy, and optic neuropathy: a clinical and pathophysiological approach to classification. p. 79. In Singermann L, Jampol L (eds): Retinal and Choroidal Manifestations of Systemic Disease. Williams & Wilkins, Baltimore, 1991

36. Keith N, Wagener H, Barker N: Some different types of essential hypertension: their course and prognosis. Am J Med Sci 197:332, 1939

37. Leishman R: The eye in general vascular disease: hypertension and arteriosclerosis. Br J Ophthalmol 41:641, 1957

38. Scheie H: Evaluation of ophthalmoscopic changes of hypertension and arteriosclerosis. Arch Ophthalmol 49:117, 1953

39. Dimmitt S, Eames S, Gosling P et al: Usefulness of ophthalmoscopy in mild to moderate hypertension. Lancet 1:1103, 1989

40. Grey R: Vascular Disorders of the Ocular Fundus. Butterworth, London, 1991

41. Hayreh S, Servais G, Verdi P: Fundus lesions in malignant hypertension. IV. Focal intraretinal periarteriolar transudates. Ophthalmology 92:60, 1985

42. Tso M, Jampol L: Pathophysiology of hypertensive retinopathy. Ophthalmology 89:1132, 1981

43. Walsh J: Hypertensive retinopathy; description, classification and prognosis. Ophthalmology 89:1127, 1982

44. Hayreh S, Servais G, Verdi P: Cotton-wool spots (inner retinal ischemic spots) in malignant arterial hypertension. Ophthalmologica 198:197, 1989

45. Apple D, Rabb M: Ocular Pathology, Clinical Applications, and Self-Assessment. Mosby-Yearbook, St. Louis, 1991

46. Hayreh S, Servais G, Verdi P: Retinal arteriolar changes in malignant arterial hypertension. Ophthalmologica 198:197, 1989

47. Hayreh S, Servais G, Verdi P: Retinal lipid deposits in malignant arterial hypertension. Ophthalmologica 198:216, 1989

48. Duke-Elder S, Dobree J: Retinopathies associated with general disease. p. 277. In Duke-Elder S (ed): System of Ophthalmology. CV Mosby, St. Louis, 1967

49. deVenecia G, Wallow I, Houser D et al: The eye in accelerated hypertension. I. Elschnig's spots in nonhuman primates. Arch Ophthalmol 98:913, 1980

50. Hayreh S, Servais G, Verdi P: Fundus lesions in malignant hypertension. VI. Hypertensive choroidopathy. Ophthalmology 93:1383, 1986

51. Pohl M: Siegrist's streaks in hypertensive choroidopathy. J Am Optom Assoc 59:372, 1988

52. Kishi S, Tso M, Hayreh S: Fundus lesions in malignant hypertension. II. A pathological study of experimental hypertensive optic neuropathy. Arch Ophthalmol 103:1198, 1985

53. Hayreh S, Servais G, Verdi P: Fundus lesions in malignant hypertension. V. Hypertensive optic neuropathy. Ophthalmology 93:74, 1986

54. Leys A: Ocular manifestations of cardiovascular and hematologic disorders. Curr Opin Ophthalmol 3:253, 1992

55. Panton R, Goldberg M, Farber M: Retinal arterial macroaneurysms: risk factors and natural history. Br J Ophthalmol 74:595, 1990

56. Elman M, Bhatt A, Quinlan P et al: The risk for systemic vascular diseases and mortality in patients with central retinal vein occlusion. Ophthalmology 97:1543, 1990

57. D'Amato R, Miller N, Fine S et al: The effect of age and initial visual acuity on the systemic and visual prognosis of central retinal vein occlusion. NZ J Ophthalmol 19:119, 1991

58. Sawle G, James C, Russell R: The natural history of non-arteritic anterior ischaemic optic neuropathy. J Neuro Neurosurg Psychiatry 53:830, 1990

59. Sperduto R, Hiller R: Systemic hypertension and age-related maculopathy in the Framingham Study. Arch Ophthalmol 104:216, 1986

60. Macular Photocoagulation Study: Krypton laser photocoagulation for neovascular lesions of age-related macular degeneration. results of a randomized clinical trial. Arch Ophthalmol 108:816, 1990

61. Jampol L: Hypertension and visual outcome in the Macular Photocoagulation Study. Arch Ophthalmol 109:789, 1991

62. Krolewski A, Canesa M, Warram J et al: Predisposition to hypertension and susceptibility to renal disease to insulin-dependent diabetes mellitus. N Engl J Med 318:140, 1988

63. Kaplan N: Systemic hypertension: therapy. p. 852. In Braunwald E (ed): Heart Disease, A Textbook of Cardiovascular Medicine. 4th Ed. WB Saunders, Philadelphia, 1992

64. Kaplan N: Clinical Hypertension. 4th Ed. Williams & Wilkins, Baltimore, 1990

65. WHO/ISH Mild Hypertension Liaison Committee: 1989 Guidelines for the management of mild hypertension. J Hypertens 7:689, 1989

66. Staessen J, Fagard R, Lijnen P et al: Body weight, sodium intake and blood pressure. J Hypertens 7:S19, 1989

67. MacMahon S, Norton R: Alcohol and hypertension: implications for prevention and treatment. Ann Intern Med 105:124, 1986

68. Weinberger M, Cohen S, Miller J et al: Dietary sodium restriction as adjunctive treatment of hypertension. JAMA 259:2561, 1988

69. Patel C, Marmot M, Terry D et al: Trial of relaxation in reducing coronary risk: four year follow-up. Br Med J 290:1103, 1985

70. Nelson L, Jennings G, Esler M et al: Effect of changing levels of physical activity on blood-pressure and haemodynamics in essential hypertension. Lancet 2:473, 1986

71. MacGregor G, Markandu N, Sagnella G et al: Double-blind study of three sodium intakes and long-term effects of sodium restriction in essential hypertension. Lancet 2:1244, 1989

72. Hagberg I, Montain S, Martin WI et al: Effect of exercise training in 60–69 year old persons with essential hypertension. Am J Cardiol 64:348, 1989

73. Stewart A, Greenfield S, Hays R et al: Functional status and well-being of patients with chronic conditions. Results from the Medical Outcomes Study. JAMA 262:907, 1989

74. Cruickshank J: Coronary flow reserve and the J curve relation between diastolic blood pressure and myocardial infarction. Br Med J 297:1227, 1988

75. Brown W, Le N, Gravanis M: Atherogenesis. p. 1. In Gravanis M (ed): Cardiovascular Disorders, Pathogenesis and Pathophysiology. CV Mosby, St Louis, 1993

76. Soukiasian S, Lahav M: Arteriosclerosis. p. 649. In Gold D, Weingeist T (eds): The Eye in Systemic Disease. JB Lippincott, Philadelphia, 1990

77. National Center for Health Statistics: Vital Statistics of the United States, 1986, Vol 11, Mortality, Part A. PHHS Pub. No. (PHS) 88-1122. Public Health Service. Washington, DC. U.S. Government Printing Office, 1988

78. Walsh J: Cardiovascular disorders. p. 22:1. In Tasman W, Jaeger E (eds): Duane's Clinical Ophthalmology. Vol. 5. JB Lippincott, Philadelphia, 1991

79. Bierman E: Atherosclerosis and other forms of arteriosclerosis. p. 1014. In Braunwald E, Isselbacher KJ, Petersdorf RG et al (eds): Harrison's Principles of Internal Medicine. 11th Ed. McGraw-Hill, New York, 1987

80. McGill H: Persistent problems in the pathogenesis of atherosclerosis. Atherosclerosis 4:443, 1984

81. Ross R: The pathogenesis of atherosclerosis. p. 1106. In Braunwald E (ed): Heart Disease, A Textbook of Cardiovascular Medicine. 4th Ed. WB Saunders, Philadelphia, 1992

82. Ross R: The pathogenesis of atherosclerosis—an update. N Engl J Med 314:488, 1986

83. Ross R, Blomset J: The pathogenesis of atherosclerosis. N Engl J Med 295:369, 1976

84. Brownstein S, Font R, Alper M: Atheromatous plaques of the retinal blood vessels: histologic confirmation of ophthalmoscopically visible lesions. Arch Ophthalmol 90:49, 1973

85. Green W: Systemic diseases with retinal involvement. p. 1034. In Spencer W (ed): Ophthalmic Pathology: An Atlas and Textbook. WB Saunders, Philadelphia, 1985

86. Michaelson I: Diseases of the retinal vessels; the hypertensive and arteriosclerotic retinopathies. p. 171. In: Textbook of the Fundus of the Eye. 3rd Ed. Churchill Livingstone, Edinburgh, 1980

87. Shelburne S: Hypertensive Retinal Disease. Grune & Stratton, Orlando, FL, 1965

88. Michaelson I: Changes in the retinal arteries. p. 89. In: Textbook of the Fundus of the Eye. 3rd Ed. Churchill Livingstone, Edinburgh, 1980

89. Appen R, Wray S, Cogan D: Central retinal artery occlusion. Am J Ophthalmol 79:374, 1975

90. Arruga J, Sanders M: Ophthalmologic findings in 70 patients with evidence of retinal embolism. Ophthalmology 89:1333, 1982

91. Braunwald E: Valvular heart disease. p. 1007. In Braunwald E (ed): Heart Disease, A Textbook of Cardiovascular Medicine. 4th Ed. WB Saunders, Philadelphia, 1992

92. Popcock W: Mitral leaflet billowing and prolapse. p. 45. In Barlow J (ed): Perspectives on the Mitral Valve. FA Davis, Philadelphia, 1987

93. Perloff J, Child J, Edwards J: New guidelines for the clinical diagnosis of mitral valve prolapse. Am J Cardiol 57:1124, 1986

94. Fontana M, Sparks E, Boudoulas H, et al: Mitral valve prolapse and the mitral valve prolapse syndrome. Curr Probl Cardiol 16:311, 1991

95. Fowler N: Mitral Valve Prolapse. Springer-Verlag, New York, 1991

96. Boudoulas H, Gravanis M: Valvular heart disease. p. 64. In Gravanis M (ed): Cardiovascular Disorders, Pathogenesis and Pathophysiology. CV Mosby, St Louis, 1993

97. Scimeca G, Magargal L: Mitral valve prolapse syndrome. p. 5. In Gold D, Weingeist T (eds): The Eye in Systemic Disease. JB Lippincott, Philadelphia, 1990

98. Savage D, Garrison R, Devereux R et al: Mitral valve prolapse in the general population. I. epidemiologic features: The Framingham Study. Am Heart J 106:571, 1983

99. Procacci P, Savran S, Schreiter S et al: Prevalence of clinical mitral valve prolapse in 1169 young women. N Engl J Med 294:1086, 1976

100. Markiewicz W, Stoner J, London E et al: Mitral valve prolapse in one hundred presumably healthy young females. Circulation 53:464, 1976

101. Levy D, Savage D: Prevalence and clinical features of mitral valve prolapse. Am Heart J 113:1281, 1987

102. Malcolm A: Mitral valve prolapse associated with other disorders. causal coincidence, common link, or fundamental genetic disturbance? Br Heart J 53:353, 1985

103. Pader E: The familial incidence of mitral valve prolapse. A report of three generations in one family. NY State J Med 84:395, 1984

104. Devereux R, Perloff J, Reicheck N et al: Mitral valve prolapse. Circulation 54:3, 1976

105. Davies M, Moore B, Braimbridge M: The floppy mitral valve. Study of incidence, pathology and complications in surgical, necropsy and forensic material. Br Heart J 40:368, 1978

106. Whittaker P, Boughner D, Perkins D, et al: Quantitative structural analysis of collagen in chordae tendineae and its relation to floppy mitral valves and proteoglycan infiltration. Br Heart J 57:264, 1987

107. Kostuk W, Boughner D, Barnett H et al: Strokes: a complication of mitral valve prolapse. Lancet 2:313, 1977

108. Walsh P, Kansu T, Corbett J et al: Platelets, thromboembolism, and mitral valve prolapse. Circulation 63:552, 1981

109. Barnett H, Boughner D, Taylor W et al: Further evidence relating mitral valve prolapse to cerebral ischemic events. N Engl J Med 302:139, 1980

110. Barnett H, Jones M, Boughner D et al: Cerebral ischemic events associated with prolapsing mitral valve. Arch Neurol 33:777, 1976

111. Caltrider N, Irvine A, Kline H et al: Retinal emboli in patients with mitral valve prolapse. Am J Ophthalmol 90:534, 1980

112. Seelenfreund M, Silverstone B, Hirsch I et al: Mitral valve prolapse (Barlow's syndrome) and retinal emboli. Metab Pediatr Syst Ophthalmol 11:119, 1988

113. von Rhee F, Blecher T, DeLepeleire K et al: Bilateral retinal artery occlusion due to mitral valve prolapse. Br J Ophthalmol 75:436, 1991

114. Young B: The significance of retinal emboli. J Clin Neuro Ophthalmol 9:190, 1989

115. Lesser R, Heenemann M, Borkowski H et al: Mitral valve prolapse and anaurosis fugax. J Clin Neuro Ophthalmol 1:153, 1981

116. Eiden S, Olivares G: Transient vision loss associated with Barlow's syndrome. J Am Optom Assoc 57:446, 1986

117. Gonder J, Magargal L, Walsh P et al: Central retinal vein obstruction associated with mitral valve prolapse. Can J Ophthalmol 18:220, 1983

118. Magargal L, Gordon J, Maher V: Central retinal vein obstruction in the young adult. Trans Pa Acad Ophthalmol Otolaryngol 37:148, 1985

119. Traboulsi E, Aswad M, Jalkh A et al: Ocular findings in mitral valve prolapse syndrome. Ann Ophthalmol 19:354, 1987

120. Beardsley T, Foulks G: An association of keratoconus and mitral valve prolapse. Ophthalmology 89:35, 1982

121. Korzeniowski O, Kaye D: Infective endocarditis. p. 1078. In Braunwald E (ed): Heart Disease, A Textbook of Cardiovascular Medicine. 4th Ed. WB Saunders, Philadelphia, 1992

122. Gold D: Endocarditis. p. 3. In Gold D, Weingeist T (eds): The Eye in Systemic Disease. JB Lippincott, Philadelphia, 1990

123. Johnson F, Darling R, Mundth E et al: The management of infected arterial aneurysms. J Cardiovasc Surg 18:361, 1977

124. Sholler G, Hawker R, Celermajer J: Infective endocarditis in childhood. Pediatr Cardiol 6:183, 1986

125. McKinsey D, Ratts T, Bisno A: Underlying cardiac lesions in adults with infective endocarditis: the changing spectrum. Am J Med 82:681, 1987

126. Pelletier L: Infective endocarditis. p. 970. In Braunwald E, Isselbacher KJ, Petersdorf RG et al (eds): Harrison's Principles of Internal Medicine. 11th Ed. McGraw-Hill, New York, 1987

127. Cowgill L, Addonizio V, Hopeman A et al: Prosthetic valve endocarditis. Curr Probl Cardiol 11:617, 1986

128. Weinstein L, Schlesinger J: Pathoanatomic, pathophysiologic and clinical correlations in endocarditis. N Engl J Med 291:832, 1974

129. Weinstein L, Rubin R: Infective endocarditis—1973. Prog Cardiovasc Dis 16:239, 1973

130. Yee J, McAllister K: The utility of Osler's nodes in the diagnosis of infective endocarditis. Chest 92:751, 1987

131. Albeit J, Krous H, Dalen J et al: Pathogenesis of Osler's nodes. Ann Intern Med 85:471, 1976
132. Kerr A, Tan J: Biopsies of the Janesway lesion of infective endocarditis. J Cutan Pathol 6:124, 1979
133. Hermans P: The clinical manifestations of infective endocarditis. Mayo Clin Proc 57:15, 1982
134. Varma M, McCluskey D, Khan M et al: Heart failure associated with infective endocarditis. A review of 40 cases. Br Heart J 55:191, 1986
135. Bayer A, Theofilopoulis A: Immunopathogenetic aspects of infective endocarditis. Chest 97:204, 1990
136. Feinstein E: Renal complications of bacterial endocarditis. Am J Nephrol 5:457, 1985
137. Churchill M, Geraci J, Hunder G: Musculoskeletal manifestations of bacterial endocarditis. Ann Intern Med 87:754, 1977
138. Salgado A, Furlan A, Keys T et al: Neurologic complications of endocarditis: a 12 year experience. Neurology 39:173, 1989
139. Williams R: Rheumatoid factors in subacute bacterial endocarditis and other infectious diseases. Scand J Rheumatol 75: S300, 1988
140. Zimet I: Nervous system complications in bacterial endocarditis. Am J Med 47:593, 1969
141. Silverberg H: Roth spots. Mt Sinai J Med 37:77, 1970
142. Erneston A, Bradford M: Clinical laboratory analysis of white-centered hemorrhages. J Am Optom Assoc 57:617, 1986
143. Kennedy J, Wise G: Clinicopathologic correlations of retinal lesions. Arch Ophthalmol 74:658, 1965
144. Dienst E, Gartner S: Pathologic changes in the eye associated with subacute bacterial endocarditis: report of five cases with autopsy. Arch Ophthalmol 31:198, 1944
145. Burns C: Bilateral endophthalmitis in acute bacterial endocarditis. Am J Ophthalmol 88:909, 1979
146. Treister G, Rothkoff L, Yalon M et al: Bilateral blindness following panophthalmitis in a case of bacterial endocarditis. Ann Ophthalmol 14:663, 1982
147. Wilson W, Geraci J, Danielson G et al: Anticoagulant therapy and central nervous system complications in patients with prosthetic valve endocarditis. Circulation 57:1004, 1978

4 Cerebrovascular Disease

BERNARD H. BLAUSTEIN

INTRODUCTION

Cerebrovascular disease refers to all disorders that affect an area of the brain permanently or transiently by ischemia or bleeding. The underlying pathologic process occurs in blood vessels that supply blood to the brain and may be due to occlusion, such as thrombus or embolus, or less commonly, hemorrhage. The threat of stroke is the major concern regarding cerebrovascular disease.

Stroke is the most common life-threatening and disabling neurologic disease of adult life and is the third-leading cause of death in the United States.[1–3] Although most patients survive the acute episode, considerable residual disability often occurs. Results of the Framingham Study indicate that 16 percent of the survivors remain institutionalized, 31 percent required long-term assistance in self-care, and 71 percent had a reduced capacity to earn a living.[4]

Many cases of cerebrovascular disease and impending stroke present with premonitory eye signs and symptoms. The optometrist often can identify patients at risk of stroke and refer them for interventional therapy. Thus, stroke may be averted.

CASE REPORT

A 66-year-old man presented with right-sided periorbital pain and recurrent episodes of right-sided transient visual loss (TVL). The pain was described as throbbing, accompanied by mild photophobia, and occurring intermittently for several weeks. The visual disturbance lasted approximately 5 minutes and was described as usually being attitudinal, as though a shade were being pulled over the eye.

The patient reported no other neurologic or constitutional symptoms but did note a generalized reduction in visual clarity with his right eye. He also reported a long history of poorly controlled hypertension and cardiac problems, which were treated with digitalis, β-blockers, calcium channel blockers, and cardiac antiarrhythmics.

The visual analysis revealed minimal refractive error with the best corrected visual acuity measuring 20/25 OD and 20/20 OS. Color vision was normal in both eyes. A photostress test revealed a 40-second delay to recovery in the right eye as compared with the left eye. The Amsler grid test revealed an equivocal distortion with the right eye.

The external ocular evaluation revealed normal ocular motility and normal visual fields to confrontation testing. The right eye revealed dilated tortuous epibulbar vessels and diffuse corneal edema (Fig. 4-1) and Plate 4-1). The right pupil was smaller than the left and was not as reactive. No evidence of an afferent pupil defect, was noted however.

All aspects of the internal ocular evaluation of the left eye were entirely normal. The right eye revealed the following pathology: grade 1 flare and cells in the anterior chamber, a fine net of neovascularization around the pupil and in the angle, a grade 1 posterior subcapsular cataract, a frond of neovascularization on the optic nerve, and mid-peripheral hemorrhages and

---

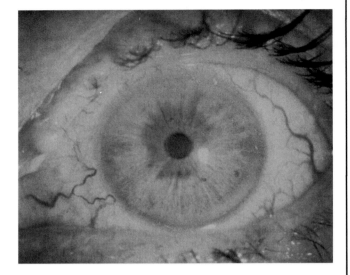

Fig. 4-1. Dilated, tortuous epibulbar vessels characterize ischemia to the anterior segment. (See also Plate 4-1).

cotton-wool spots (CWS) (Fig. 4-2 and Plate 4-2). The intraocular pressure (IOP) measured 11 mmHg OD and 15 mmHg OS.

Ophthalmodynamometry (ODM) to diastole measured 25 OD the right and 40 OS. A systolic bruit was heard along the carotid vasculature on the right, and an increased pulse was felt along the right superficial temporal artery. Blood pressure measured 150/95 mmHg in each arm. The erythrocyte sedimentation rate measured 10 mm/h. The serum cholesterol measured 270 mg/dl with a low-density lipoprotein (LDL) fraction of 165 mg/dl.

The patient was referred to a retinologist with a diagnosis of ocular ischemic syndrome secondary to carotid insufficiency. Ocular ischemia was confirmed, and ultrasound as well as angiographic studies revealed an 80 percent stenosis of the right carotid artery at the bifurcation (Fig. 4-3). The patient was considered to be at risk of stroke.

The patient underwent panretinal photocoagulation in the right eye and a right carotid endarterectomy. Subsequent follow-up revealed a white, quiet eye with regression of the rubeosis irides, retinal neovascularization, mid-peripheral hemorrhages, and CWS. Moreover, the pupillary reactions, ODM, photostress, and IOP measurements were essentially equal between the two eyes. The patient was free of all previous symptoms.

Fig. 4-2. Venous stasis retinopathy. Note the mid-peripheral blot and dot hemorrhages as well as the dilated veins. (See also Plate 4-2).

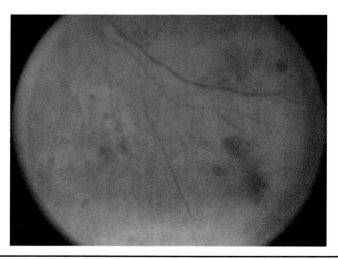

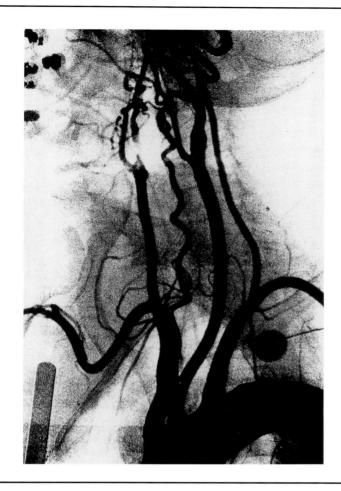

Fig. 4-3. Arteriography showing very severe stenosis of the proximal portion of the right internal carotid artery.

CEREBROVASCULAR DISEASE AND STROKE

Stroke is defined as a sudden, nonconvulsive, neurologic deficit caused by a reduction in blood flow below that which is necessary for the viability of brain cells. It is the abruptness with which the neurologic deficit occurs—seconds, minutes, hours—that marks the disorder as having a vascular cause. The term *cerebrovascular accident* is often used interchangeably with the term *stroke*. In its most severe form, stroke may cause patient to become hemiplegis or comatose. In its mildest form, stroke may cause an insignificant neurologic deficit.

The incidence of stroke has declined significantly during the past 40 years.[1] Probable reasons for the decline include better control of hypertension, diabetes mellitus, and cardiac disease as well as the public's increasing awareness of the risk of smoking and elevated serum lipids. More than 500,000 strokes occur annually in this country, however, and one in four stroke patients dies within 1 month.[5]

The incidence of cerebrovascular disease and stroke doubles with every decade of life after age 45. Men are more prone to stroke than women at all ages, and blacks are more prone to stroke than whites.[6,7]

Thromboembolic phenomena account for approximately 70 to 80 percent of all strokes.[8] Most of the remainder are caused by intracerebral or subarachnoid hemorrhage. A thrombus may lead to cerebral ischemia by the obstruction of a larger vessel with an aggregation of platelets, fibrin, calcium, and other cellular elements. An embolus, a small portion of the clot, may brake off from the parent thrombus and travel downstream to occlude a smaller vessel. If the reduction in blood flow caused by an embolus is transitory, or is not so intense as to result in cell death, neuronal function may return to normal. Such a situation is termed a *transient ischemic attack* (TIA).

TIAs are rapid in onset and commonly last from 2 to 15 minutes.[9] After the attack, the patient returns to preattack status with no apparent clinical evidence of infarct or permanent damage. The transient nature of the attack is explained by a temporary blockage of a vessel by a small embolus. The rapid fragmentation and dissolution of these microemboli preclude permanent clinical damage. However, TIAs are most often an indication that occlusive cerebrovascular disease is established.

The link between TIAs and stroke, while difficult to quantify, is well established. The general consensus is that persons who experience TIAs have an annual stroke risk of 5 to 6 percent.[7,10] One-half of all patients who have strokes in the carotid circulation report having had carotid territory TIAs.[11] The risk of major cerebral infarction is greatest within the first month following a TIA; 36 percent of infarcts occur within that time, and 50 percent occur within the first year.[7] As a general rule, following a TIA, about one third of patients will have no further symptoms, one third will have recurrent TIAs, and one third will have a stroke.[7,11] Significantly, the greatest risk following a TIA is a threefold to fourfold increase in cardiac mortality, which reflects the generalized involvement of atherosclerosis in these patients.[12]

Hemorrhagic strokes are frequently accompanied by severe, uncontrolled hypertension. Blood leaks from the vessel directly into the brain, one of the ventricles, or the subarachnoid space. The subsequent compression and displacement of the brain tissue almost always results in significant neurologic damage. Hemorrhagic strokes do not usually present with any warnings or prodromal ocular signs or symptoms. Thromboembolic strokes are most apt to present with ocular manifestations that herald their onset.

Pathophysiology of Thromboembolism

Atherosclerosis is the major pathologic process underlying ischemic cerebrovascular disease.[13] It is characterized by the deposition of lipids in the innermost layer of medium and large arteries in areas of bifurcations and curves. Atherosclerotic lesions are found most frequently at the origin of the internal carotid artery (ICA). The next most common site is the proximal portion of the vertebral arteries as they branch off the subclavian arteries.

Elevated levels of cholesterol with a concomitant elevation of LDLs encourage the deposition of lipids in the medium and large arteries. Smooth muscle cells ultimately proliferate into the intimal layer, causing the formation of a plaque, which protrudes into the lumen. The subsequent narrowing of the arterial lumen results in a relative stasis and turbulence of blood flow.

The continual deposition of lipids encourages the breakdown of the endothelial cells of the intima and leads to an ulcer. Subsequently, platelets agglutinate and stick to the roughened site, and a thrombus starts to develop. The parent vessel may occlude, or small particles of the thrombus may break off and embolize to smaller distal vessels.

Risk Factors

Risk factors for stroke include several that predispose for the development of atherosclerosis (Table 4-1).

Hypertension, both systolic and diastolic, is the most important risk factor for cerebrovascular disease and stroke.[14–16] Hypertension is present in 30 percent of the American population over age 40.[15] Hypertensive patients have an estimated stroke risk that is four times that of normotensive patients; elevated systole may be more predictive than elevated diastole.[16]

Elevated serum concentrations of lipids and cholesterol, particularly LDLs, are positively related to cerebrovascular atherosclerosis but are less closely correlated with stroke than with coronary heart disease.[17–20] The LDLs are thought to transport cho-

Table 4-1. Risk Factors for Stroke

Factors that predispose for atherosclerosis
    Hypertension
    Elevated cholesterol
    Smoking
    Diabetes
    Oral contraceptives
Factors that do not predispose for atherosclerosis
    Obesity
    Impaired cardiac function
    Migraine headaches
    Giant cell arteritis

lesterol to the intimas of medium-size arteries. Numerous studies indicate that the incidence of coronary artery disease and stroke is reduced if blood levels of total cholesterol remain at or lower than 200 mg/dl of blood and if the LDL fraction measures lower than 140 mg/dl.[21–24]

Several studies have implicated smoking as a risk factor for cerebrovascular disease and stroke. Paffenberger and Williams[25] found that smoking was one of the most important factors among college students who later had ischemic strokes. Love et al.[26] found that the risk of stroke in those who smoked more than 40 cigarettes per day was twice that of those who smoked less than 10 per day.

Diabetes is considered a risk factor for cerebrovascular disease. It is believed that diabetes increases LDL levels and accelerates the production of atherosclerosis. The risk is greater in women.[27]

Impaired cardiac function is highly correlated with stroke. Cardioembolic stroke occurs in the setting of coronary artery disease, mitral or aortic valve disease, left ventricular hypertrophy, and atrial fibrillation. At any level of blood pressure, persons with cardiac disease have more than twice the risk of stroke than those with normal cardiac function.[28–30]

The role of oral contraceptives is unclear. The American Heart Association Committee on Risk Factors could not agree on whether the use of oral contraceptives was an independent risk factor for stroke. In several retrospective studies, however, a 4- to 13-fold increase in risk for cerebral infarction was found among users of oral contraceptives.[31–33] The risk for stroke is enhanced if users are older than 35 years, or are smokers or have misgrainers or diabetes.[31–32]

Anatomic Correlates

The major blood supply to the brain arises from the aortic arch and involves two vascular systems: (1) the anterior circulatory system, fed by the carotid artery complex; and (2) and the posterior circulatory system, fed by the vertebral artery complex (Figs. 4-4 and 4-5 and Plates 4-3 and 4-4).

The common carotid artery bifurcates into the ICA and external carotid artery (ECA). The ICA enters the skull through the carotid canal of the temporal bone and then enters the cavernous sinus. As it emerges from the sinus, the ICA gives off its first branch, the ophthalmic artery, which supplies the eye and the orbit. Beyond the cavernous sinus, the ICA gives off the anterior choroidal artery to supply the optic tract and three major trunks: the anterior cerebral artery, the middle cerebral artery, and the posterior communicating artery. These three large vessels supply the ipsilateral frontal, temporal, and parietal lobes. Thus, on each side, the ICA is the major source of blood supply to the eye and the anterior cerebral hemispheres.

Carotid artery disease or a decreased perfusion within the ICA may result in decreased ophthalmic artery pressure with a concomitant ipsilateral decrease in vision and generalized ischemia to the globe. When the middle cerebral artery or its branches are specifically involved, a contralateral hemiplegia results, with the motor deficit being more pronounced in the upper extremities. The hemiplegia may be associated with a hemisensory deficit and homonymous hemianopsia. When the anterior cerebral artery is involved, a contralateral hemiplegia and an occasional hemisensory deficit may result. The defect is greater in the lower extremity.

The vertebral artery is the first branch of the subclavian artery. Each vertebral artery passes upward and posteriorly through the transverse foramina of the cervical vertebra to enter the skull through the foramen magnum. Within the skull, each artery then runs medially to unite with its fellow to form the basilar artery.

The basilar artery is a single mid-line vessel with branches to both sides of the posterior aspect of the brain. The signs and symptoms that result from ischemia to the vertebral–basilar complex may show considerable variation (Table 4-2). Unilateral, bilateral, or alternating involvement of cranial nerves III to VII may result in ophthalmoplegia or motor and sensory deficits in the face. Bilateral involvement of the medulla may have an impact on descending and ascending tracts, resulting in motor and sensory deficits in the limbs. If the descending sympathetic fibers that run along the lateral medulla are compromised, a Horner syndrome may result.

Cranial nerves housed in the medulla may suffer from ischemia, resulting in dysphagia and dysphonia. Cerebellar defects may result in vertigo or ataxia. Ischemia to the occipital cortex may result in bilateral

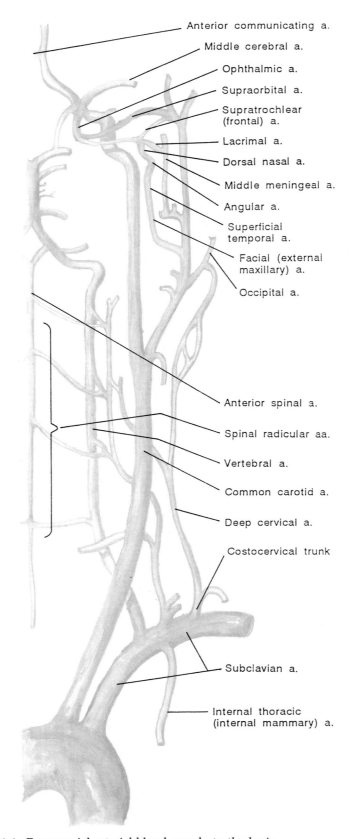

Anterior communicating a.

Middle cerebral a.

Ophthalmic a.

Supraorbital a.

Supratrochlear (frontal) a.

Lacrimal a.

Dorsal nasal a.

Middle meningeal a.

Angular a.

Superficial temporal a.

Facial (external maxillary) a.

Occipital a.

Anterior spinal a.

Spinal radicular aa.

Vertebral a.

Common carotid a.

Deep cervical a.

Costocervical trunk

Subclavian a.

Internal thoracic (internal mammary) a.

Fig. 4-4. Extracranial arterial blood supply to the brain.

Table 4-2. Signs and Symptoms of Cerebrovascular Insufficiency

Signs
  Vomiting
  Dysphagia
  Dysphonia
  Unilateral and/or bilateral motor deficits to the face
  Unilateral and/or bilateral sensory deficits to the face
  Unilateral and/or bilateral motor deficits to the limbs
  Unilateral and/or bilateral sensory deficits to the limbs
  Hemianopsias
  Ataxia
  Syncope
Symptoms
  Diplopia
  Vertigo
  Headache
  Bilateral dimming of vision

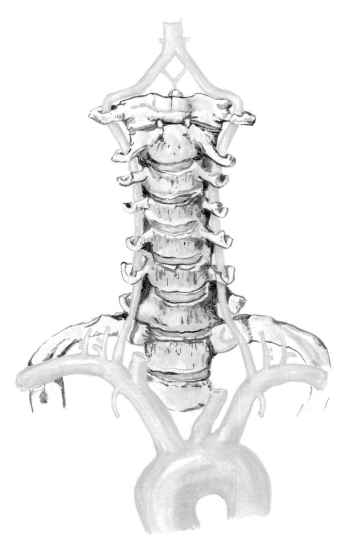

Fig. 4-5. Course of the vertebral arteries. Note that each artery meets at the midline to form the basilar artery.

heminopsia, which the patient may interpret as a bilateral dimming of vision. Finally, headache, vomiting, and syncope may occur.

Not all of the preceding signs and symptoms need occur with vertebral–basilar insufficiency. Moreover, vertigo and/or dizziness alone, without other symptoms, often are observed in older patients and do not necessarily indicate posterior circulatory ischemia.

With carotid territory TIAs, patients may experience TVL, or amaurosis fugax. TVL is a subtype of a TIA

and is defined as a transient monocular visual loss attributed to ischemia or vascular insufficiency to the retina. Typically, patients describe diminished or absent vision in one eye that lasts several minutes. The loss of vision usually begins in the upper field and often is described as a shade being pulled over the eye.

A less common variety of TVL is termed *light-induced amaurosis.* On looking at a bright light source such as the sun, patients may experience a diffuse, nondescript dimming of vision. The duration of the symptom is variable, lasting from minutes to hours and is thought to be due to poor perfusion to the retinal pigment epithelium and the outer retinal segments of the photoreceptors. As a consequence, visual pigments that have been bleached by bright light are not resynthesized at an adequate rate.[34]

DIAGNOSIS AND CLINICAL CORRELATION

The optometrist should approach the work-up of the patient suspected of manifesting cerebrovascular disease systematically. An attempt should be made to extract a thorough history and to correlate the symptoms with the observable ophthalmic and nonophthalmic signs.

History

The single most important clue to the localization of cerebrovascular disease to the carotid territory is a history of unilateral TVL. As previously noted, the visual loss is usually described as a dimming, darkening, or obscuring of vision as if a shade or curtain had fallen from above. After a few minutes, the shade lifts, leaving no permanent visual loss. The attacks of TVL are caused by decreased blood flow through the ophthalmic artery, the first tributary of the ICA (Fig. 4-5 and Plate 4-4). The lesion affects the ICA proximal to the ophthalmic artery or affects the ophthalmic artery itself.

Occasionally, patients with ocular ischemia report unilateral, short-lived spells of reduced vision after exposure to bright light. This light-induced amaurosis is thought to result from reduced retinal perfusion, which results in an inability to quickly resynthesize bleached visual pigments in the outer retina.[35] The symptom may be substantiated clinically by noting a delayed recovery to photostress.

A very important differential diagnostic consideration in patients with TVL is migraine aura. The flickering aura associated with migraine may stimulate TVL if the scintillations are followed by a central scotoma or hemianopsia. The older patient usually does not experience the pulsating, pounding headache that so often is associated with classic migraine. Typically, these migraine equivalents are characterized by zig-zag, rapidly flashing lights that start centrally and move peripherally within the visual field. The flickering phenomena lasts from 15 to 30 minutes unlike the much shorter-lived TVL.

A patient older than 60 years who notes a history of TVL and head pain must be suspect for giant cell arteritis. Such patients should be questioned as to whether they have experienced loss of appetite, weight loss, fatigue, low-grade fevers, generalized joint and muscle aches, and jaw claudication on chewing. These patients should be referred for measurement of erythrocyte sedimentation rates and for temporal artery biopsies. If the erythrocyte sedimentation rate is above 40 mm/h, or if the biopsy reveals the characteristic giant cells and destruction of the internal elastic membrane, the patients should be treated with large doses of systemic steroids.[36]

Biomicroscopy and Ophthalmoscopy

Prolonged generalized ischemia to the eye may lead to a constellation of findings in the anterior and posterior ocular segments known as the *ocular ischemic syn-*

Table 4-3. Signs of the Ocular Ischemic Syndrome

Anterior segment
    Dilated epibulbar vessels
    Corneal edema
    Flare and cells
    Poorly responsive pupil
    Iris neovascularization
Posterior segment
    Neovascularization of the disc or retina
    Venous dilation
    Cotton-wool spots
    Mid-peripheral microaneurysms and hemorrhages

drome[37] (Table 4-3). A careful biomicroscopic and ophthalmoscopic evaluation should be performed to determine whether any ocular structure reveals poor perfusion.

The anterior manifestations of the syndrome may include engorged episcleral vessels, corneal edema, mild anterior uveitis, iris neovascularization, and an irregular, poorly responsive pupil. Initially, hypotony occurs because of impaired ciliary body function. Ultimately, neovascular glaucoma may occur secondary to the iris neovascularization. Moreover, in time the iris atrophies, and diffuse cataracts develop.

The posterior manifestations may include pulsatile arterioles at the nerve head. In addition, dilated tortuous veins, CWS, and mid-peripheral microaneurysms as well as blot and dot hemorrhages may be noted. This latter entity represents venous stasis retinopathy and is an important hallmark of carotid insufficiency.

In addition, the retina may reveal the presence of plaques and infarcts. Retinal arteriolar plaques may appear as bright and glistening. These small cholesterol crystal emboli, known as Hollenhorst plaques, are highly refractile bodies that usually lodge at the bifurcations of retinal arterioles[38] (Fig. 4-6 and Plate 4-5). These emboli may rarely cause TVL but more often will fragment and pass through the retinal vasculature without incident. Solid, white nonrefractile plaques that lodge in larger vessels around the nerve head originate from calcifications on cardiac valves. These calcific emboli often are occlusive and may cause retinal infarcts.

Long dull-white plugs represent platelet emboli from the surface of atheromas. They are mobile and will

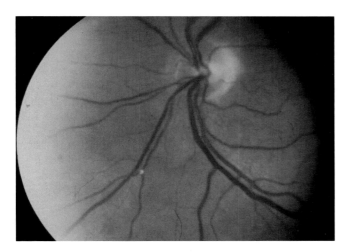

Fig. 4-6. Hollenhorst plaque lodged in the branch of a retinal arteriole. These bright, glistening particles represent cholesterol emboli from carotid atheromas. (See also Plate 4-3.)

undergo fragmentation and dissolution but can cause transient obstruction to retinal blood flow. TVL may occur. Linear white deposits within arterioles probably represent fibrin or thromboembolic material from the walls of the heart. They are less friable than platelets and may result in occlusions and subsequent infarcts.

Ancillary Clinical Procedures

Ascultation of the extracranial vessels in the neck may reveal a characteristic sound associated with turbulent blood flow through narrowed arterial lumens. The ab-normal sound, known as a *bruit*, commonly is located over the carotid bifurcation but may be heard in the supraclavicular fossa in vertebral–basilar insufficiency. These bruits suggest a hemodynamically significant arterial stenosis (i.e., a narrowing of the lumen in excess of 50 percent of the original diameter). Bruits usually are not heard if the stenosis approaches 90 percent.[39]

Clues to the patency of the ICA can also be obtained by careful palpation of the superficial temporal branch of the ECA.[40,41] When the ICA is occluded before its ophthalmic branch, the ECA may supply critical collateral vessels to the orbit via the superficial temporal artery. The pulse in the superficial temporal artery ipsilateral to the blocked ICA will be augmented compared with its fellow.

ODM is a relatively easy technique that may be very revealing. ODM is performed using an ophthalmodynamometer, a calibrated hand-held pressure sensor (Fig. 4-7). The instrument is placed on the sclera, and external pressure is gradually applied while the retinal arterioles are observed through an ophthalmoscope. When the applied external pressure exceeds the ophthalmic artery diastolic pressure, the arterioles will pulsate. When additional pressure is applied to the eye, the systolic pressure in the ophthalmic artery is exceeded, and the retinal arterioles will blanch and stop pulsating. The external pressures needed to overcome the diastolic and systolic ophthalmic artery pressures in the two eyes are then compared. Because the ophthalmic arteries are the first derivatives of the ICAs, a lower ODM on one side implies occlusive dis-

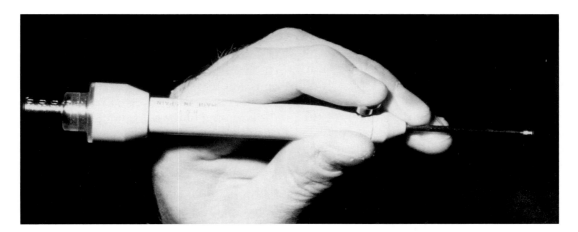

Fig. 4-7. An ophthalmodynamometer. Pressure is applied to the sclera in a tangential fashion while the retinal aterioles are observed through an ophthalmoscope.

ease in the ipsilateral ICA. A 20 percent difference in ODM between the two eyes is considered significant, but such a difference is not usually found unless a hemodynamically significant stenosis of the ICA is present.[42,43]

Sphygmomanometry should be performed on each arm. A difference of 20 mmHg in systolic pressure in each arm may indicate a reduced blood flow in the subclavian artery to the arm with the lower blood pressure. If the patient also reports symptoms of claudication and vertebral–basilar insufficiency (Table 4-2) after arm exercise, subclavian steal syndrome is manifested.[44] This syndrome is caused by an atherosclerotic stenosis of the subclavian artery just proximal to the origin of the vertebral artery. As a pressure gradient develops between the arm and the stenosed vessel, blood is diverted from the vertebral–basilar circulation and flows retrograde to supply the arm.

Noninvasive Tests

A wide variety of noninvasive tests have been used to study arterial flow to the brain. Most of these investigations have been superceded by newer ultrasound technology and neuroimaging techniques.

Oculoplethysmography is a technique in which sensing devices are placed on the corneae to measure the systolic ophthalmic artery pressures or relative arrival times of the ocular pulses in each eye. The intraocular pressures are raised simultaneously in each eye until the ocular pulse disappears. The pressures are then reduced simultaneously until the pulsations return. A delay in the pulse in one eye indicates a decreased flow to that eye. A comparison of the measurements in the two eyes is used to predict disease in the ICA–ophthalmic artery system. The technique will not reliably detect lesions that are not hemodynamically significant.[45,46]

High-resolution B-mode ultrasound scanning of the carotid bifurcation and the origin of the vertebral arteries from the subclavians can demonstrate lesions by means of sound wave reflection from the interfaces of tissues of different acoustic impedances. Use of this technique permits identification of subtle plaques and small ulcers as well as delineation of the residual lumen diameter. When compared with angiography and pathologic specimens of diseased arteries, B-mode ultrasonography has a greater than 80 percent

sensitivity and specificity for detecting significant occlusive lesions.[47,48]

Doppler sonographic systems may be used to detect direction and velocity of blood flow. Periorbital directional Doppler sonography uses high-frequency sound waves to ascertain the direction of blood flow in the periorbital arteries. The transducer is applied just below the supraorbital notch, and sound waves are transmitted to the area. The frequency of the reflected sound waves is a function of the direction of relative to the source. If red blood cells are moving toward the transducer, the frequency is increased. A hemodynamically significant stenosis at any point along the ICA will cause a reversal of blood flow in the orbital branches of the ECA.[49]

Advancing the Doppler probe along the course of the carotid and vertebral arteries while simultaneously analyzing the reflection of the projected high-frequency sound waves provides a measurement of blood flow velocity. When a stenosis is present, blood flow velocity increases, resulting in an increase in the frequency of the reflected sound waves off the moving red blood cells. This technique has an accuracy of 90 percent when compared with angiography.[50]

The combined B-mode ultrasonography and Doppler diagnostic systems are called duplex systems. These systems provide qualitative information about the arterial lumen as well quantitative data about the hemodynamic blood flow through the artery. The duplex system thus offers advantages over either B-mode scanning or Doppler analysis alone and has a 95 percent agreement with angiography.[50]

A number of newer methods have recently become available for the noninvasive determination of intracranial as well as extracranial blood flow. These include transcranial Doppler ultrasound, single photon emission computed tomography, positron emission tomography, and magnetic resonance angiography. A discussion of these techniques is beyond the scope of this chapter.

Invasive Tests

Intra-arterial angiography remains the standard and tested method of best defining the nature of vascular lesions in the extracranial and intracranial vessels and is considered the gold standard against which all other tests are judged. The technique is performed by threading a catheter into the aortic arch and selectively injecting contrast dye into individual arterial circulations. Radiographic pictures are then taken. In experienced hands, angiography reveals very valuable information and has a relatively low, but nevertheless, definable risk.[51] The risk factors are related to the general health of the patient, the severity of vascular disease, the number of injections, and the type and amount of contrast dye used.

TREATMENT AND MANAGEMENT

After the appropriate optometric work-up, the patient with ocular manifestations of cerebrovascular disease may be jointly managed by the retinologist and vascular specialist.

If iris neovascularization or retinal neovascularization (or both) is present, panretinal argon laser photocoagulation is the treatment of choice. Several hundred 500-μm diameter burns are applied to each quadrant of the fundus. The treatment extends posteriorly to 2 disc diameters from the center of the macula in the temporal quadrants and 0.5 disc diameter from the border of the optic nerve nasally. The total number of burns approximates 1,400. Additionally, focal treatment using moderate-intensity confluent burns may be applied directly to the new vessels on the retina.[52]

The panretinal photocoagulation is often followed by regression of the retinal and iris neovascularization within several days. The beneficial effects stem from the ablation of normal retinal tissue so that retinal metabolic demand decreases. The decreased perfusion to the retina that results from carotid artery disease is believed to stimulate the formation of new blood vessels on the retina and iris.

The medical approach to cerebrovascular disease concentrates on reducing the risk factors for stroke and administering specific platelet anticoagulants. All risk factors should be reduced or eliminated, if possible; as the predominate precursor of stroke, however, hypertension in particular must be controlled. In addition, particular attention must be payed to treating cardiac dysfunction.

A single dose of 325 mg of aspirin reduces the prostaglandin that induces platelet aggregation. Several studies indicate that aspirin reduces the incidence of stroke after TIAs.[53–58] Other agents that are clinically useful in reducing platelet aggregation are sulfinpyra-zone (Anturane), dipyridamole (Persantine), and the recently introduced introduced drug ticlopidine (Ticlid).[56–58]

The most common surgical approach for the remediation of reduced perfusion through the carotid vasculature is carotid endarterectomy (CEN). In this procedure, the atheromatous plaque is removed from the ICA at the bifurcation, and the defective arterial wall is patched with either a leg vein or polymer graft.

The North American Symptomatic Carotid Endarterectomy Trial (NASCET) and the European Carotid Surgery Trial (ECST) were conducted to evaluate the efficacy of CEN as compared with medical therapy in the prevention of stroke.[59,60] The data indicated that patients with symptoms such as TIAs or small strokes related to severe stenosis (70 to 99 percent) benefited from CEN when performed by selected surgeons with past low rates of complications. On the basis of the results of the NASCET and the ECST the following recommendations can now be made. Patients who have had recent symptoms within the carotid territory, have stenosis of between 70 and 99 percent, and who are otherwise fit for surgery should undergo CEN. Patients with stenosis between 30 and 69 percent should be randomized within ongoing carotid surgery trials. Patients with stenosis less than 30 percent should be treated medically.

REFERENCES

1. Adams HP, Caplan LR, Feussner JR et al: Management dilemmas in carotid artery disease. Patient Care 20:4, 1990
2. Callow A: An overview of the strobe problem in the carotid territory. Am J Surg 140:181, 1980
3. US Department of Commerce, Bureau of the Census: Statistical Abstract of the United States. 103rd Ed. Vol. 76, 1982
4. Gresham GE, Fitzpatrick TE, Wolf PA et al: Residual disability in survivors of stroke: The Framingham study. N Engl J Med 293:954, 1975
5. Stallones RA, Dyken ML, Fang HCH et al: Report of the joint committee for stroke facilities planning. Stroke 3:360, 1972
6. Kannel WB: Current status of the epidemiology of brain infarction associated with occlusive arterial disease. Stroke 2:295, 1971
7. Wolf P: Risk factors for stroke. Stroke 16:359, 1985
8. Toole JF, Patel AN: Cerebrovascular disease, 2nd Ed. McGraw-Hill, New York, 1967
9. Genton E, Barnett HJ, Fields WS: Cerebral ischemia: the role of thrombosis and of antithrombolic therapy. Report of the Joint Committee for Stroke Resources. Stroke 8:150, 1977
10. Adams HP, Kassell N, Mazuz H: The patient with ischemic attacks: is this the time for a new therapeutic approach? Stroke 15:371, 1984
11. Davis PH, Dambrosia JM, Schoenberg BS et al: Risk factors for ischemic stroke: a prospective study in Rochester, Minnesota. Ann Neurol 72:319, 1987

12. Dyken ML, Wolf PA, Barnett HJM et al: Risk factors in stroke. A statement for physicians by the Subcommittee on Risk Factors and Stroke of the Stroke Council. Stroke 15:1105, 1984
13. Ross R, Glomset JA: The pathogenesis of artherosclerosis. N Engl J Med 295:369, 1976
14. Sandercock PAG, Warlow CP, Jones LN, Starkey IR: Predisposing factors for cerebral infarction: the Oxfordshire Community Stroke. Br Med J 298:75, 1989
15. Wolf PA: Hypertension as a risk factor for stroke. p. 105. In Whisnant JP, Sandok B (eds): Cerebral Vascular Diseases. Grune & Stratton, Orlando, FL, 1975
16. Kannel WB, Wolf PA, Verter J: Epidemiological assessment of the role of blood pressure in stroke: the Framingham study. JAMA 245:301, 1970
17. Lowering blood cholesterol to prevent heart attack. Consensus conference. JAMA 254:2080, 1985
18. Lipid Research Clinics Program: The Lipid Research Clinics Coronary Primary Prevention Trial Results. I. Reduction in the incidence of coronary heart disease. JAMA 251:351, 1984
19. Kannel WB, Castelli WP, Gordon T: Cholesterol in the prediction of atherosclerotic disease: new perspective based on the Framingham study. Ann Intern Med 90:85, 1979
20. Gordon T, Castelli WP, Hjortland MC et al: High density lipoprotein as a protective factor against coronary heart disease: the Framingham study. Am J Med 62:707, 1977
21. Iso H, Jacobs DR, Wentworth D et al: Serum cholesterol levels and six year mortality from stroke in 350,977 men screened for the multiple risk factor intervention trial. N Engl J Med 320:904, 1989
22. Yano K, Reed DM, Madean CJ: Serum cholesterol and hemorrhagic stroke in the Honolulu Heart Program. Stroke 20:1460, 1989
23. Steinberg D, Parthasarthy S, Carcio TE et al: Beyond cholesterol: modification of low-density lipoprotein that increases its atherogenicity. N Engl J Med 320:915, 1989
24. Scance A, Lawin RM, Berg K: Lipoprotein (a) and atherosclerosis. Ann Intern Med 115:209, 1991
25. Paffenberger R, Williams J: Chronic disease in former college students: V. Early precursors of fatal stroke. Am J Public Health 57:1290, 1967
26. Love BB, Jones MP, Biller J et al: Cigarette smoking: a risk factor for cerebral infarction in young adults. Arch Neurol 47:693, 1990
27. Schoenberg BS, Schoenberg DG, Pritchard DA et al: Differential risk factor for completed stroke and transient ischemic attack (TIA): study of vascular disease (hypertension, cardiac disease, peripheral vascular disease) and diabetes mellitus. Trans Am Neurol Assoc 105:165, 1980
28. Wolf PA, Dawker TR, Thomas HE et al: Epidemiological assessment of chronic atrial fibrillation and risk of stroke: the Framingham study. Neurology 28:973, 1978
29. Wolf PA, Kannel WB, McGee DL et al: Duration of atrial fibrillation and imminence of stroke: the Framingham study. Stroke 14:664, 1983
30. Wolf PA, Dyken M, Barnett HJM et al: Risk in stroke. Stroke 15:1105, 1984
31. Collaborative Group for the Study of Stroke in Young Women: Oral contraceptives and stroke in young women: associated risk factors. JAMA 231:718, 1975
32. Collaborative Group for the Study of Stroke in Young Women: Oral contraceptives and increased risk of cerebral ischemia or thrombosis. N Engl J Med 288:871, 1973
33. Handin R: Thromboembolic complications of pregnancy and oral contraceptives. Prog Cardiovasc Dis 16:395, 1974
34. Roberts D, Sears J: Light-induced amaurosis associated with carotid occlusive disease. Optom Vis Sci 11:889, 1992

35. Wiebers DO, Swanson JW, Cascino TL, Whisnant JP: Bilateral loss of vision in bright light. Stroke 20:554, 1989
36. Wilkinson I, Russell R: Arteries of the head and neck in giant cell arteritis. Arch Neurol 27:378, 1972
37. Brown GC, Margaral LE: The ocular ischemic syndrome: clinical, fluorescein angiographic and carotid angiographic features. Int Ophthalmol 11:239, 1988
38. Hollenhorst RW: Significance of bright plaque in the retinal arterioles. JAMA 178:125, 1961
39. Ziegler DR, Zileli T, Dick A et al: Correlation of bruits over the carotid artery with angiographically demonstrated lesions. Neurology 21:860, 1971
40. Fisher CM: Facial pulses in internal carotid artery occlusion. Neurology 20:476, 1970
41. Caplan LR: The frontal artery sign. N Engl J Med 288:1008, 1973
42. Ackerman R: A perspective on noninvasive diagnosis of carotid disease. Neurology 29:615, 1979
43. Toole J: Ophthalmodynamometry. Arch Intern Med 112:219, 1963
44. Blaustein B: The subclavian steal syndrome. Clin Eye Vision Care 3:25, 1991
45. Gee W, Oiler D, Wylie E: Noninvasive diagnosis of carotid occlusion by ocular plethysmography. Stroke 7:18, 1976
46. Kartchner M, McRae L: Noninvasive evaluation and management of asymptomatic carotid bruit. Surgery 82:840, 1977
47. O'Donnell TF, Erdoes L, Mackey W et al: Correlation of B-mode ultrasound imaging and arteriography with pathologic findings at carotid endarterectomy. Arch Surg 120:443, 1985
48. Schenk EA, Bond G, Aretz T et al: Multicenter validation study of real-time ultrasonography, arteriography, and pathology: pathologic evaluation of carotid endarterectomy specimens. Stroke 19:289, 1988
49. Hennerici M, Freund HJ: Efficacy of CW-Doppler and duplex system examination for the evaluation of extracranial carotid disease. J Clin Ultrasound 12:155, 1984
50. Barnes RW: Continuous-wave Doppler ultrasound. p. 19. In Bernstein EF (ed): Noninvasive Diagnostic Techniques. 3rd Ed. CV Mosby, St. Louis, 1985
51. Earnest F, Forbes G, Sandok BA et al: Complications of cerebral angiography: prospective assessment of risk. AJNR 4:141, 1983
52. Johnson ME, Gonder JR, Canny CLB: Successful treatment of the ocular ischemic syndrome with panretinal photocoagulation and cerebrovascular surgery. Can J Ophthalmol 23:114, 1988
53. Mundall J, Quintero P, von Kaulla K et al: Transient monocular blindness and increased platelet aggregability treated with aspirin—a case report. Neurology 21:402, 1971
54. Harrison MJG, Marshall J, Meadows JC et al: Effect of aspirin in amaurosis fugax. Lancet 2:743, 1971
55. Fields WJ, Lemak N, Frankowski R et al: controlled trial of aspirin cerebral ischemia. Stroke 8:310, 1977
56. Barnett HJM: The Canadian Cooperative Study: a randomized trial of aspirin and sulfinpyrazone in threatened stroke. N Engl J Med 299:53, 1978
57. Fitzgerald GA: Dipyrimadole. N Engl J Med 316:1247, 1987
58. Hass WK, Easton JD, Adams HP et al: A randomized trial comparing ticlopidine hydrochloride with aspirin for the prevention of stroke in high-risk patients. N Engl J Med 321:501, 1989
59. North American Symptomatic Carotid Endarterectomy Trial (NASCET) Collaborators: Beneficial effects of carotid endarterectomy in symptomatic patients with high-grade stenosis. N Engl J Med 325:445, 1991
60. European Carotid Surgery Trialist's Collaborative Study Group: MRC European Carotid Surgery Trial: interim results of symptomatic patients with severe (70–99%) or with mild (0–29%) carotid stenosis. Lancet 1:1235, 1991

5 Rheumatologic Disease

BRIAN P. MAHONEY

Rheumatic disease is not a single entity but a group of diseases, or syndromes, that share similar clinical features. Immunologic deficiencies are a hallmark feature, and they are implicated in the initiation of inflammatory foci throughout the body. The inflammation has a predilection for articular tissue, resulting in arthritis to varying degrees. The variable joint predilection helps differentiate between the specific types of rheumatic disease. Other organ systems throughout the body, including ocular tissues, are also affected to varying degrees. Ocular manifestations can indicate a change in the level of systemic activity requiring additional intervention by the patient's rheumatologist before a vision-threatening or life-threatening event occurs. Eye care practitioners need to be able to recognize the numerous ocular manifestations of these diseases as well as the side effects of the medications used to treat these diseases. Ophthalmic practitioners need to participate in the health-care delivery for patients with rheumatic disease to ensure detection of sight-threatening changes at early stages and to provide necessary information regarding the medical management when appropriate.

CASE REPORT

A 36-year-old white woman presented for an eye examination because of a sudden decrease of vision in her left eye. She stated that she had been experiencing myalgia, fever, and soreness and swelling of her hands. She stated that her knuckles were so swollen that she could not put her rings on. She said that she had felt like this on occasion for the past year or more but had never suffered vision loss until 1 week earlier.

The results of her external examination revealed her pupils to be P4/4 round, reactive to light (RRL) (+) afferent pupillary defect (APD) OS, confrontation fields were normal, and extraocular motility revealed no diplopia and no evidence of restriction. Best corrected visual acuity was 20/20 OD and 20/100 OS. Amsler grid showed no scotoma in the right eye and a scotoma in the left eye, which was most dense centrally, extending over approximately 10 degrees. Biomicroscopic evaluation revealed no abnormalities of the lids, conjunctiva, cornea, anterior chamber angle (grade IV von Herrick, both eyes), or iris. Intraocular pressure (IOP) was measured at 13 mmHg OD and 12 mmHg OS by Goldmann applanation tonometry.

Dilated fundus findings in the right eye included clear media to the posterior pole, C/D ratio of .3 × .3 with sharp margins and healthy retinal vasculature and macular area. Peripheral retinal evaluation revealed scattered areas of paving stone degeneration. Dilated fundus findings in the left eye included clear media to the posterior pole. Optic nerve swelling was noted in the left eye with superficial hemorrhages in the peripapillary region (Fig. 5-1 and Plate 5-1). No evidence of retinal vascular occlusion was present. A foveal reflex was present in the macula with no evidence of maculopathy. The retinal periphery was similar to the right eye.

The patient tested positive for antinuclear antibody (ANA) and elevated serum complement and had a sedimentation rate of 58. Negative testing included rapid plasma reagin (RPR), rheumatoid factor (RF), and angiotensin-converting enzyme (ACE). She was referred for rheumatologic evaluation for previously undiagnosed systemic lupus erythematosus (SLE) with ischemic optic neuropathy. The patient was started on oral prednisone and was monitored over the following 6 months. Complete resolution of the disc edema was observed, but the vision recovered only to the 20/30 level with persistent Amsler grid distortion centrally.

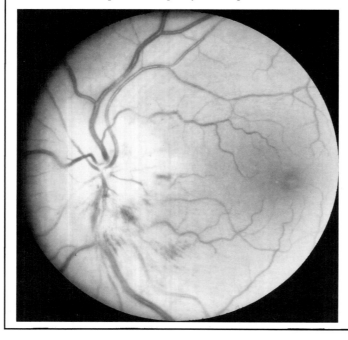

Fig. 5-1. Anterior ischemic optic neuropathy in the left eye of a patient with systemic lupus erythematosus. (See also Plate 5-1.)

OVERVIEW OF RHEUMATIC DISEASE

Altered immunologic mechanisms play a role in the associated inflammatory responses, which involve both articular (joint) and extra-articular tissues.[1] Tissue destruction results from inflammatory responses that go awry and cannot be controlled due to modified immunologic mechanisms. Anomalous immune complexes contribute to the initiation of the inflammatory reaction involving tissues in which they are found. The exact role these immunologic abnormalities play in the initiation and control of the associated inflammatory response is not fully understood. Articular and extra-articular tissue involvement is variable for patients with rheumatic disease, and therefore the expected clinical course for each entity is not the same, despite similar etiologic mechanisms. Similar mechanisms for various rheumatic diseases give rise to overlapping patient symptoms, leading to difficulty in diagnosis for some patients with rheumatologic disease. Table 5-1 lists the entities classified as both acquired connective tissue disease and seronegative spondyloarthropathies within the family of rheumatologic disease.

Table 5-1. Classification of Rheumatic Diseases

Acquired connective tissue disease
  Rheumatoid arthritis
  Systemic lupus erythematosus
  Polyarteritis nodosa
  Sjögren syndrome
  Polymyositis/dermatomyositis
  Mixed connective tissue disease
  Vasculitis
    Giant cell arteritis
    Temporal arteritis
    Takayasu's arteritis
    Hypersensitivity vasculitis
    Wegener's granulomatosis
Seronegative spondyloarthropathies
  Ankylosing spondylitis
  Reiter syndrome
  Inflammatory bowel disease
    Crohn's disease
    Ulcerative colitis
  Psoriatic arthritis

Abnormalities in the humoral immunologic system include the development of antibodies to host proteins. Antibodies to immunoglobulin (IgG) and IgM in rheumatoid arthritis (RA) patients can be detected and are referred to as *rheumatoid factors.* Antibodies to nuclear material (ANA) in SLE develop to DNA (ds-DNA) and RNA (Sm-RNA) and can be detected in the patient's serum. Antiphospholipid antibodies have been implicated in the development of retinitis in SLE.[2] Once antibodies are produced to these proteins, they are identified as foreign to the body. Unfortunately, the antibodies identify host tissues as foreign and an inflammatory reaction perpetuates, resulting in tissue destruction.

Deficiencies in cellular immune mechanisms primarily affect the T-cell function and activity. These deficiencies are linked to the loss of control of inflammation, which also contributes to tissue destruction. Initiation of the complement cascade by alternative pathways also contributes to chronic inflammation in patients with rheumatic disease (including RA and SLE). Serum levels of complement are elevated during active periods of SLE yet are normal during active RA, despite elevated levels in the synovium of affected joints.

The identification of certain human leukocyte (HLA) antigens in a group of patients with polyarthropathy, yet no rheumatoid factor, is the criteria for classification of a patient with one of the seronegative spondyloarthropathies. The clinical course of these diseases and extent of the associated arthropathy are not as severe as with RA. The presence of these antigens serves only to identify patients at high risk for the development of these diseases.

A strong association exists between the presence of HLA-B27 and ankylosing spondylitis (AS), Reiter syndrome (RS), and inflammatory bowel diseases. HLA-DR3 is a common associated finding in patients with Sjögren syndrome and systemic sclerosis. An inciting event such as enteric infection (Crohn's disease) or sexually transmitted disease (RS) appears to trigger the onset of the arthritis as well as the various systemic manifestations of the seronegative arthropathies. Before this time, the immune system does not appear to be involved in atypical inflammatory behavior.

Inflammatory arthritis is a predominant clinical feature of patients with rheumatic diseases. Synovitis results in inflammatory granulation and pannus in affected joints leading to destruction of the joint and functional impairment in patients with RA. Inflammation of the enthesis (insertion of the tendon) is a common finding in patients with seronegative spondyloarthropathy. Joint destruction is not commonly found in patients with seronegative spondyloarthropathies, therefore, less functional impairment is observed clinically. Radiographs of the affected joints help differentiate inflammatory arthritis (found in patients with rheumatic disease) from osteoarthritis (noninflammatory). Loss of joint space, erosion of the lateral aspects of the joint bones and lateral osteoporosis are frequent findings in the seronegative spondyloarthropathies. Hypertrophic synovial tissue along the surfaces of the bones of joints (with little lateral bone involvement) with surface erosion is characteristic of acquired connective tissue disease. Joint deformity and decreased function result from destruction of joint cartilage, capsule, and ligaments.

ACQUIRED CONNECTIVE TISSUE DISEASE

Rheumatoid Arthritis

RA is the most chronic form of inflammatory joint disease and results in some loss of function in 83 percent of patients.[3] Women are affected three times more frequently than men, and the average age on onset is between 35 and 50 years of age. Active synovitis affects the metacarpal joints early and, as the disease progresses, involves the feet, knees, elbows, and shoulders. Joints affected by active inflammation are swollen, hot, and tender. Joint stiffness will persist even after the articular inflammation is treated.

Joint stiffness is greatest after prolonged periods of inactivity (as in the morning) and improves with exercise. Joint deformity manifests when tissue destruction occurs in addition to the active periods of inflammation (Fig. 5-2). Only 17 percent of RA patients remain fully functional, while the remaining patients suffer from varying degrees of functional loss as the disease progresses.

Extra-articular features are seen in RA patients and reflect disease progression (Table 5-2), with 75 percent of patients manifesting two or more features.[4] Large cutaneous and subcutaneous nodules are present in approximately 25 percent of seropositive patients.[5] Nodular softening and shrinkage occur with treatment, but complete resolution should not be expected. Systemic vasculitis is rare but implies a poor

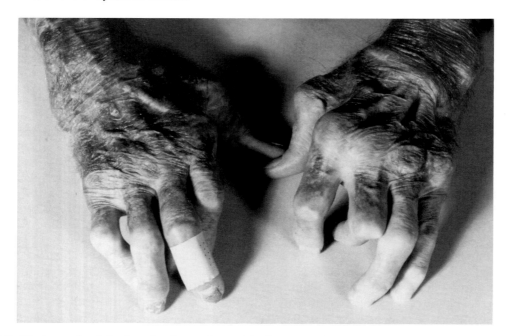

Fig. 5-2. Photograph of the hands of a patient with rheumatoid arthritis. Note the deformity involving the interphalangeal joints, which occurred over an 18-year period. This patient suffers from significant physical functional impairment.

patient prognosis when present. The tissues surrounding the inflammed vessels are affected, and focal necrosis occurs, leading to extensive tissue destruction if it is not detected and treated expeditiously. Most patients with extra-articular features (including ocular) are seropositive and have advanced disease.[6]

Ocular Sequellae

Ocular involvement can manifest at any stage of RA. The degree of ocular involvement does not parallel the severity of arthritis; however, it is more likely to be observed in the mid and later stages of RA. Ocular involvement is not exclusively inflammatory in nature, although an immunologic cause is implicated.

Table 5-2. Extra-articular Features of Rheumatoid Arthritis

Cutaneous and subcutaneous nodules
Infarction and/or hemorrhage (involving the nail folds of the hands and feet)
Anemia
Pericarditis
Pneumonitis
Vasculitis

Keratoconjunctivitis sicca is seen in 10 to 25 percent of RA patients and follows a chronically progressive course. Patients with dry eye have a compromised ocular defense mechanism, which predispose these patients to developing secondary bacterial keratitis. Topical antibiotics are not needed for all patients with keratitis sicca; however, these agents should be considered if secondary bacterial infection presents. Lubrication therapy, using nonpreserved solutions and ointments (preferred over preserved preparations), improves the integrity of the corneal epithelium and enhances patient comfort. Incomplete resolution of the corneal staining with improved tear breakup time is observed in most patients. A baseline amount of superficial keratitis is expected to be observed despite therapy. Improved epithelial integrity or patient comfort, or both, should be regarded as a therapeutic success. An optimal maintenance schedule for lubrication needs to be determined on an individual basis, considering patient symptoms and the chronicity of keratitis sicca.

Less than 2 percent of keratitis sicca patients develop filamentary keratitis. The presence of filaments is usually accompanied by acute symptoms of pain. Corneal filament stripping followed by intensive lubrication is necessary to improve patient comfort. Bandage contact lenses or pressure patching following filament re-

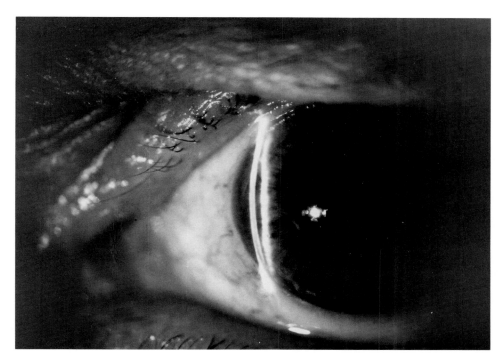

Fig. 5-3. Peripheral corneal furrowing in the same patient in Fig. 5-2. Note the thinning of the biomicroscopic beam inside the limbal area, which was present in a 360-degree area. No progression to corneal ulceration has occurred during the 8 years of follow-up care. (See also Plate 5-2.)

moval may exacerbate filament development and should be discontinued if the filaments recur immediately. Subsequent reformation of the filaments may occur following complete healing of an acute episode, which would warrant a more aggressive course of lubrication to maintain patient comfort as well as epithelial integrity. Peripheral furrowing of the corneal stroma represents a benign condition that is associated with advancing RA (Fig. 5-3 and Plate 5-2). Rarely is corneal ulceration associated with the thinning that may be caused by an immune-mediated, noninfective process, although a pathogenic cause must be excluded from the differential diagnosis.

Recurrent episcleritis can manifest before, or can parallel, systemic exacerbations of RA.[7,8] The presence of episcleritis therefore correlates better with disease activity than keratitis sicca. Recurrences can be unilateral and may involve either eye. Anterior scleritis associated with RA can be diffuse or nodular. Necrotizing scleritis (with or without significant inflammation of the eye) is observed less frequently but is a harbinger of patient mortality when present.[9] Scleromalacia perforans is associated with scleral and episcleral tissue loss, ectasia formation, and possible perforation of the globe. The presence of scleromalacia perforans

is associated with significant systemic inflammatory foci, which may be life-threatening regardless of the apparent lack of systemic symptoms. Aggressive medical management using systemic immunosuppressive therapy is indicated to enhance the likelihood of patient survival beyond 5 years. Peripheral corneal inflammation occurs in 50 to 70 percent of scleritis patients; therefore, an association with previous scleritis or presently active scleritis should be suspected when sectoral furrowing or keratolysis is observed in a patient with RA.

Treatment

The treatment of RA is individualized depending on the activity of the disease, severity of any extra-articular involvement, and the patient's level of functioning at the time of the initial evaluation.[10–14] Therapeutic modalities are considered in a sequential manner, although some medications and treatments may be selected out of sequence, considering the random nature in progression of RA (Table 5-3). Many medications used for the treatment of RA have ocular sequellae. Patients using these medications need to be monitored for the development of ocular involvement (Table 5-4).

Table 5-3. Treatment of Rheumatoid Arthritis

1. Education regarding disease
   Physical therapy/exercise
   Aspirin
   Nonsteroidal anti-inflammatory drugs
2. Steroids
       Systemic
       Intra-articular injections
   Antimalarial medications[a]
       Hydroxychloroquine
       Chloroquine (rarely)
   Oral gold[a]
3. Parenteral gold[a]
   Methotrexate[a]
4. Surgical joint replacements
   D-Penicillamine[a]
   Azathioprine[a]
5. Non-FDA approved treatment
       Sulfasalazine[a]
       Cyclophosphamide[a]
       Cyclosporine (Questionable)[a]

[a] Slow-acting anti-rheumatic drugs.

Systemic Lupus Erythematosus

SLE is a frequently encountered acquired connective tissue disease. Women of childbearing years are at highest risk of developing SLE, and black women are afflicted more frequently than white women.

Table 5-4. Frequent Ocular Side Effects From Medications Used to Treat Rheumatic Disease

NSAIDs
    Whorl keratopathy
    Optic neuropathy (possibly toxic)
    Photosensitivity
    Nystagmus
    Retinal hemorrhage
    Subconjunctival hemorrhage
Steroids
    Secondary open-angle glaucoma
    Posterior subcapsular cataract
Gold salts
    Corneal deposition (stroma)
    Lens deposition (capsular/anterior cortex)
Antimalarial agents
    Pigmentary maculopathy
    Pigmentary retinopathy
    Optic neuropathy
Methotrexate
    Punctate keratitis
    Blurred vision
Azathioprine
    Lash loss
    Possible retinal pigment epithelium disruption

The triggering mechanism for SLE is unknown, although the presence of autoantibodies directed toward nuclear components (DNA and RNA) is a predominant clinical feature. The precise role of these "anomalous" immune complexes in the initiation of systemic features is uncertain. Immune complex deposition in various tissues is implicated in the initiation of focal inflammation and subsequent tissue destruction.[15] Circulating ANAs to DNA (ds-DNA) and RNA (Sm-RNA) can be detected in the serum of 95 percent of patients with SLE.

Patients with SLE present with fatigue most commonly (more than 90 percent of the time) and have a low-grade fever with weight loss in more than 60 percent of cases.[16,17]

The arthritis associated with SLE also has an immune mechanism; however, joint predilection for the small joints of the hands and feet helps differentiate it from RA (Fig. 5-4). The progression in the articular disease does not result in as severe functional impairment. Patient mortality from the extra-articular involvement, however, is much greater.

Patients with SLE have numerous extra-articular features (Table 5-5). Approximately 40 percent of SLE patients manifest a butterfly rash in the malar region of the face at some point during the course of the disease. Central nervous system (CNS) involvement, observed in 30 percent of patients with SLE, may manifest as focal seizure activity, other sensory or motor deficits, or potentially life-threatening hematoma. Most CNS deficits probably result from a combination of mechanisms, for example, microvascular abnormalities and neuronal membrane damage from immunologic mechanisms.[18] The ophthalmic structures may be involved, giving rise to visual or ocular symptoms, or both. Cranial nerve palsies, nystagmus, other motility abnormalities, and optic neuropathies are found in SLE patients. Patients with CNS involvement may have symptoms of other neurologic diseases, which need to be considered in the differential diagnosis. Renal and cardiac involvement serve as a source for significant patient morbidity.[19,20] Systemic treatment with steroids has been the conventional treatment for renal disease, but it has no proven efficacy. The glomerular hyalinization and interstitial scarring persist despite steroid therapy and reflect a poor patient prognosis.

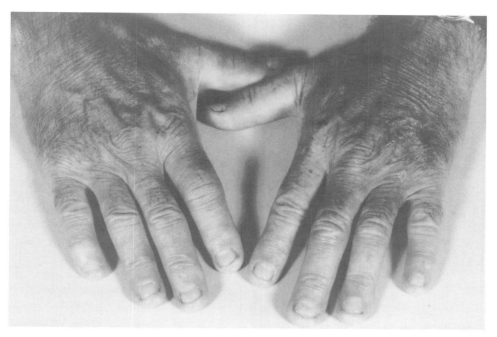

Fig. 5-4. Arthritis in a patient with systemic lupus erythematosus, with involvement of the proximal metacarpal joints. This patient presented with keratitis sicca without evidence of other ocular involvement throughout a 5-year follow-up period.

Ocular Involvement

The ocular manifestations of SLE are observed less frequently, since the medical management of lupus has improved. Vision loss does not occur frequently. External ocular structures are frequently involved, as evidenced by the development of marginal telangectasias and erythematous patches, which are seen on the eyelids. Nonspecific conjunctivitis and keratitis are observed in 3 to 20 percent of SLE patients.[21] Keratitis sicca is a common finding with SLE that contributes to the development of Sjögren syndrome. Anterior scleritis, episcleritis, and iridocyclitis are observed less frequently and usually accompany cycles of activity of the disease.

Table 5-5. Extra-articular Involvement of Systemic Lupus Erythematosus

Mucocutaneous
Central nervous system
Renal
Pulmonary
Cardiac
Musculoskeletal
Vasculitis
Hematopoesis

Inflammation of the retinal and choroidal vasculature can be seen with or without associated occlusion.[22] Retinal microinfarcts (cotton-wool spots) most frequently manifest in the posterior pole (Figs. 5-5 and 5-6, and Plates 5-3 and 5-4), without associated retinal hemorrhages, and resolve in less than 3 months. Superficial retinal hemorrhages can manifest without retinal microinfarction. Coincidental hypertension from renal involvement must be considered when retinal hemorrhages or microinfarcts are observed, yet it is rarely found. Retinal venous occlusion (central or branch) may accompany retinal arterial vasculitis.

Focal vasculitis involving the CNS and extraocular structures causes a variety of neuro-ophthalmic manifestations from SLE. Cranial nerve palsies, nystagmus, diplopia, intranuclear ophthalmoplegias, and orbital pseudotumors are among the neuro-ophthalmologic complications attributed to SLE.[23,24] Ischemic optic neuropathy, most commonly unilateral (although bilateral is possible), is associated with connective tissue disease, including SLE.[25]

Treatment

The clinical course of SLE is characterized by episodic exacerbations and remissions, requiring a combination of medications for both short- and long-term

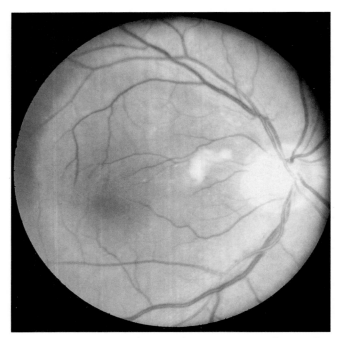

Fig. 5-5. Large microinfarct in the superior papillomacular bundle of the right eye in a patient with systemic lupus erythematosus. There was no drop in vision associated with the presence of the microinfarct. No evidence of diffuse vaso-occlusive retinopathy was appreciated. (See also Plate 5-3.)

management. No specific drug regimen is used for SLE patients with active disease because multiple foci of activity are frequently seen simultaneously. In these situations, the most serious of the complications (i.e., pericarditis, pleuritis, nephritis) are treated most aggressively with less attention delivered to the less serious complications (arthritis, dry eye, etc.).

Systemic steroids continue to be used most frequently in controlling the more serious complications from SLE. Their efficacy has not been proven in controlled studies, although significant clinical experience supports the use of systemic steroids. Short-term use of nonsteroidal anti-inflammatory drugs (NSAIDs), particularly indomethacin, is effective in treating low-grade arthralgia, myalgia, fever, pleuritis, and pericarditis. Antimalarial medications are useful in treating the dermatologic manifestations of SLE and are effective for long-term usage in reducing the frequency and severity of articular and extra-articular exacerbations. The use of immunosuppressive agents is usually reserved for patients who have a poor response to systemic steroids. Cyclophosphamide and methotrexate are the two most commonly used immunosuppressive agents for treating SLE.

Polyarteritis Nodosa

Polyarteritis nodosa (PAN) is one of the rarest collagen vascular diseases encountered clinically. It is characterized by a diffuse vasculitis involving medium and small blood vessels throughout the body. It afflicts men twice as frequently as women and is seen most commonly in people between the ages of 40 and 60. It is seen with greater frequency in patients with a history of intravenous drug abuse.

A hypersensitivity reaction to a substance or pathogen is one proposed mechanism for the development of PAN. PAN is seen at a higher rate in intravenous drug abusers. Immune complex deposition in vessel walls most likely triggers the vasculitis. Disruption in the normal anatomy of the vessel wall results in thrombosis or aneurysmal formation (or both), leading to vascular occlusion, which causes infarction and death of the surrounding tissues.

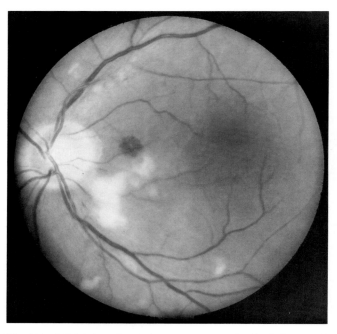

Fig. 5-6. Multiple microinfacts were seen in the left eye of the same patient in Fig. 5-5 and Plate 5-3. Note the blossom hemorrhage off the 2:30 o'clock area of the disc. This retinopathy cleared within 3 weeks after the patient was treated with oral steroids. (See also Plate 5-4.)

Table 5-6. Extra-articular Features of Polyartheritis Nodosa

Renal and cardiac involvement (70%)
Liver and gastrointestinal tract (50%)
Peripheral neuropathy (50%)
Skeletal muscle (30%)
Central nervous system (10%)
Cutaneous lesions (<50%)
Ocular involvement (<20%)

The arthritis associated with PAN affects the large joints of the lower extremities in 20 percent of cases. It responds well to treatment, and decreased patient function and mobility resulting from joint destruction are rare. Involvement of various organ systems is associated with significant patient morbidity and mortality (Table 5-6). Random foci of vessel inflammation explain the variability of subjective symptoms. These patients usually present with fever, malaise, and weight loss, which progresses rapidly. Clinically significant renal disease, peripheral neuropathy, and the presence of cutaneous lesions are all consistent with PAN. Hypertension is seen in 25 percent of PAN patients with renal disease. Patients with RA and Sjögren syndrome may manifest PAN as a complication.

Ocular sequellae

It should not be surprising that many ocular sequellae associated with PAN are similar to those associated with SLE considering similar immunologic mechanisms between the two entities. About 10 to 20 percent of PAN patients manifest ocular involvement during periods of disease activity. The ocular manifestations of PAN are predominantly characterized by an acute inflammation of the affected tissue. Episcleritis and scleritis (both diffuse and nodular types are possible) and peripheral corneal furrowing have been described. Cogan syndrome is a rare complication of PAN and comprises interstitial keratitis with audiovestibular abnormalities.[26] Deep stromal vascularization and infiltration result in corneal opacification and cause decreased vision. Other forms of sterile keratitis have been described, but their involvement is usually limited to the peripheral cornea.

Retinal vasculitis is the most frequently observed ocular finding in PAN patients. Retinal microinfarcts, superficial hemorrhages, arterial sheathing, and perivascular transudates can be observed with active vasculitis. Vaso-occlusive events may complicate the vasculitis and involve the retinal or choroidal vascula-

ture as well as the optic nerve. They can occur as an isolated entity or in conjunction with each other. Aggressive immunosuppressive therapy is warranted under these circumstances and is best done in an inpatient setting.

Treatment

The 5-year survival rate for PAN patients is 10 percent. Intravenous or oral steroids are the initial therapy of choice for PAN patients followed by a maintenance dose of oral steroids for 6 months or more, depending on patient circumstances. The use of cytotoxic or immunosuppressive agents is considered if patients have a poor response to steroids or if a significant life-threatening sequella is clinically evident. Patients treated with cyclophosphamide have a better chance of remission, and treatment with cyclophosphamide has been associated with a higher patient survival rate. Treatment for up to 1 year may be necessary, following apparent control, which will minimize recurrences.

Sjögren Syndrome

Sjögren syndrome is an immune-mediated disease that results in diffuse exocrine gland dysfunction throughout the body. Similar to other immune-related diseases, it frequently afflicts women between the ages of 40 and 60. It can occur without associated systemic disease (primary Sjögren syndrome) or as a complication of many of the collagen vascular diseases (with arthritis). RA and SLE are the most common collagen vascular diseases associated with Sjögren syndrome.

The exact mechanism initiating the lymphocytic and plasma cell infiltration of the exocrine glands throughout the body is poorly understood. Autoimmune mechanisms targeting exocrine glands cause glandular dysfunction and decreased efficiency, resulting in mucous membrane drying.[27] Mucous membrane functions, including both lubrication and immunologic defense mechanisms, are compromised. This predisposes Sjögren syndrome patients to ocular surface, nasopharyngeal, and gastrointestinal abnormalities as well as secondary infections involving these membrane surfaces.

The severity of the systemic features of Sjögren syndrome varies with any associated collagen vascular

Table 5-7. Systemic Features of Sjögren Syndrome

Glandular
    Keratitis sicca
    Nasopharyngeal drying
    Respiratory tract drying
    Parotid gland enlargement
Extraglandular
    Arthritis
    Renal (tubular acidosis)
    Dermatologic vasculitis
    Polymyopathy
    Central nervous system abnormalities
    Lymphoma
    Collagen vascular disease

---

disease. Table 5-7 lists the glandular and extraglandular features of Sjögren syndrome. Progressive drying of the affected mucous membranes is the source of significant patient symptoms. Keratitis sicca, xerostoma, epistaxis, and dysphagia are present to varying degrees in most Sjögren syndrome patients.[28,29] Parotid gland enlargement is seen in 50 percent of Sjögren syndrome patients and most frequently occurs bilaterally.[30] Other hematologic and immunologic diseases are associated with Sjögren syndrome; for example, Hashimoto's thyroiditis and acquired collagen vascular diseases are seen in a higher frequency in Sjögren syndrome patients.[31,32] The incidence of non-Hodgkin's lymphoma is 44 times greater in Sjögren syndrome patients and may develop up to 29 years after the initial onset of the syndrome.

Rheumatoid arthritis is present in about 50 percent of Sjögren syndrome patients. The inflammatory arthritis associated with Sjögren syndrome is progressive throughout the course of the disease and follows the same clinical course of the related collagen vascular disease. Only a 10 percent chance of developing arthritis exists after the first year following the onset of the sicca complex, if it has not developed by that time. One should not assume that all patients with primary Sjögren syndrome will develop secondary Sjögren syndrome with disease progression.

Cutaneous vasculitis is a rare complication of Sjögren syndrome; however, 66 percent of patients with cutaneous vasculitis have CNS abnormalities. The cranial nerve palsies and peripheral motor or sensory neuropathies may mimic multiple sclerosis or other neurologic disease. The possibility of coexisting neurologic disease must be considered when evaluating Sjögren syndrome patients.

Ocular sequellae

Ocular involvement is a dominant clinical feature of Sjögren syndrome. Keratitis sicca is the primary ocular manifestation for 90 percent of Sjögren syndrome patients.[33] Emotional tearing is not impaired unless significant lacrimal gland infiltration and destruction occurs. The symptoms of dry eye will progress in severity throughout the course of the disease and reflect the extent of conjunctival glandular damage. A noninfectious ropey discharge and papillary response of the conjunctiva develops in response to chronic irritation of the tissues due to a lack of lubrication. These findings are not indicative of an infective process and do not require antibiotic therapy. Aggressive lubrication therapy may minimize these findings, but complete resolution should not be expected (see the section, *Rheumatoid Arthritis*). Some degree of corneal opacification and pannus may result from chronic drying and exposure, despite the use of lubricating agents. Other therapeutic modalities that have proven efficacy for patients with severe keratitis sicca include temporary or permanent punctal occlusive procedures.

Staphylococcal infection of the lids, conjunctiva, or corneal surfaces occurs in 75 percent of Sjögren syndrome patients. Other pathogenic organisms may also cause infective keratitis. The presence of ulcerative bacterial keratitis requires aggressive antibiotic therapy (solution and ointment) in addition to lubrication therapy to avert corneal scar formation and possible vision loss.

The incidence of filamentary keratitis is small compared to the total number of Sjögren syndrome patients with keratitis sicca. Acute exacerbations of filamentary keratitis does occur and causes the patient to experience severe ocular pain. Removal of the filaments followed by frequent lubrication is warranted but may not be sufficient for all patients, because recurrences are possible despite previous successful treatment. No single regimen has proved successful for all patients with filamentary keratitis, and therefore a variety of measures must be considered. Some combination of filament removal with subsequent heavy lubrication, bandage contact lenses, and/or punctal obstructive measures warrants consideration, depending on patient symptomotology and previous ocular history.

Treatment

Only palliative treatments are available for Sjögren syndrome patients because no known cure exists. It is imperative that patients have a thorough understanding of their condition and realize the limited therapeutic measures available to combat this frustrating disease. This will prevent unrealistic expectations on their part and hopefully maximize patient compliance. Treatment of any associated collagen vascular disease is necessary but has little effect on the glandular disease. Enhancing the hydration and lubrication of involved mucous membranes is the goal of treatment. Increasing fluid intake and the humidity of air at home or work, in conjunction with the frequent use of mucomimetic agents can offer significant relief for patients afflicted with Sjögren syndrome.

Dermatomyositis/Polymyositis Complex

Dermatomyositis/polymyositis (DM/PM complex) is a group of inflammatory diseases that affect skeletal muscle, resulting in progressive damage to the muscle tissue. Dermatomyositis affects muscle and skin (Fig. 5-7). Polymyositis, however, primarily affects skeletal muscle tissue, although overlapping situations have been documented. DM/PM complex may occur primarily or may be associated with other diseases such as SLE, RA, scleroderma, PAN, and other malignancies. DM/PM complex is seen twice as frequently among black Americans compared with white Americans. DM/PM complex can afflict children and adults alike. Dermatomyositis is seen 2 to 20 times more frequently then polymyositis in children in the United States.

The exact cause of DM/PM complex is not fully understood. As with other rheumatic diseases, an immune-mediated response directed toward skeletal muscle has gained the most support among the proposed theories for the cause of DM/PM. Progressive muscle weakness, which may or may not be preceded by fever, typifies this complex. Elevated Westegren sedimentation rates, urinary creatine levels, and serum creatine kinase levels are common findings during acute episodes of muscle inflammation. About 90 percent of patients with polymyositis displays some abnormality on electromyographic studies.[34] Other humoral and cellular immunologic abnormalities have been described, although their relationship to the clinical manifestations is still uncertain, as is the case in most rheumatic diseases.

The use of oral corticosteroids remains the mainstay of treatment for patients with DM/PM. Mortality is approximately 30 percent in childhood DM/PM and 40 percent for adult DM/PM when patients are treated with steroids, compared to mortality rates of 38 to 60 percent, respectively, without steroid treatment.[35,36] Immunosuppressive agents have been used with lim-

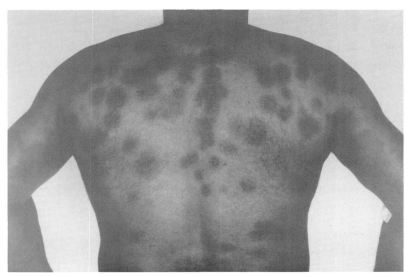

Fig. 5-7. Multiple areas of dermatologic involvement in this patient were attributed to the previous diagnosis of dermatomyositis.

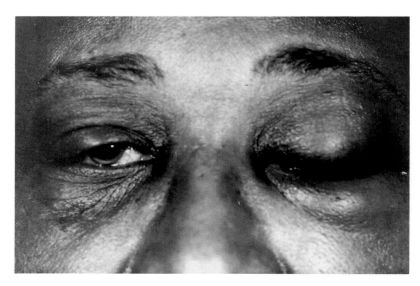

Fig. 5-8. Angioedema of the left eye of the same patient seen in Fig. 5-7. This patient presented with acute swelling of the upper lid. Neither his vision nor extraocular motility were affected. The swelling resolved within 3 days following treatment with oral steroids.

ited success. Morbidity and mortality rates are higher for adults than for children with DM/PM complex. This also holds true for patients with malignancies when compared to those with nonmalignancy-associated DM/PM complex.

Ocular involvement associated with DM/PM complex is rare. Eyelid abnormalities dominate the reported cases of ocular involvement. Eyelid tightness and palpebral lid swelling with telangectatias develop with associated edema (Fig. 5-8). The myositis may involve the orbicularis occuli and/or extraocular muscles, resulting in nystagmus, gaze palsies, and ptotic lid positions. Oral steroids are warranted in these cases when malignancy is not present.

SERONEGATIVE SPONDYLOARTHROPATHIES

Seronegative spondyloarthropathies are a group of arthritic diseases that share common clinical features (Table 5-8). The most striking is the lack of seropositive rheumatoid factors and an association with HLA antigens (primarily B27). The HLA histocompatability factors are inherited on an autosomal co-dominant basis, which explains why variants of these diseases run in families. It is not unusual for Sjögren syndrome patients to have children or siblings with AS or RS. A relationship exists between the presence of specific HLA factors and the development of arthritis, but it probably is an indirect relationship. The presence of HLA-B27 appears to reflect a predisposition for the development of this group of diseases, most notably AS and RS.

Ankylosing spondylitis, RS, and inflammatory bowel disease are triggered by an inciting infection, commonly a gut infection (*Shigella, Salmonella,* and *Klebsiella* spp.).[37-40] A reactive arthritis develops subsequent to the infection. A cross-reactivity exists between the antigens produced to the offending agent (i.e., *Chlamydia*) and articular tissues; therefore, no symptoms manifest until after the patient is exposed to the inciting agent, and antibodies are produced. These patients test positive for HLA-B27 before the onset of arthritis or other systemic symptoms.

The articular involvement in seronegative spondyloarthropathies may be indistinguishable from RA in

Table 5-8. Common Clinical Findings With Seronegative Spondyloarthropathy Syndromes

No association with rheumatoid factors
Strong HLA-B27 association with variable familial expression
Active sacroiliitis not always associated with spondylitis
Inflammatory arthritis with predilection for peripheral joints with asymmetric involvement
No rheumatoid nodules
Ocular inflammation with anterior segment predilection
Mucocutaneous ulcerations with variable expression

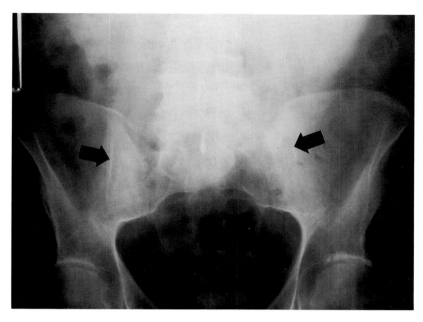

Fig. 5-9. Radiograph of the sacroiliac joint of a patient with Reiter syndrome. Note the fusion of the joint space at the arrows. Inflammation in the joint space results in eradication of the joint space. This process is frequently accompanied by pain.

the early stages. The synovitis differs from RA because different structures are involved than in RA. The inflammation is centered around the ligamentous–bony junction (entheses), cartilage, subchondral bone, capsule, and periosteum. The arthritic predilection is for the sacroiliac, intervertebral, and sternoclavicular joints. Calcification and fibrosis occur without bony destruction, which is commonly seen with RA. Fusion of the joint results in significant functional impairment for the patient (Fig. 5-9). Extra-articular involvement is variable among these disorders, but ocular involvement is common as these diseases progress.

Ankylosing Spondylitis

Ankylosing spondylitis is one of the earliest identified seronegative spondyloarthropathies and is also referred to as Marie-Strümpell disease. It affects men more frequently then women, and the onset of the disease is usually between 20 and 40 years of age. It can be seen in 1 to 2 percent of the white American population. It has the highest association with HLA-B27 and is present in 90 percent of AS patients. Approximately 20 percent of patients with HLA-B27 antigens will develop AS, and 40 percent of patients with AS will be asymptomatic.[41]

One of the offending organisms associated with the development of AS is *Klebsiella* sp. It is also seen at a higher frequency in the AS population. The sacroiliac joint is affected early in the course of the disease and progresses until obliteration of the joint space occurs. Patients with significant sacroiliac joint fusion can be asymptomatic 50 percent of the time. The pain associated with sacroiliac inflammation can involve the lower back, buttocks, hips, or upper leg.

Involvement of the vertebral column gives rise to the characteristic "bamboo" appearance seen on radiographs. The development of the intervertebral calcification, which causes this appearance, is variable and cannot be detected in most AS patients. Peripheral joints are involved less frequently and less extensively than with RA. The arthritic predilection for the axial skeleton is the hallmark feature of this disease.

Extraspinal involvement occurs in 40 percent of AS patients (Table 5-9). Ocular involvement is seen in about 20 percent of AS patients. Aortic involvement occurs in 3 to 10 percent of AS patients. A rare complication associated with AS is valvular reflux (from secondary amyloidosis) and is a source of patient mortality. Complete heart block, pericarditis, and pulmonary fibrosis are rarer complications, which

Table 5-9. Clinical Features of
Ankylosing Spondylitis

Axial skeleton joint involvement
    Sacroiliac joint
    Vertebral column
    Sternoclavicular
Peripheral joint involvement (rare)
Ocular inflammation
    Acute iridocyclitis
Anemia
Prostatitis/cervicitis
Pulmonary fibrosis
Aortic valvular disease
Cardiac
    Conduction deficits
    Pericarditis
    Amyloidosis

usually develop after age 50, can prove to be fatal in these cases.[42]

Ocular Sequellae

AS is the most frequently identified systemic disease associated with recurrent anterior iridocyclitis.[43–45] Approximately 25 percent of AS patients manifest iridocyclitis, and it is seen more frequently in HLA-B27-positive patients than HLA-B27-negative patients.[46] It is also estimated that 10 to 33 percent of all uveitis is associated with AS. The iridocyclitis may precede any patient symptoms and may be the sentinel event leading to the initial diagnosis (Figs. 5-10 and 5-11 and Plates 5-6 and 5-7). Iridocyclitis is rarely the only extraspinal manifestation. Recurrent episodes may be in the same or opposite eye or opposite eye, but bilateral involvement commonly develops with disease progression. Simultaneous presentation of iridocyclitis has also been reported. Few sequellae develop as a result of chronic inflammation except for posterior synechia, which is observed frequently (Fig. 5-12 and Plate 5-8). Angiographic confirmed macular edema may develop after multiple recurrences but is usually of such a mild degree that vision is rarely affected.

Treatment

Aggressive therapy is not warranted for most AS patients, considering the less severe nature of the arthritis and extraspinal manifestations. An exception to this philosophy is in rarer situations where life-threatening cardiopulmonary or aortic disease complicates the patient presentation.[46,47] The chronic use of NSAIDs combined with an aggressive physical therapy or exercise program remain the mainstay of therapy for AS patients. Vertebral calcification and sacroiliac joint fusion are delayed using NSAIDs on a chronic basis. The chronic use of NSAIDs may have little impact on the recurrence rate for iridocyclitis, and short-term use for acute iridocyclitis is advocated for some patients. Stronger anti-inflammatory medications and immunosuppresive agents are not commonly used, considering the less severe nature of AS disease.[48]

Topical steroids and longer lasting cycloplegic agents

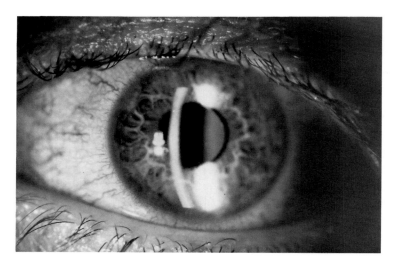

Fig. 5-10. Ankylosing spondylitis patient with active iridocyclitis in the left eye. Recurrences involved both eyes with a predilection for the left eye. Patient was successfully treated with topical medications without developing cataracts, glaucoma, or macular edema. Posterior synechia did develop. (See also Plate 5-5.)

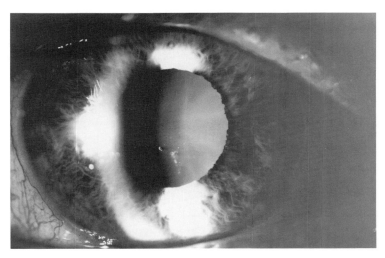

Fig. 5-11. Same patient as in Fig. 5-9 with evidence of broken posterior synechia following treatment with topical steroids and cycloplegics. (See also Plate 5-6.)

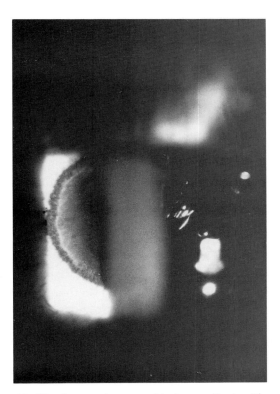

Fig. 5-12. Fixed posterior synechia in a patient with ankylosing spondylitis after recurrent episodes of iridocyclitis. Note the posterior synechia with fibrosis at the pupil border, which extended from 1:00 to 7:00 o'clock. No medical regimen was successful in breaking the synechia. (See also Plate 5-7.)

comprise the mainstay of therapy when recurrent iridocyclitis develops. Most episodes of iridocyclitis require medical intervention for a 4- to 8-week period. Oral NSAIDs may be beneficial in some cases but have not been proved to decrease the duration of therapy and have no effect on the recurrence rate of iridocyclitis. Topical NSAIDs have not been proved to be effective in treating AS associated iridocyclitis.

Reiter Syndrome

RS is another seronegative spondyloarthropathy. It is the most common arthralgia in the 20- to 35-year-old age group, affecting men five times more frequently than women. These numbers may be misleading, because active cervicitis remains occult in many women, which may lead to underestimation of the number of cases. Approximately 90 percent of all RS patients are young men. The classic triad consists of urethritis (or cervicitis), arthralgia, and ocular inflammation (conjunctivitis or iridocyclitis). Reiter syndrome is seen more frequently in white patients, consistent with the higher prevalence of HLA-B27 in whites, and it is of interest that black patients with RS are HLA-B27 positive less frequently.[49] HLA-B27 is present in 70 to 90 percent of all RS patients.

The most accepted proposed etiology of RS is a postinfectious reactive arthropathy, much like AS. *Chlamydia* and *Shigella* spp. are two identified pathogens associated with RS. The recurrent episodes of urethritis (or cervicitis) are not associated with active sexually transmitted disease. Arthritis affecting the sacroiliac joint is a predominant feature of this syndrome and can be confirmed by radiographic evaluation. A bone scan is more sensitive than a radiograph at detecting low-grade inflammation in the sacroiliac joint. A bone scan should be considered when clinical presentation is consistent with the diagnosis of RS yet radiographic evaluation is negative. Less arthritic involvement of the vertebral column is seen with RS as compared to AS. The peripheral joint involvement is more severe when compared with AS. Achilles tendenitis is a common finding and can manifest before any other extraspinal sequellae.

The clinical course of RS cannot be predicted for all patients. Acute attacks frequently run a 3-month course with quiescent periods between each cycle. The number of attacks may be finite and occur over a period of less than 5 years (self-limiting), although a significant number of patients continue to have recurrent cycles of activity for more than 10 years (chronic). More severe articular and extra-articular manifestations are seen in patients with the chronic form as compared to patients with the self-limiting form. Chronic inflammation results in more extensive functional impairment and possibly severe vision loss. Reiter syndrome can no longer be perceived as a relatively benign disease. Some studies report chronic disease in 62 to 80 percent of cases with varying follow-up periods from 2 to 15 years.[49–51] Patients who manifest the syndrome following a sexually transmitted disease are at higher risk for developing the chronic form of RS.[52] Severe physical disability that renders patients unemployable or causes them to change jobs occurs in 25 percent of RS patients.[50]

Arthritic involvement has a predilection for the weight-bearing joints of the lower extremities, particularly the hips, knees, and ankles. Polyarthropathy is seen in 96 percent of RS patients compared to 4 percent of patients who manifest monoarthritic disease. Exacerbations of the arthritis occur without symptoms of other extra-articular involvement; however, exacerbations of the extra-articular features are generally accompanied by cycles of arthritic activity. Active episodes of urethritis (or cervicitis) frequently signal the beginning of a recurrent cycle of other extra-articular inflammation. Mucocutaneous abnormalities are seen in 50 percent of RS patients and most commonly manifest as oral ulcerations, vesicular rashes involving the penis or cervix.[53] Dermatologic findings

are rarer and are usually limited to keratoderma blennorhagica of the foot or hand. Amyloidosis, complete heart block, aortic insufficiency, and pericarditis are rare complications of RA that many result in cardiac failure and death.[54–56]

Ocular Sequellae

A cyclical pattern of ocular inflammation can precede active episodes of arthritis in RS. Patients with HLA-B27 experience more frequent recurrences than HLA-B27-negative RS patients. A nonspecific conjunctivitis with mild papillae and follicles present on the palpebral conjunctiva is associated with minimal discharge or keratitis. No evidence of active infection is observed clinically, and resolution occurs over a 2-week period. Antibodies to *Chlamydia* cross-react with HLA lymphocytes, binding to conjunctival tissue, and probably contributing to the subsequent clinical presentation.[56] Decreased tear breakup time is seen coincidentally with the conjunctivitis, and these signs tend to resolve together. Acute tendenitis frequently precedes the onset of conjunctivitis by days or weeks, or it can parallel the onset of the conjunctivitis.

Reiter syndrome patients who run a chronic course frequently develop recurrent iridocyclitis (Fig. 5-13 and Plate 5-9). Other sequella from chronic iridocyclitis, including glaucoma, cataract, and macular edema, may develop. This situation differs from recurrent iridocyclitis, because low-grade inflammation may be present in the anterior chamber during quiescent periods of the disease. The dramatic nature of each recurrence places the patient at risk of developing posterior synechia, which is a very common finding. Bilateral involvement is common, and simultaneous presentation is possible with advancing articular and ocular disease. On rare occasions, optic neuritis has been a complication attributed to RS.[57]

Treatment

Like AS therapy, the mainstay of RS therapy consists of aggressive physical therapy programs and the long-term use of NSAIDs.[47] Increased amounts of medication may be considered for acute exacerbations, but stronger medications are rarely used in patients with self-limiting disease. Oral steroids and intralesion steroid injections are beneficial in controlling more aggressive forms of RS. Other immunosuppressive or cytotoxic agents are needed to control the arthritic disease for those patients who do not respond favorably to less aggressive therapeutic modalities.[47,58,59] Clinical improvement has been demonstrated using both

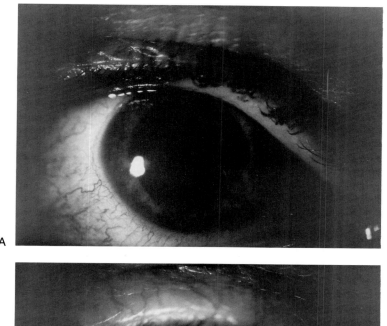

A

B

Fig. 5-13. Patient with Reiter syndrome. **(A)** Recurrent uveitis in the right eye. Patient has steroid-responding glaucoma, which complicated the treatment and management of the inflammation. This eye went on to develop macular edema, poorly controlled glaucoma, and vision loss. **(B)** Left eye. Fixed posterior synechia between 1:00 and 3:30 o'clock distorted the pupil but the decreased vision of "count fingers" was caused by cataract formation and glaucoma. These findings were evident at initial presentation years after the initial diagnosis. (See also Plate 5-8.)

methotrexate and azathioprine, although recurrences of iridocyclitis are still seen despite treatment with these agents.

Ocular lubrication is adequate to control the mild discomfort associated with the conjunctivitis of RS. Short-term topical vasoconstrictors have also been an effective treatment. Topical steroids and long-acting cycloplegics are needed to control the iridocyclitis. Periocular steroid injections or oral steroids are used to control recalcitrant forms of iridocyclitis. Cytotoxic

medications help control ocular inflammation insofar as they control the systemic disease, but these are slow-acting drugs and are not efficacious for short-term control of ocular or systemic inflammation.

Arthropathy Associated With Inflammatory Bowel Disease

Crohn's disease and ulcerative colitis share many clinical features, including a low correlation with HLA-B27 (unless associated with other rheumatic disease

Table 5-10. Clinical Characteristics of Inflammatory Bowel Disease

	Crohn's Disease	Ulcerative Colitis
Intestinal involvement	Large	Small and large
Sacroiliac involvement	Yes	Yes
Spondylitis	4%	5%
Peripheral arthropathy	25%	15%
HLA association	Rare	Rare

such as AS), colitis, arthropathy, and ocular inflammation. The initial onset is between 20 and 30 years of age, and men manifest these diseases as frequently as women. A reactive mechanism following a gut infection is likely (similar to other seronegative spondyloarthropathies). Crohn's disease and ulcerative colitis have some distinguishing characteristics, which helps differentiate between the two (Table 5-10), although many clinical features are shared.

The peripheral arthritis associated with ulcerative colitis is migrating, involving up to 10 joints, and may last for months to years before resolving. Recurrences are common, but joint destruction is uncommon. Most attacks of arthritis coincide with active colitis. It is unusual for extraintestinal involvement, including arthritis, to precede the intestinal inflammation. Spondylitis can be detected years before the colitis in some HLA-B27-positive patients, although this is not an expected finding. Active sacroiliitis is a common association with ulcerative colitis but is unrelated to the presence of HLA-B27. Progression in the articular inflammation coincides with intestinal inflammation. Pyoderma gangrenosum (ulcerative dermatitis) can be seen in up to 4 percent of cases. Arthritis and other extraintestinal sequella commonly resolve following colectomy.

The extraintestinal features of ulcerative colitis commonly precede any intestinal inflammation. The oligoarthritis of Crohn's disease involves the weight-bearing joints and resolves within weeks to months, unlike ulcerative colitis. Crohn's patients are three times more likely to have sacroiliitis at the time of diagnosis, and spondylitis may be seen in up to 25 percent of cases. The extent of articular disease does not necessarily parallel the intestinal involvement. Granulomas can be identified in the synovium of joints, which causes clubbing of the fingers, and can also be found in other tissues of the body. Pyoderma gangrenosum is rarely present with Crohn's disease,

in contrast to ulcerative colitis. Arthritis and other extraintestinal sequellae do not resolve following colectomy.

Ocular Involvement

Patients with ulcerative colitis and spondylitis are more likely to have iridocyclitis than patients without spondylitis. Acute iridocyclitis is the most common ocular manifestation associated with ulcerative colitis, and it is seen in about 4 percent of patients. Other ocular findings include episcleritis and immune-mediated keratopathies[60] (Fig. 5-14 and Plate 5-10). Patients with Crohn's disease who have extensive joint disease (particularly from granuloma formation) are at higher risk of developing ocular involvement.[61] Acute iridocyclitis is seen in about 13 percent of cases. Episcleritis and peripheral keratitis are seen less frequently.

Treatment

The mainstay of treatment for inflammatory bowel disease includes systemic corticosteroids, which have proven to be very effective in controlling the colitis. The extraintestinal involvement is usually well controlled once bowel inflammation is successfully treated. Colectomy has been very effective in controlling both the intestinal and other systemic manifestations of ulcerative colitis. It has not proven to be as effective for patients with Crohn's disease.

Physical therapy and exercise are the first treatment modality for patients with inflammatory bowel disease (particularly those with spondylitis and/or sacroiliitis). Control of the peripheral articular disease includes using low-dose NSAIDs, which have proven to be very effective considering the mild nature of these agents. Intra-articular steroid injections may be needed in rare cases when a chronic inflammation affects a joint.

Topical steroids are effective in controlling episcleritis and noninfective (immune-mediated) keratitis. Short-acting cycloplegics, in addition to topical steroids, are used to control recurrent episodes of acute iridocyclitis. Posterior synechia, glaucoma, cataracts, and macular edema rarely complicate the clinical presentation of these patients. The use of periocular steroid injections, systemic steroids, or cytotoxic agents is not indicated given the less aggressive nature of the iridocyclitis associated with inflammatory bowel disease.

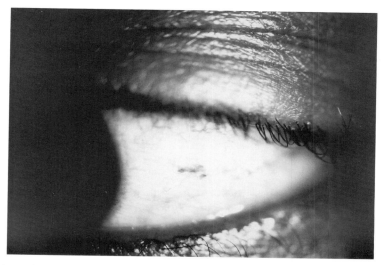

Fig. 5-14. Episcleritis of the left eye in a patient with Crohn's disease. Note the sectoral injection in a triangular shape pointing away from the limbus. The recurrent episodes occurred prior to the onset of colitis four times over a 2-year period. Topical steroids were necessary to control the episcleritis and the colitis responded very well to systemic steroid therapy. (See also Plate 5-9.)

CONCLUSION

The ocular side effects of rheumatic disease and treatment continue to challenge our clinical abilities on a regular basis. Despite advances in treatment with the use of steroids immunosuppressive and cytotoxic agents, there is no known cure. The associated arthropathy and oculopathy contribute to significant functional impairment for many patients with rheumatic disease. Many aspects of rheumatologic disease cannot be explained. The particular role that immunologic mechanisms and mediators play in the inflammatory process and why specific tissues are targeted in the natural course of these diseases are not fully understood. Significant ocular morbidity is associated with rheumatic disease. Manifestations such as keratitis sicca or recurrent iridocyclitis reflect natural disease progression despite systemic therapy. The ramifications of other manifestations (such as necrotizing scleritis) include not only potential vision loss but, more importantly, impending loss of life if aggressive therapeutic measures are not taken. Patients with rheumatic disease must be monitored for ocular sequella from both their disease and medications. Eye care practitioners play an integral role in the health care of these patients. Full eye examinations need to be performed regularly to determine the exact status of the patient's ocular health, considering the diagnosis and specific treatment regimen. Coordination of care with the patient's rheumatologist or internist offers the best opportunity to detect serious complications at an early stage and to minimize the possibility of vision loss, functional impairment, or loss of life.

REFERENCES

1. Panush RS: Principles of Rheumatic Disease. John Wiley & Sons, New York, 1982
2. Snyders B, Lambert M, Hardy JP: Retinal and choroidal vaso-occlusive disease in systemic lupus erythematosus associated with antiphospholipid antibodies. Retina 10:254, 1990
3. Bell CL, Rothenberg RJ: Rheumatoid arthritis. p. 269. In Graziano FM, Lemanske RF (eds): Clinical Immunology. Williams & Wilkins, Baltimore, 1989
4. Harris ED: Clinical features of rheumatoid arthritis. p. 874. In Kelly WN, Harris ED, Ruddy S, Sledge CB (eds): Textbook of Rheumatology. WB Saunders, Philadelphia, 1993
5. Harris ED: Etiology and pathogenesis of rheumatoid arthritis. p. 833. In Kelly WN, Harris ED, Ruddy S, Sledge CB (eds): Textbook of Rheumatology. WB Saunders, Philadelphia, 1993
6. Lotz M, Vaughn JH: Rheumatoid arthritis. p. 1365. In Samter M (ed): Immunological Disease. Vol. 2. Little, Brown, Boston, 1988
7. Watson P: Diseases of the scleral and episclera. p. 4. In Duane TD, Jaeger E (eds): Clinical Ophthalmology. HarperCollins, Hagerstown, MD, 1987
8. McGavin DD, Williamson J, Forrester JV et al: Episcleritis and scleritis. A study of their clinical manifestations and their association with rheumatoid arthritis. Br J Ophthalmol 60:192, 1976
9. Rao NA, Marak GE: Necrotizing scleritis. Ophthalmology 92:1542, 1985
10. Sanz II, Alboukrek D: Treatment of rheumatoid arthritis: traditional and new approaches. p. 99. In Fischbach M (ed): Rheumatoid arthritis. Churchill Livingstone, New York, 1991
11. Boers M, Ramsden M: Long acting drug combinations in rheumatoid arthritis: a formal overview. Rheumatol 18:316, 1992
12. Clements PJ, Paulus HE: Nonsteroidal anti-inflammatory drugs

(NSAIDs). p. 700. In Kelly WN, Harris ED, Ruddy S, Sledge CB (eds): Textbook of Rheumatology. WB Saunders, Philadelphia, 1993

13. Fauci AS, Young KR: Immunoregulatory agents. p. 797. In Kelly WN, Harris ED, Ruddy S, Sledge CB (eds): Textbook of Rheumatology. WB Saunders, Philadelphia, 1993

14. Rynes RL: Antimalarial drugs. p. 731. In Kelly WN, Harris ED, Ruddy S, Sledge CB (eds): Textbook of Rheumatology. WB Saunders, Philadelphia, 1993

15. James DG, Graham E, Hamblin A: Immunology of multiystem ocular disease. Surv Ophthalmol 30:155, 1985

16. Stahl JI, Klippel JH, Decker JL: Fever in systemic lupus erythematosus. Am J Med 67:933, 1979

17. Schur PH: Clinical features of systemic lupus erythematosus. p. 1017. In Kelly WN, Harris ED, Ruddy S, Sledge CB (eds): Textbook of Rheumatology. WB Saunders, Philadelphia, 1993

18. Woods VL: Pathogenesis of systemic lupus erythematosus. p. 999. In Kelly WN, Harris ED, Ruddy S, Sledge CB (eds): Textbook of Rheumatology. WB Saunders, Philadelphia, 1993

19. Stevens MB: Systemic lupus erythematosus and the cardiovascular system. p. 707. In Lahita RG (ed): Systemic Lupus Erythematosus. Churchill Livingstone, New York, 1992

20. Rubin LA, Urowitz MB, Gladman DD: Mortality in systemic lupus erythematosus—the bimodal pattern revisited. Q J Med 55:87, 1985

21. Gold DH, Morris DA, Henkind P: Ocular findings in systemic lupus erythematosus. Br J Ophthalmol 56:800, 1972

22. Snyders B, Lambert M, Hardy JP: Retinal and choroidal vaso-occlusive disease in systemic lupus erythematosus associated with antiphospholipid antibodies. Retina 10:254, 1990

23. Rosenstein ED, Sobleman J, Kramer N: Isolated third nerve palsy as initial manifestation of systemic lupus erythematosus. J Clin Neuro Ophthalmol 9:285, 1989

24. Rosenbaum JT: Systemic lupus erythematosus. p. 206. In Fraunfelder FT, Roy FH (eds): Current Ocular Therapy. WB Saunders, Philadelphia, 1990

25. Miller NR: Anterior ischemic optic neuropathy. p. 212. In: Walsh and Hoyt's Clinical Neuro-ophthalmology. 4th Ed. Williams & Wilkins, Baltimore, 1984

26. Chisholm DM, Waterhouse JP, Mason DK: Lymphocytic sialadenitis in major and minor glands: a correlation in post mortem studies. J Clin Pathol 23:690, 1970

27. Bloch KJ, Buchanan WW, Wohl MJ, Bunim JJ: Sjögren's syndrome. A clinical, pathological and serological study of sixty two cases. Medicine 44:187, 1965

28. Fox RI, Kang HI: Sjögren's syndrome. p. 931. In Kelley WN, Harris ED, Ruddy S, Sledge CB (eds): Textbook of Rheumatology. WB Saunders, Philadelphia, 1993

29. Mikulicz JJ: Concerning peculiar symmetrical disease of the lacrimal and salivary glands. Med Classics 2:165, 1937

30. Preston SJ, Buchanan WW: Rheumatic manifestations of immune deficiency. Clin Exp Rheumatol 7:547, 1989

31. Mattison PJ: Dry eyes: Autoimmunity and relationship to other systemic disease. Trans Ophthalomol Soc UK 104:458, 1985

32. Tala N: Sjögrens syndrome and connective tissue disease with other immunologic disorders. p. 810. In McCarty DJ (ed): Arthritis and Allied Conditions. Lea & Febiger, Philadelphia, 1989

33. Friedlaender MH: Arthritic and connective tissue disorders. p. 226. In Friedlaender MH (ed): Allergy and Immunology of the Eye. HarperCollins, Hagerstown, MD, 1993

34. DeVere R, Bradley WG: Polymyositis: it's presentations, morbidity and mortality. Brain 98:637, 1975

35. O'Leary PA, Waisman M: Dermatomyositis. Arch Dermatol 41:1001, 1940

36. Schuermann H: Dermatomyositis. Ergeb Inn Med Kunderheilkd 10:428, 1958

37. Keat AC: Reiter's syndrome and reactive arthritis in perspective. N Engl J Med 309:1606, 1983

38. Keat AC, Thomas B, Dixey J, et al: Chlamydia trachomatis and reactive arthritis: the missing link. Lancet 1:72, 1987

39. Geczy AF, et al: Possible role of enteric organisms in the pathogenesis of the seronegative spondyloarthropathies. p. 129. In Ziff M, Cohen SB (eds): Advances in Inflammation Research. Vol. 9. Raven Press, New York, 1985

40. Saag MS, Bennett JC: The infectious etiology of chronic rheumatic diseases. Semin Arthritis Rheumatol 17:1, 1987

41. Calin AC, Fries JF: Striking prevalence of ankylosing spondylitis in "healthy" W27 positive males and females; a controlled study. N Engl J Med 293:835, 1975

42. Wollheim FA: Ankylosing spondylitis. p. 943. In Kelly WN, Harris ED, Ruddy S, Sledge CB (eds): Textbook of Rheumatology. WB Saunders, Philadelphia, 1993

43. Kimura SJ, Hogan MJ, O'Connor GR, Epstein WV: Uveitis and joint disease: a review of 191 cases. Trans Am Ophthalmol Soc 64:301, 1966

44. Rahi AHS: HLA and eye disease. Br J Ophthalmol 63:283, 1979

45. Saari R, Lahti R, Matti Sari K et al; Frequency of rheumatic diseases in patients with acute anterior uveitis. Scand J Rheumatol 11:121, 1982

46. Brewerton DA, Hart FD, Nichols A, et al: Ankylosing spondylitis and HL-A27. Lancet 1:904, 1973

47. Hardin JG, Longnecker GL: Drug therapy of specific rheumatic diseases. p. 175. In: Handbook of Drug Therapy in Rheumatic Disease. Little, Brown, Boston, 1992

48. Dougados M, Boumier P, Amor B: Sulfasalazine in ankylosing spondylitis: a double-blind controlled study in 60 patients. Br Med J 293:911, 1986

49. Calin A: Reiter's syndrome. p. 119. In Calin A (ed): Spondyloarthropathies. Grune & Stratton, Orlando, FL, 1984

50. Fox R, Calin A, Gerbo RC et al: The chronicity of symptoms and disability in Reiter's syndrome: an analysis of 131 consecutive patients. Ann Intern Med 91:190, 1979

51. Csonka GW: The course of Reiter's syndrome. BMJ 1:1088, 1958

52. McClusky OE, Lordon RE, Arnett FC, et al: HLA 27 in Reiter's syndrome and psoriatic arthritis: a genetic factor in disease susceptability and expression. J Rheumatol 1:263, 1974

53. Khan MA, Skosey JL: Ankylosing spondylitis and related spondyloarthropathies. In Samter M, Talmage DW, Frank MM, et al (eds): Immunologic Diseases. 4th Ed. Little, Brown, Boston, 1988

54. Fan PT, Yu DTY: Reiter's syndrome. p. 961. In Kelly WN, Harris ED, Ruddy S, Sledge CB (eds): Textbook of Rheumatology. WB Saunders, Philadelphia, 1993

55. Bleehen SS, Everall JD, Tighe JR: Amyloidosis complicating Reiter's syndrome. Br J Venereal Dis 42:88, 1966

56. Wakefield D, Penny R: Cell mediated immune response to chlamydia in anterior uveitis: the role of HLA-B27. Clin Exp Immunol 51:191, 1983

57. Oates JK, Hancock JAH: Neurologic symptoms and lesions occurring in the course of Reiter's disease. Am J Med Sci 238:79, 1959

58. Burns T, Marks S, Calin A: A double-blind, placebo controlled, cross over trial of azathioprine (AZA) in refractory Reiter's syndrome. Arthritis Rheum 26:539, 1983

59. Lally EV, Ho G: A review of methotrexate therapy in Reiter's syndrome. Semin Arthritis Rheumatol 15:139, 1985

60. Ferry AP: The eye and rheumatic diseases. p. 507. In Kelly WN, Harris ED, Ruddy S, Sledge CB (eds): Textbook of Rheumatology. WB Saunders, Philadelphia, 1993

61. Hopkins DJ, Horan E, Burton IL et al; Ocular disorders in a series of 332 patients with Crohn's disease. Br J Ophthalmol 58:732, 1974

6 Neuromuscular Disease

ANDREW S. GURWOOD

INTRODUCTION

Optometry has always possessed an intimate relationship with neurology. The diagnosis of many neurologic diseases may be based on the signs and symptoms in the eyes. A significant percentage of nerve fibers within the central nervous system are directly concerned with visual function. Furthermore, the nerve fibers that innervate the extraocular muscles compose a significant portion of the brain stem and, like the visual fibers, travel through the brain in a lengthy, circuitous route. The course of all these fibers brings them in close proximity to many important neurologic landmarks, such that abnormalities in or adjacent to these structures will influence the visual or ocular motility system.

The neuromuscular system, with its complicated anatomic structure and plethora of integrated neurologic connections, can serve as an indicator to beginning, advancing, or impending neurologic disease. This chapter explores neuromuscular dysfunction as it relates to neurologic disease by discussing the salient anatomy, then characterizing a selection of neuromuscular dysfunctions in a logical fashion so the eye care practitioner can interrelate the neutralities with other aspects of neuro-ocular disease. Data collection and appropriate laboratory testing are stressed so the practicing optometrist can establish the differential diagnosis and participate in the management of these entities.

CASE REPORT

A 42-year-old white man presented to the clinic for routine eye examination, with a chief complaint of general fatigue, intermittent diplopia, and what he described as "eyelids that liked to close." On further questioning, he revealed that the symptoms were transient, with good days and bad. He further volunteered that his symptoms were always worse at the end of the day. With the exception of marginal systemic hypertension controlled by diet, the rest of the patient's history was unremarkable and noncontributory.

Best corrected visual acuities were OU 20/20 at distance and near. External examination revealed a slight ptosis of the left eyelid which seemed to become retracted momentarily on gaze (Cogan's lid twitch sign). No appreciable contralateral lid retraction was noted. Photophobia was mild but not overly disconcerting. Myasthenia gravis was suspected on the basis of the patient's history and other objective signs, and the obicularis oculi muscle of the left eye was checked for weakness and compared to the strength of the right eye by forceful opening. All other external examination findings were normal; no evidence of afferent pupillary defect was noted.

Refraction revealed hyperopia with astigmatism and presbyopia. Slit lamp examination was unremarkable

---

with normal applanation pressures, measured at OU 16 mmHg. Dilated fundus examination revealed normal nerves and an absence of posterior or peripheral pathology.

A complete blood count, erythrocyte sedimentation rate, fasting blood glucose, and 120-point automated visual field screening were ordered to assess overall health. All tests were negative for disease.

The patient was promptly referred to the neurologist with the suggestion that ocular and systemic myasthenia gravis should be ruled out. The neurologist ordered an acetylcholine-receptor antibody assay and proceeded with both the ice pack and endrophonium chloride (tensilon) test.

The results were positive for myasthenia gravis, confirming the diagnosis. Treatment was initiated with 60 mg of pyridostigmine (mestinon) and 30 mg of oral prednisone. Ocular lubricants were prescribed to protect the cornea from exposure keratitis, and alternate intermittent patching was used to control the sporadic, shifting episodes of diplopia. Finally, sunshields were prescribed for light sensitivity.

At last report, the patient was much improved and doing well. Vitamin D supplements will be considered if the systemic anti-inflammatory medications begin to have an osteoporetic effect.

ANATOMY

The human nervous system contains approximately 10 billion neurons.[1] These building blocks of the nervous system allow transmission of signals to be passed from one area of the body to another. The standard unit of the nervous system is the axon. Axons possess dendrites, which extend from the cell body and arborize extensively. Through these dendrites, axons communicate with other axons, gathering impulses to carry to the next destination. The first portion of the axon is called the *initial segment*. The axon ends in a number of synaptic knobs called *terminal buttons*. These knobs contain granules, or vesicles, that store the synaptic neurotransmitter secreted by the nerve. The neurotransmitter in all synaptic endplates of the neuromuscular junction of skeletal muscle is acetylcholine and called the *cholinergic system*. In smooth muscle and cardiac muscle, there is a dual innervation. Some of the motor endplates contain cholinergic neurotransmitters or *acetylcholine* whereas others are noradrenergic and contain a different neurotransmitter called *norepinephrine*.

The purpose of the neurotransmitter is to propagate the electrical signal from axon to axon or from axon to tissue endplate. Once the neurotransmitter is released, it causes an action. Whether that action is signal propagation or muscular contraction, it is stopped by special enzymes in the junction that break down the neurotransmitter. This enzyme in the cholinergic system is called *acetylcholinesterase*. The enzyme designed to degrade norepinephrine in the adrenergic system is called *monoamine oxidase*.[1–5]

The neuron is surrounded by supportive cells called *Schwann cells*. Many layers of Schwann cells form a protein–lipid complex, which insulates the axon, speeding up signal transmission, called *myelin*.[1] The myelin sheath envelops the axon except at its end and at intermittent streaks called nodes of Ranvier. Not all neurons are myelinated. Some are surrounded by Schwann cells, without the wrapping of the Schwann cell membrane around the axon that produces myelin. In the central nervous system of mammals, most neurons are myelinated, but the cells that form the myelin differ from the cells that form the myelin in the peripheral nervous system and are called *oligodendrogliocytes*. Unlike Schwann cells, which form myelin between two nodes of Ranvier, oligodendrogliocytes stimulate multiple processes that form myelin on many neighboring axons.[1,2]

In multiple sclerosis, patchy destruction of myelin in the central nervous system occurs, with associated failure in the normal conduction in the affected neurons.

The preceding terminology applies well to spinal neurons and interneurons but is somewhat unconventional for other types of neuron. Therefore, the dendritic zone of the neuron is typically referred to as the *receptor membrane* with the axon serving to deliver the signal to the next destination.

Nerve cells have a low threshold for excitation. Stimuli that excite the nerve may be electrical, chemical, or mechanical. The impulse is normally conducted along the axon to its termination. Nerve tissue, however, is a poor conductor. In the nerve tissue, conduction is an active process requiring great amounts of energy.[1,2]

With respect to neuromuscular disease, transmission of activity across the neuromuscular junction is the first intramuscular process involved in muscle excitation. Skeletal muscle fibers contract in response to action potentials, which travel over the muscle plasma membranes. These action potentials originate at the endplates, in response to activity in the nerve terminals. The extraocular muscles are included in the category of skeletal muscles, which are neurogenic, requiring neural input to originate their activity.[3-5] This differs from smooth muscle, or myogenic muscle, from which activity arises spontaneously.

The muscle action potential spreads out in all directions. Skeletal muscle comprises individual muscle fibers, the building blocks of the muscular systems in the same manner that neurons are the building blocks of the nervous system. These fibers are divisible into fibrils, which are composed of filaments of contractile proteins. As the impulse travels over the fiber, it initiates events within the fiber that leads to contraction.[3-5]

Any form of trauma, toxicity, restriction, infiltration, compression, demyelination, degeneration, or infection that causes damage to the extraocular muscles, nerves, or neuromuscular junction and its neurotransmitters will result in intermittent or permanent neuromuscular dysfunction.

NEURO-OPHTHALMIC EXAMINATION

The ocular system is an interesting set of anatomic structures with many integrated and interdigitated neurologic connections. The structure, posture, functional ability and neuro-ophthalmic connections should be scrutinized for normalcy. In many ways the eyes can serve as the optometrists' informant to beginning, advancing, or impending neurologic disease.

Patients who present with neuromuscular dysfunction, whether by chief complaint or clinical observation, warrant immediate attention. The neuro-ophthalmic examination emphasizes history taking[6]

Table 6-1. Elements of the Neuro-ophthalmic History

Optometric physician objectives
    Is the problem the result of organic or functional disorders?
    Where is the lesion?
    What is the cause?
Questions to include
    The time of onset for symptoms and recurrences
    History of present illness
    Previous radiologic or electrophysiologic examination
    History of past and present medication
    Review of past and present ocular history
        Any transient loss of vision
        Qualitative loss of vision
        Scotomas
        Photophobia
        Metamorphopsia
        Diplopia
    Review of neurologic history and symptoms
    Family history
    Social and occupational history
    Observation
    Evaluation of the "other" cranial nerves
Questions of localization: Diagnosis of neuro-ophthalmic lesions
  by the evidence and data
    Is this a lesion of the muscle?
    Is this a lesion of the neuromuscular junction?
    Is this a lesion of the nerve?
    Is this a lesion of the brain?

(Table 6-1). The optometrist should proceed logically, attempting to answer questions concerning cause and localization. Once rapport is established, the eye care practitioner will elicit the necessary information. Patients often fail to identify pertinent signs and symptoms, possibly because they are not trained observers or they consider a particular condition long-standing and normal. The optometrist must identify the important issues, rank them in order of importance, and proceed to accumulate information regarding onset, duration, exacerbating factors, and alleviating factors. The history should include present and past illness, present and past ocular status, medications, family history, and social and occupational experience.

MYASTHENIA GRAVIS

The diagnosis of myasthenia gravis can often be straightforward but on other occasions may be elusive. Despite well-publicized ocular signs, myasthenia ranks high on the list of "missed diagnoses," principally because optometrists are unaware of its variations in presentation.[7] Furthermore, skill and experience are required to examine patients for subtle clinical signs such as unusual ocular motility disturbances with or without ptosis in the presence of normal pupillary responses.[7,8]

Glaser and Bachynski[7] characterize myasthenia gravis as muscular weakness without other signs of neurologic deficit, such as loss of reflex, sensory loss, or muscle atrophy, with variability of muscle function within minutes, hours, or weeks.[7] Remissions and exacerbations may occur and sometimes are triggered by sickness or trauma with a predilection for affecting extraocular, facial, and oropharyngeal muscles.[7]

The term *myasthenia gravis* is Greek in origin and means "muscle weakness from gravity."[8] It has an incidence of 2:20,000 persons with a slight predilection for women over men (3:2).[7,8] The onset of myasthenia may occur at any age, but onset before the age of 40 is more common in women. Neonatal forms are rare. Cases diagnosed in children demonstrate a wider variety of myasthenic syndromes.[7–10] Up to 90 percent of patients with myasthenia gravis present with some type of ocular sign or symptom. A small percentage of individuals presents with purely ocular myasthenia. When a patient presents with signs of diplopia, ptosis, or lid retraction, myasthenia gravis should be ruled out.[7–11]

Myasthenia is associated with thymoma, dysthyroidism, and collagen vascular disorders. Association with thymoma is well known and occurs in approximately 10 percent of myasthenic patients.[12] Dysthyroidism is found in approximately 5 percent of patients. In patients with this combination, ocular signs can be mixed (ptosis with exophthalmos), making diagnosis more difficult.

Myasthenia is known to be an autoimmune disorder characterized by a reduction in available postsynaptic acetylcholine receptors at the endplates of the neuromuscular junctions of skeletal muscles (Fig. 6-1). Anti-acetylcholine-receptor antibody has been isolated in 80 percent of patients with generalized disease and in approximately 50 percent of patients with ocular myasthenia.[13,14] Although recoverable antibody titers correlate poorly with the severity of the disease, Drachman et al.[15] demonstrated that the antibodies accelerate acetylcholine-receptor degradation and increase the receptor blockade.[15]

The cause of the autoimmune attack on the acetylcholine receptors is still unknown. The source of these maverick antibodies appears to be within or at least linked to the thymus gland, which regularly shows epithelial cell tumoral growth. These epithelial cells resemble skeletal muscle on a histologic level and are hypothesized to stimulate an antigenic response.[7]

The most obvious ocular manifestation of myasthenia gravis is ptosis, brought on by weakness within the muscles responsible for keeping the eyelids open. This includes both the obicularis oculi and levator palpebrae superioris.[11,13–16] Myasthenia gravis and ocular myasthenia are hypothesized to affect the levator and obicularis most because of their increased blood

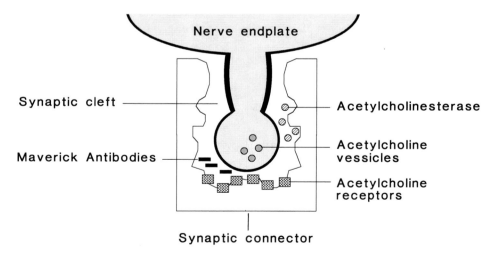

Fig. 6-1. Schematic representation of the anatomy of the neuromuscular junction in myasthenia gravis. (Drawing, Andrew S. Gurwood)

supply from the internal carotid artery and corresponding increased serum antibody exposure.[13]

Osserman[17] concluded that ocular muscle involvement eventually occurs in 90 percent of all myasthenia patients, with 75 percent presenting with ocular symptoms as their chief complaint.[17] Bever and co-workers[18,19] found that 49 percent of ocular myasthenia remains strictly ocular. Of the remaining patients who developed systemic myasthenia, 82 percent did so within 2 years of their ocular diagnosis.[7,18]

Ocular Manifestations

Myasthenia gravis is often classified by pediatric and adult varieties. The symptoms tend to follow diurnal variations and last for weeks and months with exacerbations and remissions[20] (Table 6-2).

The four outstanding ocular signs associated with myasthenia gravis are ptosis, the paradoxical sign or lid retraction, diplopia, and obicularis weakness.[11,12] The ptosis can be pharmacologically exacerbated by antibiotics such as neomycin, polymyxin B, gentamicin, and tetracycline.[21] β-Blockers (topical and systemic), phenothiazines, alcohol, and quinine derivatives have also been shown to exacerbate ptosis in patients with myasthenia gravis.[22,23] Patients with facial signs always possess obicularis weakness. This can result in exposure keratitis. Decreased corneal sensitivity is also a common finding and should be checked in suspected patients. Environmental factors

may also escalate symptoms. These include bright lights, heat, infection, stress, or trauma.[8]

Lid retraction or paradoxical sign[11] is often diagnosed when mild contralateral ptosis is overlooked. Three types of eyelid retraction are observed in myasthenia. Patients with ptosis secondary to myasthenia gravis often develop eyelid retraction that lasts only a few seconds following a saccade from downgaze to the primary position. This is termed Cogan's lid twitch sign.[11,24,25] Some patients may develop transient eyelid retraction lasting from seconds to minutes after prolonged upward gaze. This occurs because both superior rectus and levator muscles, innervated by the superior branch of cranial nerve III, receive excessive stimulation during prolonged upward gaze, leaving the levator in a slight state of tetany.[11] The third type of lid retraction in patients with myasthenia gravis results from exerted attempts at elevating the contralateral ptotic lid.[11,26]

The usual explanation for eyelid retraction in myasthenia gravis is Hering's law of equal and opposite innervation.[11,26] According to this principle, patients who have myasthenic ptosis in the right eye need increased levels of neurologic activity to keep it open. This increased innervation is subsequently received by the levator of the nonptotic left eye. Because the left eye is less involved in the disease process than the right, it rises above its normal position, appearing retracted.[11,25] When the suspected ptotic lid is covered or manually lowered, the contralateral retraction subsides or disappears. The eye care practitioner

Table 6-2. Myasthenia Gravis Summary Table

Classification	Incidence in patients with MG (%)	Onset	Signs/Symptoms
Pediatric			
Neonatal	10–20, mother positive	At birth	Resolution within 6 weeks
Congenital/juvenile	15–20, mother negative	Birth thru life	Severe ocular signs
			Mild generalized disease
Adult			
Ocular myasthenia	15–20	Variable	Mild signs; good prognosis
Mild and generalized	15–20	Slow onset	Gradual skeletal muscle weakness
			Moderate response to medicines
Moderate and generalized	15–20	Slow onset	Slowly progressive; respiratory distress possible
Acute fulminating	15–20	Rapid onset	Severe generalized disease
			Moderate response to severe signs occur within 6 months; high mortality; poor response to drugs
Late severe	15–20	Slow onset	Sudden onset of severe symptoms

(Modified from Gurwood,[20] with permission as adapted from Rodgin.[8])

should also observe the patient's forehead. The patient may attempt to raise the ptotic eyelid by activating the frontalis. In this case, the brow may show excessive wrinkling. To expose this, the optometrist can place a hand on the patient's forehead and manually prohibit it from working.

The hallmark signs of myasthenia gravis are exacerbations and remissions brought on by variable amounts of activity. Although some degree of ptosis is invariable, it is typically noticed unilaterally. This ptosis may shift from eye to eye. Clinically, the ptosis can be made more apparent by requesting the patient to undergo repeated eyelid closure or sustained upgaze.[7,27]

Intermittent diplopia should be discussed for completeness. This symptom usually results from affected muscles (predominantly medial rectus) on convergence or superior rectus in upgaze.[8,11,28] The diagnostic evaluation for patients with either ptosis or lid retraction begins with extraocular muscle evaluation to rule out nerve palsy or mechanical restrictions. The eye care practitioner should also take care to measure the palpebral fissures for future reference.

Diagnostic Testing

Diagnostic testing usually prescribed for patients suspected of having myasthenia gravis is endrophonium chloride (tensilon) injection.[27,29] This anticholinesterase is preferred because of its rapid onset of action and brief duration.[8] The customary method is to load 1 ml (or 10 mg) into a syringe. Venipuncture should be performed, and a 0.2-ml test dose should be administered. If no improvement is perceived, the remaining 0.8 ml should be slowly administered over 30 seconds, watching for signs of improvement in muscle functioning.[29] Optometrists may choose to rule out functional disorders by first injecting a saline placebo. If improvement is noticed following placebo injection, the disorder is termed *neuroasthenia* and classified as functional.

Tensilon testing can produce false-negative results in the early stages of the disease and in cases of ocular myasthenia gravis. If the eye care practitioner remains suspicious, the patient should be retested.[8]

The ice pack test is a noninvasive alternative to tensilon testing. Ptosis has been shown to improve after administration of an ice pack. Ice wrapped in a towel is used to lower the surface skin temperature to 29°C. Acetylcholinesterase is reduced by cooling, whereas neurotransmitted release is increased by cooling.[7,25] The recommended time for holding the ice pack to the patient's eye is 2 minutes.[7,25]

Therapy

Laboratory testing is essential in patients who are suspected of having myasthenia gravis. The association between thyroid disease and myasthenia is well documented.[30] Chest radiographs, computed tomography (CT) scans, magnetic resonance imaging (MRI), and thyroid function tests should be considered. As documented by Oosterhuis[13] and others, the treatment of choice for 10 to 20 percent of myasthenic patients with thymus neoplasm is surgical removal of the thymus (thymectomy).[7,13,25] Blood glucose testing and purified protein derivative testing (for tuberculosis) should also be considered, because steroid regimens used in the treatment of myasthenia gravis patients can activate or exacerbate diabetes and tuberculosis.[8]

Treatment for myasthenia gravis should be relegated to the neurologist. The two current treatment modalities include anticholinesterases that block the degradation of acetylcholine in the neuromuscular junction and steroids. Current anticholinesterase medications include pyridostigmine (mestinon) and neostigmine (prostigmine). Topical anticholinesterases such as phospholine iodide may provide some resolution of myasthenia gravis.[8] Prudence is advised when using these medications; they possess a high degree of toxicity to skeletal muscle.[8]

Oral steroids suppress the immune reaction in myasthenia gravis and relieve symptoms in up to 80 percent of patients. Improvement of ptosis and diplopia are often accomplished within 2 weeks of the first administration. This is the treatment of choice for strictly ocular cases.[8] Steroidal therapy is generally continued for 1 year, then discontinued to check for spontaneous remission. Therapy can be re-established if symptoms recur. In cases of extensive systemic weakness, corticosteroid usage is controversial, because corticosteroids have been implicated in causing respiratory weakness and exacerbation of symptoms.[7,8]

Other supportive therapies include sunshades to minimize discomfort from orbicularis oculi strain, occlusion therapy, ptosis crutch, and the use of a fresnel press-on prism for diplopia.[7,8] When diplopia cannot be eliminated by the use of prism, a patch or opaque lens should be attempted.

EATON-LAMBERT SYNDROME

Eaton-Lambert syndrome is a disorder of the neuromuscular junction that produces proximal limb weakness resembling myasthenia gravis. In contrast to myasthenia gravis, ocular, facial, and oropharyngeal muscles are spared with a temporary increase in muscle power evident after brief exercise. The key to diagnosis is the absence of deep tendon reflexes.[7]

In patients in whom Eaton-Lambert syndrome is suspected, electromyographic testing is essential. Eliciting the characteristic incremental response to repetitive exercise (opposite the response of myasthenia gravis) is essential to diagnosis.[31]

Although the mechanism of the syndrome is poorly understood, it is believed to be the result of presynaptic events that impair the release of acetylcholine.[31] Approximately 70 percent of Eaton-Lambert patients harbor malignant neoplasms of the lungs, bronchogenic carcinoma.[32]

Ocular involvement is extremely rare. In fact, the determination of ocular involvement practically excludes the Eaton-Lambert syndrome.[7]

Pharmacologic agents such as D-penicillamine have been documented to produce ocular signs and symptoms similar to that of myasthenia gravis.[33,34] A number of antibiotics, including the polypeptide polymyxin B and the aminoglycosides neomycin and streptomycin, have been reported as possible causes of muscular weakness resembling myasthenia gravis.[35] Other medications that can decrease transmission at the neuromuscular junction are antiarrhythmics (procainamide), anticonvulsants (phenytoin), β-blockers (timolol, propranolol), lithium, and chloroquine.[7]

Ocular signs similar to myasthenia include ptosis, external ophthalmoplegia, muscle paresis, facial palsies, and lagophthalmus. They must be investigated along with myasthenia gravis in the differential diagnosis.

Ocular treatment includes removal of the exacerbating agent, when possible, along with supportive therapies such as ptosis crutches.

DYSTHYROID OPHTHALMOPATHY

Thyroid eye disease, Graves ophthalmopathy, dysthyroid ophthalmopathy, and Graves orbitopathy, Graves disease are all synonymous terms. The disease is characterized clinically by eyelid retraction, proptosis, injection and chemosis of the conjunctivae, corneal compromise secondary to exposure, extraocular muscle fibrosis, and, in severe cases, slight loss resulting from compressive optic neuropathy within the orbit[29,36–38] (Table 6-3).

With respect to the eye, it is primarily an orbital disease, hypothesized to be of autoimmune origin.[29,36] Thyroid eye disease may occur at any age and is most often found in persons with a strong familial history of thyroid dysfunction. Females are generally affected more than males, by a ratio of $2.3:1$.[38] Whereas ocular thyrotoxicosis is one of the common clinical entities of the optometric and ophthalmic clinical picture, ophthalmopathy typically occurs in only 25 to 50 percent of cases.[35]

McKenzie[38] is cited in the literature as providing the most pragmatic definition for Graves disease.[30,39] He states that Graves disease is a multisystem disorder of unknown cause, characterized by one or more of the following: (1) hyperthyroidism associated with diffuse hyperplasia of the thyroid gland; (2) infiltrative ophthalmopathy; and (3) infiltrative dermopathy (localized pretibial myxedema: focal swelling and infiltration of the connective tissues of the skin).[39]

Some interesting notations regarding thyroid dysfunction include that ocular findings may occur independently from systemic dysthyroid function. That is, ocular findings may be more severe, less severe, or match the system condition. Euthyroid Graves ophthalmopathy is a common clinical syndrome in which the characteristic ophthalmic manifestations of Graves disease exist in the presence of a clinically and biomedically normal thyroid.[30]

The pathophysiology, laboratory testing, common eye signs, and treatment modalities for Graves disease are discussed in detail in Chapter 1. Patients suspected of having thyroid disease should be examined promptly and carefully. The differential diagnosis for Graves disease includes orbital mass, inflammatory processes, and vascular abnormalities.[30,36–39]

Table 6-3. Thyroid Eye Disease Quick Reference

Class	Signs and Symptoms	Treatment
0	No ocular signs; patients may undergo weight loss with increased appetite, nervousness, palpitation, tachycardia at rest and systolic hypertension	Referral to general practitioner for blood work; rule out systemic hypertension, diabetes; no ocular modalities
1	Systemically, patients may suffer from increased anxiety; ocularly, mild periorbital edema, startled or staring look; mild corneal stippling inferiorly	Copious artificial tear solutions and ointments; monitor for progression
2	Lid retraction (Darymple's sign), increased stare, possibly unilateral proptosis, lid lag (von Graefe's sign), dry eye with gritty sensation, more corneal compromise	Copious artificial tear solutions and ointments; more ointment may now be necessary; supportive patient education; consult general practitioner for possibility of initiating systemic therapy
3	Proptosis, positive >22 mm, increased lid retraction; restrictive myopathy; positive forced duction test; difficulty everting eyelid (Gifford's sign); decreased blink posture (Stellwag's sign)	Copious artificial tear solutions and ointments; depending on the severity of the blink posture, moisture chamber patches, blindfolds, or lid taping may be required
4	Extraocular muscle involvement increases; more restriction leads to intermittent diplopia, which is slowly progressive; positive forced duction testing; intraocular pressure rises by ≥4 mm on upward gaze; positive "30 degree" test on A- B-scan ultrasound	Referral to general practitioner to initiate systemic corticosteroid therapy (40–80 mg/day); fresnel press on prisms or occlusive therapy to eliminate diplopia; consider partial surgical removal of thyroid
5	Corneal epithelium is compromised and threatened by proptosis; ulceration is possible; severe dryness	More corneal support; may require antibiotic ointments; if dryness threatens to provoke permanent visual disability, consider tarsorraphy; may try increased steroid dosage (40–100 mg)
6	Compressive sight loss secondary to orbital congestion; central, paracentral, and arcuate scotomata apparent	Surgical innervation required; supervoltage orbital irradiation (1,600–2,000 rads) directed toward the orbital apex; orbital decompression as a last resort using Krönlein, Ogura, or Two Wall procedures

(From Gurwood,[20] with permission.)

HORNER SYNDROME

Horner syndrome is a fairly common abnormality, the causes of which range from such benign problems as migraine headache to serious conditions such as tumor, infarction, aneurysm, and trauma. Occasionally, the history in combination with the physical examination will determine the etiology, although more often, the cause is not readily discernible (Table 6-4).

The pupillodilator fibers are controlled by the sympathetic nervous system. The neuronal arc consists of three neurons. The first neuron originates in the posterolateral hypothalamus.[40] Fibers course through the brain stem to synapse in the intermediolateral portion of the C8 through T2 level of spinal cord, known as the ciliospinal center of Budge. Second-order axons continue from the latter cord levels and exit the ventral root. They ascend to cross the apex of the lung and course (without synapse) to the stellate ganglion, inferior cervical ganglion, around the subclavian artery, and through the middle cervical ganglion.[40] These second-order fibers synapse in the superior cer-

Table 6-4. Horner Syndrome Quick Reference

Pupillodilator fibers under control of the sympathetic nervous system have a three neuron pathway
    Fibers originate in the hypothalamus
    Second-order axons emerge from the spinal cord at the T1 level in the ventral root
    Third-order fibers synapse in the superior cervical ganglion and form the final common pathway to the pupillodilator

The patient presents with ptosis, miosis, and facial anhidrosis

Anosocoria is greater in dim illumination than bright illumination

The 5–10% cocaine test (blocks reuptake of norepinephrine) results in poor pupillary dilation and confirms the presence of Horner syndrome
    The cocaine test confirms or denies the presence of Horner syndrome

The 1% hydroxyamphetamine (Paredrine) test (releases norepinephrine) can separate third order Horner syndrome from second and first order

First and second order Horner syndrome may only be differentiated by associated brainstem (first order) or spinal cord and lung (second order) signs and symptoms

vical ganglion at the level of the angle of the mandible and bifurcation of the carotid at C3 through C4. Third-order neurons originating from the superior cervical ganglion form the final pathway to the pupillodilator muscles.[40] These nerve fibers follow the carotid into the cavernous sinus, where they travel with the ophthalmic division of the trigeminal nerve (V) and emerge with the nasociliary branch and long ciliary nerves to the dilator of the iris. The neurotransmitter released at the dilator is norepinephrine.[40]

Any dysfunction or damage to the sympathetic chain will decrease the output of norepinephrine in the synaptic cleft of the dilator and Müller's muscle. All patients with Horner syndrome have ptosis, miosis with preservation of the light, and near reflex.[40] Facial anhidrosis is another clinical sign because the sweat glands of the face and forehead are innervated by sympathetic postganglionics below the level of the bifurcation of the carotid.[41] Rosenberg[40] described a method for determining the presence of asymmetric facial sweating by subjectively observing the relative difference in friction while rubbing a prism bar against one side of the forehead and then the other. The procedure is simple. The forehead and prism bar are cleaned with an alcohol swab, allowed to dry, the bar is held against the forehead above the eyebrow with the axis perpendicular to the floor, and the bar is allowed to slide downward.[41] Compare the friction of one side to the other. The results of this study correlate well with starch-iodine testing. This finding is significant because lesions above the carotid bifurcation will not affect facial sweating.[41]

Two additional tests are useful in diagnosing and localizing the presence of a Horner syndrome. The cocaine test is the primary means of confirming or denying the presence of Horner syndrome. A drop of 5- to 10-percent ophthalmic cocaine solution is placed in both eyes and repeated 1 minute later. Sympathetic damage at any level will result in a pupil that dilates poorly to cocaine.[40,42] Cocaine blocks reuptake of neuroepinephrine at the synaptic cleft. Damage to any neuron of the arc will give a positive result.[40] Kardon et al.[41] demonstrated with confidence that Horner syndrome can be effectively diagnosed by measuring the amount of postinstallation anisocoria,[42] 50 to 60 minutes after initiating the test. Kardon et al.[42] concluded that postcocaine anisocoria of at least 1 mm is required to make the diagnosis.

The paredrine test, or hydroxyamphetamine 1 per-

cent ophthalmic drop test, is used to differentiate first- and second-neuron defects from third-neuron dysfunction.[40] When the first and second neurons in the sympathetic arc are damaged, the final pathway, remaining intact, continues to produce, store, and transport norepinephrine. Paredrine releases available norepinephrine from the vesicles into the synaptic cleft. Therefore, when it is instilled into a normal eye or a known Horner eye with a viable third neuron, the pupil will dilate. Failure to dilate usually indicates a third-order (superior cervical ganglion or postganglionic) problem.[40,43] The cocaine test identifies the existence of Horner syndrome, the paredrine test differentiates third-neuron Horner syndrome from first- and second-neuron syndromes. The only way to identify first neuron disorders like brain stem disease and stroke from second neuron disorders like spinal cord disease, carotid artery dissection, and Pancoast's tumor (tumor of the apex of the lung) is by the associated clinical testing.[40]

The cause of adult-onset, acquired Horner syndrome is often idiopathic. Conditions known to produce Horner syndrome include tumors, inflammatory processes, aneurysms, cluster headaches, and injuries following surgery to correct carotid artery disease.[44] Horner syndrome with ipsilateral cranial nerve VI palsy localizes the lesion to cavernous sinus. In 1988, Striph and Burde[45] documented two cases of lesions within the cavernous sinus producing Horner syndrome with ipsilateral cranial nerve VI palsy. Lyme disease has been found to produce reversible Horner syndrome in untreated cases and should be considered within the differential diagnosis.[46] The facial nerve is the most commonly involved cranial nerve, but lesions of every cranial nerve have been documented.[45] The syndrome will resolve when the underlying lesion is treated.

Horner syndrome in temporal arteritis[47] and contralateral trochlear nerve (IV) paresis is also possible as is ipsilateral Horner syndrome[48] and Horner syndrome in children.[49] Horner syndrome in temporal arteritis has been identified as a rare but viable complication secondary to the granulomatous inflammation of the vessels surrounding the internal carotid or vasa nervorum. Patients in the correct age range with acquired ptosis or Horner syndrome in the presence of significant symptoms should be examined for temporal arteritis and other vascular diseases.[47] Patients with paresis of the trochlear nerve (IV) contralateral to the eye with a Horner syndrome should be suspected for brainstem lesions. Coppeto in 1983[50] documented that cases of this type provide localizing signs to caudal lesions of the dorsal mesencephalon.[48] Horner syndrome in children is most often the result of birth trauma to the lower brachial plexus.[49] Recent studies have reported neuroblastoma as a causative factor in all cases of Horner syndrome onset within the first year of life. Horner syndrome in children, especially when the onset is within the first year of life, must be investigated with chest radiographs, CT scanning of the head and neck, and 24-hour urinary catecholamine assay.[49]

The two most common forms of treatment for acquired Horner syndrome ptosis is to remove the underlying cause or to perform a Müller's muscle–conjunctival resection procedure.[51] Typically, the surgeon instills either 2.5 or 10 percent phenylephrine into the superior fornix of the ptotic eye. The surgeon compares postinstillation posture to preinstillation posture and then resects the amount of standard tissue required by that reference value.[51]

MUSCULAR DYSTROPHIES

The term *muscular dystrophy* refers to the group of genetically determined disorders that cause progressive weakness and wasting of skeletal muscles, affecting muscle cells directly. Some forms cause death after 20 years of life, whereas others are compatible with normal life expectancy.[27]

Congenital Muscular Dystrophies

Fukuyama-Type Congenital Muscular Dystrophy

Patients with symptoms reported at birth, variable clinical course, and dystrophic muscle pathology are considered to possess congenital muscular dystrophy (CMD).[52] CMD is not rare and represents approximately 16 percent of childhood muscular dystrophies.[53] Patients with CMD show generalized muscle involvement at birth. Muscle atrophy and weakness are typically symmetric. Neither ptosis nor ophthalmoplegia has been observed in patients with CMD with the exception of Fukuyama-type CMD.[54-57]

Patients with Fukuyama syndrome have CMD with central nervous system involvement, mental retardation, convulsions, and impaired motor development.

The average life span for children who suffer from Fukuyama-type CMD is 8 to 10 years.[27]

Fukuyama-type CMD is transmitted as an autosomal recessive trait without predilection for sex. Ocular involvement is often severe and extensive.[55,57,58]

Ocular involvement includes high myopic refractive error, anterior polar, and nuclear cataracts, optic nerve hypoplasia and atrophy, obicularis weakness, gross abnormalities of the retina, displaced foveas, irregularities of the retinal pigment epithelium, and retinal detachment.[57,58]

Little treatment is available for the ocular consequence of Fukuyama CMD. The patients are often cognitively limited with limited motor capacity.[58] The eye care practitioner's goal should be to guard the health of the cornea and provide supportive therapies.

Congenital Myotonia

Myotonia is a phenomenon in which muscle fibers have pathologically persistent activity after contraction or are continuously active when they should be relaxed.[27] This condition is thought to occur from a disorder of the muscle membrane and conducting system.[27,59]

Congenital myotonia is a heredofamilial disease that becomes apparent during the early years of life. It is characterized by delayed relaxation of the voluntary muscle, increased muscle signs, and mental retardation. Becker[27,60] classified the disease into two subtypes, according to mode of inheritance: autosomal recessive and autosomal dominant. The autosomal recessive forms are more common and usually more severe.[27,60]

The pathologic findings are confined to the skeletal muscles. In fact, neither the peripheral nervous system nor other organs of the body change. The onset of ocular symptoms occur in infancy and become accentuated at puberty. The primary ocular manifestation of congenital myotonia is blepharospasm, a voluntary or involuntary narrowing of the upper and lower lids brought about by obicularis contraction.[61] Burde et al.[61] states that it is invariably associated with elevation of the lower lid and a lowering of the brow. Blepharospasm is frequently accompanied by visible twitching of the obicularis.[61] Myokymia is a similar but benign anomalous function that occurs most often in young and middle-aged adults. It is described as an episodic, involuntary twitching of the obicularis muscle and is not a true blepharospasm.

Paramyotonia congenita is an autosomal dominant form of congenita myotonia. It is far less severe, usually manifesting as ocular symptoms of ptosis. Unlike its autosomal recessive counterpart, it is not progressive and may improve as the patient grows older. No treatment is available for congenital myotonia other than supportive therapies.

Myotonic Dystrophy

The most frequent and disabling of the myotonic diseases is myotonic dystrophy. Myotonic dystrophy is separated from the other forms of muscular dystrophy because it is the only one in which myotonia is accompanied by dystrophic changes in other tissues and organs.[27]

Myotonic dystrophy is a genetic disorder that presents with an autosomal dominant inheritance pattern. The incidence is 4.5 to 5.5/100,000 population, with men and women affected equally.[27]

Myotonic dystrophy is a rare but interesting cause of symmetric external ophthalmoplegia. The etiology of the disease is poorly understood. Myotonic muscles apparently have abnormal membranes; neither nerve block nor destruction abolishes the characteristic muscle contractility.[7] The disease typically possesses cardiac respiratory, smooth muscle, skeletal bone, and gastrointestinal involvements as well. Many, but not all, patients with myotonic dystrophy present with mental retardation.

The myotonia is variable within the course of the day, often being worst in the morning. It can be increased by excitement, fatigue, hunger, and menstruation. It can often be brought out by asking a patient to shake hands. Affected individuals will continue the hand clasp after an attempt has been made to release the grasp.

The ocular changes in myotonic dystrophy include ptosis, obicularis weakness, infrequent blinking, and difficulty in closing the eyes.[27] Abnormalities of eye movements have been documented by von Norden,[62] Walton and Natress,[63] and Lessel et al.[64] In its mildest form, oculomotor involvement consists of slow saccades with normal motility ranges and no visual complaints. In its more severe forms, patients present with varying degrees of ophthalmoparesis without restriction (negative forced duction test).[27]

The most common clinical entity found in these patients are cataracts. Virtually all patients with myotonic dystrophy possess spoke-like subcortical opacities.[65] These cataracts are unique in that they contain globular-shaped, red, green, and blue crystals in a stellate pattern.[27]

Other documented ocular abnormalities include sluggish miotic pupillary responses that respond poorly to mydriatics and react poorly to the near reflex, vascular abnormalities of the iris, dark-adaptation abnormalities, pigmentary retinopathy involving the macula, decreasing vision, and abnormalities in visual-evoked potentials in the absence of retinal abnormalities.[27] Fields are usually normal without constriction.

Treatment of patients with myotonic dystrophy is supportive. When infrequent blinking causes corneal compromise, artificial tears and tear ointments may be dispensed for frequent use. If incomplete closure of the eyes occurs during sleep, lid taping or the use of a blindfold along with ointment may help. In many cases these patients do not possess any visual complaints. When ptosis becomes a problem, referral to an oculoplastics specialist or the use of ptosis crutches should be considered. When cataracts reduce vision, surgical removal should be considered.

In cases of prominent pigmentary degeneration, the eye care practitioner should realize that the cause of this degeneration differs completely from the pigmentary degeneration seen in retinitis pigmentosa. Regardless of appearance, the retinopathy is not as severe and does not cause blindness.

Oculopharyngeal Dystrophy

Oculopharyngeal dystrophy is a hereditary condition that is typically autosomal dominant. First described by Taylor[66] in 1915, it is characterized by progressive dysphagia and ptosis.[27,66] The disease, as noted by Murphy and Drachman,[67] has a predilection for attacking individuals of French-Canadian stock in the fourth to sixth decade of life.[7,27,67,68] Classically, the dysphagia precedes the ptosis by several years. The ptosis usually begins unilaterally but often progresses to a symmetric bilateral ptosis. External ophthalmoplegia is not an uncommon finding in affected patients. Patients often present with the Hutchison face, head tilted back with overaction of the frontalis to compensate for the ptosis. This condition is not considered rare; patients with oculopharyngeal muscular dystrophy make up approximately 33 percent of all patients who acquire ptosis.[69] The strategy for managing these patients is similar to those previously mentioned.

Progressive External Ophthalmoplegia

Sometimes classified as forms of muscular dystrophy, chronic progressive external ophthalmoplegia (CPEO) and CPEO-plus (or Kearns-Sayre-Daroff syndrome) are a mixture of myopathy and neuropathy.[7] Morphologic changes in skeletal muscle cause the characteristic red-ragged muscle fibers seen in CPEO and CPEO-plus diseases.

CPEO is a category of diseases characterized by mitochondrial dysfunction. Walsh and Hoyt,[27] together with contributing authors, state "it should be clear . . . that this is simply a clinical sign and does not, in and of itself, represent the nosologic entity." First categorized by von Graefe in 1868[70] as a neurogenic disorder, others such as Kiloh and Nevin[71] have maintained that CPEO is of myopathic origin. Drachman,[72,73] in 1968, united both schools through showing that patients with CPEO reveal a variety of neurologic and muscular abnormalities. He therefore classified the disease as a multisystem disorder and termed it CPEO-plus.[27,72] Drachman's description of CPEO-plus includes progressive limitation of ocular motility with clinical sparing of pupillary function, as seen with a variety of disorders.[27,72] Ptosis is usually the first sign of involvement and may precede ophthalmoparesis by months or years. The ptosis is characterized as bilateral, slow, and progressive, often becoming complete over time. Kearns-Sayre-Daroff syndrome is a clinical entity that was first described by Kearns and Sayre in 1958[74] as CPEO, retinitis pigmentosa, and complete heart block.[74]

The major ocular manifestations of CPEO-plus are childhood progressive external ophthalmoplegia and retinal pigmentary degeneration. Heart block, ragged-red muscle fibers, elevated cerebrospinal fluid protein, and marked vacuolization of the brain stem are among the systemic problems.

Therapy for CPEO and CPEO-plus disorders includes management of ptosis and strabismus and in some cases, pharmaceutical therapy. Although no pharmacologic relief is available for weak muscles, the administration of coenzyme Q-10 (a component of the mitochondrial transport system) has been shown to normalize pyruvate and lactate levels known to be abnormal in ragged-red muscle fibers as well as to improve atrioventricular block and ophthalmoplegia.[7] Patients suspected of having Kearns-Sayre-Daroff syndrome should be under the care of a cardiologist because swift neurologic and cardiac deterioration can occur.

Conditions Similar to Chronic External Ophthalmoplegia

Extraocular muscle paresis and ptotic lid position, the hallmark signs of CPEO, are almost always present for any lesion of the oculomotor nucleus, fasicle, or nerve. The subnucleus that serves levator function is a midline structure located at the caudal end of the oculomotor nuclear complex. Because of the proximity of structures, other signs often accompany ptosis with this etiology including exotropia, skew deviations, and pupillary dilation.[7,27]

Oculomotor nerve palsy and ptosis from involvement of the oculomotor fascicle or nerve are usually unilateral and associated with intracranial aneurysm, meningioma, expanding intracranial mass, or meningitis.[27] In oculomotor nerve palsy, the eye becomes fixed in a down and out position.[75,76] A patient with compression of the oculomotor nerve in the subarachnoid space by berry-type aneurysms of the posterior communicating artery (PCA) almost always presents with intractable headache, ptosis, mydriasis, and extraocular muscle paralysis.[77,78]

Good[77] reported a case of oculomotor palsy by compression of the PCA for which ptosis and headache alone were the only presenting signs. He advises that cases of isolated ptosis without pain are rarely compressive. However, the association of ipsilateral headache with acquired ptosis, as found in standard cases of cranial nerve III palsy, should alert one of the possibility of an intracranial aneurysm.[77] Prompt and careful follow-up with diagnostic testing is essential. Although CT scans and MRI are effective, angiography is the only definitive test for identifying this lesion.[76,77]

Ophthalmoplegic migraine can produce similar symptoms and even involve the pupil. Presentation, however, is usually repetitive, with an onset before the age of 10.[76,77] Ophthalmoplegic migraine has been reported in infants as young as 8 months of age.[76,77] Migraine, in such cases, is strictly a diagnosis of exclusion. Finally, in cases of acquired ptosis and painless cranial nerve III palsy, diabetes and myasthenia gravis should be appropriately ruled out.

The treatment for PCA aneurysm is referral to neurosurgery. The neurosurgeon will clip the neck of the aneurysm.[76] The prognosis for recovery is proportional to the entering deficit. Partial palsies almost always completely recover; more severe palsies tend to recover less.[76] Surgery within 10 days of diagnosis is crucial to prognosis.[76]

Miscellaneous Causes of Ptosis and Partial Ophthalmoparesis

Other miscellaneous causes of ptosis and partial ophthalmoparesis include neurogenic ptosis, apraxia of lid opening, postsurgical traumatic ptosis, blepharospasm, and lesions of cranial nerve VII.

Neurogenic ptosis is most commonly caused by involvement of the oculomotor nerve of oculosympathetic pathway. Many varied and complex mechanisms are causative.

Apraxia of lid opening is an interesting type of supranuclear insufficiency. Patients with this disorder have difficulty initiating eyelid opening because levator neurons are abnormally inhibited. The cause is thought to be consistent with extrapyramidal syndromes such as Parkinson's disease.

Postsurgical traumatic ptosis has several mechanisms. Most often occurring after blepharoplasty surgery, the levator complex may become damaged by way of deep dissection into the upper eyelid. Resultant ptosis can be caused by direct injury or as a secondary sequellae from edema and hematoma,[27,37] which weigh the eyelid down. This type of ptosis is often temporary and resolves as the swelling dissipates.

In general, these conditions should be included in the differential diagnoses for acquired ptosis, extraocular muscle paresis, and neuromuscular disease. Typically, they are treated by eliminating the underlying cause. When surgery is considered for the correction of ptosis, contraindications should be discussed at length, including the risks of diplopia, corneal exposure, and pseudoptosis by overcorrection. Ptosis crutches can be considered when surgical correction is either contraindicated or denied.

Blepharospasm. In the presence of bilateral, involuntary eyelid closure, the optometrist must evaluate the patient for elements of bilateral blepharospasm.[27,78] The most obvious cause of bilateral ocular blepharospasm is painful and irritative ocular disease and inflammation.[27,79] Bilateral uveitis, dry eye, foreign body (including chemicals) and keratitis are all commonly causative. Ocular forms of blepharospasm must be excluded before neurologic forms are considered.

Bilateral blepharospasm is a documented feature of both the postencephalitic and idiopathic forms of parkinsonism.[61,79] These patients demonstrate reflex eyelid spasms whenever their lids or brows are touched.[61] They must often simply wait for their lids to open or use a head thrust to catalyze opening, because mechanical attempts only facilitate additional spasms.[61]

Other documented causes of blepharospasm include stress; fatigue, Gilles de la Tourette's disease or Tourette syndrome; Huntington's chorea (fourth decade, muscle spasticity and mental fatigue); and idiopathic essential blepharospasm (no other associated neurologic findings).[61,79]

Essential blepharospasm is a bilateral condition characterized by spasmodic eyelid closure and accompanied face and tongue contortion. Occurring predominantly in women (75 percent), the onset is usually in the fourth decade of life. The condition often worsens in sunlight and in stressful environments. The condition may become so intense it will render patients functionally blind. These patients are often labeled as hypochondriacs or emotionally disturbed. When associated with dystonic facial movements (prolonged contracture), the disease is termed Meige syndrome.[27,61]

Lagophthalmus is the generic term for the inability to voluntarily close the eyelids. This may result in poor blink posture, sleeping with the eyes open, and an inferior superficial exposure keratitis. Lagophthalmus has many secondary causes, including orbital proptosis and lid scarring; the most severe and ominous cause is paralysis of cranial nerve VII.[7,79–81]

Common causes of cranial nerve VII palsies include poliomyelitis, measles, chicken pox, infectious mononucleosis, tuberculosis, and diphtheria.[78] Intracranial sarcoid and Hodgkin's disease are associated with intracranial complications, some involving cranial nerve VII, in approximately 5 percent of patients.[78] Melkenson syndrome (recurrent swelling of the face and lips that becomes chronic and results in scarring with paralysis) and trauma secondary to blows around the mastoid process should not be ignored.[78] In cases with no history of previous facial palsy, a vermiform or worm-like spastic paretic facial contracture may be observed.[61] This undulating contraction of the obicularis oculi and other facial muscles is known as pathologic myokymia.[61] This condition differs from benign myokymia in that it is usually secondary to pontine neoplasm, multiple sclerosis, or compression of the medulla by tumor.[61,82] This supranuclear lesion renders cranial nerve VII hyperexcitable, causing the pathoneumonic vermiform appearance.[82] The three major masqueraders of spastic paretic facial contracture are facial contracture as part of an aberrant regeneration syndrome of the facial nerve, spastic facial contracture associated with multiple sclerosis, and hemifacial spasm.[80]

Hemifacial spasm is characterized by unilateral, involuntary bursts of tonic activity within the muscles of facial expression. It usually occurs in young adults.[81] The episodes have no clear-cut precipitants and occur randomly, even in sleep.[61] Patients with this disorder typically present without signs of facial palsy or pathologic myokymia. Diagnosis is based on electromyographic studies.

Gardner and Sava[83] postulated that compression of cranial nerve VII, either by tumor or injury, produces increased neuroirritability and firing. The synkinesis is explained as a type of "domino" effect (ephatic transmission): impulses flowing in one direction set off similar neuronal firings in adjacent fibers, so that one set of neurons excites other sets of muscle groups as well as its own. Although cerebellopontine angle tumors and brain stem lesions have been described in association with hemofacial spasm, they are considered rare.[83] In most cases, the cause is believed to involve the compression of cranial nerve VII by a stiff and tortuous cerebral vessel, the anterior inferior cerebellar artery, or the posterior inferior cerebellar artery.[83]

In its early stages, hemifacial spasm may be confused with facial epilepsy. The diagnosis of focal epilepsy must be ruled out with electroencephalographic testing.[84] Best treated by a neurologist, some cases remit without treatment.

Hemifacial spasm may be treated aggressively with surgery (suboccipital craniotomy and the placement of a sponge between cranial nerve VII and the indenting vessel at the lower pons) or by administration of oral carbamazepine.[84] If resolution is incomplete, supportive therapy must be given. Artificial tear ointments, solutions, moisture chamber patches, and even tarsorraphy should be considered.[84]

Bell's Palsy. If the patient has no history of trauma, and biomicroscopic examination is negative, the diagnosis of facial weakness must be considered. The most common cause of acquired facial weakness is Bell's palsy. It usually affects young men (approximately 75 percent) with an incidence of 20 in 100,000.[85,86] It is described as a sudden loss of function as a result of unknown inflammatory processes in the vicinity of the petrous bone portion of the seventh cranial nerve.[86] The condition may reflect postviral demyelination secondary to herpes simplex virus infection; the onset of sarcoidosis; Paget's disease; and in patients 40 years or older, the onset of diabetes, which is found in 20 percent of these patients.[85] In the recovery phase of a lower motor neuron Bell's palsy, facial muscles on the involved side become slightly contracted. On attempted voluntary movement—the patient can be asked to smile—paresis will be apparent on the affected side.[84,85]

Depending on the proximity of the lesion, taste (anterior two-thirds of the tongue), salivary as well as lacrimal output, and occasionally auditory function are affected via the stapedus nerve, producing hyperacusis.[85] A typical Bell's palsy produces a pseudo-lid retraction, with the mouth pulled over and a loss of facial wrinkles on the involved side (Fig. 6-2).

Clinically, all patients with Bell's palsy should be assessed for tear production and corneal compromise by Schirmer tear test strips and sodium fluorescein staining. Corneal evaluation should be completed with attention to blink quality and rate. Symptoms may range from scratchiness and dry eye to epiphora from exposure and iridocyclitis.[86]

Treatment includes complete supportive therapy with lanolin-based ointments, copious tear solutions, moisture chamber patches (Guibora eye patch), or the taping the lid closed. When taste centers are involved, some optometrists prescribe oral steroids. Usually, Bell's palsy resolves without treatment, initial gains are seen after the sixth week. Delayed recovery is con-

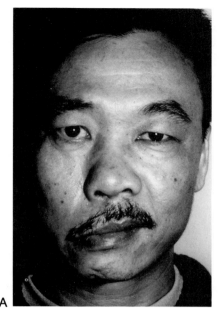
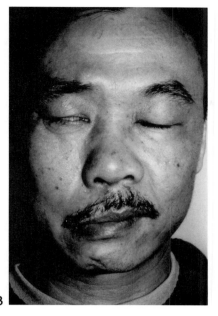
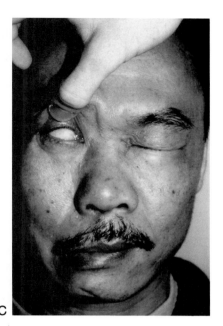

Fig. 6-2. (A–C) Bell's palsy with right facial and right orbicularis weakness.

sidered evident after 12 weeks and usually indicates that an incomplete recovery or anomalous reinnervation (jaw wink) is in process.[82,85]

Misdirection of the facial nerve occurs in approximately 25 percent of the cases of Bell's palsy that do not reach complete recovery. It is characterized by co-contraction of the facial muscles and obicularis oculi when stimulated by closure or movement of the mouth.[80] When associated with Bell's palsy, this is termed misdirection of the facial nerve. When noted congenitally, however, it is often termed Marcus Gunn jaw-wink phenomenon.

First described by Marcus Gunn[84] as maxillopalpebral synkinesis in 1883, the jaw-winking phenomenon represents anomalous innervation between the motor division of cranial nerve V (innervation to muscles and mastication) and the ipsilateral levator palpebrae-superioris.[84,87] The typical presentation includes lid elevation with opening of the mouth, jaw movement to the opposite side, and jaw movement to the same side. Atypical presentations exist and include elevation of the lid on protrusion of the jaw, protrusion of the tongue, swallowing, clenching of the teeth, and smiling.[88] Amblyopia, strabismus, and ptotic lid posture are the common clinical findings. The management of Marcus Gunn phenomenon requires aggres-

sive amblyopia therapy, strabismus correction, and the surgical correction of ptosis. Surgery should be considered only after patients reach an age at which they can discuss the risk/benefit ratios of repair.[84]

In addition, Mobius syndrome (frequent, congenital findings of bilateral cranial nerve VI and VII palsy), acquired thiamine deficiency, multiple sclerosis, lead poisoning, and hypertensive crisis with hemorrhage into the facial canal are potential causes of pseudoptosis secondary to involvement with cranial nerve VII. In each case, treatment of the underlying cause will usually be curative.

MULTIPLE SCLEROSIS

Multiple sclerosis is a chronic disease of unknown origin that causes demyelination and sclerosis of the central nervous system.[89,90] Predominantly, the disease occurs in young adults, with an onset between the ages of 20 and 40. Multiple sclerosis characteristically affects women more than men and increases in prevalence with each latitude further from the equator.[89]

Ocular symptoms occur commonly and are found in approximately 85 percent of patients diagnosed with multiple sclerosis.[91] Ocular findings include motility disturbances, disturbances of the pupillary light reflex,[90] optic or retrobulbar optic neuritis,[92] abnormalities in the visual-evoked potentials, myokimia, Sjögren syndrome,[93] and granulomatous uveitis.[89]

Patients presenting with retrobulbar optic neuritis automatically qualify for consideration of a diagnosis of multiple sclerosis. Typically, these patients have accompanying symptoms such as muscle weakness and Utoff sign (muscle weakness brought on by increases in body temperature, usually through exercise or immersion in hot water). In cases such as these, management is straightforward.

Occasionally, however, patients present with signs and symptoms not usually associated with multiple sclerosis. The differential diagnosis of granulomatous iridocyclitis typically includes sarcoidosis, toxoplasmosis, tuberculosis, lupus, syphilis, Fuchs' hederochromic iridocyclitis,[89] and Vogt-Koyanagi-Harada syndrome (a disorder of the uveal tract, retina, and meninges of autoimmune origin).[89,94] Lim and coworkers[89] clearly demonstrate that patients who test negatively for these diseases with conventional laboratory testing should be examined by MRI. When patients present with chronic recurrent granulomatous iridocyclitis of undetermined origin, multiple sclerosis should be considered and ruled out. Leys and associates[92] advocate early and continued monitoring of the visual-evoked potentials of patients suspected to have multiple sclerosis. They point out that patients who continue to have abnormal visual evoked potentials after the apparent resolution of optic neuritis are at a higher risk of developing multiple sclerosis.[92]

Sjögren syndrome is defined as dry eyes and/or dry mouth (keratoconjunctivitis sicca and xerostomia) and polyarticular arthritis. Ocular confirmation is usually accomplished through Schirmer tear testing, tear break-up time, and by observation of a visibly thin tear prism and corneal compromise on sodium fluorescein or Rose Bengal staining.

Elleman et al.[93] and others[95,96] have documented a high prevalence of central nervous system involvement in patients with Sjögren syndrome. The manifestations of Sjögren syndrome may be subtle and easily overlooked.[93] Patients with Sjögren syndrome should be tested for multiple sclerosis, and patients with multiple sclerosis should be monitored for Sjögren syndrome.

The systemic treatment of multiple sclerosis is best performed by the neurologist. Treatment for the optic neuropathies requires corticosteroid therapy and should be managed by the neuro-ophthalmologist. Treatment for uveitis is managed in the standard way using atropine 1 percent twice daily to achieve mydriasis and cycloplegia along with aggressive topical anti-inflammatory therapy such as Pred Forte every 2 hours to four times per day, as the circumstances merit. Sjögren syndrome is best managed with topical supportive therapies such as artificial tears and tear ointments.

MISCELLANEOUS FORMS OF NEUROMUSCULAR DYSFUNCTION

Traumatic myopathy is one of the more common causes of isolated extraocular muscle damage. When the injury is not associated with orbital fracture, oculomotor dysfunction may result from the intramuscular edema and hemorrhage.[27]

The term *Myositis* may be used for any disorder in which inflammation affects muscle tissue.[26] Inflammation confined to a single muscle or diffuse throughout the orbit has the potential for creating ptotic lid posture. Generally, inflammation of the orbit has two causes, idiopathic and infectious.[27] These entities are usually painful and result in ptosis from lid chemosis. One example of idiopathic myositis is the acquired form of Brown superior oblique tendon sheath syndrome; inflammation and scarring occur, either within the superior oblique or its tendon, causing restriction.

Ophthalmoplegia may result from muscle tumors and from the congestion of blood caused by carotid cavernous fistulas. Toxic and drug-induced myopathies can occur from exposure to snake venom, botulism, anticholinesterases, phenothiazines, and chloroquine.[27]

A number of disorders of uncertain pathogenesis have been noted in association with defects of neuromuscular transmission. These disorders include amyotrophic lateral sclerosis, poliomyelitis, and syringomyelia. Neuromuscular transmission deficits have been recorded in patients with peripheral neuropathies from various diseases including diabetes mellitus, alcoholism, malnutrition, and drug dependency.

REFERENCES

1. Ganong WF: Excitable tissue: nerve. p. 32. In: Review of Medical Physiology. 12th Ed. Lange, Los Altos, CA, 1983
2. Burgess C: Synaptic transmission. p. 47. In Brown AM, Stubbs DW (eds): Medical Physiology. John Wiley & Sons, New York, 1983
3. Ganong WF: Excitable tissue: muscle. p. 45. In: Review of Medical Physiology. 12th Ed. Lange, Los Altos, CA, 1983
4. Ganong WF: Synaptic and functional transmission. p. 62. In: Review of Medical Physiology. 12th Ed. Lange, Los Altos, CA, 1983
5. Baker RD, Moore LE: Skeletal Muscle. p. 69. In Brown AM, Stubbs DW (eds): Medical Physiology. John Wiley & Sons, New York, 1983
6. Miller NR: Topical diagnosis of lesions in the visual sensory pathway. p. 108. In: Walsh and Hoyt's Clinical Neuro-ophthalmology. Vol. 1. 4th Ed. Lea & Febiger, Philadelphia, 1985
7. Glaser JS, Bachynski B: Infranuclear disorders. p. 361. In Glaser JS (ed): Neuro-opthalmology. 2nd Ed. JB Lippincott, Philadelphia, 1990
8. Rodgin SG: Ocular and systemic myasthenia gravis. J Am Optom Assoc 61:384, 1990
9. Seybold ME, Lindstrom JM: Myasthenia gravis in infancy. Neurology 31:476, 1981
10. Manz F, Schmidt D: Diagnostik der okularen Myasthenie im Kindesalter. Klin Monatsbl Augenheilkd 157:173, 1970
11. Kansu T, Subutay N: Lid retraction in myasthenia gravis. J Clin Neuro-ophthalmol 7:145, 1987
12. Seybold ME: Myasthenia gravis: a clinical and basic science review. JAMA 250:2516, 1983
13. Oosterhuis HJ: The ocular signs and symptoms of myasthenia gravis. Doc Ophthalmol 52:363, 1982
14. Soliven BC, Lange DJ, Penn AS: Seronegative myasthenia gravis. Neurology 78:514, 1978
15. Drachman DB, Adams RN, Josifek LF, Self SG: Functional activities of autoantibodies to acetyolcholine receptors and the clinical severity of myasthenia gravis. N Engl J Med 307:769, 1982
16. Clemente CD: Gray's Anatomy. 13th Ed. Lea & Febiger, Philadelphia, 1985
17. Osserman KE: Ocular myasthenia gravis. Invest Ophthalmol 6:277, 1967
18. Grob D, Arsura EL, Brunner NG, Namba T: The course of myasthenia gravis and therapies affecting outcome. Ann NY Acad Sci 505:472, 1987
19. Bever CT, Abdias VA, Penn AS: Prognosis of ocular myasthenia. Ann Neurol 114:516, 1983
20. Gurwood A: The eyelid and neuro-ocular disease. p. 438. In Blaustein B (ed): Ocular Manifestations of Neurologic Disease. Vol. 4. JB Lippincott, Philadelphia, 1992
21. Martens EL, Awsink BJ: A myasthenia-like syndrome and polyneuropathy: complications of gentamicin therapy. Clin Neurol Neurosurg 81:241, 1979
22. Shaivitz SA: Timolol and myasthenia gravis. JAMA 242:1611, 1979
23. Acres TE: Ocular myasthenia gravis mimicking pseudo-internuclear ophthalmoplegia and variable esotropia. Am J Ophthalmol 88:319, 1979
24. Cogan DG: Myasthenia gravis: a review of the disease and description of lid twitch as a characteristic sign. Arch Ophthalmol 74:217, 1965
25. Sethl KD, Riuner MH, Swift TR: Icepack test for myasthenia gravis. Neurology 37:1383, 1987
26. Francis IC, Nicholson GA, Kappagoda MB: An evaluation of signs in ocular myasthenia gravis and correlation with acetylcholine receptor antibodies. Austral NZ J Ophthalmol 13:395, 1985
27. Miller NR: Myopathies and disorders of neuromuscular transmission. p. 785. In: Walsh and Hoyt's Clinical Neuro-ophthalmology. Vol. 2. 4th Ed. Lea & Febiger, Philadelphia, 1985
28. Katz JL, Lesser RL, Merikangas JR, Silerman JD: Ocular myasthenia gravis after D-penicillamine administration. Br J Ophthalmol 73:1015, 1989
29. Seybold ME, Daroff RD: The office tensilon test for ocular myasthenia gravis. Arch Neurol 43:842, 1986
30. Sergott RC, Glaser JS: Grave's ophthalmopathy: a clinical and immunologic review. Surv Ophthalmol 26:1, 1981
31. Molenaar PC, Newsom-Davis J, Polak RL, Vincent A: Eaton-Lambert syndrome: acetylcholine and choline acetyltransferase in skeletal muscle. Neurology 32:1061, 1982
32. O'Neill JH, Murray NMF, Newsom-Davis J: The Lambert-Eaton myasthenic syndrome. Brain 111:577, 1988
33. Vincent A, Newsom-Davis J, Martin V: Anti-acetylcholine receptor antibodies in D-penicillamine-associated myasthenia gravis. Lancet 1:1254, 1978
34. O'Keefe M, Morley KD, Haining WM, Smith A: Penicilline-induced ocular myasthenia gravis. Am J Ophthalmol 99:66, 1985
35. McQuillen MP, Cantor HE, O'Rourke JR: Myasthenic syndromes associated with antibiotics. Arch Neurol 18:402, 1969
36. McGarvey EJ: Thyroid eye disease: review and case reports. J Am Optom Assoc 61:689, 1990
37. Hamed LM, Lingua RW: Thyroid eye disease presenting after cataract surgery. J Pediatr Ophthalmol Strabis 24:10, 1990
38. Grove AS: The eyelids and lacrimal system. p. 47. In Pavan-Langston D (ed): Manual of Ocular Diagnosis and Therapy. 3rd Ed. Little, Brown, Boston, 1991
39. McKenzie JM: Humoral factors in the pathogenesis of Graves' disease. Physiol Rev 48:252, 1968
40. Wray SH: Neuro-ophthalmology: visual field, optic nerve and pupil. p. 327. In Pavan-Langston D (ed): Manual of Ocular Diagnosis and Therapy. 3rd Ed. Little, Brown, Boston, 1991
41. Rosenberg ML: The friction sweat test as a new method for detecting facial anhidrosis in patients with Horner's syndrome. Am J Ophthalmol 108:443, 1989
42. Kardon RH, Denison CE, Brown CK, Thompson S: Critical evaluation of the cocaine test in the diagnosis of Horner's syndrome. Arch Ophthalmol 108:384, 1990
43. Cremer SA, Thompson S, Digre KB, Kardon RH: Hydroxyamphetamine mydriasis in Horner's syndrome. Am J Ophthalmol 110:71, 1990
44. Haskes LP, Oshinskie LJ: Transient acquired ptosis. J Am Optom Assoc 60:668, 1989
45. Striph GG, Burde RM: Abducens nerve palsy and Horner's syndrome revisited. J Clin Neuro-ophthalmol 8:13, 1988
46. Glauser TA, Breynan P, Galetta SL: Reversible Horner's syndrome and Lyme disease. J Clin Neuro-ophthalmol 9:225, 1989
47. Bromfield EB, Slakter JS: Horner's syndrome in temporal arteritis. Arch Neurol 45:604, 1988
48. Guy JG, Day AL, Schatz NJ: Contralateral trochlear nerve paresis and ipsilateral Horner's syndrome. Am J Ophthalmol 107:73, 1989
49. Woodruff G, Buncic JR, Morin JD: Horner's syndrome in children. J Pediatr Ophthalmol Strabis 25:40, 1988
50. Coppeto JR: Superior oblique paresis and contralateral Horner's syndrome. Ann Ophthalmol 15:681, 1983
51. Glatt HJ, Putterman AM, Fett DR: Muller's muscle—conjunctival resection procedure in the treatment of ptosis in Horner's syndrome. Ophthalmic Surg 21:93, 1990
52. Howard R: A case of congenital defect of the muscular system (dystrophica muscularis congenita) and its association with congenital talipes equinovarus. Proc R Soc Med 1:157, 1908
53. Deffeminis RHA, Vincent D, Silva GE et al: [Pure congenital muscular dystrophy. Nosological location, incidence, clinical and development aspects and classification.] Acta Neurol Latinoam 18:20, 1972
54. Fukuyama Y, Kawazura M, Haruna H: A Peculiar form of con-

genital progressive muscular dystrophy: report of 15 cases. Paediatr Univ Tokyo 4:5, 1960

55. Kukuyama Y, Osawa M, Suzuki H: Congenital progressive muscular dystrophy of Fukuyama type—clinical genetic and pathological considerations. Brain Dev 3:1, 1981

56. McMenamin JB, Becker LE, Murphy EG: Fukuyama-type congenital muscular dystrophy. J Pediatr 101:580, 1982

57. Yoshioka M, Kuroki S, Kondo T: Ocular manifestations in Fukuyama-type congenital muscular dystrophy. Brain Dev 12:423, 1990

58. Tsutsumi A, Uchida Y, Osawa M, Fukuyama Y: Ocular findings in Fukuyama-type congenital muscular dystrophy. Brain Dev 11:413, 1989

59. Astrom KE, Adams RD: Myotonic disorders. p. 266. In Mastaglia FL, Walton J (eds): Skeletal Muscle Pathology. Churchill Livingstone, Edinburgh, 1982

60. Becker PE: Syndromes associated with myotonia: clinical-genetic classifications. In Rowland LP (ed): Pathogenesis of Human Muscular Dystrophies. Excerpta Medica, Amsterdam, Holland, 1977

61. Burde RM, Savino PJ, Trobe JD: Incomitant ocular misalignment. p. 247. In: Clinical Decisions in Neuro-ophthalmology. CV Mosby, St. Louis, 1985

62. von Norden GK, Thompson HS, Van Allen MW: Eye movements in myotonic dystrophy: an electro-oculographic study. Invest Ophthalmol 3:314, 1964

63. Walton JN, Natress FJ: On the classification, natural history and treatment of myopathies. Brain 77:169, 1974

64. Lessel S, Coppeto J, Samet S: Ophthalmoplegia in myotonic dystrophy. Am J Ophthalmol 71:1231, 1971

65. Vos TA: Twenty-five years of dystrophia myotonica. Ophthalmologica 141:37, 1961

66. Taylor EW: Progressive vagus-glossopharyngeal paralysis with ptosis: contribution to group of family diseases. J Ment Dis 42:129, 1915

67. Murphy SF, Drachman DB: The oculopharyngeal syndrome. JAMA 203:1003, 1968

68. Bray GM, Kaarsoo M, Ross RT: Ocular myopathy with dysphasia. Neurology 15:678, 1965

69. Johnson CC, Kuwabara T: Oculopharyngeal muscular dystrophy. Am J Ophthalmol 77:872, 1974

70. von Graefe A: Verhanolungen Arztucher Gesellschaften. Berlin Klin Wochenschr 5:125, 1868

71. Kiloh LG, Nevin S: Progressive dystrophy of external ocular muscles (ocular myopathy). Brain 74:115, 1951

72. Drachman DA: Ophthalmoplegia plus: the neurodegenerative disorders associated with progressive external ophthalmoplegia. Arch Neurol 18:654, 1968

73. Drachman DA: Progressive external ophthalmoplegia: a finding associated with neurodegenerative disorders. p. 124. In Smith JL (ed): Neuro-ophthalmology. Vol. 4. CV Mosby, St. Louis, 1968

74. Kearns TP, Sayre GP: Retinitis pigmentosa: external ophthalmoplegia and complete heart block. Arch Ophthalmol 60:280, 1958

75. Gottlob I, Cataland RA, Reinecke RD: Surgical management of oculomotor nerve palsy. Am J Ophthalmol 111:71, 1991

76. Kyriakides T, Aziz TZ, Torrens MJ: Post-operative recovery of third nerve palsy due to posterior communicating aneurysms. Br J Neurosurg 3:109, 1989

77. Good EF: Ptosis as the sole manifestation of compression of the oculomotor nerve by an aneurysm of the posterior communicating artery. J Clin Neuro-ophthalmol 10:59, 1990

78. Baker AB, Joynt RJ: Clinical Neurology: Disorders of the Brainstem and its Cranial Nerves. Vol. 3. Harper Collins, New York, 1988

79. Roy FH: Ocular Differential Diagnosis. 4th Ed. Lea & Febiger, Philadelphia, 1989

80. Smith JL: Neuro-ophthalmology Focus 1982: Spastic Facial Contracture. Vol. 22. Masson, New York, 1982

81. May M, Galetta S: The facial nerve and related disorders of the face. p. 239. In Glaser JS (ed): Neuro-ophthalmology. 2nd Ed. JB Lippincott, Philadelphia, 1990

82. Nunery WR, Cepala M: Levator function in the evaluation and management of blepharoptosis. Ophthalmol Clin North Am 4:1, 1991

83. Gardner WJ, Sava GA: Hemifacial spasm: a reversible pathophysiological state. J Neurosurg 19:240, 1962

84. Miller NR: Anatomy and physiology and abnormal eyelid position and movement. p. 932. In: Walsh and Hoyt's Clinical Neuro-ophthalmology. 4th Ed. Vol. 2. Lea & Febiger, Philadelphia, 1985

85. Norden LC: The eyelids. p. 279. In Barresi BJ (ed): Ocular Assessment: The Manual of Diagnosis for Office Practice. Butterworths, Boston, 1984

86. Wesley RE, Jackson CG, Tiepeken P, Glasscock M: Reconstruction of the eyelid after facial nerve paralysis. Ophthalmol Clin North Am 4:47, 1991

87. Gunn RM: Congenital ptosis with peculiar associated eye movements of the affected lid. Trans Ophthalmol Soc UK 3:283, 1883

88. Eve RF: Pterygoid-levator synkinesis: the Marcus Gunn jaw-winking phenomenon. J Clin Neuro-ophthalmol 7:61, 1987

89. Lim JI, Tessler HH, Goodwin JA: Anterior granulomatous uveitis in patients with multiple sclerosis. Ophthalmology 98:142, 1991

90. Van Diemen HAM, Van Dongen MMM, Nauta JJP et al: Pupillary light reflex latency in patients with multiple sclerosis. Electroencephalography and clinical neurophysiology 82:213, 1992

91. Poser CM, Alter M, Sibley WA, Scheinberg LC: Demyelinating diseases. p. 593. In Rowland EP (ed): Merritt's Textbook of Neurology. 7th Ed. Lea & Febiger, Philadelphia, 1984

92. Leys MMJ, Candaele CMJ, DeRouck AF, Odom JV: Detection of hidden visual loss in multiple sclerosis: a comparison of pattern-reversal visual evoked potentials and contrast sensitivity. Doc Ophthalmol 77:255, 1991

93. Ellemann K, Krogh E, Arlien-Soeborg P: Sjögren's syndrome in patients with multiple sclerosis. Acta Neurol Scand 84:68, 1991

94. Hedges TR: Consultation in Ophthalmology. C Decker, Toronto, 1987

95. Noseworthy JH, Bass BH, Vanderwoort MK et al: The prevalence of primary Sjögren's syndrome in a multiple sclerosis population. Ann Ophthalmol 25:95, 1989

96. Miro J, Peja-Sagredo JL, Berciano J et al: Prevalence of Sjögren's syndrome in patients with multiple sclerosis. Ann Neurol 27:582, 1990

7 Metabolic Disease

NICKY R. HOLDEMAN

INTRODUCTION

As optometry continues to expand its emphasis on primary care, the identification of patients with systemic disease is becoming increasingly important. Many disorders are widely prevalent and have well-known ocular manifestations (e.g., diabetes mellitus, hypertension, and thyroid abnormalities). In comparison, other diseases are relatively rare and have lesser known eye findings (e.g., a-β-lipoproteinemia, homocystinuria, and Wilson's disease). Although less common, these latter diseases are often treatable but if undetected may be associated with a high incidence of morbidity and early mortality. Consequently, health providers should have a basic understanding of meta-bolic diseases to ensure a prompt diagnosis, appropriate treatment, and comprehensive counseling.

This chapter focuses on representative diseases associated with disorders of amino acid metabolism, lipid metabolism, and mineral metabolism. Carbohydrate and collagen-vascular abnormalities are covered in separate chapters. In addition, this chapter is not intended to be encyclopedic. Only the more clinically relevant diseases in each category are discussed, whereas much rarer genetic disorders such as the liposomal storage abnormalities, the sphingolipidoses, the mucolipidoses, the urea cycle abnormalities, and the mucopolysaccharidoses have been intentionally excluded[1-5] (Table 7-1).

CASE REPORT

An 11-year-old Puerto Rican boy presented with a chief complaint of poor vision in both eyes since childhood. The history revealed that the parents had noted a nystagmus shortly after birth, but no action was taken at that time. The remainder of the ocular history was unremarkable. The patient's medical history disclosed an easy bruisability, an episode of prolonged bleeding following a routine dental procedure, and several reported instances of epistaxis, but none required medical intervention. The family stated that the child had no known systemic illnesses, no hospitalizations, and no major operations. The patient was not using any medications and had no evidence of drug allergies.

The family history indicated no consanguineous relationship between the father and mother. No immediate family members, including a younger brother, had any ocular or systemic diseases. Previous eye examinations of the parents had shown both to be healthy with normal fundi.

The social history was noncontributory, and a review of systems failed to elicit any additional symptoms. Specifically, no cardiorespiratory, gastrointestinal, or urologic problems were noted.

General inspection revealed an apparently healthy 11-year-old boy with dark hair but somewhat lighter cutaneous pigmentation than his mother (Fig. 7-1 and Plate 7-1). No petechiael hemorrhages were noted in the skin or the oral mucosa. A horizontal nystagmus was present, but the eyes appeared orthophoric by cover test. The patient's best corrected visual acuities were 20/200 OD, OS, and OU. Pupillary testing was normal, and no restrictions of ocular movement in the cardinal positions of gaze were noted. Biomicroscopy demonstrated moderately pigmented irides with transillumination defects and severe photophobia

(Fig. 7-2 and Plate 7-2). The remainder of the anterior segment as well as applanation tonometry were within normal limits. Ophthalmoscopy revealed an albinotic fundus with prominent choroidal vessels (Fig. 7-3 and Plate 7-3). The optic discs and retinal vessels were normal. Foveal hypoplasia was observed in both eyes, and no foveal reflex was elicited. Ancillary testing showed normal rod and cone function on the electroretinogram (ERG) and normal color discrimination by the D-15 panel. Stereoscopic vision was absent as assessed by the Titmus stereo fly test.

Laboratory studies including a complete blood count, platelet count, prothrombin time, and partial thromboplastin time were all within normal limits. The patient's bleeding time, however, was prolonged and was found to exceed 11 minutes (normal, 3 to 9.5 minutes).

Based on the examination and laboratory investigation, a diagnosis of Hermansky-Pudlak syndrome (HPS) was made. The patient was counseled about his condition and advised to abstain from contact sports and aspirin-containing compounds, which could initiate or exacerbate his hemostatic defect, respectively. The patient was instructed to avoid prolonged exposure to the sun and to wear dark glasses, opaque clothing, and high-index skin-protection factor sunscreens to reduce photophobia and the chances of actinic skin damage. The patient was referred to the low vision clinic for advice on various optical aids and to an internist for a complete physical examination, chest radiograph, and electrocardiogram—all of which were normal. To this point, no evidence indicates the presence of ceroid-like deposition in any organ system, which is part of the triad of HPS. With time, however, this substance likely will be detected and will adversely affect the function of the involved organs.

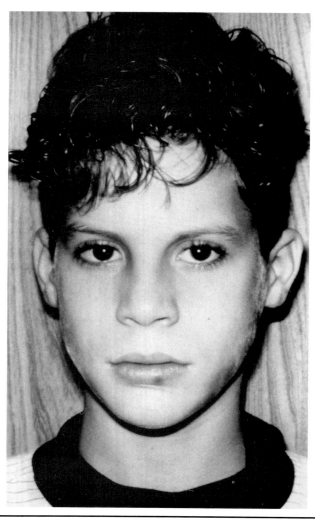

Fig. 7-1. Healthy 11-year-old boy with dark hair but somewhat lighter cutaneous pigmentation than his mother. (See also Plate 7-1.)

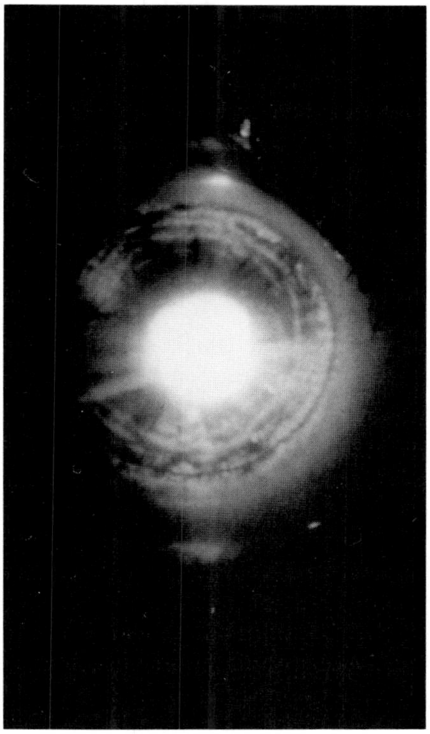

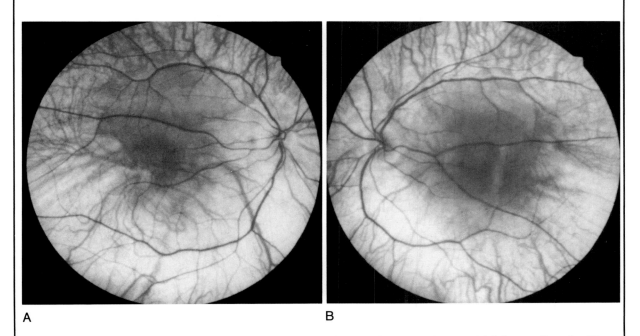

Fig. 7-2. Pigmented irides with transillumination defects and severe photophobia. (See also Plate 7-2.)

A   B

Fig. 7-3. Albinotic fundus with prominent choroidal vessels. **(A)** Right eye, **(B)** left eye. (See also Plate 7-3.)

Table 7-1. Metabolic Diseases

Disorder	Defect/Deficiency	Inheritance	Manifestations
Amino acid abnormalities			
Albinism	Tyrosinase	Recessive or X-linked	Light eyes, diaphanous irides, decreased visual acuity, nystagmus, strabismus, foveal hypoplasia, pale fundus, photophobia, generalized albinism, mesodermal dysgenesis, absence of stereovision, refractive errors
Homocystinuria	Cystathionine β-synthetase	Recessive	Ectopia lentis, secondary glaucoma, cystic degeneration of the retina, Marfanoid appearance, myopia, cardiovascular abnormalities, vascular thrombosis, mental retardation, cataract, optic atrophy, skeletal abnormalities
Cystinosis	Renal amino acid transport	Recessive	Late pigmentary retinopathy, proteinuria due to glomerulonephritis, nephrolithiasis, corneal and conjunctival crystals, maculopathy
Alkaptonuria	Homogentisic acid oxidase	Recessive	Brownish scleral deposits, discoloration of ear cartilage (ochronosis), osteoarthritis, black urine, valvular heart disease, atherosclerosis
Phenylketonuria	Phenylalanine hydroxylase	Recessive	Depigmentation of the iris, mental retardation, neurologic changes, eczema, partial albinism, seizures, blue sclera, corneal opacities, cataracts, macular atrophy
Gout	Uric acid metabolism disorder	Dominant	Hyperuricemia, recurrent acute arthritis, renal calculi, renal failure, conjunctivitis, episcleritis, scleritis, band keratopathy
Familial dysautonomia (Riley-Day syndrome)	Dopamine-β-hydroxylase	Recessive	Alacrimia, poor corneal sensation, corneal ulcers, exotropia, optic atrophy, failure to thrive, spontaneous fractures
Tyrosinemia	p-Hydroxyphenylpyruvic acid hydroxylase	Recessive	Hepatosplenomegaly, aminoaciduria, Fanconi syndrome, hepatic cirrhosis, hepatic failure
Histidinemia	Histidase (L-histidine ammonia lysase)	Recessive	Speech defect, retardation, neurologic manifestations, sometimes asymptomatic
Hyperprolinemia I	Proline oxidase	Recessive	Renal defects, retardation, sometimes asymptomatic
Hyperprolinemia II	δ-1-Pyrroline-5-carboxylic acid dehydrogenase	Recessive	No manifestations
Branched chain ketoaciduria	Branched chain keto-oxidase	Recessive	Episodic acidosis, vomiting, urine odor, retardation, neurologic changes
Hyperlysinemia	Lysine-ketogluterate reductase	Recessive	Ectopia lentis, spherophakia, muscle weakness, retardation
Hyperornithinemia	Ornithine keto acid transaminase		Gyrate atrophy of the retina and choroid
Hypophosphatasia	Alkaline phosphatase		Band keratopathy, proptosis, papilledema, skeletal abnormalities
Lowes syndrome	?	X-linked	Cataract, glaucoma, miosis, corneal dystrophy, retardation, hypotonia, renal abnormalities
	Sulfite oxidase deficiency		Ectopia lentis, optic atrophy
Tyrosinemia	Tyrosine aminotransferase	Recessive	Corneal ulcers
Maple syrup urine disease	Branched chain keto acid decarboxylase	Recessive	Hypertonicity, odor of urine and sweat, convulsions, coma, death
Valinemia	Valine aminotransferase	Recessive (?)	Retardation
Isovaleric acidemia	Isovaleryl CoA dehydrogenase	Recessive (?)	Vomiting, lethargy, acidosis, retardation, neonatal death
β-Hydroxyisovaleric aciduria	β-Methylcrotonyl-CoA carboxylase		Retardation, muscle atrophy, unpleasant urine odor
Methylacetoacetate accumulation	Acetyl-CoA thialase (?)		Acidosis, coma, retardation
Cystathioninemia	Cystathionase	Recessive (?)	Retardation (?) may be benign trait without symptoms

(Continued)

Table 7-1. *(Continued)*

Disorder	Defect/Deficiency	Inheritance	Manifestations
Glycinemia (nonketotic)	Glycine cleavage enzyme system		Convulsions, retardation
Methylmalonic acidemia	Methymalonyl-CoA mutase	(?)	Acidosis, lethargy, coma, mental and physical retardation
Propionic acidemia	Propionyl-CoA carboxylase	Recessive	Acidosis, lethargy, coma, mental and physical retardation
Hypersarcosinemia	Sarcosine dehydrogenase	Recessive	Mental retardation (?)
β-Alaninemia	β-Alanin-a-ketogluterate aminotransferase		Seizures, somnolence, death
Hyperprolinemia	Proline oxidase	Recessive	Hereditary nephritis, nerve deafness (?)
Hydroxyprolinemia	Hydroxyproline oxidase	Recessive	Mental retardation, central nervous system symptoms
Lysine intolerance	Lysine: NAD oxidoreductase		Vomiting, coma
Saccharopinuria	Aminoadipic semialdehydeglutamate reductase		Retardation
Glutamicacidemia	?		Mental and physical retardation, seizures, trichorrhexis nodosa
Pyroglutamic acidemia	?		Episodic vomiting, retardation
Lipid abnormalities			
Type I HLP	Chylomicronemia	Recessive	Lipemia retinalis, xanthomas, adult-onset Coat's disease, fat intolerance, lipid keratopathy, pancreatitis, hepatosplenomegaly
Type II HLP	Hyper-β-lipoproteinemia	Dominant	Xanthelasma, corneal arcus, accelerated atherosclerosis, tendon and tuberous xanthomas
Type III HLP	Abnormal β-lipoprotein, elevated triglycerides	Recessive	Xanthelasma, corneal arcus, lipemia retinalis, accelerated atherosclerosis, diabetes mellitus, planar xanthomas, tuboeruptive and tendon xanthomas
Type IV HLP	Hyperpre-β-lipoproteinemia, elevated triglycerides	Sporadic	Palpebral eruptive xanthomas, lipemia retinalis, glucose intolerance, hyperuricemia, hepatospenomegaly, possible accelerated atherosclerosis
Type V HLP	Hyperchylomicronemia, hyperpre-β-lipoproteinemia		Palpebral eruptive xanthomas, lipemia retinalis, retinal and choroidal xanthomas, pancreatitis, hepatosplenomegaly, sensory neuropathy, hyperuricemia, glucose intolerance
A-β-lipoproteinemia (Bassen-Kornzweig disease)	Reduction in plasma lipids Low vitamin A	Recessive	Pigmentary retinopathy, progressive ophthalmoplegia, acanthocytosis, anemia, malabsorption syndrome, ptosis, cataract, optic nerve pallor, muscle weakness, cardiac dysrhythmias, areflexia
Refsum's disease	Phytanic acid α-hydroxylase	Recessive	Pigmentary retinopathy, cataract, miosis, partial deafness, cerebellar ataxia, ichthyosis, ophthalmoplegia, glaucoma, neuropathy, cardiomyopathy
Lecithin cholesterol acyltransferase disease	Lecithin cholesterol acyltransferase		Corneal deposits, corneal arcus
Tangier disease	α-Lipoprotein	Recessive	Corneal stromal opacities
Mineral abnormalities			
Wilson's disease	Ceruloplasmin	Recessive	Cirrhosis, jaundice, splenomegaly, esophageal varices, ascites, spasticity, rigidity, dysarthria, tremors, Kayser-Fleischer ring, sunflower cataract, psychotic episodes
Hemochromatosis	Excessive intestinal absorption of ingested iron	Recessive (?)	Cirrhosis, diabetes mellitus, increased skin pigmentation, splenomegaly, congestive heart failure, arrhythmias, hyperpigmentation of eyelids and bulbar conjunctiva, conjunctival and retinal microaneurysms, slate-blue fundus

(Continued)

Table 7-1. *(Continued)*

Disorder	Defect/Deficiency	Inheritance	Manifestations
Lysosomal storage abnormalities			
Type II glycogenosis (Pompe's disease)	1,4-Glucosidase	Recessive	Myopathy, cardiomyopathy
GM₁ gangliosidosis (general gangliosidosis)	Acid β-galactosidase A, B, C	Recessive	Corneal clouding, cherry red macula, retinal hemorrhages, retardation, seizures, blindness, optic atrophy
Tay-Sachs disease (GM₂ gangliosidosis)	Hexosaminodase A	Recessive	Cherry red macula, optic atrophy, retardation, seizures
Sandhoff's disease	Hexosaminodase A, B	Recessive	Cherry red macula, optic atrophy (?)
Krabbe's disease	Galactocerebroside β-galactosidase	Recessive	Optic atrophy, cortical blindness, retardation, leukodystrophy
Metachromatic leukodystrophy	Arylsulfatase A	Recessive	Cherry red macula, optic atrophy, retardation, leukodystrophy, psychosis, variable corneal clouding
Niemann-Pick disease	Sphingomyelinase	Recessive	Cherry red macula, retardation, seizures, ataxia, hepatomegaly, optic atrophy (?)
Gaucher's disease	β-Glucocerebrosidase	Recessive	Pigmented pingueculas, strabismus, retardation, spasticity, ataxia, hypersplenism
Fabry's disease	Galactosidase A	X-linked recessive	Corneal whirl deposits, tortuous conjunctival and retinal vessels, painful neuropathy, cataracts, angiokeratomas, renal failure, giant telangiectasias
Aspartylglycosaminuria	Aspartylglycosamine amidase	Recessive	Mental retardation, lens opacity, short stature
Lactosyl ceramidosis	Lactosyl ceramide galactosyl hydrolase β-Galactosidase	Recessive	Optic atrophy, macular grayness or redness
Farber's disease	Ceramidase	Recessive	Gray macula
Mucopolysaccharidosis			
MPS IH (Hurler syndrome)	α-Iduronidase	Recessive	Corneal clouding, pigmentary retinopathy, mental retardation, cardiovascular lesions, bone lesions, stiff joints, coarse facies, optic atrophy, deafness, dwarfism, subnormal ERG
MPS IS (Scheie syndrome)	α-Iduronidase (partial)	Recessive	Same as MPS IH although may have normal intellect
MPS II (Hunter syndrome)	Iduronosulfate sulfatase	X-linked Recessive	Pigmentary retinopathy, corneal stromal opacity, mental retardation, bone lesions, dwarfism, retinal degeneration, optic atrophy, subnormal ERG
MPS IIIA (San Filippo syndrome A)	Heparin sulfate sulfatase	Recessive	Pigmentary retinopathy, mental retardation, optic atrophy, retinal vascular narrowing
MPS IIIB (San Filippo syndrome B)	N-acetyl-α-D-glucosaminidase	Recessive	Pigmentary retinopathy, mental retardation, optic atrophy
MPS IV (Marquio syndrome)	Excess production of keratosulfate	Recessive	Corneal clouding, skeletal dysplasia, optic atrophy
MPS VI (Maroteaux-Lamy syndrome)	Maroteaux-Lamy corrective factor	Recessive	Corneal clouding, skeletal dysplasia
MSP VII (Sly syndrome)	β-Glucuronidase	Recessive	None

(Continued)

Table 7-1. *(Continued)*

Disorder	Defect/Deficiency	Inheritance	Manifestations
Mucolipidoses			
Lipomucopoly-saccharidosis (MLS I)	?	Recessive	Corneal clouding, cherry red macula
Mucolipidosis type II	?β-Galactosidase + others?	Recessive	Corneal opacities, glaucoma(?)
Mucolipidosis type III	?	Recessive	Corneal opacities
Goldberg-Cotlier syndrome	β-Galactosidase	Recessive	Corneal clouding, cherry red macula
Sea blue histiocytic syndrome	?	Recessive	Macular grayness or cherry red spot
Mannosidosis	Mannosidase	Recessive	Macroglossia, flat nose, large head and ears, skeletal abnormalities, hepotosplenomegaly, storage material in retina
Urea cycle abnormalities			
Hyperammonemia I	Ornithine transcarbamylase	X-linked	Fatal in infancy, episodic NH_3 toxicity in heterozygotic adults, retardation, vomiting, lethargy
Hyperammonemia II	Carbamyl phosphate synthatase	Recessive	Fatal in infancy, NH_3 toxicity, vomiting, lethargy, seizures, coma
Citrullinemia	Argininosuccinate synthatase	Recessive	Variable retardation, seizures, NH_3 toxicity
Argininosuccinicaciduria	Argininosuccinase	Recessive	Variable retardation, seizures, NH_3 toxicity
Argininemia	Arginase	Recessive	Variable retardation, seizures, NH_3 toxicity, spasticity

Abbreviations: ERG, electroretinogram; CoA, coenzyme A; NAD, nicotinamide adenine dinucleotide; MPS, mucopolysaccharidosis; MLS, mucolipidosis.
(Data from Cahill,[1] Block and Henkind,[2] Ramsey et al.,[5] Fredrickson,[4] Berkow,[48] and Kelley and Limbeck.[49])

AMINO ACID METABOLISM DISORDERS

Albinism

Albinism describes a group of genetically inherited conditions caused by defective melanin production. The biosynthesis of melanin by melanocytes requires the oxidative enzyme tyrosinase. In albinism, the tyrosinase system appears to be defective. The disorder may be generalized, affecting the eyes, skin, and hair (oculocutaneous albinism), or localized, affecting primarily the eyes (ocular albinism). Oculocutaneous albinism may be tyrosinase-negative or tyrosinase-positive, depending on the ability of a hair bulb plucked from the patient and incubated in tyrosine solution to synthesize melanin.[6] This test may not prove accurate until a child is 3 to 5 years of age; thus, ascertaining the type of albinism when the patient is younger than age 3 may be difficult.[7]

Witkop recognizes 10 different types of oculocutaneous albinism (OCA) and 4 types of ocular albinism.[8] Of these, tyrosinase-positive OCA is the most common form of albinism with normal tyrosinase activity.

In general, the ocular manifestations are less severe than in tyrosinase-negative albinism; with age, tyrosinase-positive albinos may acquire pigmentation with the potential for improved vision.[9]

Tyrosinase-negative OCA is the classic form of albinism and is the second most common type.[6] The tyrosinase-negative groups develop no melanin, thus retaining both ocular and cutaneous hypopigmentation throughout life.[10] These individuals tend to have more severe visual disabilities, with a visual acuity of 20/200 or worse, marked nystagmus, and a 90 percent incidence of strabismus.[6]

The Case Report described a patient with HPS, which is the third most common type of albinism. HPS is a triad consisting of (1) tyrosinase-positive OCA, (2) a mild bleeding diathesis that is due to platelet dysfunction, and (3) ceroid storage disease.[11] Although HPS has been reported in many different nationalities, it occurs most commonly in Puerto Ricans.[6] As in other OCA disorders, HPS has an autosomal recessive pattern of inheritance. Pigmentation of the integument can range from nearly amelanotic, resembling tyrosinase-negative OCA, to nearly normal, as in our patient. Ocular manifestations include decreased visual acuity (average, 20/200), nystagmus, diaphanous iridis, albinotic fundus, and foveal hypoplasia.[9] The hemorrhagic diathesis seen in HPS is secondary to platelet dysfunction. Electron microscopy of platelets in these patients reveals a decreased number of "dense bodies." These dense bodies contain serotonin, adenine nucleotides, epinephrine, and calcium, which are important factors in platelet aggregation and hemostasis.[11] Clinically, patients with HPS often relate a history of easy bruisability, epistaxis, or prolonged bleeding following surgical procedures. Death may result from uncomplicated child birth, trauma, or peptic ulcer disease.[6] Laboratory studies typically reveal normal blood counts, platelet counts, prothrombin time, and partial thromboplastin time. Bleeding time is usually prolonged. HPS patients should avoid medications containing aspirin-type compounds and may require platelet transfusions before surgery.

A granular compound resembling ceroid lipofuscin has been observed to accumulate in the kidney, gastrointestinal tract, lung, bone marrow, liver, spleen, and heart.[6] Deposition of this material may result in pulmonary fibrosis, colitis, gingivitis, renal failure, and cardiomyopathy.

Another potentially fatal form of albinism is the Chédiak-Higashi syndrome (CHS). This disorder is characterized by tyrosinase positivity, susceptibility to infection, peripheral neuropathy, and giant peroxidase-positive lysosomal granules in leukocytes.[6] Consequently, when examining a child with albinism, questioning the family about bleeding disorders and immunodeficiency is important so that a suspect patient may be referred for a complete medical evaluation.

All forms of true albinism may have several common ocular characteristics. These features are listed in Table 7-2.[12] Many of the features cited in Table 7-2 are interrelated. For example, photophobia is secondary to the hypopigmentation of the uveal tract and retina. The reduction in visual acuity is attributable to photophobia, nystagmus, and foveal hypoplasia, which limits the improvement of acuity through refraction. The hypoplastic development of the fovea and decussation defects at the optic chiasm lead to the nystagmus and strabismus seen in albinism.[13] The absence of stereopsis is also related to the develop-

Table 7-2. Ocular Anomalies in Albinism

Decreased visual acuity
Photophobia with blepharospasm
High incidence of refractive errors
Congenital nystagmus
Iris translucency
Decreased retinal pigment
Foveal hypoplasia
Absence of stereo vision
Strabismus (mainly exotropia)
Axenfeld's anomaly
Mild protanopia

(Data from McHam and Fulton,[6] Haefemeyer and Kruth,[7] and Kritzinger and Wright.[12])

mental disorder of the nerve fiber pathways. In albinos, the axons from the central temporal retina, which normally remain ipsilateral, decussate at the chiasm and synapse in the contralateral lateral geniculate nucleus (Fig. 7-4). Consequently, because a maximum of 20 to 25 percent of axons remain uncrossed from each retina, as compared to 45 percent in normal persons, representation from the retina to the occipital cortex is aberrant. This misrouting anomaly precludes the development of stereovision.[6,7]

Albinism may also be associated with anterior segment dysgenesis of the Axenfeld type and minor color vision abnormalities.[6] Axenfeld's anomaly is the combination of posterior embryotoxin with iridocorneal adhesions to or beyond Schwalbe's line. Progression to glaucoma has been observed in some patients with this disorder (Axenfeld's syndrome). Advanced color vision testing may elicit a mild protan defect in a significant number of albinistic patients.

It is important to make the diagnosis of albinism as early as possible and to openly discuss the features and prognosis of the disorder with the patient and parents. The family should be informed that there is no cure but that individuals with this disorder can live a fairly normal life with appropriate support.

The vision specialist should provide tinted lenses to relieve glare intolerance and various low-vision aids, in conjunction with the patient's best visual correction, to allow sufficient vision for daily activities. Gonioscopy must be performed to disclose any abnormalities of the anterior segment, and color vision testing should be conducted to detect chromatic defects. A dermatologist can provide instruction on skin protection and regular examinations for cutaneous disorders

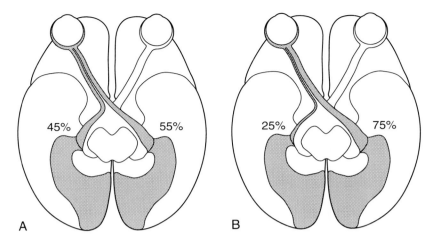

Fig. 7-4. In albinism, the axons from the central temporal retina decussate at the chiasm and synapse in the contralateral lateral geniculate nucleus. **(A)** Normal. **(B)** Albinism.

and malignancies. The albinotic patient should receive a complete history and physical to detect any associated conditions such as a hemorrhagic diathesis (HPS) or immunodeficiency (CHS). Finally, the patient and family should receive genetic counseling, and any misconceptions about the disorder should be alleviated. Some patients may require or benefit from social and psychological counseling as well. Professionals may also assist their patients with albinism by directing these individuals to support groups such as the National Organization of Albinism and Hypopigmentation (NOAH) for additional information and resources.

Homocystinuria

Homocystinuria is an autosomal recessive disorder and is the second most common inborn error of metabolism. Homocystinuria is due to a deficiency in cystathionine β-synthetase resulting in an increased concentration of homocystine and its dietary precursor, methionine, in blood and other body fluids.[14] Ectopia lentis is the most notable eye finding. The patient with untreated homocystinuria, however, is typically asymptomatic in infancy but subsequently develops mental retardation, skeletal disorders, and thromboembolism in addition to numerous ocular complications.[15] The abnormal lens zonules responsible for the ectopia lentis are part of a widespread systemic defect of connective tissue. The increased levels of homocystine inhibits cross-linkage in collagen and elastic tissue, thus predisposing these individuals to lens zonule degeneration and skeletal abnormalities such as

scoliosis, arachnodactyly, and pectus excavatum. The skeletal manifestations often make differentiation from Marfan syndrome difficult.[16] The diagnosis of homocystinuria is established by amino acid electrophoresis and chromatography of urine and plasma.[2]

Patients with homocystinuria are also susceptible to thromboembolic episodes involving both arteries and veins. Consequently, these patients are subject to premature deaths from myocardial infarctions, pulmonary emboli, and cerebrovascular accidents.[2] Thromboembolic disease has also resulted in central retinal artery occlusions leading to severe visual impairment.[17,18] Other ocular features of this disorder include microcystic peripheral retinal degeneration, secondary pupillary block glaucoma, retinal detachment, myopia, cataract, strabismus, optic atrophy, spherophakia, iris atrophy, uveitis, and keratitis.[10,12,15,17] Surgeons must be aware that affected patients experience a greater incidence of postoperative thromboembolism with general anesthesia; surgical procedures therefore are best performed under local anesthesia, if possible.[2,16]

Homocystinuria is one of the few metabolic disorders for which therapy is available. The risk of ocular complications seems to be substantially reduced in patients administered pyridoxine (vitamin B_6) in combination with dietary restriction of methionine within 6 weeks of birth.[2,16] Data indicate, however, that ocular changes continue to progress despite biochemical control in late-detected cases.[16]

Cystinosis

Cystinosis is a rare inborn error of amino acid metabolism with autosomal recessive inheritance, occurring in three clinical forms, infantile, adolescent, and adult, all of which have some ocular involvement.[2,10] The enzymatic defect is unknown, but the biochemical pathology is characterized by the intracellular accumulation of free cystine crystals within the lysosomes of all tissues, especially the liver, spleen, bone marrow, kidneys, and eyes.[19] The most severe type of cystinosis is the infantile or nephropathic form. Infantile cystinosis is characterized by Fanconi syndrome with growth failure, renal rickets, metabolic acidosis, and progressive renal failure requiring renal transplantation by 10 to 13 years of age.[20] Ocular features of nephropathic cystinosis include tinsel-like crystals in the conjunctiva, cornea, sclera, iris, ciliary body, and lens. A dense deposition of these cystine crystals may result in photophobia, pupillary block glaucoma, posterior synechia, and decreased visual function.[2,15,20] A retinopathy consisting of retinal pigment epithelial mottling and peripheral depigmentation is nearly universal in patients with infantile cystinosis.[20] The milder variants of the disease, "adolescent" and "benign adult" cystinosis, both have deposition of crystals in the conjunctiva and cornea, yet the fundi seem free of abnormalities. Of all the ocular findings, the pigmentary retinopathy may be responsible for the degradation of visual functioning.[21]

Although the retinopathy associated with cystinosis is irreversible, treatment of the renal and corneal complications is possible. Cysteamine, an agent capable of depleting cystine from body tissues, has been used orally to improve renal function and delay renal failure.[22] Unfortunately, systemic administration of cysteamine has not demonstrated an effect on crystalline deposits in the cornea.[19] Topical 0.5 percent cysteamine drops instilled hourly during waking hours, however, apparently has no significant ocular toxicity and may yield excellent clearance of corneal crystals even in severely affected individuals.[23] Compliance is a well-recognized problem with this medication as frequent and chronic instillations are necessary, and topical cysteamine is a malodorous, foul-tasting substance.[20] Corneal transplantation has been employed for intractable symptoms, yet crystals may again accumulate in the graft as early as 6 weeks after keratoplasty.[24]

Alkaptonuria

Alkaptonuria is a rare autosomal recessive disorder caused by a deficiency of the enzyme homogentisic acid oxidase. This enzyme deficiency results in defective tyrosine metabolism and the accumulation of homogentisic acid in tissues and urine.[10] The elevated levels of homogentisic acid in the urine with oxidation results in a dark brown-black color, and the initial diagnosis may result from observation of discolored urine.[25] Homogentisic acid that is not excreted in the urine will polymerize to form a black pigment deposited in cartilage and other connective tissues.[26] Visible pigmentary deposition may occur in the face, nose, ears, and eyes and is referred to as *ochronosis*. Ochronotic changes in the eye affect both sexes and tend to occur most commonly in the sclera near the insertion of the horizontal rectus muscles.[10] Scleral pigmentation secondary to alkaptonuria must be differentiated from an age-related hyaline plaque, choroidal melanoma, nevi, melanosis, and foreign body.[27] To aid in the diagnosis, one should consider the clinical triad of (1) black urine with increased levels of homogentisic acid, (2) ochronosis, and (3) degenerative arthritis.[25] Most of these patient's will experience deterioration of articular cartilage involving the intervertebral discs, knees, shoulders, and hips, which can be visualized radiographically.[26]

Unfortunately, no specific treatment is available for alkaptonuria. The onset of the disease is in the first few days of life, and pigmentation tends to slowly progress with time. In addition to extensive osteoarthritis, these patients may experience valvular heart disease and atherosclerosis, which may all lead to early morbidity and mortality.[9]

Phenylketonuria

Phenylketonuria (PKU) is the most common inborn error of amino acid metabolism,[2] characterized by a diminished activity of the enzyme phenylalanine hydroxylase and thus an elevation of plasma phenylalanine. The symptoms of hyperphenylalaninemia are usually absent in the newborn, but ultimately result in a blonde, blue-eyed child with light complexion, eczema, and mental retardation. Seizures and behavioral problems frequently result. These children often manifest a "mousy" odor, which is caused by phenylacetic acid in the urine and sweat.[28] Because of the severe consequences and relative prevalence of this disorder, programs designed for early detection of high plasma phenylalanine levels are now conducted in most newborn nurseries.[28] Fortunately, the eye care specialist is not likely to encounter a patient with undiagnosed phenylketonuria. In undetected PKU, the ocular findings may include a blue sclera, photophobia, corneal opacities, cataracts, partial ocular albinism, and macular atrophy.[9]

The effects of PKU are prevented through early identification and treatment. Therapy is aimed at limiting the phenylalanine intake of the child so that essential amino acid requirements are met but not exceeded. This approach allows normal growth and development but prevents accumulation of phenylalanine and its abnormal end products. Dietary restrictions will not reverse or improve existing mental retardation but if instituted before age 2 months, the child has a significant chance of attaining normal intelligence.[28] Blood phenylalanine levels must be monitored regularly to ensure that plasma levels are kept within a tight range (3 to 10 mg/dl). Opinion differs as to when phenylalanine restriction can be safely discontinued. Some believe that the diet should be maintained for life; others believe that food restraints may be terminated when myelinization of the brain is virtually complete, at about 5 to 6 years of age.[29] Certain foods containing phenylalanine (i.e., NutraSweet brand sweetner) provide disclosure to phenylketonurics regarding the ingredients of their products.

Gout

Gout is a disorder of uric acid metabolism, and its prevalence is closely linked to the serum concentration of uric acid. Classically, hyperuricemia and gout has been separated into primary and secondary disease. Primary disease is attributable to a genetic abnormality of purine metabolism.[30] The secondary form can result from increased cellular turnover, as seen in patients with psoriasis or myeloproliferative disorders or from decreased renal excretion of uric acid.[9]

Overt gout is manifested clinically by recurrent episodes of exquisitely painful monoarthritic attacks. Any joint may be affected, but the most common initial site of involvement is the first metatarsophalangeal joint (podagra). Recurrent attacks may also involve the ankle, heel, knee, fingers, and wrists.[2] Within hours of onset, the involved joint becomes inflamed, swollen, warm, and tender and may be mistaken for cellulitis or septic arthritis.

The ocular complications of gout are infrequent but may occur simultaneously with an acute attack of gouty arthritis. Conditions such as conjunctivitis, scleritis, episcleritis, uveitis, band keratopathy, and ocular motor disturbances have all been reported.[9,10]

Gout is inherited by an autosomal dominant mode, and there is a male preponderance of 20:1.[2] The complications of chronic disease include bony erosions with joint deformities, renal failure, and the deposition of tophi in locations such as the pinna of the ear, myocardium, pericardium, aortic valves, and extradural spinal regions. In addition, several associated conditions frequently seen in gouty patients include hypertension, diabetes mellitus, obesity, and hypertriglyceridemia, all of which contribute to a high incidence of cardiovascular disease.[30]

Treatment of a patient with gout is directed toward both the acute and chronic phases of the disease. Acute gouty arthritis is typically treated with nonsteroidal anti-inflammatory agents. Colchicine may also be used for acute episodes but is not the drug of choice because of its frequent gastrointestinal side effects. When the distinction between septic and gouty arthritis is not firmly established, however, treatment with colchicine is frequently helpful because it will not mask the periarticular inflammation of joint sepsis. For chronic gout, overproducers of uric acid are treated with allopurinol, which blocks the enzymatic conversion of soluble xanthine to insoluble urate. Underexcreters of uric acid may be treated with uricosurics such as probenecid or sulfinpyrazone, which block the renal tubular reabsorption of urate.[30] In the absence of clinical findings, asymptomatic hyperuricemia need not be treated unless the risk of incipient gout or nephropathy is high.

LIPID METABOLISM DISORDERS

Hyperlipoproteinemias

Interest in plasma lipids stems from their strong relationship to atherosclerosis. Because the complications of atherosclerotic disease can be reduced, health care providers should be knowledgeable of the diagnosis, manifestations, and treatment of the major abnormalities of lipoprotein metabolism.

In 1967, Fredrickson et al.[31] classified the hyperlipoproteinemias into five types, based on the elevation of specific lipids and lipoproteins. This section uses

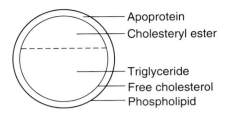

Fig. 7-5. Lipoprotein composition.

the Fredrickson classification scheme to discuss each phenotype, all of which show ocular abnormalities. The Fredrickson system, however, does not reflect pathophysiologic mechanisms responsible for the lipid elevations. Furthermore, this system was constructed before it was known that the level of high-density lipoproteins is inversely associated with cardiovascular risk. Consequently, the term *dyslipoproteinemias* is now preferred over the term *hyperlipoproteinemias,* because the former is more descriptive of either high or low lipoprotein levels.[32]

The principle circulating lipids in humans are (1) triglycerides, (2) free cholesterol, (3) cholesteryl esters, and (4) phospholipids. The plasma lipids do not circulate free but rather are transported from sites of absorption and synthesis to sites of use as spheric macromolecular complexes, termed *lipoproteins.* The lipoproteins have an inner core of hydrophobic lipids (triglycerides and cholesteryl esters) and are encased by a membrane composed of various apoproteins and hydrophilic lipids (free cholesterol and phospholipids)[32] (Fig. 7-5).

The major lipoproteins are (1) chylomicrons, (2) very low-density (pre-β) lipoproteins (VLDLs), (3) intermediate-density (slow pre-β) lipoproteins (IDLs), (4) low-density (β) lipoproteins (LDLs), and (5) high-density (α) lipoproteins (HDLs). The plasma lipoproteins are isolated and identified by either ultracentrifugation or electrophoresis. In addition to differences in density and electrophoretic mobility, lipoproteins also vary in size and by lipid and apoprotein composition.[2]

An excess or deficiency of certain lipoproteins constitutes a dyslipoproteinemia and can result from a primary genetic disorder or may be secondary to an acquired metabolic dysfunction. Secondary causes of lipoprotein disorders include diabetes mellitus, hypothyroidism, obesity, anorexia nervosa, pregnancy, acute myocardial infarction, nephrotic syndrome, renal failure, primary biliary cirrhosis, smoking, alcohol intake, stroke, hypertension, infections, and various drugs.[32,33] A primary disorder should be suspected if there is a strong family history of atherosclerotic disease or lipid abnormalities. Family screening often leads to identification of other (possibly asymptomatic) hyperlipoproteinemic subjects.

If measurement of lipoprotein levels is to be useful, one must be aware of the following[33]:

1. The concentrations of lipids and lipoproteins increase with age. A normal value in one age group may be quite abnormal for another.
2. Fasting for 12 to 16 hours is desired before a test specimen is collected, especially for triglyceride assays.
3. Lipoprotein concentrations are under dynamic metabolic control and are readily affected by diet, illness, drugs, posture, and weight changes as well as other secondary conditions as listed above.
4. If an abnormal measurement is obtained, confirmatory measurements should be obtained before selecting therapy.
5. When dyslipoproteinemias are due to a secondary cause, treatment of the underlying disorder will usually help correct the abnormality.

An increase in one or more of the lipoproteins forms the basis for classifying the five clinical types of primary hyperlipoproteinemias (HLPs). These "types" should not necessarily be considered disease entities but are useful for discussing the clinical manifestations and for determining a rational treatment plan.

Type I

Type I HLP (hyperchylomicronemia) is a rare autosomal recessive condition characterized by massive chylomicronemia when a patient is eating a normal diet, with disappearance of the chylomicrons a few days after fat is eliminated from the diet. The underlying defect of this disorder appears to be due to a congenital deficiency of lipoprotein lipase, which controls the catabolism of glycerides. Chylomicrons are particularly rich in triglycerides, and lipemia retinalis may be seen when serum triglycerides exceed 2500 mg/dl. Because cholesterol accounts for as much as 10 percent of the weight of chylomicron particles, the patient's serum cholesterol may also be elevated. At this time, however, no evidence shows that this form of HLP predisposes to atherosclerosis.

Pancreatitis is the major hazard, with bouts of abdominal pain recurring during periods of fat indulgence.

Pancreatic lipase is suspected to act on triglycerides in pancreatic capillaries, resulting in the formation of toxic fatty acids that cause inflammation. Avoidance of dietary fat will prevent serious sequelae.[32]

Besides pancreatitis, the major clinical features are hepatosplenomegaly, eruptive xanthomas, and fat intolerance. Ocular signs include lipemia retinalis, adult-onset Coat's disease, lipid keratopathy, and rarely palpebral, iris, and retinal xanthomas.[2,9,10]

Type II

Type II HLP (hyperbetalipoproteinemia) is the most common hyperlipoproteinemia resulting from defective LDL cell receptors, thus interfering with the clearance of β-lipoproteins. This disorder is transmitted in an autosomal dominant fashion. Serum cholesterol (LDL) may be as much as two to three times higher than normal, while triglyceride levels are within normal limits.

Systemic manifestations include an accelerated atherosclerosis, early myocardial infarction, and the presence of tendon xanthomas. Ocular signs show xanthelasma; retinal, choroidal, and conjunctival xanthomas; lipid keratopathy; and corneal arcus.[2,9,10]

Treatment is directed at lowering cholesterol by dietary and medicational means. Oral administration of bile acid sequestrants or nicotinic acid, or both, is often employed in this condition.[32]

Type III

Type III HLP (dysbetalipoproteinemia) is a rare disorder resulting from the absence of the apoprotein E-3, causing an accumulation of IDL remnants. Blood chemistry analysis reveals an excess of both triglycerides and cholesterol. This is a recessively inherited disorder occurring predominately in early adulthood in males but later in females, because estrogens seem to reduce accumulation of the "remnant" particles. These patients are often obese and may show a mild glucose intolerance and hyperuricemia. Clinical symptoms include planar (palmer) xanthomas, premature artherosclerosis, and peripheral vascular disease. Ocular signs are xanthelasmas, xanthomas of the lids, corneal arcus, lipemia retinalis, and crystalline corneal dystrophy.[2,9,10]

Treatment to lower both cholesterol and triglycerides may be particularly gratifying in type III disease. Di-

etary measures aimed at weight reduction and restriction of dietary cholesterol may produce marked improvement. The addition of clofibrate or niacin usually normalizes the blood lipid levels.

Type IV

The pre-beta lipoproteins are excessive in type IV HLP (hyperprebetalipoproteinemia), which is of uncertain genetic pattern. It is a common condition, characterized by variable elevations in serum triglycerides and often associated with caloric excess, obesity, hyperuricemia, stress, alcoholism, mildly abnormal glucose tolerance, and dietary indiscretion. This lipemia may be associated with premature coronary artery disease. Ocular findings include lipemia retinalis and palpebral xanthomas. Treatment is directed at weight reduction in the obese by avoiding high carbohydrate, fat, or alcohol intake, and caloric excess. Niacin and clofibrate may further reduce the lipemia in certain cases.[2,9,10]

Type V

Type V HLP (mixed hyperlipidemia) is a rare disorder characterized by excessive pre-β-lipoproteins and chylomicrons. Onset is usually in early adult life, and the clinical manifestations are a combination of those found in types I and IV (i.e., recurrent abdominal pain, pancreatitis, hepatosplenomegaly, eruptive xanthomas, and glucose intolerance). Like type I, this HLP shows little predilection to atherosclerosis. This disorder is aggravated by increased amounts of dietary fat and by alcohol excess. The ocular findings consist of lipemia retinalis, palpebral xanthomas, and rarely retinal and choroidal xanthomas. Therapy is similar to that for type IV, except that fat restriction is especially necessary, as in type I.[2,9,10]

Recently, several investigators have noted correlations between plasma lipid levels and diabetic retinopathy. From a small patient sample, Dodson and Gibson[34] concluded that hyperlipidemia and hypertension may be associated with the development of exudative maculopathy in diabetics. In a similar pilot study, Gordon et al.[35] found that aggressive therapy to lower plasma lipids in diabetic patients with hyperlipidemia resulted in an improvement in background retinopathy. Six of six patients had a documented improvement in hard exudates, while four of six showed a decrease in microraneurysms.

By contrast, Orlin et al.[36] did not find arteriolarsclerotic changes in the retinal arterioles of patients with hyperlipidemia when compared with normal control patients. The presence of hyperlipidemia without concomitant risk factors such as hypertension or advanced age apparently does not increase the chances of retinal arteriolar changes. Although examining the retina may not be helpful in detecting many hyperlipidemic states, eye care specialists should encourage diabetic patients to seek control of concurrent conditions (e.g., elevated lipoproteins, hypertension, etc.) as well as blood glucose levels, to reduce both ocular and systemic complications.

A-β-lipoproteinemia

A-β-lipoproteinemia (Bassen-Kornzweig syndrome) is a rare congenital disorder transmitted as a recessive trait and results from an inability to synthesize apolipoprotein B. In a-β-lipoproteinemia, LDL (β-lipoprotein) is absent, as are VLDL and chylomicrons.[2] Absorption of fats is markedly impaired, and the first obvious abnormalities are usually steatorrhea and abdominal distention during infancy. Alterations in membrane function secondary to the metabolic lipid abnormality leads to demyelination of nerves and results in the development of sensory ataxia between the ages of 5 and 10.[37] An atypical retinitis pigmentosa ensues as the primary ocular finding, although lens opacities, choroiditis, ophthalmoplegia, ptosis, nystagmus, optic nerve pallor, macular degeneration, dyschromatopsia, and angoid streaks have also been reported.[2,9,12,38,39]

A-β-lipoproteinemia should be considered in a patient who manifests a mild malabsorption in association with retinal degeneration and neurologic dysfunction. A diagnosis may be confirmed by examination of a blood smear to detect acanthocytes (erythrocytes with spiny projections of the membrane) and electrophoretic or ultracentrifugal studies to detect lipid abnormalities. By early adulthood, most patients have a decreased visual acuity, field defects, and night blindness. Both the ERG and dark adaptometry reveal diminished rod function.[2,39] Treatment is mainly empiric, although the administration of fat-soluble vitamins, especially vitamins E and A, may stabilize the neurologic manifestations and help prevent visual loss from the retinopathy.[40,41]

Refsum's Disease

Refsum's disease is a rare autosomal recessive disorder of lipid metabolism associated with marked accumulation of phytanic acid in the plasma and tissues, especially the liver, kidneys, heart, and central nervous system. The onset is usually between 4 and 7 years of age and is due to the absence or deficiency of phytanic acid hydroxylase, an enzyme needed for the metabolism of phytanic acid.[2,9] Typically insidious, yet progressive, systemic manifestations are present, including cerebellar ataxia, peripheral neuropathy, deafness, central nervous system degeneration, ichthyosis, wasting of extremities, and complete heart block.[2,9,12] Death is usually secondary to cardiac failure or respiratory paralysis.

Ocular findings include miosis, nystagmus, retinitis pigmentosa, cataracts, optic atrophy, ophthalmoplegia, ptosis, glaucoma, and corneal opacities.[2,9,10,12,42]

A-β-lipoproteinemia and Refsum's disease are two metabolic disorders in which retinitis pigmentosa is a major ocular manifestation. If a pigmentary retinopathy is detected, however, the optometrist should be aware that numerous entities may be associated with this particular retinal finding. Table 7-3 lists several diseases and syndromes that may show retinal pigmentary-like changes in addition to other ocular and systemic manifestations.[43,44] Consequently, if one were to detect retinal pigment epithelium disturbances, a comprehensive eye examination and medical referral may both be appropriate.

Table 7-3. Diseases and Syndromes Associated With Pigmentary Retinopathy

A-β-lipoproteinemia
Alström syndrome
Bardet-Biedl syndrome
Batten-Mayou disease
Cockayne syndrome
Dialinas-Amalric syndrome
Frenkel syndrome
Friedreich's disease
Hallgren syndrome
Hunter syndrome MPS II
Kearns-Sayre syndrome
Laurence-Moon-Bardet-Biedel syndrome
Ophthalmoplegic-retinal degeneration
Refsum's disease
Sanfillippo syndrome (MPS III)
Sjögren-Larssen syndrome
Syphilis
Usher syndrome

(Data from Coles[43] and Geeraets.[44])

MINERAL METABOLISM DISORDERS

Wilson's Disease

Wilson's disease (hepatolenticular degeneration) is an autosomal recessive inherited error of copper metabolism. The excretion of copper into bile appears to be defective in Wilson's disease, leading to an accumulation of excess copper, especially in the erythrocytes, liver, kidney, brain, and eyes. Symptoms generally appear in late childhood and by 10 to 15 years of age, most affected individuals have experienced symptoms that are due to either neurologic or hepatic disease.[2,45] Hepatic dysfunction is usually manifested by cirrhosis, jaundice, splenomegaly, esophageal varices, spider nevi, and ascites. When hepatic copper-binding sites are saturated, copper is released from the liver and incorporated into erythrocytes, which may produce an associated hemolytic anemia. Neurologic symptoms include tremors, spasticity, rigidity, gait disturbances, dysarthria, and personality changes. In addition to the liver, copper is typically concentrated in the lenticular nucleus of the basal ganglia, thus the term *hepatolenticular degeneration*.

The pathognomonic clinical feature of Wilson's disease is the Kayser-Fleisher ring, a thin green-brown crescent of pigmentation just inside the corneal limbus. This ring consists of copper granules in Descemet's membrane and is found in all cases with neurologic involvement.[45] Copper granules may also deposit on the lens capsule, producing the classic "sunflower cataract" similar to the lenticular opacity produced by an intraocular copper foreign body.[2,9,12] Obviously, the eye care practitioner can play a key role in detecting and diagnosing this disorder.

The exact pathogenesis of Wilson's disease is unclear. The main laboratory test abnormalities are a decreased serum ceruloplasmin (a globulin that binds most serum copper), decreased serum copper, and increased urinary excretion of copper. These patients may also show amino-aciduria, glycosuria, and uricosuria, which indicates diffuse renal damage by excessive copper.[2,45] Rarely, a liver biopsy may be necessary to establish the diagnosis by demonstration of elevated hepatic copper content.

Untreated disease is invariably fatal, with death usually resulting from hepatic failure. Prevention of further copper accumulation is achieved by avoiding foods high in copper (organ meats, shellfish, nuts, whole grain cereals, chocolate, etc.) and using drugs to lessen the absorption of copper and to promote its excretion. Pharmacologic therapy has included the use of the copper-chelating agent penicillamine, potassium sulfide, and zinc acetate. Treatment, which must be extended indefinitely, usually results in an improvement to the extent that most patients can live relatively normal lives.[2,45]

Hemochromatosis

Hemochromatosis (bronze diabetes) is a rare disorder of iron metabolism characterized by excessive accumulation of iron in various tissues and organs. The proximate cause is an excessive intestinal absorption of iron without a corresponding increase in excretion. As iron overload progresses, abnormal amounts of iron are deposited in the liver, joints, gonads, pancreas, heart, and skin. Because many years are required to amass significant body stores of iron, clinical symptoms are not generally seen before patients are 40 to 60 years of age.[2,46] This disease occurs 10 times more often in men than women. This male preponderance was initially believed due to menstruation, pregnancy, and lactation.[2] These small losses of iron are now considered insignificant; the X chromosome may actually suppress expression of the hemochromatosis gene.[47]

The classic clinical characteristics of hemochromatosis consists of hepatic cirrhosis, diabetes mellitus, and increased skin pigmentation (bronze diabetes). Involvement of other organs may also result in hypogonadism, thyroid disease, arthropathy, arrythmias, and cardiomyopathy.[47] Ocular manifestations are few, but eyelid hyperpigmentation, background diabetic retinopathy, slate blue retinal pigmentation, and conjunctival hyperpigmentation have all been observed.[2,9,10]

Early diagnosis is critical, because patients treated before diabetes or cirrhosis develops have a normal life expectancy. Laboratory testing will show an elevated transferrin saturation value and an elevated serum ferretin.[47] The usual treatment involves removal of excess iron by regular phlebotomies. This treatment does not resolve the underlying disorder, and the patient will continue to absorb excess amounts of iron from food. Consequently, phlebotomies will be required periodically for life.[46,47] If anemia develops during venesection, deferoximine (a chelating agent for iron) may further reduce iron stores through urinary iron excretion without exacerbating the anemia.

Although the diseases discussed in this chapter are relatively uncommon, each disorder has ocular manifestations such that the eye care specialist may play a significant role in the detection and diagnosis. In most cases, a comprehensive case history, an extended review of systems, and a thorough examination will ensure that individuals with metabolic disease receive prompt therapy and counseling.

REFERENCES

1. Cahill GF Jr: Genetics and inborn errors of metabolism. Section 9, Ch. IV. In Rubenstein E, Federman DD (eds): Scientific American Medicine. Scientific American, Inc, New York, 1987
2. Block RS, Henkind P: Ocular manifestations of endocrine and metabolic diseases. Ch. 21, p. 1. In Tasman W (ed): Duane's Clinical Ophthalmology. Vol. 5. JB Lippincott, Philadelphia, 1991
3. Vinger PF, Sachs BA: Ocular manifestations of hyperlipoproteinemia. Am J Ophthalmol 70:563, 1970
4. Fredrickson DS: Hereditary systemic diseases of CV metabolism that affect the eye. p. 9. In Mausolf FA (ed): The Eye and Systemic Disease. CV Mosby, St. Louis, 1975
5. Ramsey RC, Benson WE, Day DK: Metabolic diseases affecting the retina. p. 65. In: Retina and Vitreous, Basic and Clinical Science Course. Section 4. American Academy of Ophthalmology, San Franciso, 1987–1988
6. McHam LM, Fulton A: Albinism. p. 185. In Jakobiec FA, Azar D (eds): International Ophthalmology Clinics, Pediatric Ophthalmology. Vol. 32. Little, Brown, Boston, 1992
7. Haefemeyer JW, Kruth JL: Albinism. J Ophthalmic Nurs Technol 10:55, 1991
8. Witkop CJ Jr, Quevedo WC Jr, Fitzpatrick TB, Begudet AL: Albinism. p. 2905. In Scriver CR, King RA (eds): The Metabolic Basis of Inherited Disease. 6th Ed. McGraw-Hill, New York, 1989
9. Roy EH: Ocular Syndromes and Systemic Diseases. 2nd Ed. WB Saunders, Philadelphia, 1989
10. Collins JF (ed): Ophthalmic Desk Reference. Raven Press, New York, 1991
11. Suzuki T, Ohga H, Katayama T et al: A girl with Hermansky-Pudlak syndrome. Acta Ophthalmol 69:256, 1991
12. Kritzinger EE, Wright BE: The Eye and Systemic Disease. Year Book Medical Publishers, Chicago, 1984
13. Collewijn H, Apkarian P, Spekreijse H: The oculomotor behavior of human albinos. Brain 108:1, 1985
14. Rubenstein E: Thromboembolism. Section 1, Ch. XVIII. In Rubenstein E, Federman DD (eds): Scientific American Medicine. Scientific American Inc, New York, 1992
15. Roy EH: Ocular Syndromes and Systemic Disease. 2nd Ed. WB Saunders, Philadelphia, 1989
16. Burke JP, O'Keefe M, Bowell R, Naughten ER: Ocular complications in homocystinuria—early and treated. Br J Ophthalmol 73:427, 1989
17. Berg Wvd, Verbraak FD, Bos PJM: Homocystinuria presenting as central retinal artery occlusion and longstanding thromboembolic disease. Br J Ophthalmol 74:696, 1990
18. Wilson R, Ruiz R: Bilateral central retinal artery occlusion in homocystinuria. Arch Ophthalmol 82:267, 1969
19. Dufier JL, Dhermy P, Gubler MC et al: Ocular changes in long term evaluation of infantile cystinosis. Ophthalmic Paediatr Genet 8:131, 1987
20. Richler M, Milot J, Quigley M, O'Regan S: Ocular manifestations of nephropathic cystinosis. Arch Ophthalmol 109:359, 1991
21. Kaiser-Kupfer MI, Caruso RC, Minkler DS, Gahl WA: Long term ocular manifestations in nephropathic cystinosis. Arch Ophthalmol 104:706, 1986
22. Gahl WA, Reed GF, Thoene JG et al: Cysteamine therapy for children with nephropathic cystinosis. N Engl J Med 316:971, 1987
23. Jones NP, Postlethwaite RJ, Nobel JL: Clearance of corneal crystals in nephrophatic cystinosis by topical cysteamine 0.5%. Arch Ophthal 109:311, 1991
24. Katz B, Melles RB, Schneider JA: Recurrent crystal deposition after keratoplasty in nephropathic cystinosis. Am J Ophthalmol 104:190, 1987
25. Carlson DM, Helgeson MK, Hiett JA: Ocular ochronosis from alkoptonuria. J Am Optom Assoc 62:854, 1991
26. Robinson DR: Osteoarthritis. Section 15, Ch. X. In Rubenstein E, Federman DD (eds): Scientific American Medicine. Scientific American Inc, New York, 1991
27. Roy FH: Ocular Differential Diagnosis. 4th Ed. Lea & Febiger, Philadelphia, 1989
28. Robinson A, Goodman SI, O'Brien D: Genetic and chromosomal disorders, including inborn errors of metabolism. p. 1015. In Kemp HC, Silver HK, O'Brien D (eds): Current Pediatric Diagnosis and Treatment. 8th Ed. Lange Medical, Los Altos, CA, 1984
29. Kosek MS: Medical genetics. p. 1045. In Krupp MA, Schroeder SA, Tierney LM (eds): Current Medical Diagnosis and Treatment. Appleton & Lange, Norwalk, CT, 1987
30. Krane SM, Harris ED Jr: Crystal-induced joint disease. Section 15, Ch. IX. In Rubenstein E, Federman DD (eds): Scientific American Medicine. Scientific American Inc., New York, 1992
31. Fredrickson DS, Levy RI, Lee RS: Fat transport and lipoproteins—an integrated approach to mechanisms and disorders. N Engl J Med 276:32, 1967
32. Fortmann SP, Maron DJ: Disorders of lipid metabolism. Section 9, Ch. II. In Rubenstein E, Federman DD (eds): Scientific American Medicine. Scientific American Inc, New York, 1991
33. Cooper GR, Myers GL, Smith SJ, Schlant RC: Blood lipid measurements, variations and practical utility. JAMA 267:1652, 1992
34. Dodson PM, Gibson JM: Long term follow up and underlying medical conditions in patients with diabetic exudative maculopathy. Eye 5:699, 1991
35. Gordon B, Chang S, Kavanagh M et al: The effects of lipid lowering on diabetic retinopathy. Am J Ophthalmol 112:385, 1991
36. Orlin C, Lee K, Jampol LM, Farber M: Retinal arteriolar changes in patients with hyperlipidemias. Retina 86, 1988
37. Gray GM: Diseases producing malabsorption and maldigestion. Section 4, Ch. XI. In Rubenstein E, Federman DD (eds): Scientific American Medicine. Scientific American Inc, New York, 1988
38. Carr RE: Abetalipoproteinemia and the eye. Birth Defects 12: 385, 1976
39. Duker JS, Belmont J, Bosley TM: Angoid streaks associated with abetalipoproteinemia. Arch Ophthalmol 105:1173, 1987
40. Gouras P, Carr RE, Gunkel RD: Retinitis pigmentosa in abetalipoproteinemia: effects of vitamin A. Invest Ophthalmol 10:784, 1971
41. Runge P, Muller PR, McAllister J et al: Oral vitamin E supplements can prevent the retinopathy of abetalipoproteinemia. Br J Ophthalmol 70:166, 1986
42. Dick AD, Jagger J, McCartney ACE: Refsum's disease: electron microscopy of an iris biopsy. Br J Ophthalmol 74:370, 1990

43. Coles WH: Ophthalmology—A Diagnostic Text. Williams & Wilkins, Baltimore, 1989
44. Geeraets WJ: Ocular Syndromes. 2nd Ed. Lea & Febiger, Philadelphia, 1969
45. Cutler RWP: Degenerative and hereditary diseases. Section 11, Ch. IV. In Rubenstein E, Federman DD (eds): Scientific American Medicine. Scientific American Inc, New York, 1984
46. Gregory PB: Cirrhosis of the liver. Section 4, Ch. IX. In Rubenstein E, Federman DD (eds): Scientific American Medicine. Scientific American Inc, New York, 1986
47. Schrier SL: Anemia: Blood loss and disorders of iron metabolism. Section 5, Ch. II. In Rubenstein E, Federman DD (eds): Scientific American Medicine. Scientific American Inc, New York, 1991
48. Berkow R (ed): The Merck Manual of Diagnosis and Therapy. 14th Ed. Merck, Rahway, NJ, 1982
49. Kelley VC, Limbeck GA (eds): Metabolic Endocrine, and Genetic Disorders of Children. Hagerstown, MD, Harper & Row, 1974

8 Endocrine Disease

ANDREW S. GURWOOD

INTRODUCTION

The endocrine system consists of ductless glands that produce chemical messengers called *hormones*, which pass directly into the circulatory system and are carried to all portions of the body.[1-6] Included within this body system are the pancreas, thyroid gland, parathyroid gland, pineal gland, adrenal glands, and pituitary gland.[1-6] Of the systemic diseases affecting the eye, endocrine dysfunction is among the three most often causing ocular consultation.[6] Disorders of the endocrine pancreas, thyroid gland, parathyroid gland, pineal gland, adrenal glands, and pituitary gland all produce distinct and discernible ocular complications. Endocrinologic disease is a broad and encompassing topic. Any disease, combination of diseases, or condition that affects the anatomy, health, and/or physiology of endocrine glands, endocrine blood supply, or related or supportive organs will result in endocrinologic dysfunction. The prominent endocrinologic diseases with ocular manifestations have therefore been selected for discussion. These include diabetes mellitus, thyroid eye disease, parathyroid, pinealoma, dorsal midbrain syndrome, Cushing's disease, neuroblastoma, pheocromocytoma, Addison's disease, and pituitary gland disease. Medical treatment is available for each of these clinical entities when early detection and diagnosis are provided.

CASE REPORT

A 32-year-old white woman presented for a routine eye examination, with a chief complaint of dry, irritated eyes that seemed to be worsening during the last 2 months. After further questioning, the patient denied having discharge or debris present but described the discomfort as a sensation much like the having "sand" in the lower eyelids of both eyes. The rest of her personal history was unremarkable. The only positive finding of interest was familial history of goiter (her maternal grandmother). She denied using medications of any kind and reported no known allergies.

Her best corrected entering visual acuities were 20/20 OU at distance and near. External examination revealed a slight bearing of the inferior sclera in both eyes. Schirmer tear testing was negative, revealing 10 mm of wetting after 5 minutes. Eyelid to globe congruity was normal, and the lacrimal lake appeared adequate. Hertel exophthalmometry measured 23 mm OU. Extraocular muscle motilities were normal and without restriction. No evidence of relatively afferent pupillary defect was noted. All other external findings were normal and unremarkable. No obvious signs of lid lag (von Graefe sign) were noted. All lymph nodes were normal to palpation.

Biomicroscopy revealed a slight superficial punctate keratitis over the inferior one-third of both corneas. A grade I injection was also observed over the medial and lateral recti of both eyes; however the patient had no history of pain on eye movement. The rest of the eye was calm and quiet. The intraocular pressure was found to be 18 mmHg OU by Goldmann applanation tonometry. The dilated fundus examination was normal, revealing healthy nerves, maculae, and fundi in both eyes, without evidence of posterior pole or peripheral pathology.

Further questioning of the patient elicited a description of additional symptoms: a feeling of "a lump in her throat" along with fatigue and diarrhea. Although palpation was negative for frank masses or nodules, she was referred back to her primary physician with the suggested laboratory testing of triiodothyronine (T_3), thyroxine (T_4), and thyrotropic hormone (also known as thyroid-stimulating hormone [TSH]), with consideration radioactive iodine testing to rule out thyroid dysfunction. We also suggested a visual field screening to rule out compressive or restrictive disorders.

This testing was completed, along with ultrasound of the thyroid gland. The results revealed normal levels of T_3 and T_4, slightly elevated levels of TSH, and high concentrations of antimicrosomal antibodies. Ultrasonography demonstrated multinodular goiter with two "hot" thyroid nodules. Based on these results and a consultation from an endocrinologist, the diagnosis of Hashimoto's thyroiditis was made.

Treatment was administered conservatively, using 1 mg/day of levothyroxine orally to prevent the growth of additional nodules, shrink existing nodules, and prevent the onset of hypothyroidism. Ophthalmically, treatment was dispensed for the sequelae of already present hypothyroidism and stage I Graves ophthalmopathy. The patient was given artificial tears to use on an as-needed basis and instructed to sleep with a blindfold to prevent exposure keratitis. At the last office visit, the patient was enjoying good vision with good comfort.

PANCREAS AND DIABETES MELLITUS

The pancreas is a long, soft, greyish-pink digestive gland. It extends across the posterior abdominal wall, posterior to the stomach, from the duodenum to the spleen.[2] The pancreas is both an exocrine and an endocrine gland. It produces an external secretion called *pancreatic juice,* which enters the duodenum via the pancreatic duct, and internal secretions called *glucagon* (sugar-releasing hormone) and insulin (sugar-storage hormone), which enter the bloodstream.

Generally speaking, diabetes mellitus is a genetically influenced heterogeneous group of diseases with glucose intolerance. Diabetes is characterized as a disorder of metabolic regulation, resulting from either a relative or absolute deficiency of insulin. In its fully developed clinical form, diabetes displays acute metabolic disturbances marked by fasting hyperglycemia, muscle wasting, hyperlipemia, and ketosis. Chronic complications include large vessel disease, small vessel disease, and retinal vascular disease.[2–4,6–12]

The prevalence of diabetes in the American population (approximately 2 percent) coupled with the high incidence of retinal microvascular changes (approximately 50 percent) allow the optometrist to participate in the care of patients referred from internists and general medical practitioners.[6–8]

Diabetes remains a severe problem. Some studies estimate that 5 percent of the population has diabetes, with only 50 percent of cases diagnosed.[8] More than 600,000 new cases are diagnosed each year, with estimates that numbers double every 15 years.[8]

The American Diabetes Association states that diabetic eye disease is the number one cause of new blindness in people between the ages of 20 and 74 in this country, and each year more than 5,000 Americans lose their sight because of diabetes.[8] Diabetic ocular changes are responsible for 12 percent of the blind population of the United States.[8] Clearly, the development of vision-threatening diabetic retinopathy increases in incidence with age and is related to the degree of control in the early phases of its systemic process.[6–8]

The incidence of blindness from diabetes peaks between the ages of 30 and 50. Diabetics are 25 times more prone to blindness, 17 times more prone to renal disease, 20 times more prone to gangrene, and 2 times more prone to myocardial infarction or stroke than nondiabetics.[8–11]

OCULAR MANIFESTATIONS OF DIABETES MELLITUS

Fluctuating Refractive Error

A frequent ocular sign of diabetes mellitus is fluctuating refractive error.[6] This typically occurs when blood sugar is not adequately controlled. Tonicity within the cells of the lens increases as glucose and sorbitol (sugar alcohol of glucose) accumulate. Differences in the lens and serum osmolarity cause the crystalline lens to shrink and swell, causing refractive changes. Typically, as blood sugar increases, relative myopia ensues. Conversely, as blood sugar falls, relative hyperopia is involved. These symptoms can be eliminated by controlling and stabilizing blood sugar. Clinicians should be reminded that glasses or contacts should not be prescribed until blood sugar levels remain stable for at least 3 weeks.[6,12]

Cataract

Some evidence suggests that diabetic patients develop cataracts earlier and more rapidly than nondiabetics. In fact, even if blood sugar is abruptly lowered after it has been elevated for a significant period, acute crystalline lens swelling and opacification may occur as a result of osmotic stress. "True diabetic cataracts, as opposed to early nuclear sclerosis, may occur when blood glucose levels increase. Even in well-regulated diabetics, osmotic stress and toxicity of crystalline lens cells secondary to glycosylation (adding glucose to proteins covalently) causes premature lens opacification[6,13] (C. M. Wormington, personal communication, 1994). The process usually begins as snow-white areas of cortex and posterior subcapsular opacities, which eventually coalesce to cloud the entire lens.[6,13] Diabetic cataracts are usually more visually debilitating than naturally occurring nondiabetic cataracts because they are often bilateral.[13]

Diabetic Retinopathy

The genesis of diabetic retinopathy seems to stem from microscopic changes that occur in the basement membrane of the capillary walls. This, in combination with sticky blood, produces capillary nonperfusion, hypoxia, and altered vascular structure.[8-12]

Approximately two-thirds of diabetics will present with retinopathy after they have had the disease for 15 years.[6,13] Surprisingly, control plays only a minor role in the prevention and onset of diabetic retinopathy once the processes of nonperfusion, hypoxia, altered vascular structure, changes in blood viscosity, and other complications of microangiopathy have begun.[13] In fact, juvenile diabetics typically develop severe proliferative diabetic retinopathy within the first 25 years of life, despite good control.[6,13]

To consider background diabetic retinopathy (BDR) relatively benign is misleading.[8] The retinal vascular components attributed to BDR are microaneurysms, deep dot and blot intraretinal hemorrhages, and the formation of hard exudates. Together, these sequellae possess the ability to initiate severe and lasting changes that may alter the vision of an individual for a lifetime.

Microaneurysms are balloon entities that occur along the walls of weakened capillaries. These microaneurysms are structurally weak and leaky and often are the sources of excess fluid exudation (leakage) that causes the retinal edema that spreads to the macula and affects vision.[6,8,12-17]

Deep dot-blot intraretinal hemorrhages represent ruptures in weakened capillary walls.[8] Hemorrhages indicate the presence of deep intraretinal edema.[8] Hemorrhages that encroach into the foveal avascular zone (FAZ) indicate edema encroaching on the FAZ and should be considered an immediate threat to vision.[8,12-17]

Hard exudates represent areas of lipid deposition that are a sign of chronic retinal edema secondary to leaking microaneurysms or choroidal neovascular nets.[8] Although the exudates themselves are benign, they indicate the presence of long-standing chronic edema.[8] Often, exudates circle the area of leakage. When they surround the macula, they are often collectively called *circinate maculopathy*[8] (Fig. 8-1 and Plate 8-1). Because exudates signal the presence of chronic edema, their presence in and around the FAZ indicates a poor prognosis for return of good vision.[6,8,11,13-17]

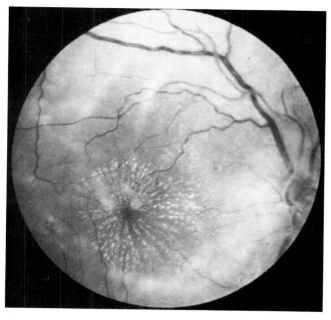

Fig. 8-1. Circinate background diabetic maculopathy. (See also Plate 8-1.)

Recognition of the signs of preproliferative and proliferative diabetic retinopathy is crucial in the management of the diabetic patient. BDR leads to compromise of retinal arterioles, producing microaneurysms, small intraretinal hemorrhages, edema, exudates, and nerve fiber layer infarcts (cotton-wool patches). This is the severe hypoxic form of BDR that is the precurser to the release of vasoproliferative substance and is termed the *preproliferative stage*. The components of microaneurysms, exudates, intraretinal edema, hemorrhages, and nerve fiber layer infarcts along with tortuous shunting capillaries are collectively called intraretinal microvascular abnormalities (IRMA).[6,8,12–17]

IRMA represents the retina's relocation system, attempting to compensate for areas with severe capillary nonperfusion.[8] IRMA forms in an attempt to drain areas of stasis and is neither leaky nor a threat to vision.[8] IRMA, as an indicator of stasis and retinal hypoxia, is not itself dangerous, but is thought to represent the germination bed of retinal neovascularization.[8] It should be followed at 3- to 4-month intervals after intravenous fluorescein angiography (IVFA) has been performed to rule out neovascularization.[8]

Proliferative diabetic retinopathy (PDR) is estimated to effect more than 5 percent of patients with diabetic fundus changes.[6] If left untreated, approximately 50 to 60 percent of eyes with PDR become legally blind (visual acuity less than 20/200) after 5 years.[6,8,17]

The components of PDR include neovascularization of the disc (NVD), neovascularization elsewhere (NVE), fibrotic proliferation accompanying the neovascularization, tractional retinal detachment, and vitreous hemorrhages.[6,8,12–17] Every component of PDR has the potential to create blindness.[8]

NVD occurs in approximately 25 percent of patients with PDR.[8] NVD and NVE both typically delay their appearance until 15 years after the onset of diabetes mellitus.[8] This neovascularization is believed to be the response to hypoxia of retinal tissue. Both seem to progress more rapidly in younger patients. Fine networks arise, increasing the likelihood of tractional retinal detachment, vitreous hemorrhage, retinal hypoxia with rubeosis irides (neovascularization of the iris), and neovascular glaucoma.[6,8,17]

NVE arises from similar circumstances and takes a similar course. NVE is thought to sprout out of beds of IRMA, perforate the internal limiting membrane, and proliferate along the vitroretinal interface. NVE

Table 8-1. Quick Reference for Causes of Retinal Neovascularization

Diabetes mellitus
Central retinal vein occlusion (ischemic > nonischemic)
Carotid artery disease and carotid artery occlusion (ocular ischemic syndrome)
Carotid cavernous fistula
Sickle cell disease
    SS type = worst systemic sequelae
    SC type = worse ocular sequelae
Retinopathy of prematurity
Ocular trauma
Retinal detachment
Temporal arteritis
Collagen vascular diseases

adheres to the vitreal hyloid membrane and grows rapidly.[8] Coupled with vitreous syneresis and vitreous collapse, selected pockets can produce vitreous hemorrhage and retinal detachment.[8] Table 8-1 lists some of the causes of retinal neovascularization.

Treatment

BDR requires no ocular treatment. Patients should be educated and encouraged to follow the instructions of their internist. Follow-up care consists of an extended dilated fundus examination using Hruby, 90, 78, and 20 indirect ophthalmoloscopy at 6- to 12-month intervals. The critical changes that dictate the necessity for treatment in cases that do not involve neovascularization are encroachments on the macula known as clinically significant macular edema (CSME).[8,12–17] CSME is probably the single largest cause of vision loss in diabetics. It is apparent to the clinician on binocular funduscopic examination with the observable characteristics of (1) blunted foveal reflex, (2) blurred and indistinct choirdal vasculature, (3) decreased retinal transparency, and (4) decreased retinal pigment epithelium granularity.

The diagnosis of CSME is not related to visual acuity and is based on finding any one of three criteria: (1) thickening of the retina at or within 500 μm of the center of the macula; (2) hard exudates at or within 500 μm of the center of the macula, if associated with thickening of adjacent retina; or (3) a zone or zones of retinal thickening 1 disc area or larger, any part of which is within 1 disc diameter of the center of the macula[12,15,16] (Table 8-2). When CSME is diagnosed by the ocular physician, the patient should be instructed to obtain a prompt consultation with a retinologist. In addition, IVFA may be suggested along

Table 8-2. Quick Reference for Diagnosing Clinically Significant Macular Edema (Treatable Diabetic Retinopathy)

Thickening of the retina at or within 500 μm of the center of the macula

Hard exudates at or within 500 μm of the center of the macula, only if associated with thickening of the adjacent retina (not included are residual hard exudates remaining after the disappearance of retinal thickening)

A zone or zones of retinal thickening 1 disc area or larger, any part of which is within 1 disc diameter of the center of the macula

(From Early Treatment of Diabetic Retinopathy Study Research Group,[15] with permission.)

with focal or grid laser photocoagulation.[12,15,16] (For more specifics regarding diabetes, see Ch. 9.)

Pre-PDR requires no ocular treatment. The ocular physician, however, should monitor patients with these funduscopic changes more closely than those who have simple BDR. Prudent management includes patient education along with close observation for funduscopic changes using extended dilated procedures, at 3-month intervals. The five signs of pre-PDR include (1) cotton-wool spots (nerve fiber layer infarction), (2) venous tortuosity, (3) capillary closure, (4) arteriolar abnormalities, and (5) IRMA. A retinology consultation is indicated if any three of these five signs are apparent.[8,17]

PDR requires ocular treatment, if it meets the criteria found in the Diabetic Retinopathy Study Research Group report number 14.[12] The two retinal criteria that represent high-risk characteristics include (1) neovascularization of the disc larger than ½ disc diameter and (2) neovascularization of the disc or neovascularization elsewhere with any vitreous hemorrhage[12,17] (Table 8-3). When PDR is diagnosed, the

Table 8-3. Quick Reference for the Criteria of Treating Proliferative Diabetic Retinopathy

Background diabetic retinopathy without clinically significant macular edema: monitor at 3–4-month intervals

Preproliferative diabetic retinopathy with cotton-wool spots, flame-shaped hemorrhages, venous beading, venous tortuosity, arteriolar narrowing, and intraretinal microvascular abnormalities: monitor at 3–4-month intervals for the formation of proliferative retinopathy

Proliferative diabetic retinopathy requires panretinal photocoagulation when there is neovascularization of the disc (NVD) that is ½ disc diameter or greater or if there is NVD or neovascularization elsewhere in the presence of vitreous hemorrhage

(From Diabetic Retinopathy Study Research Group,[12] with permission.)

patient should be educated that a prompt referral for a consultation with a retinologist is in order. IVFA and panretinal photocoagulation (PRP) may be suggested so that visual losses may be minimized, stabilized, or prevented.[8,12,17] Other factors that warrant consideration with respect to initiating laser PRP include the presence of vitreous or preretinal hemorrhage, anterior segment neovascularization, severe intraretinal lesions, vitreoretinal relationships (traction), macular edema, systemic factors, and past course.[12] (For more specifics regarding diabetes mellitus, see Ch. 9.)

Neuro-ocular Sequellae

Acute-onset isolated third, fourth, or sixth cranial nerve palsies are frequently seen in middle-aged or elderly diabetics.[6] Isolated cranial nerve II (ocular motor nerve) palsy may be the initial symptom in a previously undiagnosed case of diabetes mellitus.[6]

Third cranial nerve palsy accounts for up to 40 percent of diabetic neuro-ocular disease. Uniquely, diabetic third cranial nerve palsies often leave the pupil completely spared. This presumably occurs because the ischemic vascular elements of the disease tend to affect the core of the nerve rather than peripheral portions, where the pupillary fibers are located. The pupil has been reported to be involved in no more than 30 percent of patients who present with diagnosed diabetic ophthalmoplegia.[6] Because pain almost always occurs in diabetic oculomotor nerve palsy, the distinct feature of a working pupil distinguishes it from aneurysm and other compressive lesions.[6] Although pain is common in diabetic cranial nerve III palsies, it is not common in cases of diabetic cranial nerve IV palsy (20 percent of diabetic ophthalmoplegias) or diabetic cranial nerve VI palsy (40 percent of diabetic ophthalmoplegias).[6]

All forms of diabetic ophthalmoplegia show significant spontaneous improvement within 4 to 6 weeks of their onset. Complete resolution often occurs within 3 months. The key is consistent, successful control of the systemic facets of the disease. As the diabetic's control fluctuates, ophthalmoplegia may return. Simultaneous involvement of more than one cranial nerve, however, must be viewed as suspicious and ominous. Any diabetic patient with multiple cranial nerve palsies, optic neuropathy, or retinal artery occlusion should be suspected of having mucormycosis (a fungal infection) of the pananasal sinuses, orbit, or cavernous sinus.

Open-angle glaucoma and neovascular glaucoma are more common in diabetics than in the general population. Furthermore, some have speculated that diabetic small vessel disease increases the risk of the development of glaucomatous optic nerve damage.[6] (For more information on diagnosis, prognosis, and management of diabetes mellitus, see Ch. 9.)

DISORDERS OF THE THYROID AND PARATHYROID GLANDS

The endocrine glands or ductless glands are often grouped together because they share the common characteristic of not having ducts and of discharging their specific secretions (hormones) directly into the bloodstream.[18,19] These glands of the body include the thyroid, parathyroid, pituitary, superadrenal, paraganglia, and pineal glands. Endocrine ophthalmopathy is associated with Graves hyperthyroidism in 90 percent of cases.[20,21] Since its first descriptions more than 150 years ago, Graves disease, or thyrotoxicosis, with its complex manifestations and unpredictable clinical course, has fascinated, perplexed, and frustrated internists, surgeons, ophthalmologists, optometrists, and immunologists alike.[22–27]

Because of its many facets, thyroid-related eye disease continues to remain an enigma despite the current research and the more than 40 theories promulgated regarding its pathogenesis. Although certain histopathologic features have been documented, the mechanisms (systemic and/or ocular) that are precisely responsible remain unclear. In fact, the ocular condition characteristic of Graves disease may exist in the absence of clinical or biochemical evidence of thyroid dysfunction. Furthermore, when systemic and ocular conditions exist simultaneously, they may follow completely different clinical courses.[22,25,28]

The eye, with its plethora of integrated and interdigitated structures may serve as the first diagnostic indicator of impending, beginning, or progressing systemic and/or ocular thyroid disease. Clinicians should therefore be well informed and skilled in its detection, differential diagnosis, and management.

Anatomy and Physiology

Thyroid Gland

The thyroid gland develops from the median diverticulum of the ventral wall of the pharynx and first appears in approximately the fourth week of life.[18] A highly vascularized organ situated in the anterior triangle of the neck, the thyroid consists of right and left lobes connected across the mid-line by a narrow portion of tissue called the *isthmus* (L. Lombardi, personal communication, 1993). Its weight is variable but typically approximates 30 g. The lateral, superficial surface is convex and covered by the muscles of the neck and skin. The deep, medial surface is molded over the trachea, cricoid muscles, the esophagus and deep muscles, and the nerves and vasculature of the throat.[20]

The thyroid gland secretes two significant hormones: T_4 and T_3. These chemicals have the profound effect of increasing the body's metabolic rate. Thyroid hormone secretion is controlled primarily by TSH, which is secreted by the anterior pituitary gland. TSH levels are regulated by a substance known as thyrotropin-releasing hormone (TRH), which is secreted by the nerve endings in the median eminence of the hypothalamus (Fig. 8-1).

Approximately 90 percent of the hormone secreted by the thyroid gland is T_4, whereas only 10 percent is T_3.[19] These two hormones have basically the same function; however, they differ in rapidity and intensity of action, with T_3 being approximately four times more potent.

To form normal quantities of thyroxine, the body requires 1 mg/wk of iodides. This can be found in iodized table salt, which contains 1 part sodium iodide to every 100,000 parts of sodium chloride. The formation of these hormones is accomplished through complicated biochemical reactions that occur in the gland itself. To maintain normal levels of metabolic activity in the body precisely, the proper amount of thyroid hormones must be secreted at all times. This is accomplished through a feedback loop involving T_3, T_4, TSH, and TRH[18,19] (Fig. 8-2).

Changes in temperature, emotional reactions (e.g., anxiety, stress and excitement)—conditions that stimulate the sympathetic nervous system—can all affect the hypothalamus and TRH production, increasing

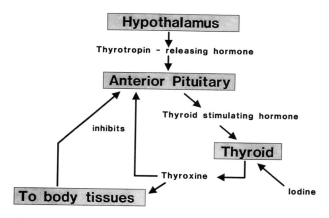

Fig. 8-2. Schematic representation of thyroid secretion

or decreasing thyroid-related activity. Among other things, cold stimulates TRH production and consequently activates the thyroid gland, whereas heat—whether generated from anxiety, excitement or stress—acts to inhibit TRH production and slow thyroid activity.[19]

The thyroid gland has a profound effect on carbohydrate metabolism, fat metabolism, plasma and liver fat levels, vitamin metabolism, basal metabolic rate, body weight, heart rate, cardiac contractility, cardiac output, respiratory rate, muscle tone, and most notably, the function of the other endocrine glands.[19]

Parathyroid Gland

The small round parathyroid glands are situated between the dorsal borders of the lateral lobes of the thyroid gland. These tiny columns of richly vascularized chief cells secrete parathyroid hormone (PTH), which is necessary for calcium metabolism. Although the parathyroid glands have little direct effect on the ocular system and function, they may cause systemic effects if damaged secondary to disease of the thyroid gland or treatment of thyroid disease.[18,19] Although rare, band keratopathy may occur as a presenting sign of the condition known as *hyperparathyroidism*. Band keratopathy associated with hyperparathyroidism presents with corneal changes that include diffuse, superficial, milky opacities of the Bowman's membrane and superficial stroma. These opacities are intracellular calcium salts. These calcium salts differ from those that exist in patients with renal disease. The condition is easily recognizable, with observable whitish flecks and glass-like crystals seen running concentrically across the cornea from the nasal limbal

junction.[29] The treatment of band keratopathy ranges from chelation removal using topical ethylendiaminateracetic acid (EDTA) spread on the lesion with a cotton-tipped applicator to supportive therapy with patient education and copious lubrication. Supportive therapies may include artificial tear solutions, applied on an as-needed basis; artificial tear ointments, applied twice daily; and hypertonic solutions or ointments, applied two to four times daily.

Hypothyroidism

A relatively common disorder that increases in frequency with age, hypothyroidism has three principle forms: primary hypothyroidism (an intrinsic defect in thyroid structure or function), secondary hypothyroidism (secondary to insufficient TSH caused by pituitary failure), or tertiary hypothyroidism (inadequate TSH levels from a normal pituitary secondary to insufficient secretion of thyrotropin-releasing hormone (TRH) from the hypothalamus).[30,31]

Primary hypothyroidism is the most common form of thyroid inadequacy, occurring in approximately 1: 4,000 to 6,000 births, irrespective of geographic location.[31] As with all thyroid disease, hypothyroidism affects women more commonly than men. The other common causes of hypothyroidism are destruction of the gland by infection, virus, other processes, and ablation via radiation or removal surgical procedures.

The classic signs and symptoms of hypothyroidism are cold intolerance, thickened dry skin, anemia, hypercholesterolemia, decreased sweating, periorbital edema (primarily the lower eyelids), lethargy, thick tongue, and constipation. Collectively, these symptoms associated with severe thyroid deficiency are termed *myxedema*[30,31] (Table 8-4).

Patients with hypothyroidism may present to the ocular physician with ocular signs that may include swelling of the eyelids (with a preponderance for swelling in the lower eyelids); facial swelling; signs of hypercholesterolemia such as arteriole knicking, banking and broadened light reflex; and funduscopic microvascular changes similar to those associated with anemia. A definite association between hypothyroidism and uveitis also exists. Although mechanisms are still somewhat unclear, hyperthyroidism and uveitis have little association.[32]

The diagnosis of primary hypothyroidism is

Table 8-4. Systemic Signs and Ocular Sequelae of Hypothyroidism (Myxedema)

Common systemic signs of hypothyroidism (myxedema)
  Fatigue
  Dry coarse skin
  Lethargy/depression
  Slow speech/thick tongue
  Decreased sweating
  Hoarseness
  Memory impairment
  Constipation
  Hair loss (alopecia)
  Cold intolerance/bradycardia
Common ocular sequelae
  Decreased sweating on the brow and face
  Facial/periorbital edema
  Edema of the eyelids (most prominent in the lower eyelids)
  Sequelae of hypercholesterolemia
    Atherosclerotic vessel changes
    Microvascular abnormalities in the fundus

straightforword; however, it is often missed because the symptoms are vague and nonspecific. The practicing eye care physician should refer suspected patients to an internist or an endocrinologist for measurement of plasma T_4 and plasma TSH levels. Marked low levels of plasma T_4 or high levels of TSH (the body's attempt to compensate) are positive for diagnosis of hypothyroidism.

Primary hypothyroidism is a rewarding disease to treat. Systemic therapy is simple and efficacious. Unfortunately, many patients wait too long to seek therapy or avoid or discontinue therapy and sink into a profound state of myxedema. For this reason, continual follow-up and reinforcement of the need for thyroid hormone are necessary.

Commercially available forms of thyroid hormone are T_4 (100 μg), desiccated thyroid or purified thyroglobulin (65 mg) and T_3 (25 μg). Therapy is almost always given orally, because these preparations are readily absorbed in the gut.[30,31]

The only serious danger in treating primary hypothyroidism with thyroid hormone (levothyroxine) is that patients susceptible to cardiac stress or patients with coronary artery disease may have a greater demand placed on the heart, possibly causing myocardial infarction or arrhythmias. Finally, in standard cases, 100 to 200 μg of levothyroxine daily will suffice as sufficient replacement therapy. Occasionally, patients require 300 μg of levothyroxine to complete adequate

replacement. The literature clearly recognizes cases in which patients develop evidence of thyrotoxicosis (hyperthyroidism) when receiving of thyroid hormone doses exceeding 100 μg. The practitioner should keep this in mind and monitor accordingly.

Secondary and tertiary hypothyroidism are so similar to primary hypothyroidism that no clear differentiation can be made on clinical grounds alone.[30,31] Patients with hypopituitarism typically produce very low levels of TSH and have small thyroid glands. The most useful diagnostic course in cases such as these is to refer the patient to an internist or endocrinologist for measurement of plasma T_4 and TSH levels. In cases of secondary and tertiary hypothyroidism, TSH levels, which are high in primary hypothyroidism, will be markedly low. Internists and endocrinologists use TRH injection to differentiate between secondary hypothyroidism (pituitary difficulty) and tertiary hypothyroidism (hypothalamic difficulty). Theoretically, if the problem is caused by pituitary destruction or disease, the levels of TSH will not rise when TRH is introduced. If the difficulty is hypothalamic in nature, however, TSH will rise when TRH is injected.

Treatment for secondary and tertiary hypothyroidism is TSH and adrenocortical replacement therapy. The ocular management is identical to that for primary hypothyroidism.

Nontoxic Goiter

Nontoxic goiter is the most common endocrine disease.[30] It is classified and characterized as thyroid enlargement that is not associated with either thyrotoxicosis or thyroid neoplasm.[30] Surveys conducted in iodine-sufficient regions reveal that an estimated 4 percent of the world's population has nontoxic thyroid enlargement. It is six times more common in women than men. Often, nontoxic goiter is categorized as *endemic*, meaning very prevalent in a certain geographic area (10 percent or more of the population).[30,31] The term *sporadic nontoxic goiter* is used to indicate that the disease affects only a small portion of the population (10 percent or less of the population).[30,31] Susceptibility to goiter is inherited and thought to result from one or more biosynthetic defects in thyroid hormone synthesis or secretion.

Endemic goiter is most prevalent in underdeveloped areas of the world where public health practices are limited and food sources local. The primary cause of endemic goiter is deficient dietary intake of iodine, which interrupts the normal synthesis of thyroid hormone.

Confusion can occur in the diagnosis of endemic and sporadic nontoxic goiter because goiter is common in nonendemic regions and is an inherited trait. In any case, these patients will often present with hypothyroid symptomatology and must be referred to an internist or endocrinologist for thyroid function studies and measurement of plasma T_4 concentrations, plasma T_3 concentrations and TSH levels.[30,31] If treatment is delayed, the glands may become disfiguring, sometimes exceeding 1 kg in weight.[30]

The optimal treatment for endemic goiter is prophylaxis. Great care must be exercised when considering the addition of iodine to iodine-deficient diets. Epidemiologic studies have documented a transient pronounced increase in the incidence of thyrotoxicosis when iodine supplementation is introduced to iodine-deficient areas.[30]

Treatment of sporadic nontoxic goiter involves gently suppressing TSH concentration. This is accomplished through careful administration of low dosages of thyroid hormone (L. Lombardi, personal communication, 1993). The eye care professional must monitor these patients for therapeutic compliance and the recurrent ocular signs of hypothyroidism and hyperthyroidism.

Thyroid Neoplasms

Thyroid cancer remains a controversial topic in medicine, with no clear consensus on the proper approach to the problem. Two facts remain: (1) death from thyroid cancer is rare and (2) clinically, single thyroid nodules are common. Statistics compiled by the National Cancer Institute indicate that the mortality rate from thyroid cancer in the United States has remained stable at 0.6/100,000.[20] On the other hand, single thyroid nodules that are considered suspicious and potentially malignant occur in 2 to 4 percent of the population (2,000/100,000).[31]

Given the marked difference between the prevalence of a single thyroid nodule and the mortality rate from thyroid cancer, it is clear that few patients with thyroid nodules will die from malignancy. The prevalence of malignancy increases in some ethnic groups. Occult thyroid carcinomas are found in approximately

25 percent of all Japanese, yet the mortality rate from thyroid cancer in Japanese is no higher than in non-Japanese. Because the current recommended treatment of thyroid carcinoma is considered somewhat risky, the risk of therapy may be higher than the risk of untreated disease. These processes can cause ocular signs ranging from hypothyroidism to hyperthyroidism, and the practicing optometrist should be aware of their systemic signs and symptoms.

In general, thyroid malignancies exhibit a broad spectrum of behavior, from clinically insignificant papillary carcinomas to relentlessly progressive anaplastic cancers. Thyroid cancer may be caused by low-dose irradiation of the gland (200 to 2,000 rads, usually done for an enlarged thymus or enlarged tonsils); may be familial, as in the case of medullary carcinoma; or as in most cases, is of unknown cause. It typically presents as a thyroid nodule that may or may not produce local symptoms. Diagnosis of malignancy is difficult and often considered inconsistent.[30,31] Despite these inconsistencies, patients have a good prognosis. Iodine-131 scanning and serum thyroglobulin levels serve as excellent follow-up indicators.[31]

Papillary Carcinoma

Papillary carcinoma is a well-differentiated thyroid malignancy that accounts for one-half of the clinical thyroid cancers. Its pathologic features include papilliform arrangement of cells, atypical nuclei with cytoplasmic inclusions, and psammoma bodies, which can be detected on biopsy.

Papillary carcinoma is the most common malignancy in childhood, and its incidence also increases in older adults.[31] It is multifocal in 20 percent of cases and typically spreads into adjacent structures by extension or through regional lymphatics.[31] Metastases to the lungs are distant sites of progressively malignant thyroid disease, with no cases of metastases to the choroid of the eye reported.[30,31] Patients older than age 40 who contract the disease have a poorer prognosis for recurrence and death secondary to pulmonary and extensive lymph node involvement. These tumors are typically treated with hemithyroidectomy of the lobe containing the nodule. If evidence of remaining cancer is found, eradication of all thyroid tissue through large doses of radioactive iodine is recommended. Because the papillary tumors usually concentrate iodine well, the tumor can be retreated with iodine-131 if necessary.[31]

Follicular Carcinoma

Less than one-sixth of thyroid cancers have what is known as a follicular appearance and account for approximately 15 percent of thyroid carcinomas.[30] Follicular carcinoma occurs most commonly in the middle-aged and elderly. In addition to local invasion and regional lymphatic spread, these malignancies metastasize, particularly to lung and bone.[31] Distant metastases have been shown to concentrate iodine, making radioactive treatments a possibility. No cases of metastases to the choroid have been reported. Typically, prognoses is poor.

Anaplastic Carcinoma

Anaplastic carcinomas are undifferentiated thyroid tumors that grow rapidly and cause serious problems, both locally and with invading metastases.[30] These rare tumors represent less than 5 percent of all thyroid cancers. Except for occasional reports of success with combinations of radiation and chemotherapies, prognosis is poor with no effective treatment.

Medullary Carcinoma

Medullary carcinoma an unusual tumor, derived from calcitonin-secreting parafollicular thyroid cells, constitutes approximately 5 percent of thyroid malignancies.[30] Medullary carcinomas may develop from an inherited dominant autosomal trait and may be associated with functional tumors of the adrenal medulla and hyperparathyroidism. They usually cause excessive secretion of calcitonin. Unless there is a known family history, a preoperative diagnosis is unlikely. The pentagastrin test is primarily used to provoke high levels of plasma calcitonin levels to identify family members who may be at risk. High-risk patients should be reevaluated every 1 to 2 years, with thyroidectomy considered at the appropriate time.[30]

Lymphoma and Other Thyroid Malignancies

Lymphoma may involve the thyroid gland primarily or as part of systemic disease. Thyroid lymphoma is most frequently encountered in patients with pre-existing autoimmune thyroiditis. Squamous cell carcinoma may arise from or secondarily involve the thyroid gland. Typically, the presence of these malignancies is diagnosed from a needle biopsy.[31]

Ocular Sequelae of Thyroid Neoplasms

In general, these entities do not cause eye disease or ocular signs and symptoms. The clinical practitioner should act as a keen observer, promptly referring patients who present with signs and symptoms to an endocrinologist.

Table 8-5. Common Causes of Hypothyroidism

Postablative process by radiation or surgery
Thyroiditis
Subacute (de Quervain)
Lymphocytic (postpartum)
Autoimmune
Drug induced (blockade of hormone release secondary to iodine, lithium, and others)
Secondary lack of TSH stimulation

The best treatment for well-differentiated thyroid carcinoma and its ocular symptoms is generous excision. Partial thyroidectomy remains controversial, with total thyroidectomy preferred. Radioactive iodine scanning and therapy complete the treatment. Postoperative thyroid hormones prevent secondary side effects and aid in preventing tumor recurrence. The treatment of thyroid carcinoma and its ocular sequelae are the same as those for Graves ophthalmopathy and should be managed on a case-by-case basis.[31] The primary care optometrist should be aware of the signs and symptoms of systemic thyroid disease as well as the ocular sequelae. Prompt referral to an endocrinologist will expedite the correct diagnosis and aid in facilitating swift treatment[19,25] (Table 8-5).

Thyroiditis

The term *thyroiditis* indicates thyroid inflammation. The pathologic, clinical, and laboratory features of various forms of thyroiditis are poorly and only partially understood. Thyroid inflammation may cause local neck symptoms, constitutional complaints, and abnormalities of thyroid hormone production.

Subacute thyroiditis is believed to be caused by viral infection of the thyroid gland and is often preceded by prodromal upper respiratory syndrome. The cardinal symptom of subacute thyroiditis is pain, which may be referred to the throat, ear, or lateral neck. Constitutional symptoms include fever, sweating, fatigue and malaise. The thyroid gland is typically enlarged, firm, and tender and often induces transient hyperthyroidism.

Hashimoto's thyroiditis is a disease now thought to be almost identical to Graves disease as far as immunohereditary mechanisms are concerned. Hashimoto's thyroiditis, however, is not commonly associated with hyperthyroidism. Furthermore, exophthalmos, if found at all, is mild and transient. In this disease, T_4 levels become marginally high at first but then subside as the inflammatory crisis causes a shutdown of iodine uptake. The result is Graves orbitopathy, which is otherwise characteristically present on computed tomography (CT) scanning and ultrasonography.[19,28,30]

The diagnosis of subacute thyroiditis is confirmed by detection of abnormal thyroid hormone concentrations, elevated laboratory levels of the erythrocyte sedimentation rate (ESR, Westergren method) and markedly decreased thyroidal radioactive uptake.

The condition is best left to run its course. Typically, the thyroid dysfunction is not treated and in most cases, returns to normal once the event has passed. The inflammatory and constitutional signs are best treated with supportive therapies that include aspirin (600 mg every 4 to 6 hours), nonsteroidal anti-inflammatory agents (indomethacin, 50 mgs TID PO) and in rare cases, systemic steroids (prednisone, 20 mg BID PO).[31]

Hyperthyroidism and Graves Ophthalmopathy

Thyroid eye disease, Graves ophthalmopathy, dysthyroid ophthalmopathy, and Graves orbitopathy are all synonymous terms.[22] Thyroid eye disease may occur at any age and is most often found in persons with strong familial histories of thyroid dysfunction. Females are generally affected more than males by a ratio of 2.3:1.[31] Graves ophthalmopathy is one of the most common clinical entities seen in the practice of optometry and ophthalmology; however, clinically apparent ophthalmopathy occurs in only 25 to 50 percent of cases.[33] Differential diagnosis includes orbital mass, inflammatory processes, and vascular abnormality.

Graves ophthalmopathy is the most common cause of true eyelid retraction.[34] This retraction is due to fibrotic contracture of Müller's muscle and the levator.[22,33–38] Primarily an orbital disease and hypothesized to be of autoimmune etiology,[22,33,39–43] Graves ophthalmopathy may be clinically characterized by eyelid retractions, proptosis, conjunctival injection and chemosis, corneal compromise, secondary dry-

eye syndrome, extraocular muscle fibrosis, and decreased vision resulting from compressive optic neuropathy within the orbit[22,33–38,44,45] (J. Wurzel, personal communication, 1993).

Definition

Ocular findings may occur independently from systemic dysthyroid function. In other words, ocular findings may be more severe, less severe, or match the systemic condition. Euthyroid Graves ophthalmopathy is the common clinical syndrome in which the characteristic ophthalmic manifestations of Graves disease exist in the presence of a clinically and biomedically normal thyroid.[22,42] During the disease stages, most of the patients manifest hyperthyroidism. Standard laboratory testing includes measurement of T_3 and T_4 levels as well as TSH profiles[22] (J. Wurzel, personal communication, 1993). McKenzie is cited in the literature[22] as providing the most pragmatic definition for Graves disease: a multisystem disorder of unknown etiology characterized by one or more of the following: (1) hyperthyroidism associated with diffuse hyperplasia of the thyroid gland, (2) infiltrative ophthalmopathy, and/or (3) infiltrative dermopathy (localized pretibial myxedema).[22]

Pathophysiology

The thyroid gland, skin, extraocular muscles, and orbital fat are infiltrated by lymphocytes, macrophages, and mast cells. The skin changes resulting from excessive mucopolysaccharides are termed *pretibial myxedema*.[46] Excess mucopolysaccharide (hyaluronic acid) within the extraorbital fat and muscles with interstitial edema and inflammatory cellular reaction cause the increased mass of the orbital contents.[22,33,45] This pathologic proptosis leads to corneal exposure, diplopia, contracture of extraocular muscles, and eventually, compressive optic neuropathy[18–22,33,39] (Figs. 8-3 and 8-4).

Patients not exhibiting signs or symptoms of ocular thyroidopathy will often display systemic clues indicating the onset of Graves disease. Weight loss despite increased appetite, nervousness, palpitations, tachycardia at rest, systemic hypertension, and hyperreflexia are indicators of potential onset[22,30,31,33] (Table 8-6).

Ocular Sequelae and Differential Diagnosis

The American Thyroid Association along with Werner[47] have classified the stages of orbital Graves disease. The classes range from 0 to 6 and can easily

Normal orbital anatomy

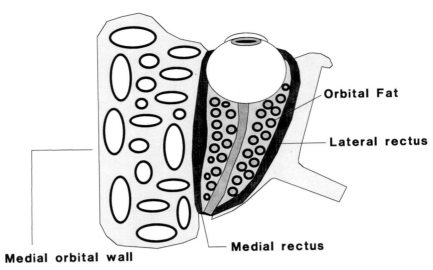

Fig. 8-3. Normal ocular anatomy within the orbit.

be remembered with the mnemonic NO SPECS[22,47] (Table 8-7).

The common ocular signs associated with thyroid eye disease multiply and progress over the course of the disease. The earliest signs include conjunctival injection and mild corneal stippling. As the disease advances, the conjunctiva becomes chemotic, the eyelids become edematous, and extraocular muscle involvement ensues, causing secondary eyelid retraction (Dalrymple sign)[22,25,30,31] and upper lid lag on down gaze (von Graefe sign).[22,25,29,31] In addition, tremor of the closed eyelid (Rosenbach sign)[21,25,30,31] and infrequent blinking (Stellwag sign)[21,24,29] (L.

Graves ophthalmopathy

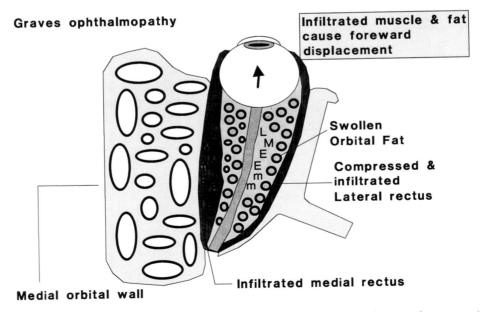

Fig. 8-4. Abnormal, congested contents of mucopolysaccharide-laden extraocular muscles as seen in Graves ophthalmology. M, mucopolysaccharides; m, macrophages; L, lymphocytes; E, edema.

Table 8-6. Common Causes and Signs/Symptoms of Thyrotoxicosis

Common causes of thyrotoxicosis (in decreasing frequency)
  Graves disease
  Toxic nodular goiter
  Thyroiditis
  Coinet's disease (iodine-induced thyrotoxicosis)
  Excessive gonadotropin secretion (choriocarcinoma)
  Excessive TSH secretion
Common signs and symptoms
  Nervousness
  Sweating/heat intolerance
  Goiter
  Eye signs
  Palpations/tachycardia/forceful cardiac impulse
  Fatigue
  Weight loss
  Increased appetite
  Brisk reflexes
  Systemic hypertension
  Gynecomastia

Table 8-8. Eye Signs Commonly Associated With Graves Ophthalmopathy

Name	Definition
Ballet sign	Paralysis of one or more extraocular muscles
Dalrymple sign	Upper eyelid retraction
Enruth sign	Edema of the lower eyelid
Gifford sign	Difficulty with upper eyelid eversion
Griffith sign	Lower lid lag on upward gaze
Knie sign	Uneven pupil dilation in dim illumination
Kocher sign	Spasmatic retraction of the upper eyelid during prolonged fixation
Means sign	Increased superior scleral show upgaze
Payne/Trousseau sign	Dislocation of globe
Rosenbach sign	Tremor of gently closed eyelids
Suker's sign	Inability to maintain fixation on extreme lateral gaze
Stellwag sign	Incomplete and infrequent blinking
von Graefe sign	Upper eyelid lag on downgaze

(Adapted from Char,[25] with permission.)

Lombardi, personal communication, 1993) may be present along with other signs[22,25,30,31] (Table 8-8).

The etiology and evolution of the eyelid lag and associated orbitopathy are well understood. Enlargement of the retrobulbar tissues, adenexal fat, and muscles result in forward distension of the globe (proptosis).[22,33–39,45]

Several other notable entities also can produce proptosis. The optometrist should be careful to exclude orbital neoplasm, inflammatory pseudotumor, vascular anomalies (carotid cavernous sinus fistula), and orbital encephalocele.[22]

Because there are several causes of eyelid retraction, differential diagnosis is essential. Included in the differential diagnosis are Graves ophthalmopathy, aber-

rant regeneration of cranial nerve III, unilateral ptosis with contralateral overaction of the levator, and Parinaud syndrome, sometimes referred to as *dorsal midbrain syndrome* or *sylvian aqueduct syndrome* with eyelid refraction on downgaze, known as Collier's lid sign (Table 8-9).

Dorsal midbrain syndrome develops secondary to lesions of the subcortical brain centers for vertical gaze. The most common cause is tumor of the pineal gland.[45] The lesion is associated with inability to converge,[45] bilateral lid retraction without lag on downgaze, Collier's lid sign,[22,45] convergence retraction nystagmus on attempted upward gaze[22] and middilated pupils, fixed to light but reactive to the near synkinesis. This characteristic is never found in

Table 8-7. Mnemonic for Orbital Graves Disease

Numerical Class	Mnemonic Letter	Definition
0	N	No signs, no symptoms
1	O	Only signs, no symptoms
2	S	Soft tissue involvement
3	P	Proptosis
4	E	Extraocular muscle involvement
5	C	Corneal involvement
6	S	Sight loss secondary to optic nerve involvement

Table 8-9. Non-neoplastic Conditions with Eye Signs that May Mimic Thyroid Ophthalmopathy

Myopia
Dorsal midbrain syndrome (Parinaud syndrome); posterior commisure lesions
Congenital anomalies
Side effects of systemic medication (e.g., steroids or lithium)
Hydrocephalus
Cushing syndrome
Chronic obstructive pulmonary disease
Uremia
Sympathomimetic medications (e.g., cocaine)
Cranial nerve III lesions
Status after eyelid surgery

Grave's ophthalmopathy. The vertical gaze impairment is supranuclear in nature. This allows reflex pathways such as Doll's head rotations or Bell's reflex phenomenon to move the eyes.[22] This sign has tremendous diagnostic value because patients with thyroid eye disease have mechanical eye restrictions. Therefore, they cannot move their eyes either voluntarily or reflexively.

The mechanical restrictions affecting the musculature also affect the elastic soft tissues of the orbit. This makes moving the eye by force (mechanical forced duction testing) and eversion of the eyelid (Gifford sign) difficult[22] (Fig. 8-5).

As previously mentioned, the optometrist should complete a thorough examination with extensive history, extraocular muscle motilities, pupil testing, color vision (acquired deficits may indicate compressive optic neuropathy), confrontational visual fields, tonometry (an elevation of 4 mm in upgaze is positive for Graves ophthalmopathy, secondary to congestion),[22] and dilated fundoscopy.

Any pertinent findings regarding extraocular muscles or subjective complaints of diplopia must be quantitatively recorded. This is evaluated most easily using traditional prism-cover testing.[22] If necessary, forced

duction testing may be completed by administering topical anesthesia and then placing either cotton-tipped applicators or forceps on the conjunctiva over the lateral recti and attempting movement of the eyes. The optometrist should take care to "feel" for, as well as observe restriction.

Evaluation of the eyelids should include measurement of the palpebral fissures and notes on lid lag, lagophthalmus, and restrictions. One method of determining the nature of eyelid posture is by comparing present observations to old photographs or a driver's license. Proptosis should be accurately measured by Hertel or Lute exophthalmometry. Readings greater than 22 mm or asymmetry greater than 3 mm are positive. Sergott and Glaser[22] suggest taking two readings, the first with the patient seated and the second with the patient supine. Normal eyes settle into the orbit by approximately 3 mm. Graves eyes do not settle more than 1 mm[22] (Fig. 8-6).

Anterior segment findings associated with Graves ophthalmopathy include conjunctival injection, punctate-type keratitis, exposure keratopathy, and decreased lacrimal gland function. Schirmer's tear test should be performed. This procedure is best done by instilling one drop of topical anesthetic into both eyes, then placing the tear strips into the inferior palpebral

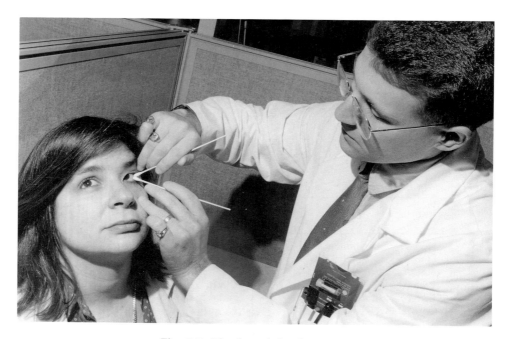

Fig. 8-5. The forced duction text.

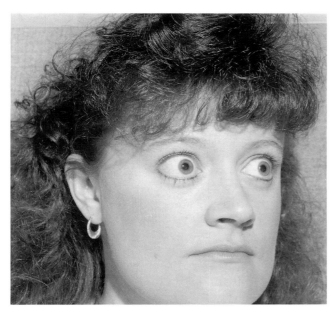

Fig. 8-6. The pathoneumonic eyelid stare of Graves ophthalmopathy and exophthalmometry.

fissure for 5 minutes.[22,33] Positive results at levels measured at under 7 mm indicate a lack of wetting. If compressive ophthalmopathy is suspected, Goldmann or automated threshold visual fields should be obtained. Paracentral, arcuate, or enlarged blind-spot scotomas are considered positive findings.[22,33]

Myasthenia gravis is often associated with, or mimics, thyroid disease. In appropriate cases, ice pack testing or tensilon injection should be considered. CT scanning and magnetic resonance imaging (MRI) are extremely useful in viewing enlarged orbital muscles.[22,33,36,37,44,45,48] Typically, the posterior third of the muscular belly is enlarged near the orbital apex. This can lead to compression of the optic nerve as it exits the optic foramen. The optometrist should order axial and coronal views of the brain and orbit, in 1- to 1.5-mm sections, near the apex.[33]

A- and B-scan ultrasonography are also useful, noninvasive, diagnostic modalities by which extraocular muscle changes may be documented.[22,35] Clinically involved eyes show enlarged muscles, whereas non-Graves eyes do not. The enlarged muscles can be consistently measured with A-scan ultrasonography.[35] This is extremely useful for distinguishing patients with proptosis secondary to thyroid eye disease from patients with intraorbital mass or fistula.[22] A specific

test for evaluating the optic nerve for increased fluid and infiltration is called the *30-degree test*,[33] in which B-scan ultrasonography is performed with the patient's eye turned approximately 30 degrees. In Graves ophthalmopathy, the nerve may appear larger, infiltrated, and swollen. This is considered a positive 30-degree test. Typically, solid masses do not provide this appearance, giving a negative 30-degree test.

Finally, consideration should be given to other disease entities that may result in unilateral or bilateral exophthalmos and ocular motility restriction. The differential diagnoses include adjoining sinus cavity tumors invading the orbit by direct extension, orbital pseudotumor, Hashimoto's thyroiditis, superior orbital fissure syndrome of the Tolosa Hunt type (acute inflammatory syndrome with painful ophthalmoplegia), and idiopathic myositis (Table 8-9).

Stages of Graves Ophthalmopathy

Graves ophthalmopathy presents with a wide spectrum of clinical manifestations. The symptoms may be as mild as dry eye and the "Graves stare" or as severe as vision loss from optic nerve compression. A further source of confusion is the sometimes equivocal role of the thyroid gland, compounded by various complications of therapies.

Class 0

Patients in class 0 have diagnosed Graves disease without signs of ophthalmopathy. Why some patients are spared ophthalmic complications is poorly understood, but these patients are not assured of such absence from signs forever. Even with the absence of symptoms over the course of years, ophthalmopathy may eventually develop.[22]

Classes 1 and 2

Typically, classes 1 and 2 merge without distinct criteria for separation. Upper eyelid retraction may be present in one or both eyes, exposing the superior corneoscleral limbis. This gives these patients the characteristic "stare" or startled appearance. When the eyes pursue a slowly downwardly moving target, the eyelid (or eyelids) will "lag" behind. This is called *von Graefe sign*. The presence of these signs is highly suggestive of Graves ophthalmopathy. Symptomatology includes chronic intermittent tearing, infrequent blinking, foreign body sensation, and a dry or gritty sensation exacerbated by sleep.[22]

Class 3

Class 3 Graves ophthalmopathy signifies the first appearance of proptosis. It is marked by any exophthalmometry measurement greater than or equal to 22 mm in either eye. Typically, the proptosis is not an isolated finding but is accompanied by restrictive myopathy, lid retraction, and other congestive signs.[22]

Accurate quantitative assessment of proptosis can be accomplished by using either a Hertel or Lute exophthalmometer. Assessment can be difficult if the degree of proptosis is small. Sergott and Glaser[22] suggest that the method of choice for discerning smaller amounts of proptosis is by gentle displacement of the globes or by viewing the corneal apices from above the brow. Retrodisplacement and asymmetry between the orbits should also be assessed. Haver[49] suggested that exophthalmometry should be done with the patient in the seated and supine positions.[49] In the supine position, the globes settle into orbits as much as 3 mm.[22,49] This will not occur in the presence of orbital tumor and ophthalmopathy. Exophthalmometers are more useful for serial examinations of patients with proptosis.[22]

Asymmetric proptosis of more than 6 mm is extraordinary in Graves ophthalmopathy and suggests a unilateral retrobulbar tumor.[50]

Class 4

Class 4 ophthalmopathy typically requires a therapeutic program. Infiltration and inflammation of the extraocular muscles cause slowly progressive vertical or oblique diplopia. Occasionally, a mildly painful "pulling" sensation is noted on upgaze, especially during acutely active inflammatory phases.[22] Yoshikawa and co-workers[36] have noted that the four rectus muscles tend to exhibit the results of inflammation, with the inferior and medial rectus affected most frequently. They found a positive correlation between the enlargement of the recti and the occurrence of various eye signs and symptoms.[36]

An extremely helpful diagnostic physical finding is enlargement and injection of the extraocular muscle insertions. Proptosis at this stage is variable, with no notable correlation between the amount of proptosis and extent of extraocular myopathy. The crucial diagnostic test for class 4 ophthalmopathy is the forced duction test.[22,51,52] In this test, the optometrist either takes hold of the globe with forceps or pushes the globe with a cotton-tipped applicator, attempting to move the eye.

Another associated sign of class 4 disease is increased intraocular pressure in upward gaze as compared with the reading in straight gaze. This can be present even in eyes without ductional deficits. A rise of 4 mmHg or greater is a positive finding.[22,52]

Because carotid cavernous sinus fistula and orbital mass may cause similar signs and symptoms, radiographic or echographic studies should be considered. CT scanning, MRI, and ultrasonography have proven to be powerful diagnostic tools for the differentiation of Graves ophthalmopathy from clinical masqueraders such as carotid cavernous sinus fistula, mass lesions, and orbital hemangiomas.[22,53]

Class 5

In class 5 disease, proptosis approaches moderate-to-severe levels, and the cornea becomes threatened by chronic exposure keratitis. Lid retraction, infrequent blinking, poor tear adherence, and inability to close the lids even during sleep compound the difficulties. Corneal involvement may range from chronic dry eye to ulceration.[22]

Class 6

Class 6 ophthalmopathy is characterized by visual loss secondary to optic nerve involvement or permanent severe corneal disease.[22] The optometrist must make use of color perception, pupillary responses, and visual field analysis to obtain the correct diagnosis. Resultant field defects from class 6 disease are characterized by central scotomas (with reduced acuity) and inferior arcuate bundle defects. The optic disc may appear normal, edematous, or even pale in neglected cases.[22]

Ocular Therapies

The therapy for Graves ophthalmopathy classes 1 to 3 is supportive. Copious tear solutions and ointments will increase patient comfort and lubricate ocular structures. Patients with Graves disease who experience incomplete blinking or incomplete lid closure during sleep should wear a blindfold to bed, wear a Guibora moisture chamber patch, or tape the eyelid closed after the instillation of ointment. If excessive drying or corneal irritation persists, bandage contact lenses can be used.[33] One must be cautious to monitor the patient for compliance, because an unclean contact lens and compromised corneal epithelium make for a risky situation.

The common problem in class 4 thyroid eye disease is diplopia. This should be managed creatively and effectively after consultation with the patient. The alternatives range from fresnel press on prisms and single-vision yoked prism glasses for patients with patterned (A or V) syndromes to occlusion and lens frosting.[22]

Patients with class 5 thyroid eye disease present with proptosis and severe corneal involvement and must be managed with prudence. The chronically exposed cornea runs the risk of ulceration or opacification secondary to extreme dryness.[33] The ulcers that develop in these patients tend to be central and visually devastating. Prophylactic antibiotic ointments can be applied, in the morning and again at bedtime, to moisten, lubricate, and protect the cornea from microbial invasion, whereas drops are used throughout the daytime four times a day as needed.

Controlled destruction of the thyroid gland by radioactive iodine-131 is another means of thyroid regulation.[22,33,54,55] Radiotherapy may also be aimed at the extraocular muscles in an attempt to shrink their size and reduce orbital symptoms. This therapy, however, is not without risk. Miller, Goldberg, and Bullock[56] reported a case of a 65-year-old woman who had undergone orbital irradiation and developed radiation retinopathy, with intraretinal hemorrhages, cotton-wool infarcts, and exudation following the procedure.[56]

Whenever radiation is used on the thyroid, careful monitoring of thyroid status is critical because patients may develop *hypo*thyroidism, necessitating permanent thyroid replacement.[57,58]

In another study by Tallstedt and co-workers, radioactive iodine-131, was more likely to be followed by or precipitate exacerbation of Graves ophthalmopathy than other modes of antithyroid therapy.[57]

In acutely inflamed and uncomfortable orbital situations, extraocular muscular inflammation may be reduced with oral corticosteroids or surgery. Currently, no nonsteroidal anti-inflammatory regimen provides equivocal coverage. Oral corticosteroids are often most beneficial during their initial trial. Generally, they are not used until class 4 is diagnosed. Careful and tedious follow-up with slow reduction and dosage tapering must ensue. The typical initial dosage is 60 mg of prednisone daily. Improvements are often difficult to achieve after initial therapies despite larger dosages.[22] When improvements do come, they are generally seen within 4 to 12 weeks. Prolonged high-dose corticosteroid therapy therefore is ill advised and generally not done.[22]

Ironically, the best therapy, if possible, is supportive only. Despite the initial severity of advanced signs and symptoms, the inflammation tends to regress after 12 and 24 months.[22] Sergott and Glaser[22] suggest "that it is not inappropriate to simply let the orbitopathy spontaneously burn itself out."[22] This decision will ultimately require good eye care and health-care communications. Surgical removal of the thyroid is the final alternative. When corticosteroid therapies fail and spontaneous regression fails to occur, justification for surgical modalities is clear.

Supervoltage orbital irradiation (1600 to 2000 rads delivered to the orbital apex) offers the first and least-invasive alternative for patients who do not respond to steroids or patients who cannot use steroids (e.g., diabetics, hypertensives).[22]

Older[37] advocated a surgical approach for the treatment of thyroid-related eyelid retraction. With greater degrees of eyelid retraction, corneal exposure is increased, especially at night, leading to symptoms of epiphora and irritation. As corneal compromise approaches critical levels, visual acuity may become threatened or lost. The surgical principle for the correction of eyelid retraction is to weaken the elevating forces of Müller's muscle and the levator palpebrae superioris by recessing the levator aponeurosis and Müller's muscle through a lid crease incision. During this type of procedure, patients are not sedated and can sit up. This way, final eyelid position can be determined using the patient's natural posture. This type of surgical technique has virtually eliminated overcorrections and undercorrections.[37,58,59]

In extreme cases, when vision is threatened and all other modalities fail, surgical decompression of the orbit is used. The Krönlein (lateral orbitotomy) procedure, with controlled floor fracture is the most commonly performed procedure.[22] The floor removal, ethmoidal fracture, and maxillary sinus (Ogura) approach is a rarely used alternative.[22] Although surgical decompression is seemingly radical, visual recovery following these procedures is well documented. A new method of two-walled decompression may be on the horizon. Leone et al[48] have obtained some excellent outcomes using this new procedure, which enters the orbit through the eyelid, with far fewer complications. The principle complication associated with bony orbital decompressions is ocular dystopia (displacement) with inferomedial displacement caused by movement of the muscle cone and orbital connective tissue into the maxillary and ethmoidal sinuses.[44–69] Fortunately, there are surgical techniques and procedures that minimize and correct for this complication.[69,70]

Systemic Management

The systemic management of thyrotoxicosis lies within the domain of the neurologist and the endocrinologist.[68] Medical, radionuclear, and surgical therapies are three approaches to the management of hyperthyroidism. The medical approach uses agents that block the synthesis of thyroid hormone, such as propylthiouracil (Tapazole). Propranolol (Inderal) is often used adjunctively to control the hypermetabolic symptoms.

Other medical treatment modalities operate on the assumption that the disorder is a consequence of an autoimmune process.[30,60,61] Under these auspices, treatment attempts to modify the autoimmune response. Various therapeutic trials have been reported, including systemic corticosteroids,[46,63] retrobulbar steroids,[46,62] supervoltage orbital radiation,[22,42,64] azathioprine,[39,65] cyclophosphamide,[39,66] cyclosporine,[39,67] plasmapheresis, and thyroid ablation.[39,68]

The effectiveness of combination treatment involving corticosteroids and orbital irradiation cannot be disputed; however, this therapeutic approach sometimes fails because of unacceptable side effects. Several investigators have reported promising results in the treatment of Graves ophthalmopathy with high doses of intravenous γ-globulin.[39] The mechanisms by which intravenous γ-globulin works are unclear. Hypotheses include blockade in the course of inflamma-

Table 8-10. Thyroid Eye Disease Quick Reference

Class	Signs and Symptoms	Treatment
0	No ocular signs; patients may undergo weight loss with increased appetite, nervousness, palpitation, tachycardia at rest, and systolic hypertension	Referral to GP for blood work; rule out systemic hypertension, diabetes; no ocular modalities
1	Systemically, patients may suffer from increased anxiety; ocularly, mild periorbital edema, startled or staring look; mild corneal stippling inferiorly	Copious artificial tear solutions and ointments; monitor for progression
2	Lid retraction (Darymple sign), increased stare, possibly unilateral proptosis, lid lag (von Graefe sign), dry eye with gritty sensation, more corneal compromise	Copious artificial tear solutions and ointments; more ointment may now be necessary; supportive patient education; consult GP for possibility of initiating systemic therapy
3	Proptosis, positive >22 mm, increased lid retraction; restrictive myopathy; positive forced duction test; difficulty everting eyelid (Gifford sign); decreased blink posture (Stellwag sign)	Copious artificial tear solutions and ointments; depending on the severity of the blink posture, moisture chamber patches, blindfolds, or lid taping may be required
4	Extraocular muscle involvement increases; more restriction leads to intermittent diplopia that is slowly progressive; positive forced duction testing; intraocular pressure rises by ≥4 mm on upward gaze; positive 30-degree test on A-B scan	Referral to GP to initiate systemic corticosteroid therapy, 40–80 mg/daily; Fresnel press on prisms or occlusive therapy to eliminate diplopia; consider partial surgical removal of thyroid
5	Corneal epithelium is compromised and threatened by proptosis; ulceration is possible; severe dryness	More corneal support; may require antibiotic ointments; if dryness threatens to provoke permanent visual disability, consider tarsorrophy; may try increased steroid dosage 40–100 mg)
6	Compressive sight loss secondary to orbital congestion; central, paracentral, and arcuate scotomata apparent	Surgical innervation required; supervoltage orbital irradiation (1,600–2,000 rad) directed toward the orbital apex; orbital decompression as a last resort, Krönlean, Ogura, two wall[48]

Abbreviation: GP, general practitioner.

tion, provision of an undetected antibody that counteracts the causal agent in Graves disease, or suppression of the immune system by anti-iodotype antibodies[39] (Table 8-10).

DISORDERS OF THE PINEAL GLAND

The pineal gland (pineal epiphysis) is an endocrine gland that is shaped like a pine cone and arises from the roof of the third ventricle under the posterior portion of the corpus callosum and is connected by a stalk to the posterior commisure[71,72] (Fig. 8-7). The gland itself is currently under investigation for its purpose and function. Some have hypothesized that it plays a role in delaying the onset of puberty; however, most current research focuses on the gland's production of melatonin.[72] Melatonin is present in cerebrospinal fluid and in plasma but has no established function in mammals.[72]

The pineal gland becomes calcified around age 13 in humans, producing small concretions of calcium, phosphate, and carbonate called *pineal sand*.[72] Because these concretions are radiopaque, the pineal gland is visible on radiographs of the skull in 75 percent of adults.[71] This allows the pineal gland to serve as a useful neuroradiologic and neurosurgical landmark.[71,72] Charts that reveal its usual position on lateral skull radiographs are used to diagnose its displacement in patients with suspected expanding intracranial lesions.[71,72]

Pinealoma and Dorsal Midbrain Syndrome

Pinealoma is a tumor growth of the pineal gland resulting in a collection of symptoms, commonly known as the dorsal midbrain syndrome (Parinaud syndrome and Sylvian aqueduct syndrome are terms synonymous with dorsal midbrain syndrome).[70] Marked by internal neuromuscular mechanisms, this disease causes hypertonicity and paresis of pupillary constriction, paresis of accommodation, weakness of convergence, restriction of vertical gaze with globe retraction, upbeat nystagmus on upgaze, and Collier's eyelid retraction.[73-75]

Pinealoma is the most common lesion producing the "Parinaud-plus" syndrome, characterized by hypocephalus, headache, and papilledema.[73,74] Mass lesions involving the periaqueductal gray matter arise from the third ventricle quadrigeminal plate, supracollicular subarachnoid space, or falcotentorium.[73] As the mass enlarges, the aqueduct becomes obstructed, internal hydrocephalus develops, and headache and papilledema appear.[43] In addition to pinealoma, other neoplasms, vascular occlusions, arteriovenous malformation, demyelinating disease, aqueductal stenosis, aneurysms of the posterior fossa inflammations, infections, and trauma have all been associated with the dorsal midbrain syndrome.[73,74]

Patients who present with dorsal midbrain syndrome may range from adolescent to adult.[73,75] They often present with a chief complaint of frequent headache

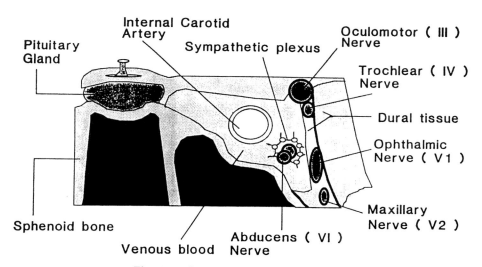

Fig. 8-7. Cavernous sinus anatomy.

and diplopia on upward gaze. On examination, the optometrist should be sure to carefully check extraocular muscle motilities. In dorsal midbrain syndrome, upward gaze is typically affected, with complete preservation of downward movement.[69] This helps to rule out other causes of ophthalmoplegia such as Graves disease, myasthenia gravis, and verticle supranuclear ophthalmoplegias associated with metabolic disorders such as Niemann-Pick and Wilson's disease.[73] Attempts at upward saccades produce variable degrees of convergence and retraction nystagmus. Examination and evaluation of the pupils reveal a mid-dilated pupillary posture that is sluggish to respond to light but constricts to near-point stimuli. This is called *light-near dissociation response*.[73,75] This should be differentiated from the small, irregularly shaped, unreactive, Argyll-Robertson pupils associated with syphilis. Other diseases that cause Argyll-Robertson-like pupils include long-standing diabetes mellitus, brain stem encephalitis, and chronic alcoholism.[75] Finally, Glaser and Bachynski[73] identify "pseudo-abducens palsy," which has a potential finding of slower movement of the abducting eye than the adducting eye during horizontal saccades.

Diagnosis and Treatment

The diagnosis of dorsal midbrain syndrome is effectively made using techniques of neuroimaging. Vascular, infections, and inflammatory etiologies may be uncovered with standard blood testing. Radiographs, CT, and MRI are all effective. These syndromes require the removal of the underlying cause. Referral to the neurosurgeon is the most appropriate course of action. Tumors are typically shrunk by radiation. Aneurysms and arteriovenus malformations are surgically clipped, whereas infections, inflammations and other etiologies (e.g., vascular) are treated with combinations of medical therapies.

DISORDERS OF THE ADRENAL GLANDS

The adrenal glands (paired suprarenal glands) are small, 3 to 5 cm long, triangular organs that lie on each side of the vertebral column against the upper pole of the corresponding kidney.[2,76–78] Each gland consists of two parts, the cortex and the medulla, each with its own specific function. The cortex is regulated by adrenocorticotropic hormone (ACTH), which is secreted by the adenopophysis of the pituitary gland and is responsible for producing three classes of steroids. Glucocorticoids (e.g., hydrocortisone), mineralocorticoids (e.g., aldosterone), and the sex steroids (e.g., androgens and estrogens) are synthesized by the adrenal cortex.[76] The adrenal medulla is largely controlled by the sympathetic nervous system and is responsible for the secretion of the catecholamines epinephrine and norepinephrine.[76]

Cushing Syndrome

An adrenal cortex that becomes hyperactive in its secretion of the glucocorticoids will give rise to the clinical state of hypercortisolism, known as Cushing syndrome.[75–80] There is no predilection for age; however, women seem to be more affected than men.[3] Patients who present with Cushing syndrome are characterized by their unique attributes which include truncal obesity, round, moon faces, muscle weakness, muscle wasting, hirsutism, acne, osteoporosis, purple striae and systemic hypertension.[75–78] Accompanying metabolic disorders include sodium retention, potassium loss, and impaired glucose tolerance (overt diabetes mellitus).[76] The disease is not usually associated with pituitary neoplasm, but rather, with a poorly understood malfunction at both ends of the pituitary axis. Functioning adrenal and pituitary tumors may also give rise to the disorder.

Several consistent ocular features are associated with Cushing syndrome. Increased intraocular pressure occurs in up to 25 percent of the Cushing syndrome population. This may represent an inherited sensitivity to the effects of systemic steroids and increases the risk of glaucomatous losses.[76,81] There is some controversy in this area. Although Haas and Nootens,[81] Robbin and Haas,[82] and others[83,84] have reported cases of increased intraocular pressure and glaucomatous damage in association with Cushing syndrome, Jonas and co-workers[85] suggest that is less frequently encountered. Surprisingly, although posterior subcapsular opacities are well-documented complications of long-term exogenous corticosteroid therapy, they are not commonly associated complications of Cushing syndrome.[75,76] Exophthalmos, along with dry-eye related irritations have been reported in 6 to 9 percent of Cushing syndrome patients.[76,86,87] Dry-eye related symptoms are associated with these ocular proptosis rather than lack of tear production.

The most severe of the ocular complications result from the onset of systemic diabetes and hypertension

Table 8-11. Hypertensive Retinopathy

Stages
1. Arteriole narrowing, beginning arteriosclerosis changes
2. Localized vessel dilation and constrictions, marked changes at vessel crossings, flame-shaped hemorrhages, and dot and blot hemorrhages, exudates, mascular star appearance
3. Hemorrhages and lipid exudates, cotton-wool spots
4. All signs of grade III plus papilledema

Quick reference of ocular and systemic sequelae
Kidney disease
Diabetes
Venous occlusive disorders
Collagen vascular conditions
Vitreous hemorrhage
Cerebrovascular disease
Stroke

(Table 8-11). The most obvious complication of systemic hypertension is hypertensive retinopathy.[88] Arteriolar changes are produced because of increased intraluminal pressure. This results in the vessels' narrowing, sometimes to a diameter so thin they appear thread-like. Arteriolosclerosis, or fibrosis and scarring of the vessel walls and perivascular tissues, occurs as a secondary complication to increased vascular stress, throughout the fundus and body.[88] As this sclerosis proceeds, the ocular vessels encounter focal attenuations and constrictions and change color, to provide the often referred to "copper wire" or "silver wire" appearance; these vessels eventually either break, causing familiar flame-shaped hemorrhages, or impinge on veins, causing venous occlusions.[88] As small vessel narrowing progresses, additional flame-shaped nerve fiber layer hemorrhages will become apparent along with ischemic nerve fiber layer infarcts, known as cotton-wool spots.[88] The culmination of severe, malignant hypertension is neuroretinal edema. This is an ocular emergency. However, it is a rare occurrence in patients with Cushing syndrome, because these patients are often diagnosed and managed long before this level of severity. The neuro-ocular symptoms of hypertension such as oculomotor, trochlear, and abduscens nerve palsy therefore are often avoided. (For more information on the ocular manifestations of hypertension, see Ch. 13.)

Management for the ocular complications of Cushing's disease is removal of the underlying cause. A referral should ultimately be made to an endocrinologist. The diagnosis of Cushing syndrome is made by measuring the amount of metabolized cortisol (17-OHCS) in the urine using the Porter-Silber method.

Patients with Cushing syndrome have elevated levels that are greater than 16 mg/24 hr (normal, 3 to 10 mg/24 hr).[3] The administration of 1 mg of dexamethasone orally at 11 to 12 PM with measurement of plasma cortisol at 7 to 8 AM the following morning is a group screening test for Cushing syndrome and is called the dexamethasone suppression test.[3] In most normal patients, the levels of plasma cortisol are suppressed, whereas patients with Cushing syndrome continue to secrete undiminished levels of cortisol.[3]

The endocrinologist will direct therapy at correcting the hyperfunction at the appropriate level in the pituitary axis (the pituitary gland or adrenal cortex).[3] The precise approach will depend on the exact physiologic abnormality but may range from pituitary irradiation to the removal of diseased adrenal tissue.[3]

Neuroblastoma

Neuroblastoma is a malignant tumor of the adrenal medulla.[76] It is one of the more common malignancies of infancy and childhood.[76] Most of these tumors arise from the adrenal medulla and present initially as abdominal masses. They tend to metastasize early by circulatory and lymphatic routes, making it common for a distant lesion to be the first evidence of the disease. The site of metastasis usually determines the symptoms; most patients note a pale color, fever, diarrhea, weight loss, and pain in the bones. Many of these tumors cause excessive secretion of catecholamines resulting in systemic hypertension.

Neuroblastoma is of concern to the eye physician because metastasis to the orbit occurs in 35 to 55 percent of cases.[76,89,90] The most frequent presenting sign is proptosis. A more unique clinical sign, however, is unexplained, unilateral eyelid ecchymosis (present in 50 percent of cases).[76] This is caused by tumor tissue that is highly vascular and necrotic. When this combination of signs presents in the absence of more common possibilities, such as trauma and blood disease, neuroblastoma should be ruled out. Horner syndrome (ptosis, melosis, facial anhydrosis) in an infant younger than 2 years of age is also suggestive of neuroblastoma arising from the upper thoracic or cervical sympathetic ganglia.[76,90] Finally, hypertensive retinopathy, optic atrophy, and papilledema, especially in the young, are additional signs of metastasis to the orbit or skull.[76,89]

The optometrist's responsibility, whenever intracranial mass is on the list of differential diagnoses, is to gather data using the available techniques. This includes extraocular muscle motilities, observing for restrictions; visual field testing, looking for atrophic or compressive field cuts; exophthalmometry, measuring for any proptosis (abnormal readings are greater than 22 mm or 6 to 8 mm of difference between the two eyes); and dilated fundus observation, using direct and indirect ophthalmoscopy to look for suspicious, pigmented, or raised lesions.

General laboratory testing should include standard blood work, neuroimaging, and urine analysis. A helpful diagnostic test to rule out neuroblastoma is the measurement of urinary catecholamines, particularly vanillylmandelic acid (VMA). This can be done directly by the ocular physician or coordinated through a doctor of internal medicine. Generally, when diagnosed, the prognosis is guarded. The treatment for neuroblastoma is chemotherapy using vincristine and cyclophosphamide.[3]

Pheochromocytoma

Pheochromocytoma is a less than common tumor that arises from chromaffin cells of the sympathetic nervous system and is mainly found (80 percent) in the adrenal medulla.[3,76] These tumors may appear at any age but are most common in the third to sixth decades. There is no predilection for sex; they are bilateral (both glands) in 10 percent of adults and in 20 percent of children; they are benign 95 percent of the time.[3,76] Pheochromocytomas vary in size, averaging only 5 to 6 cm in diameter. The clinical presentation is caused by increased catecholamine secretion and includes bouts of sweating, palpitations, tachycardia, headache, tremors, and pale skin color.[3,76] Arterial hypertension is the major clinical sign and may occur at either intermittent or sustained patterns.[3,75,76]

Ocular findings in patients with pheochromocytoma are essentially those of hypertensive retinopathy, such as flame-shaped hemorrhages, exudates, cotton-wool spots, engorged, irregular veins, narrowed, tortuous arteries, and in severe cases, papilledema.[3,75,76] These changes are mainly observed in patients with the sustained patterns of hypertension.

Pheochromocytoma has a significant incidence of association with most of the phakomatoses, which present with a plethora of ocular manifestations. The associated phakomatoses include neurofibromatosis (von

Recklinghausen's disease, found in 5 percent of patients with pheochromocytoma, characterized by multiple tumors of the skin, central nervous system, café-au-lait spots and tumors of the optic nerve); Sturge-Weber disease (marked by port wine angiomas of the skin and infantile glaucoma); angiomatoses retinae (von Hippel-Lindau syndrome characterized by sixth-decade dilation and tortuosity of retinal vessels resulting in angiomas of the retina, massive exudation, and retinal detachment); and tuberous sclerosis (Bourneville's disease, marked by adenoma sebaceum, central nervous system tumors, retinal tumors, and renal tumors).[3,13,75,76]

Any patient who presents with severe hypertensive retinopathy or any of the phakomatoses should be tested for pheochromocytomas. The diagnosis is usually not apparent on physical examination. Urine analysis testing for urinary metabolic produces of norepinephrine and epinephrine such as metanephrines and VMA is diagnostic.[3,76] Radiography and neuroimaging have some localizing value but should be carefully ordered by an expert. The treatment of choice is surgical removal of the tumor or tumors.[3] As catecholamine levels fall, hypertensive fundus changes tend to reverse and resolve.[3,76]

Addison's Disease

Addison's disease is a progressive disease resulting from adrenocortical hypofunction.[3,4,77] Nearly 70 percent of cases are due to idiopathic atrophy of the adrenal cortex. The remaining 30 percent of cases are the result of partial destruction of the gland by granuloma (e.g., tuberculosis), neoplasm, amyloidosis, or inflammation.[3,4,77]

Addison's disease manifests many symptoms as a result of aldosterone deficiency. Presenting signs and symptoms include weakness, fatigue, increased pigmentation, and excessive tanning; black freckles over the forehead, face, and neck; areas of vitiligo; weight loss; and hypotension.[3,4,77] The only associated ocular finding is papilledema, which results on rare occasions from raised intracranial pressure. Therefore, Addison's disease should be ruled out in patients who present with similar clinical signs and disc edema.

Diagnosis is typically based on skin hyperpigmentation, blood chemistries, hematologic testing, and radiographs that reveal adrenal calcifications or evidence of a small heart. Referrals to the endocrinologists or doctor of internal medicine are appropriate. Prognosis is excellent when diagnosis is provided early. The treatment for Addison's disease is hormone substitution therapy. As the systemic disease is controlled, ocular signs and symptoms will begin to show improvement.[3,75]

DISORDERS OF THE PITUITARY GLAND

Anatomy

The pituitary gland (hypophysis) is a 0.5-g mass of tissue that lies within a concavity of the sphenoid bone called the *sella turcica* (Latin, *Sella*, "saddle"; hence, Turkish saddle) and is connected to the base of the brain by a thin piece of tissue called the pituitary stalk[5,71,76,91] (Fig. 8-7). Inferiorly, the gland is separated from the sphenoid sinuses by a thin layer of bone. Laterally, the walls of the sella turcica adjoin the cavernous sinuses, each of which contains an internal carotid artery, sympathetics, and cranial nerves III, IV, V (V1 and V2), and VI.[91] Superiorly, the roof of the sella turcica is formed by the diaphragma sellae, an extension of the dura mater.[91] The optic chiasm lies superiorly to, or above the pituitary gland and 8 to 13 mm above the diaphragma sellae. Therefore, in addition to changes that result from endocrinologic disease, any lesion of the pituitary that affects the optic chiasm or cavernous sinus by compression, lateral extension, invasion, or inferior extension will result in ophthalmic and neuro-ocular sequelae.[6,71, 76,91–102]

Visual Pathway

A complete understanding of the visual pathway and anatomy of the optic chiasm is necessary to completely comprehend the opthalmic sequellae associated with space-occupying pituitary lesions (Fig. 8-8). The visual field has an inverted relationship to its anatomic components. That is, retinal and optic nerve axons located superiorly are associated with the inferior visual field, whereas axons located inferiorly are associated with the superior visual field. Those axons located nasally are associated with the temporal visual field, and axons located temporally correspond to the nasal visual field.[14,95]

The approximately 1.1 million retinal axons from each eye join to form the optic nerves. The optic nerves exit the globe through the posterior scleral foramina and course 25 to 30 mm through the muscle cone and superior optical fissure to join its counterpart at the optic chiasm.[92,95] The optic chiasm is the "crossroads" of the visual sensory system, containing approximately 2.2 to 2.4 million afferent axons. No other portion of the visual pathway offers a better opportunity for exact correlation between anatomy and function. The very architecture of the nerve fiber patterns is responsible for the characteristic changes seen in visual fields that are pathonomonic for this area alone. Binocular vision begins in the chiasm; hence, it is the first portion of the visual pathway, where a single lesion produces simultaneous defects in both visual fields.[94] The chiasm therefore is closely concerned with study of five major medical disciplines: neurosurgery, neurology, endocrinology, ophthalmology, and optometry. The inferior portion of the chiasm is usually 8 to 13 mm above the diaphragma sellae or clinoid processes. It is therefore important to stress that mass lesions of the pituitary gland need not necessarily extend into the confines of the chiasm itself.[93] The corollary is, that small tumors of the pituitary and associated tissues may only offer the signs of unilateral optic nerve damage or endocrinologic symptoms.[93] Furthermore, the presence of chiasmal visual field defects indicates the presence of a mass with advanced supersellar extension.[93]

The chiasm serves as a decussation for afferent retinal axons. Following this crossing, the visual pathway continues with the optic tract. Each optic tract contains visual fibers that represent both eyes. The right optic tract contains the temporal axons of the right eye (right nasal field) and the nasal axons of the left eye (left temporal field). The left optic tract contains the temporal axons of the left eye (left nasal field) and the nasal axons of the right eye (right temporal field). Using this description, one can see that lesions that include the chiasm and lesions posterior to the chiasm produce visual field defects that occur in both eyes simultaneously. As an example, a lesion of the left optic tract would produce a right homonymous hemianopia (left temporal axons, right nasal field loss, left eye, right nasal axons, right temporal field loss, right eye).

Finally, each optic tract courses along the base of the hypothalamus gland posteriorly to its corresponding lateral geniculate nucleus. Before synapsing there, approximately 20 percent of these fibers detour to the midbrain, where they aid in controlling the pupil. Cell bodies from the lateral geniculate nuclei give rise to

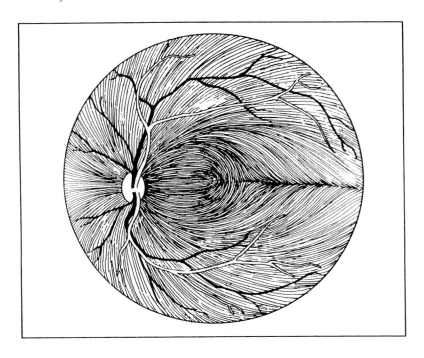

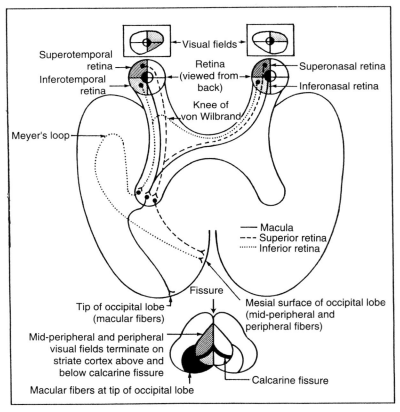

Fig. 8-8. Schematic of the visual pathway.

the geniculocalcerine tracts and optic radiations, which fan into portions of the temporal and parietal lobes while coursing posteriorly to Broadmann areas 17, 18, and 19 in the occipital cortex.[91-95]

Pituitary Physiology

The pituitary gland is composed of two divisions that are distinct in embryonic origin, histologic composition, and functional relationship to the hypothalamus.[5,104] The neurohypophysis (posterior lobe) is composed primarily of neural tissue and is separated from the adenohypophysis (anterior lobe) by a residual lumen known during development as Rathke's pouch.[5,104] The two principle hormones secreted from the neurohypophysis are antidiuretic hormone (ADH), sometimes called vasopressin, and oxytocin. ADH plays an important role in maintaining fluid and electrolyte homeostasis, whereas oxytocin causes the initiation of milk ejection from the breast and uterine smooth muscle contraction.[5,103,104]

The adenohypophysis secretes seven prominent hormones. ACTH, TSH, follicle-stimulating hormone (FSH), and leutenizing hormone (LH) work by targeting other endocrine glands and initiating them to start or stop a particular action. Growth hormone (GH) and prolactin effect body growth and sexual characteristics, and melanocyte-stimulating hormone (MSH) effects pigment-containing melanocytes of the epidermus.

The hypothalamic–pituitary axis (Fig. 8-9) is governed by the central nervous system through a wide variety of environmental and internal stimuli. In the presence of overproduction, underproduction, a lack of feedback control, or an absence of one of these chemical messengers, a wide variety of interrelated abnormalities produce disease, symptoms, and sequellae.[5,97,104] In general, diseases of the pituitary gland precipitate two types of symptomatic disturbances. The first is mechanical, for example, compression or invasion of structures adjacent to the gland. The second is hormonal, such as an increase or decrease in the secretory activity of the gland, with corresponding effects on target organs. This section concentrates on ocular sequellae of these hormonal effects on target organs.

Tumors That Affect the Pituitary Gland

Craniopharyngioma

Craniopharyngiomas are a group of tumors arising from the epithelial remnants of Rathke's pouch (80 percent of the population is estimated to have such remnants) and are characteristically seen between the ages of 10 and 25 years.[92,94] Occasionally, however, they are found in adults in the fifth and sixth decades of life.[92,94] They usually suprasellar (above the sella turcica); however, they are occasionally intrasellar. The signs and symptoms associated with craniopharyngiomas vary tremendously with the age of the patient and the exact location of the tumor as well as its growth rate.[92] Suprasellar craniopharyngiomas typically cause asymmetric chiasmal compressions, resulting in asymmetric bitemporal visual field defects. Optic disc edema is another associated finding. Pituitary deficiency may result, and involvement of the hypothalamus may cause systemic disturbances such as diabetes insipidus or stunted growth.[92] Treatment consists of removal where possible. In many cases, evacuation of the growing cystic contents is the only possible treatment.

Suprasellar Meningiomas

The most frequent tumors affecting the anterosuperior aspect of the optic chiasm are the meningiomas. These tumors may arise from the olfactory groove, tuberculum sellae (sella turcica), or lesser wing of the sphenoid bone.[94] Small meningiomas, pituitary adenomas, craniopharyngiomas and astrocytomas may arise from the intracranial lip of the optic foramen, causing unilateral superiorly inferior or lateral optic nerve compression, producing bizarre, monocular temporal hemianopias.[94,96] These patients typically present with relative afferent pupillary defects (RAPDs) on the affected side.[96] Other clinical signs and symptoms that may help in localization are indications of involvement with the nearby cranial nerves III, IV, V, VI and the presence of newly acquired unilateral exophthalmus.[94]

Olfactory groove meningiomas are not uncommon. They typically arise in the mid-line and tend to extend straight back into the anterior chiasmal angle, producing a symmetric bitemporal hemianopia, beginning in the lower quadrants (these tumors typically project to the chiasm from above). When the tumors grow along one nerve back to the chiasm, the visual field defects are more asymmetric. The classic Foster-Kennedy syndrome of the optic atrophy in the eye on the side of the tumor and papilledema in the contralateral eye may be seen in these cases.[94]

Tuberculum sellae meningiomas may produce symmetric or asymmetric bitemporal hemianopia, de-

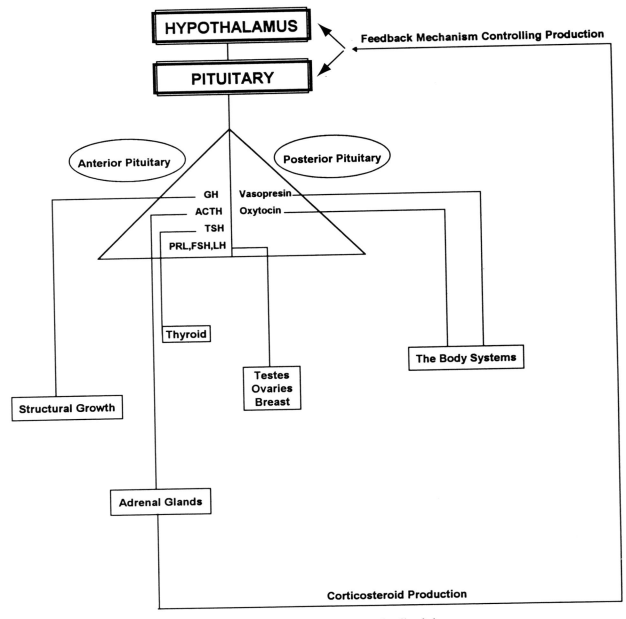

Fig. 8-9. The hypothalamic–pituitary feedback loop.

pending on where they impact on the chiasm. Junctional scotomas with contralateral temporal visual field loss caused by optic nerve compression are not uncommon and may result in bitemporal hemianopia, altitudinal hemianopia, and even homonymous hemianopia.[94]

Meningiomas of the lesser wing of the sphenoid bone are laterally situated with respect to the chi-asm and as a result produce the most irregular but symmetric of the visual fields from chiasmal compression.[94]

Treatment for meningiomas is surgical removal. The amount of recovery each patient experiences depends on the specific site of the lesion, the size of the lesion, the invasiveness of the lesion, and the time frame in which it was diagnosed.

Glioma of the Optic Chiasm

Optic chiasm glioma is a relatively rare disorder of children that sometimes occurs as part of the clinical presentation of neurofibromatosis.[92] They usually develop within the first two decades of life and may grow forward into the optic nerves or downward into the sella, causing pituitary-endocrine disturbances such as diabetes insipidus, obesity, skin changes, and infantilism.[94] The resultant visual field changes are usually irregular, asymmetric bitemporal hemianopias.[92,94] Treatment is surgical removal.

Nonspecific Granulomas of the Pituitary

Granulomatous lesions of the pituitary gland are rare.[98] They tend to affect the posterior lobe of the pituitary gland, resulting in posterior lobe insufficiency. This is often followed by anterior lobe dysfunction.[98] These tumors can produce severe and rapid deteriorations of visual acuity more predominant in one eye than in both. The vision loss is often marked by a reduction in the ability to discriminate light and dark. Visual field defects may range from bitemporal hemianopia to bilateral central scotoma.[98] Therefore, surgery is as much for diagnostic purposes as it is for curative purposes.[98]

Pituitary Apoplexy

Pituitary apoplexy is characterized by a sudden massive degeneration with hemorrhagic necrosis of the gland. It is often signaled by the abrupt onset of headache, vomiting, meningeal irritation, sight loss, diplopia, drowsiness, and confusion.[99,105] In practice, the condition is commonly misdiagnosed as an expanding intracranial aneurysm or subarachnoid hemorrhage.[99] The condition affects a variable portion of patients with pituitary adenoma that is confined either to the pituitary fossa or that has an extrasellar extension.[99] The term pituitary apoplexy has also been used to describe sudden infarction of a previous normal pituitary gland.

The ocular sequellae of pituitary apoplexy are quite variable from patient to patient. Typically, as the condition begins, visual acuity drops off rapidly. In fact, the apoplexy patient may present with visual acuity of hand motion or less.[99]

Visual field presentations are equally unique. Although central scotomas are common, bitemporal hemianopia and monocular hemianopia have been reported. Even cases with full visual fields in both eyes have been reported.[99]

Externally, ocular motility disturbances are common. In one study, cranial nerve III palsy was most common, followed by cranial nerve VI palsy and cranial nerve IV palsy.[99] Internally, the most frequently finding is some type of optic disc abnormality, which may range from unilateral optic atrophy and bilateral optic atrophy to bilateral papilledema.[99]

Pituitary apoplexy, along with its signs and symptoms, is considered to be a reversible condition. When properly diagnosed and treated, using conservative medical management—which includes the administration of high-dose steroids, radiotherapy and surgery—visual acuity and ocular motility deficits return to virtually predisease levels.[99] Treatment is best left to the neurosurgeon.

Pituitary Adenoma

The anterior lobe of the pituitary gland is a common site of origin for pituitary tumors.[76,92] Three types of cells are normally present (basophils, eosinophils, and neutrophils), and any one type may predominate in a tumor. Eosinophilic adenomas affect the chiasm less frequently than other tumors. Basophilic adenomas rarely enlarge beyond the confines of the sella turcica.[76] The most common pituitary tumor, likely to result in some type of symptomatic chiasmal impairment is the chromophobe adenoma.[6,76,92,94] Chromophobe adenomas are characterized by enlargement of the sella turcica, erosion of the clinoids, depression of libido, depression of sexual function, alterations in skin, alterations of the hair, weight gain, and adiposity. They are mid-line chiasmal compressions that are slow growing, producing visual field defects that begin in the upper temporal quadrants of both eyes, progressing slowly downward.[94] Previously, pituitary adenomas were classified on the basis of hematoxylin and eosin staining as either chromophobic, acidophilic, or basophilic. This type of classification, however, did not correlate well the secretory and clinical presentations of the tumors. A new classification system is now in use and is based on immunocytochemical analysis of tumor tissue, serum hormone concentrations, and clinical manifestations.[91]

The most common of the secreting tumors are the prolactinomas. They may cause amenorrhea (no menstruation) and galactorrhea (excessive flow of milk) in women and impotence, decreased libido, infertility, and occasionally gynecomastia and galactorrhea in men. Next in the prevalence of secreting tumors are GH-secreting adenomas. These tumors may cause gigantism in children and acromegaly in adults. The next most prevalent tumors that are secreting by nature, are the ACTH-secreting adenomas. These tumors can cause Cushing's disease. The most common of the secreting pituitary tumors are TSH-, LH-, and FSH-secreting adenomas.[91] Finally, pituitary adenomas are classified by their size. Tumors measuring 10 mm or less in diameter and confined to the sella are called *microadenomas*. Tumors measuring 10 mm or more and extending beyond the sella are categorized as *macroadenomas*. Microadenomas are rarely encountered by ocular physicians because they usually only produce endocrine symptoms. Conversely, macroadenomas are frequently detected by eye care practitioners because they produce visual symptoms. Nonsecretory chromophobe adenomas are the most common of the macroadenomas, followed by prolactin-secreting and GH-secreting adenomas.[91]

Treatment

Three therapeutic options are available for pituitary adenomas: surgery, radiotherapy, and medication. The standard surgical procedure for removing most pituitary adenomas is transsphenoidal microsurgery, although under some conditions, transfrontal craniotomy is performed instead.[91] The transsphenoidal technique involves entry under the upper lid and movement along the nasal septum with entry into the sphenoidal sinus and then up through the floor of the sella turcica.[91,100–102] In most cases, visual improvement begins within 24 hours of the procedure; however, in other cases it takes months.[91,100–102]

Conventional radiotherapy is usually used as an adjunctive treatment to prevent tumor growth. The preferred method of irradiation is with a linear accelerator, delivering daily, low-dose treatments. When combined with surgery, the recurrence rate decreases to 2 to 17 percent.[91] Also, visual field loss after the use of combined therapy is extremely rare but can be caused by tumor regrowth.

Medical therapy is an alternative to surgical and radiation modalities, especially for cases of prolactin-secreting microadenomas. Bromocriptine, an ergot derivative and dopamine agonist, has been successful in reducing tumor size, suppressing prolactin secre-

tions, restoring normal pituitary function, and improving visual function.[91] One serious drawback of this type of therapy is that cessation of the drug often results in rapid tumor enlargement. Other medications sometimes used include pergolide mesylate and cyproheptadine.[91]

Diagnosis and Management

Patients who suffer from neuroendocrinologic disorders present with a myriad of systemic, ocular, and neuro-ocular signs.[75,76,91–104] In 77 percent of cases, patients present with dull frontal headaches. Ironically, the headaches subside when the tumors break through the diaphragma sellae. When a patient presents with suspicious unexplained headache, the optometrist should consider further assessment by probing again through the history and considering additional testing, such as visual field testing (perimetry). All patients with unexplained vision loss, suspicious confrontational visual fields, and/or headache should be asked about endocrinologic symptoms. The history should include questions regarding changes in appearance and changes in sexual function (amenorrhea, gynecomastia, decreased libido, or impotence). The optometrist should also observe the patient for signs and symptoms of acromegaly, Cushing's disease, or Addison's disease.

In 7 to 38 percent of cases, diplopia is the presenting complaint. In cases in which cranial nerves are compressed (cranial nerve palsy), paretic diplopia is seen. Nonparetic diplopia, however, may result when classic bitemporal hemianopias break down fusional stability, causing an exophoric posture with vertical as well as horizontal displacement. This phoric decompensation results in a diplopia known as the *hemifield-slide* phenomenon.[91]

In up to 67 percent of pituitary adenoma cases, decreased vision or visual field impairment is present. Interestingly, a significant number of patients who have visual involvement are unaware of it.[91] These patients may provide indirect clues to these conditions by reporting a string of strange collisions with people or doorways. They may report complaints of difficulty with peripheral vision while driving or problems with keeping their place while reading. They may report simple hallucinations from compression of the tumor in the temporal lobes, which is typically a late-stage development.[91]

In 1 to 6 percent of cases, lateral compression of cranial nerves III, VI, and IV occurs as the tumor expands into the cavernous sinus. Involvement with cranial nerve III is most common, followed by involvement with VI and rarely with IV.[91] Oculomotor nerve (cranial nerve III) paresis is usually pain free and almost never complete. Almost all patients with cranial nerve palsies complain of diplopia or visual confusion.[91] See-saw nystagmus is a rare but reported finding in patients with pituitary adenoma. This abnormality involves a synchronous, alternating extorsion and depression of both eyes. When associated with bitemporal hemianopia, see-saw nystagmus is usually caused by chiasmal neoplasms, such as pituitary adenoma. Without the concurrent bitemporal defect, it is usually caused by a vascular lesion in the brain stem.[91]

A sudden onset of ophthalmoplegia, severe headache, vision loss, nausea, vomiting, and depression of consciousness may indicate pituitary apoplexy. This condition is an acute hemorrhagic infarction of the pituitary gland and is a neurosurgical emergency.[91,99]

Because the chiasm lies just above the pituitary gland, it is susceptible to compression from upward growth of a pituitary adenoma. However, although pituitary adenomas are the most common of the compressive chiasmal lesions (50 to 55 percent), craniopharyngioma (20 to 25 percent), meningiomas (10 percent), and gliomas (7 percent) should be included in the differential diagnosis.[91]

Ophthalmoscopy and Visual Fields

Direct ophthalmoscopy and binocular indirect ophthalmoscopy using the binocular indirect ophthalmoscope and slit lamp with Hruby lens, 60 D, 78 D or 90 D lens, should be used to assess the optic disc and nerve fiber layer. Frequently, retrograde axonal degeneration (optic atrophy) is the earliest detectable change and can be observed as defects in the nerve fiber layer using red-free indirect slit lamp ophthalmoscopy. Early damage to the nerve can be seen as partial atrophy of the nasal and papillomacular fibers.[91,100]

Progression of optic atrophy leads to increased pallor of the disc. Up to 66 percent of patients with pituitary adenoma exhibit some form of total, temporal, or nasal pallor. Some patients develop a horizontal band of atrophy across each optic disc, called *Bow-tie* or *Butterfly* optic atrophy.[91] Visual prognosis is significantly better for eyes without optic atrophy than for eyes with optic atrophy.[91,100–102]

The single most important visual diagnostic tool for detecting pituitary adenomas is visual field testing. Although this may include confrontational testing, tangent screen testing, Goldmann perimetry and automated perimetry, for reliability and maximum sensitivity for earliest detection, automated static threshold perimetry is recommended.[91,101]

Depending on the tumor location, location of its growth, and relative position of the optic chiasm, visual field defects may range from central bitemporal hemianopias, homonymous hemianopia (6 percent), bitemporal hemianopias (57 percent), and junctional syndromes (20 percent) (decreased acuity in one eye with a superior temporal cut in the other eye) to monocular hemianopia and monocular central scotoma (9 percent).[91]

Because the hallmark of the chiasmal lesion is the bitemporal hemianopia that respects the vertical meridian, any defect that is detected in the temporal visual field that stops at the vertical meridian should be regarded as a chiasmal lesion until proven otherwise.[91] Furthermore, any unexplained loss of visual acuity in one eye should be followed up with a check for a superior temporal loss in the fellow eye to rule out the presence of a junctional scotoma and lesion.[91]

Neuroradiologic and Other Testing

A number of tests warrant consideration when pituitary adenoma or similar diseases are suspected. Confirmation of suspected visual field defects can be obtained comparing red stimuli and color saturation between the two eyes. The patient is asked to compare the redness of two red targets presented simultaneously on either side of a fixation point. If bitemporal color desaturation is found, a chiasmal lesion is suggested.[91] Also, because pituitary adenomas can produce a compressive optic neuropathy, brightness-sense and brightness-comparison are useful and effective tests as well.[91] Differences in brightness can be graded subjectively (e.g., 100 percent OD versus 60 percent OS) or quantitatively by using neutral density filters over the better eye to abolish the difference.[91]

Color vision testing may also be a useful test for detecting compressive optic neuropathy. A higher incidence of color vision defects has been noted with prechiasmal compressions. The typical defect is a type II, acquired, red–green defect.[91]

Pupil testing may reveal the effects of pituitary adenoma and similar diseases. Suprasellar compressions from pituitary adenoma extensions have the potential to cause cranial nerve III paresis. If the iris sphincter is affected, a pupil that is dilated and reacts poorly to light will be observed. If the oculosympathetic pathway is affected, the pupil may appear smaller than the opposite pupil as well as less reactive to light.[91] Finally, if asymmetric optic neuropathy is present, a relative afferent pupillary defects may be apparent on the swinging flashlight test.[91]

Effects on depth perception have been reported in cases of pituitary adenoma, especially in cases with complete bitemporal hemianopia. This occurs because fixational movements cause the two blind, temporal hemifields to overlap beyond the point of fixation. This results in an expanding wedge of blindness beyond the fixation point, leading to problems with depth perception.[91]

Whenever a pituitary adenoma or similar disease (based on history, visual examination or visual field testing) is suspected, referral of the patient for neuroradiologic examination is required. MRI is considered the state-of-the-art neuroradiologic test. MRI has several advantages over CT. First, risk to the patient is reduced because ionizing radiation is not used; second, direct scanning in either sagittal or coronal planes can be accomplished without loss of resolution or uncomfortable patient positioning; and third, no artifacts secondary to bone imaging result.[91]

REFERENCES

1. Moore KL: Overview of Anatomy. p. 1. In: Clinically Oriented Anatomy. 2nd Ed. Williams & Wilkins, Baltimore, MD, 1985
2. Moore KL: The abdomen. p. 149. In: Clinically Oriented Anatomy. 7th Ed. Williams & Wilkins, Baltimore, MD, 1985
3. Berkow R, Talbott JH: Endocrine disorders. p. 1243. In: The Merck Manual of Diagnosis and Therapy. 13th Ed. Merck, Sharp & Dohme, Rahway, NJ, 1977
4. Ganong WF: Endocrinology and metabolism: energy, balance, metabolism and nutrition. p. 225. In: Review of Medical Physiology. 12th Ed. Lange Medical, Los Altos, CA, 1983
5. Ritchie AK: Neuroendocrinology. p. 741. In Brown AM, Stubbs DW (eds): Medical Physiology. John Wiley & Sons, New York, 1983
6. Hedges TR: Endocrinology problems. p. 15. In: Consultation in Ophthalmology. BC Decker, Philadelphia, 1987
7. Stubbs DW: The endocrine pancreas. p. 813. In Brown AM, Stubbs DW (eds): Medical Physiology. John Wiley & Sons, New York, 1983
8. Alexander LJ: Retinal vascular disorders. p. 69. In: Primary Care of the Posterior Segment. Appleton & Lange, East Norwalk, 1989
9. Dryer MS, Melton LJ, Ballard DJ et al: Incidence of diabetic retinopathy and blindness: a population based study in Rochester, Minnesota. Diabetes Care 189:316, 1985
10. Klein R, Davis MD, Moss SE et al: The Wisconsin epidemiological study of diabetic retinopathy. Adv Exp Med Biol 189:321, 1985
11. Klein R, Klein BE, Moss SE et al: Retinopathy in young-onset diabetic patients. Diabetes Care 8:311, 1985
12. The Diabetic Retinopathy Study Research Group: Indications for photocoagulation treatment of diabetic retinopathy: Diabetic Retinopathy Study report, No. 14. Int Ophthalmol Clin 27:239, 1987
13. Vaughan D, Asbury T: Ocular disorders associated with systemic disease. p. 232. In: General Ophthalmology. 10th Ed. Lange Medical, Los Altos, CA, 1983
14. Harrington DO: Diabetes of the retina. p. 159. In: The Visual Fields: A Textbook and Atlas of Clinical Perimetry. CV Mosby, St. Louis, MO, 1981
15. Early Treatment of Diabetic Retinopathy Study Research Group: Photocoagulation for diabetic macular edema: Early Treatment Diabetic Retinopathy Study report 1. Arch Ophthalmol 103:1796, 1985
16. Murphy RP, Ferris FL: Photocoagulation for diabetic macular edema: Early Treatment Diabetic Retinopathy Study. Contemp Ophthalmic For 4:25, 1986
17. The Diabetic Retinopathy Study Research Group: The four risk factors for severe visual loss in diabetic retinopathy; third report from the Dibaetic Retinopathy Study. Arch Ophthalmol 97:654, 1979
18. Clemente CD, Gray H: Anatomy of the Human Body. 13th Ed. Lea & Febiger, Philadelphia, 1985
19. Guyton AC: The thyroid metabolic hormones. p. 831. In: Textbook of Medical Physiology. 8th Ed. WB Saunders, Philadelphia, 1991
20. Salvi M, Zhang ZG, Haegert M et al: Patients with endocrine ophthalmopathy not associated with overt thyroid disease have multiple thyroid immunological abnormalities. J Clin Endocrinol Metab 70:89, 1990
21. Frilling A, Goretzki PE, Grubenporf M et al: The influence of surgery on endocrine ophthalmopathy. World J Surg 14:442, 1990
22. Sergott RC, Glaser JS: Grave's ophthalmopathy: a clinical and immunologic review. Surv Ophthalmol 26:1, 1981
23. Graves RJ: Newly observed affection of the thyroid gland in females. London Med Surg J 7:516, 1835
24. Parry CH: Diseases of the heart. Elements Pathol Theory 2: 111, 1825
25. Char DH: The ophthalmopathy of Grave's disease. Med Clin North Am 75:97, 1991
26. Clifton-Bligh P: Thyroid eye disease. Aust N Z J Ophthalmol 18:233, 1990
27. Fells P: Management of dysthyroid eye disease. Br J Ophthalmol 75:245, 1991
28. Carter JE: Ocular manifestations of neurological disorders. p. 2167. In Stein JH (ed): Internal Medicine. 2nd Ed. Little, Brown, Boston, 1987
29. Smith RE, Lee JS: The Cornea in systemic disease. p. 1. In Duane TD, Jaeger EA (eds): Clinical Ophthalmology. Vol. 4. No. 15. Harper & Row, Philadelphia, 1989
30. Greer M: Disorders of the thyroid. p. 1918. In Stein JH (ed): Internal Medicine. 2nd Ed. Little, Brown, Boston, 1987
31. Ladenson PN: Disorders of the thyroid. p. 901. In Harvey AM, Johns RJ, McKusick VA et al (eds): The Principles and Practice of Medicine. 2nd Ed. Appleton & Lange, Norwalk, CT, 1988
32. Char DH, Schlaegel TF: General factors in uveitis. p. 1. In

Duane TJ, Jaeger EA (eds): Clinical Ophthalmology. Vol. 4. No. 39. Harper & Row, Philadelphia, 1989

33. McGarvey EJ: Thyroid eye disease: review and case reports. J Am Optom Assoc 61:689, 1990

34. Kansu T, Subutay N: Lid retraction of myasthenia gravis. J Clin Neuroophthalmol 7:145, 1987

35. Arora R, Verma L, Sihota R: Echographic measurement of extraocular muscle thickness in proptosis. Ann Ophthalmol 24:106, 1992

36. Yoshikawa K, Higashide T, Nakase Y et al: Role of rectus muscle enlargement in clinical profile of dysthyroid ophthalmopathy. Jpn J Ophthalmol 35:175, 1991

37. Older JJ: Surgical treatment of eyelid retraction associated with thyroid eye disease. Ophthalmic Surg 22:318, 1991

38. Khalid BAK: Thyroid eye disease: medical or surgical therapy? Ann Acad Med Singapore 20:273, 1991

39. Antonelli A, Saracino A, Alberti B et al: High-dose intravenous immunoglobulin treatment in Grave's ophthalmopathy. Acta Endocrinol 126:13, 1992

40. Perros P, Kendall-Taylor P: Antibodies to orbital tissues in thyroid-associated ophthalmopathy. Acta Endocrinol 126:137, 1992

41. Perros P, Kendall-Taylor P: Biological activity of antibodies from patients with thyroid-associated ophthalmopathy: in vitro effects on porcine extraocular myoblasts. Q J Med 84:691, 1992

42. Kandror V, Birjukova M, Kryukova I et al: Some immunological correlations between thyroid pathology and ophthalmopathy. Exp Clin Endocrinol 97:212, 1991

43. Boucher A, Bernard NF, Zhang ZG et al: Nature and significance of orbital autoantigens and their corresponding autoantibodies in thyroid-associated ophthalmopathy. Autoimmunity 13:89, 1992

44. Hamed LM, Lingua RN: Thyroid eye disease presenting after cataract surgery. J Pediatr Ophthalmol Strabismus 27:10, 1990

45. Grove AS: Orbital disorders. p. 57. In Pavan-Langston O (ed): Manual of Ocular Diagnosis and Therapy. 3rd Ed. Little, Brown, Boston, 1991

46. Imai Y, Odajima R, Shimizu T, Shishiba Y: Serum hyaluronan concentration determination by radiometric assay in patients with pretimbial myedema and Grave's ophthalmopathy. Endocrinol Jpn 37:749, 1990

47. Werner SC: Modification of the classification of the eye changes in Grave's disease. Am J Ophthalmol 83:725, 1977

48. Leone CR, Piest KL, Newman RJ: Medial and lateral wall Decompression for Thyroid Ophthalmopathy. Am J Ophthalmol 108:160, 1989

49. Haver J: Additional clinical signs of unilateral endocrine exophthalmos. Br J Ophthalmol 53:210, 1969

50. Havard CWH: Endocrine exophthalmos. Br Med J 1:360, 1972

51. Goldstein JH: The intraoperative forced duction test. Arch Ophthalmol 72:647, 1964

52. Lyons DE: Postural changes in intraocular pressure in dysthyroid exophthalmos. Trans Ophthalmol Soc UK 91:799, 1971

53. Shammas HJF, Mickler DS, Ogden C: Ultrasound in early thyroid ophthalmopathy. Arch Ophthalmol 98:277, 1980

54. DeGroot LJ, Mangklabruks A, McCormick M: Comparison of RA ^{131}I treatment protocols for Grave's disease. J Endocrinol Invest 73:111, 1990

55. Barth A, Probst P, Burgi H: Identification of a subgroup of Grave's disease patients at higher risk for severe ophthalmopathy after radioiodine. J Endocrinol Invest 14:209, 1991

56. Miller ML, Goldberg SH, Bullock JD: Radiation retinopathy after standard radiotherapy for thyroid-related ophthalmopathy. Am J Ophthalmol 112:600, 1991

57. Tallstedt L, Lundell G, Torring O et al: Occurrence of ophthalmology after treatment for Grave's hyperthyroidism. N Engl J Med 326:1733, 1992

58. Smith M: Ophthalmology: The orbit, eyelids and lacrimal system. In: Basic and Clinical Science Course, Section 9. American Academy of Ophthalmology, San Francisco, 1985

59. Anderson RL: Upper lid retraction. p. 207. In Stewart WD (ed): Ophthalmic Plastic and Reconstructive Surgery. American Academy of Ophthalmology, San Francisco, 1984

60. Older JJ: Surgical treatment of eyelid retraction associated with thyroid eye disease. Ophthalmic Surgery 22:318, 1991

61. Wall JR: Autoimmunity and Grave's ophthalmopathy. p. 103. In Gorman CA, Waller RR, Dyer JA (eds): The Eye and Orbit in Thyroid Disease. Raven Press, New York, 1984

62. Bartalena L, Marcocci C, Bogazzi F: Use of corticosteroids to prevent progression of Grave's ophthalmopathy after radioiodine therapy for hyperthyroidism. N Engl J Med 321:1349, 1989

63. Werner SS: Prednisone in the emergency treatment of malignant exophthalmos. Lancet 1:1004, 1966

64. Garber MI: Methylprednisone in the treatment of exophthalmos. Lancet 1:958, 1966

65. Donaldson SS, Bagshaw MA, Kriss JP: Supervoltage orbital radiotherapy for Grave's ophthalmopathy. J Clin Endocrinol Metabol 37:276, 1973

66. Burrow GN, Mitchell MS, Howard RO: Immunosuppressive therapy for the eye changes of Grave's disease. J Clin Endocrinol Metabol 31:307, 1970

67. Bigos ST, Nisula BC, Daniels GH et al: Cyclophosphamide in the management of advanced Grave's ophthalmopathy: a preliminary report. Ann Intern Med 90:921, 1979

68. Prummel MF, Mourits MP, Berghout A et al: Prednisone and cyclosporine in the treatment of severe Grave's ophthalmopathy. N Engl J Med 321:1353, 1989

69. Catz B, Perzik SL: Subtotal vs. total surgical ablation of the thyroid, malignant exophthalmos and its relation to remnant thyroid. p. 1183. In Cassano C, Andreoli M (eds): Current Topics in Thyroid Research. Academic Press, Orlando, FL, 1965

70. Goldberg RA, Shorr N, Cohen MS: The medial orbital strut in the prevention of post decompression dystopia in dysthyroid ophthalmopathy. Ophthalmic Plast Reconstr Surg 8:32, 1992

71. Moore KL: The head. p. 794. In: Clinically Oriented Anatomy. 7th Ed. Williams & Wilkins, Baltimore, MD, 1985

72. Ganong WF: Other organs with established or suggested endocrine functions. p. 376. In: Review of Medical Physiology. 12th Ed. Lange Medical, Los Altos, CA, 1985

73. Glaser JS, Bachynski B: Intranuclear disorders of eye movement. p. 361. In Glaser JS (ed): Neuroophthalmology. 2nd Ed. JB Lippincott, Philadelphia, 1990

74. Poppen JL, Marino R: Pinealomas and tumors of the posterior portion of the third ventricle. J Neurosurg 28:355, 1968

75. Hedges TF: Pupillary abnormalities. p. 299. In: Consultation in Ophthalmology. BC Decker, Philadelphia, 1987

76. Bloch RS, Henkind P: Ocular manifestations of endocrine and metabolic diseases. p. 1. In Duane TJ, Jaeger EA (eds): Clinical Ophthalmology. Vol. 5. No. 21. Harper & Row, Philadelphia, 1993

77. Hall CE: Adrenal glands. p. 843. In Brown AM, Stubbs PW (eds): Medical Physiology. John Wiley & Sons, New York, 1983

78. Ganong WF: The adrenal medulla and adrenal cortex. p. 293. In: Review of Medical Physiology. 12th Ed. Lange Medical, Los Altos, CA, 1985

79. Shirley JE, Schteingart DE, Tandon R et al: EEG Sleep in Cushing's disease and Cushing's syndrome: a comparison with patients with major depressive order. Biol Psychiatry 32:146, 1992

80. Shirley JE, Schteingart DE, Tawdon R, Starkman MN: Sleep architecture and sleep apnea in patients with Cushing's disease. Sleep 16:514, 1992

81. Haas J, Nootens R: Glaucoma secondary to benign adrenal adenoma. Am J Ophthalmol 78:497, 1974

82. Robin DS, Haas JS: A 16 year follow-up in a corticosteroid-sensitive patient with glaucoma secondary to a benign adrenal adenoma. Am J Ophthalmol 107:293, 1989
83. Tatar J, Glaukom Bei M: Cushing. Graefes Arch Clin Exp Ophthalmol 139:793, 1938
84. Radnot M: Der Augenbefuno bei Chushingscher Krankheit. Ophthalmologica 104:301, 1942
85. Jonas JB, Huschle U, Kuniszewski G et al: Intraocular pressure in patients with Cushing's disease. Graefes Arch Clin Exp Ophthalmol 228:406, 1990
86. Slansky H, Kolbert G, Gartner S: Exophthalmos induced by steroids. Arch Ophthalmol 77:577, 1967
87. Plotz C, Knowlton A, Ragan C: The natural history of Cushing's syndrome. Am J Med 13:1950, 1952
88. Sowka JW: What you can do to manage hypertension. Rev Optometry 131(1):77, 1994
89. Albert D, Rubenstein R, Scheie H: Tumor metastasis to the eye: II. Clinical study in infants and children. Am J Ophthalmol 63:726, 1967
90. Alfano J: Ophthalmological aspects of neuroblastomatosis: a study of 53 verified cases. Trans Am Acad Ophthalmol Otolaryngol 72:829, 1968
91. Wormington CM: Pituitary adenoma: diagnosis and management. J Am Optom Assoc 60(12):929, 1989
92. Vaughan D, Asbury T: Neuro-ophthalmology. p. 202. In: General Ophthalmology. 10th Ed. Lange Medical, Los Altos, CA, 1983
93. Glaser JS: Topical diagnosis: the optic chiasm. p. 171. In: Neuro-ophthalmology. 2nd Ed. JB Lippincott, Philadelphia, 1990
94. Harrington DO: Chiasm. p. 267. In: The Visual Fields: A Textbook and Atlas of Clinical Perimetry. 5th Ed. CV Mosby, St. Louis, MO, 1981
95. Gurwood AS: A smarter way to decipher defects. Optom Manage 28:39, 1993
96. Hershenfeld S, Sharpe JA: Monocular temporal hemianopia. Br J Ophthalmol 77:424, 1993
97. Roy M, Collier B, Roy A: Dysregulation of the hypothalmo-pituitary-adrenal axis and duration of diabetes. J Natl Eye Inst Natl Inst Alcohol Abuse Alcoholism 218, 1991
98. Deckler RCT, Rise K: Non-specific granulomas of the pituitary: report of six cases treated surgically. Neurosurg Rev 14:185, 1991
99. McFadzean RM, Doyle D, Rampling R et al: Pituitary apoplexy and its effect on vision. Neurosurgery 29:669, 1991
100. Marcus M, Vitale S, Calvert PC, Miller NR: Visual parameters in patients with pituitary adenoma before and after transsphenoidal surgery. Aust N Z J Ophthalmol 19:111, 1991
101. Hudson H, Rissel C, Gauderman WJ, Feldon SE: Pituitary tumor volume as a predictor of postoperative visual field recovery. J Clin Neuro-Ophthalmol 11:280, 1991
102. Sullivan LJ, O'Day J, McNeill P: Visual outcomes of pituitary adenoma surgery. J Clin Neuro-ophthalmol 11:262, 1991
103. Ing EB, Sullivan TJ, Clarke MP, Buncic JR: Oculomotor nerve palsies in children. J Pediatr Ophthalmol Strabismus 29:331, 1992
104. Ganong WF: The pituitary gland. p. 329. In: Review of Medical Physiology. 12th Ed. Lange Medical, Los Altos, 1983
105. Friel JP (ed): Dorland's Illustrated Medical Dictionary. 26th Ed. WB Saunders, Philadelphia, 1985

9 Diabetes

BRIAN P. MAHONEY

INTRODUCTION

Diabetes is a complex group of diseases whose characteristic clinical feature is hyperglycemia. Significant strides in clinical research over the years have contributed to a better understanding of the complexity of diabetes. Appreciation of this complexity is evidenced by the frustration felt by both patients and health-care practitioners involved in the long-term care of diabetic patients. The chronic complications result in significant visual and physical debilitation, which serves as a major source of morbidity and mortality in patients afflicted with diabetes. Ten percent of Americans age 60 and 20 percent of those age 80 suffer from diabetes.[1] The Centers for Disease Control has reported that diabetes was responsible for 1.8 percent of deaths and contributed to an additional 8.4 percent of deaths in the United States.[2] Chronic complications are also responsible for the greatest loss of potential years of life for diabetic patients. Diabetes consumed 2 percent of the total health-care costs in the United States in

1980 when all the various complications are considered. These costs have also been increasing over the past 14 years.

Early diagnosis and treatment is necessary to maximize the quality of life for diabetic patients. Ocular involvement is commonly the presenting sign; therefore, ophthalmic practitioners frequently recognize the symptoms of diabetes leading to an initial diagnosis. Progressive ocular involvement correlates well with advancing systemic disease, thus warranting a critical review of an individual patient's medical therapy and management. Ophthalmic practitioners need to participate in the health-care delivery for all diabetic patients to ensure detection of sight-threatening changes at early stages and to provide necessary information regarding the treatment and management for these high-risk patients. It is essential for eye care practitioners to recognize the various manifestations of diabetes and to understand their implications for the health care of each diabetic patient.

CASE REPORT

A 54-year-old white man requested an eye examination to evaluate recurrent episodes of blurred vision he had been experiencing for the past year. The episodes lasted for more than 30 minutes and were not accompanied by other subjective motor or sensory deficit. He also described a gradual decrease in vision with his present glasses over the same period. His ocular history was remarkable for mild hypertension, previous myocardial infarct, and elevated triglyercide and cholesterol levels. His present medications included diltiazem and propranolol.

The external examination revealed smooth ocular motilities without restriction. Pupillary responses were

P4/4 round reactive to light (RRL) with no afferent pupillary defect (APD). Confrontation field evaluation revealed no detectable defect. Best corrected visual acuity was 20/20 OD and 20/30 OS. Amsler grid evaluation revealed an area of metamorphopsia approximately 2 degrees OD and 5 degrees OS. Biomicroscopy was remarkable for arcus senilus in both eyes and Goldmann tonometry was measured at 14 mmHg OD and 15 mmHg OS. Equally clear fundus views were obtained after dilation with direct ophthalmoscopy and 90 D lens evaluation. Fundus evaluation revealed a 0.2/0.25 cup to disc (CD) ratio OU with sharp optic nerve head margins. Scattered deep retinal hemorrhages with some exudation without microinfarcts were seen

---

in both eyes. Thickening of the macular tissue was observed in both eyes but to a greater degree in the left eye. Cystoid degeneration was present in the peripheral retina in both eyes with an isolated vitreoretinal traction tuft present at 4 o'clock in the right eye without associated retinal break or tear.

His blood pressure was measured at 148/82 mmHg. The differential diagnosis included undiagnosed diabetes. The patient reported increased frequency of urination and a weight gain of 27 pounds over the past year. His fasting blood sugar was 328, and he was hospitalized for acute control of his diabetes. Fluorescein angiography confirmed subclinical macular edema in the right eye and clinically significant macular edema in the left eye. The patient was referred to a retinologist, who successfully treated the patient for macula of the left eye with focal argon laser.

CLASSIFICATION OF DIABETES

The National Diabetic Data Group and the National Institutes of Health in addition to the World Health Organization worked to change the classification of diabetes in the late 1970s and early 1980s (Table 9-1). This classification systems reflects the pathophysiology and clinical course of each type of diabetes more accurately than the previous classification system. A thorough discussion of each type is beyond the scope of this text; this discussion therefore is limited to type I and type II diabetes, because they are the types of diabetes most frequently encountered by eye care practitioners.

Type I, insulin-dependent diabetes mellitus (IDDM), has unique clinical features. β-Cell dysfunction with obliteration is frequently seen by age 20. Clinical research supports an immune mechanism as the etiology of β-cell dysfunction.[3,4] A high correlation with human leukocyte (HLA) antigens D-related 3 and 4 (DR3 and DR4) has been found.[5-7] Few clinical symptoms are seen in the early stages because the β-cell loss is gradual. After a critical level of islet cell damage occurs, the demand for insulin exceeds the supply, and hyperglycemia results. Cellular dysfunction and death occur in tissues throughout the body, resulting in an acute hyperglycemic event and possible diabetic shock.[4] Hospitalization for the acute episode of ketoacidosis and hyperglycemia often results in the initial diagnosis.[8] The patient is committed to lifelong therapy with exogenous insulin to best control the hyperglycemia.

Type II diabetes, non-insulin-dependent diabetes mellitus (NIDDM), primarily results from insulin resistance and is seen most frequently in patients after the age of 40.[9] Inadequate insulin receptor binding and suboptimal cellular response to insulin occur despite normal or possibly elevated levels of insulin. Diabetic shock characterized by acute hyperglycemia and ketoacidosis does not occur with type II. Obesity is implicated in the development of insulin resistance. Type II diabetic patients usually exceed their ideal body weight by 20 percent, which has been implicated in changing the insulin-receptor configuration on the cell membrane. The subsequent cellular responses that would normally occur cannot be triggered; therefore, hyperglycemia results. Weight loss enhances the bonding affinity of the insulin receptor and therefore is necessary for optimal glucose control in the NIDDM patient. Diet, exercise, and the use of oral hypoglycemic agents are the mainstay of treatment of patients with type II diabetes.

CLINICAL FEATURES

An imbalance in the homeostatic mechanisms involved with glucose regulation remains the hallmark clinical feature of diabetes (Table 9-2). A breakdown

Table 9-1. Classification of Diabetes

Insulin dependent
Non-insulin dependent
Gestational
Impaired glucose tolerance

Table 9-2. Conditions Associated with Hyperglycemia

Impaired β-cell function
    Inflammatory destruction (viral and/or autoimmune)
    Toxic destruction (drug)
    Reversible drug induced
    Poor proinsulin conversion
    Hormonal abnormalities
Poor insulin action
    Anti-insulin antireceptor antibodies
    Excessive glucagon
Tissue defects
    Insufficient number of insulin receptors
    Inadequate cellular response to insulin

in the various components of glucose regulation and metabolism accounts for hyperglycemia. Adequate insulin production and release in response to a glucose load do not occur in type I diabetes, thus resulting in elevated serum glucose levels. Normal or elevated insulin levels are present in patients with type II diabetes, yet deficiencies in the binding ability of insulin and subsequent cellular responses exist. This insulin resistance causes glucose to collect in extracellular spaces, leading to hyperglycemia.

The physiologic responses in cells are affected by hyperglycemia, resulting in decreased activity and tissue death. All of the mechanisms responsible for tissue damage are not fully understood, although an integral relationship appears to exist with hyperglycemia. Histopathologic abnormalities affect most tissues throughout the body to varying degrees. Progression of these changes is related to the severity and duration of hyperglycemia. Short-term fluctuations in glucose levels are frequently associated with acute symptoms (e.g., refractive error fluctuations) and are directly influenced by glucose levels on a daily basis. The development of long-term abnormalities (retinopathy and cardiovascular disease), which are slowly progressive, correlates with long-term stability of serum glucose levels. The clinical implications for both short- and long-term complications pose various challenges for any practitioner involved in the health care of diabetic patients.

HYPERGLYCEMIC-ASSOCIATED ABNORMALITIES

Much controversy still exists concerning the exact mechanisms responsible for tissue damage and dysfunction in diabetes. Hyperglycemia plays a direct role in some tissue damage, but indirect mechanisms are also involved. Hyperglycemia has a direct effect on tissues, as evidenced by pericyte death in vessel walls. Indirect damage to tissues also occurs as a result of altered physiologic responses to elevated glucose levels, as evidenced by damage to nervous tissue contributing to motor, sensory, and autonomic neuropathy. The mechanisms by which pathologic changes occur in tissues and how these mechanisms can be influenced by glucose control are not fully understood. Increased blood flow rates in the retina and kidney cannot be restored to normal when glucose levels are near normoglycemic. The long-term complications associated with diabetes will develop

despite apparent good control of hyperglycemia. The etiologic mechanisms must be influenced by factors other than hyperglycemia alone. The results of the Diabetes Control and Complications Trial (DCCT) confirmed the direct association between good glycemic control and decreased severity of retinopathy, nephropathy, and neuropathy.[10–14] A similar relationship is suspected but has not been proven between good glycemic control and macrovascular disease.

Nonenzymatic protein glycosylation effects red blood cells, vascular endothelium, plasma proteins, collagen fibers, lens proteins, myelin, and other protein structures throughout the body. This results in altered structure and function of the effected protein. A baseline amount of glycosylation occurs, with normal glycemic levels, and is of little clinical significance. Increased amounts of glycosylation with irreversibility are associated with sustained hyperglycemia. The levels of a specific glycosylated protein (i.e., hemoglobin A_{1C}) correlate with the severity of hyperglycemia and provide some measurement of the success of medical management when compared to normoglycemic protein levels. Hemoglobin molecules that have been glycosylated do not bind or release oxygen easily. Glycosylation of tissues is implicated in the vasculopathy and tissue damage associated with diabetes.

The polyol pathway of glucose metabolism is used by diabetics to a greater extent than in nondiabetics. Byproducts of this reaction, primarily sorbitol and fructose, accumulate in tissues and alter cellular osmolarity. This contributes to cell dysfunction and death. Sorbitol accumulation in the crystalline lens contributes to cataract formation. Sorbitol and fructose have been detected in peripheral nervous tissues of diabetic rats and are implicated in the development of diabetic neuropathy.

Red blood cell abnormalities in diabetics include elevated erythrocyte sedimentation rates (about 30 to 40 as measured by Westergren method), decreased oxygen-carrying capacity, decreased deformability, increased aggregates, and increased cell membrane adhesiveness. These altered properties of erythrocytes contribute to impaired blood flow and thrombotic formation,[15,16] which contribute to vascular occlusive processes in the smaller caliber vessels throughout the body after a significant amount of time. The exact relationship of these changes to diabetic vasculopathy remains uncertain, but these changes contribute to the development of vasculopathic changes in the microvasculature in the long term and play no role in the development of macrovascular changes.

Hemodynamic abnormalities occur even before endothelial damage. The rate of blood flow in retinal and renal capillaries increases.[17] This increased flow rate in kidney glomerulii is associated with damage from hyperfiltration. The increased flow rate contributes to endothelial damage in the retinal capillary beds early in the stages of diabetic retinopathy. Strict glucose regulation appears to have a positive influence on the altered flow rates in these tissues and slows damage. Various hypercoagulation abnormalities contribute to vascular disease by increasing thrombotic formation where only minimal endothelial damage is found. Increased platelet aggregation, platelet adhesiveness, and circulating platelet groups as well as decreased fibrinolysis and decreased platelet life have all been implicated in the development of diabetic vascular disease. The exact role that each of these abnormalities play in the development of vascular disease is uncertain.

Immunologic abnormalities are also described in diabetic patients. A high association exists between the presence of HLA-DR3 and -DR4 and IDDM.[5-8] This implicates an immunologic role in the disease development; however, a direct correlation between the presence of these HLA haplotypes and the development of IDDM does not exist. No immune-mediated mechanisms are associated with the development of NIDDM, although a genetic link is more likely, given the high concordance in the development of diabetes in sets of twins. The presence of immunologic abnormalities in diabetics may indicate widespread tissue damage, reflecting the body's inability to remove the high amounts of circulating abnormal immune complexes when significant microvascular diseases are present. Elevated levels of immune complexes correlate well with proliferative retinopathy.

Diabetic Vasculopathy

Diabetic vasculopathy comprises both vessel wall disease and altered hemodynamic elements, both of which alter tissue perfusion, resulting in decreased function and possible death. Diabetic vessel wall disease occurs at a higher rate in diabetics than nondiabetics.

Large, medium, and small vessels throughout the body are affected. No direct correlation between large and small vessel disease can be made, however, because the factors influencing the development of sclerosis in each size vessel differs. Small vessel disease is related more closely to the severity of hyperglycemia reflecting a direct association between hyperglycemia and vessel wall damage.[17] Large vessel disease is related more closely to the amount of sclerosis, lipid deposition, and loss of vessel wall flexibility. Elevated triglyceride and low-density lipoprotein (LDL) cholesterol and decreased high-density lipoprotein (HDL) cholesterol levels are related to enhanced deposition and accelerated vessel wall disease (with large and medium-size vessel disease).[16] Elevated levels of endothelin-1 in aortic endothelial cells results from hyperglycemia and results in the loss of normal vasoconstrictive ability.[18] This phenomenon suggests a correlation between pericyte death and hyperglycemia. The most frequently observed macrovascular complications include peripheral vascular disease (with lower extremity predilection), carotid artery disease, and coronary artery disease.

Microvascular disease affects renal and retinal vessels as well as the vasovasorum of peripheral nerves, although not uniformly. Microangiopathy of the retinal and renal tissues appears to be influenced more significantly by altered blood flow rate, hyperglycemia-induced endothelial cell death, and increased thrombus formation. Because differences in the vessel wall structure and the mechanisms for vessel wall disease exist, smaller blood vessels are at a higher risk of suffering damage from hemodynamic factors rather than sclerotic disease. Sclerotic vessel wall disease also manifests in the retina with diabetes progression as branch or central vein occlusion.

A direct correlation does not exist between the severity of microangiopathy in vessels of similar caliber in various organs. The degree of retinal vascular disease is not equal to the amount found in the kidney. The structure and function of the vasculature varies in each organ. The vessels in each organ are not affected in the same manner or at the exact same rate. Histopathologic changes in both retinal and kidney vasculature is evident before the manifestation of symptoms or clinical signs. Clinically evident retinopathy (by ophthalmoscopy or fluorescein angiography) develops before clinically evident nephropathy (elevated blood urea nitrogen [BUN] and createnine levels). Patients with advanced retinopathy are at moderate risk of nephropathy; conversely, patients with nephropathy are at high risk of retinopathy. Pirart[14] found that 24 percent of patients with retinopathy had nephropathy and that 86 percent with nephropathy had retinopathy. Proteinuria is found in 58 percent of patients with severe retinopathy[20]; and patients with microalbuminuria are at high risk of the development of proliferative retinopathy. Proteinuria, elevated BUN levels, or elevated creatinine levels can be seen in 35 percent of diabetics with symptomatic retinopathy.[21]

Type II diabetics will manifest clinical nephropathy after 20 years of diabetes.[22] Significant renal disease is a complicating factor in the deaths of greater than 40 percent of type I diabetics. The vascular abnormalities and organ damage decreases with stabilization of glucose levels. Concurrent hypertensive and diabetic disease associated with chronic renal failure can be seen in Kimmelstiel-Wilson syndrome. A combination of severe diabetic and hypertensive vasculopathy in the retina is suggestive of this condition. These patients require aggressive co-management with a nephrologist and internist well trained in diabetic disease.

Diabetic neuropathy is seen in types I and II diabetics. No one etiologic factor explains all of the findings associated with this phenomenon.[23–25] Compromise of the vasovasorum of nervous tissue and accumulation of polyol pathway products (particularly sorbitol and fructose) play undetermined roles in nervous tissue damage. Any nerve is at risk, including motor, sensory, or autonomic nerves. Symptoms associated with the deficit depends on the function of the affected nerve. Associated symptoms can be of acute onset and last for a finite period, for example, diplopia from extraocular muscle palsy lasting for approximately 90 days and resolving gradually during that time. Diabetic neuropathy can also be of insidious onset and run a chronic course. Impaired gait resulting from a motor deficit (i.e., foot drop) may be combined with a sensory deficit (peripheral sensory neuropathy) and may persist, which contributes to functional impairment. Involvement of the autonomic nervous system, affecting cardiac function, will manifest symptoms resembling systemic hypotension and vertebrovasilar disease and should therefore be considered in the differential diagnosis of bilateral transient vision loss in patients with advanced diabetes. Poor bladder control and impotence also cause significant distress and embarrassment for diabetic patients.

Hypertension is encountered in diabetic patients at a two to three times higher rate than in nondiabetics.

Systemic sclerosis and increased vessel wall rigidity are associated with hypertension. However, hypertension can be a complication of renal involvement, which is progressive throughout the course of the disease. Elevated systolic hypertension and progressive retinopathy has been reported, yet a causal relationship is not established.[26,27] It is suspected that the retinopathy and hypertension are both complications from diabetes progression and that a causal relationship therefore does not exist.

Diabetic Oculopathy

A significant amount of research and attention have been directed toward the pathogenesis and treatment of diabetic retinopathy. This is justifiable, considering the severity of vision loss resulting from its progression. The effects of diabetes are not restricted to the retinal vasculature; involvement of various structures in the anterior and posterior segments has been well described (Table 9-3). Abnormal physiologic and electrophysiologic findings include impaired dark adaptation, abnormal electroretinogram (ERG), contrast sensitivity, and visual-evoked potential.

A variety of neuro-ophthalmic manifestations have been associated with diabetes. Focal demyelinization of the cranial nerves with subsequent recovery appears to be the mechanism for development of cranial nerve palsies (Fig. 9-1). Involvement of the VI, III, and IV cranial nerves is acute in onset and accompanied by some level of pain, ranging from mild to severe. Diabetes is not the sole cause of a pupil-sparing cranial nerve III palsy, but it is the most common is-

Table 9-3. Common Ocular Associations of Diabetes

Abnormal electrophysiological findings
Cranial nerve palsy
Anterior segment
    Poor corneal healing
    Decreased corneal sensitivity
    Open-angle glaucoma
    Neovascular glaucoma
    Iridoplegia
    Poor pupillary dilation
Crystalline lens
    Cataract
    Refractive error shifts
Retina
    Diabetic retinopathy
    Central retinal vein occlusion
Optic nerve papilopathy

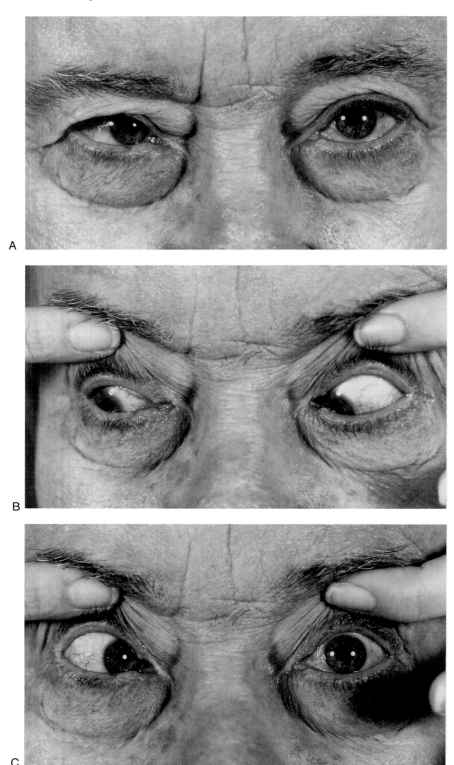

Fig. 9-1. (A–C) Left cranial nerve VI palsy in a 62-year-old type II diabetic patient. The patient had sudden onset of diplopia 3 days earlier. Note the esotropic posture of the right eye, not the left eye. The patient was fixating with the paretic eye. Versions to right field demonstrate full abduction of the right eye. Versions into the left field of gaze showed an inability to abduct the left eye with no restrictions of the right eye.

chemic vascular cause. Other forms of ischemic vascular disease must be considered, particularly those of vasculitic etiology. Cases involving compressive lesions or aneurysms effecting the subarachnoid region of cranial nerve III must be excluded. Diabetic patients can manifest one cranial nerve palsy, which possibly recurs with time. Simultaneous nerve palsies at the time of clinical presentation should be viewed with skepticism, and etiologies other than diabetes need be considered (i.e., cavernous sinus syndrome).[28] Complete or partial ophthalmoplegias can also be caused by diabetes. Resolution of cranial nerve palsies and ophthalmoplegias normally occur within 90 days. Aberrant regeneration can occur, and is frequently seen with cranial nerve III palsies.[28]

Pupillary abnormalities include a tonic pupillary response (partial iridoplegia) with sectoral paresis. Poor pupillary dilation results from autonomic neuropathy involving sympathetic tissues of the iris and is less related to myopathy.[29,30] The degree to which the pupil poorly dilates correlates well with the severity of the retinopathy and systemic disease.[29,31] The pupillary responses do not normally recover well enough to reestablish good pupillary dilation or responses.

Optic nerve involvement is a rarer manifestation of diabetes (Fig. 9-2 and Plate 9-1). Benign disc swelling in young diabetics has been described with little or no associated retinopathy.[32–35] Unilateral or bilateral (in 50 percent of cases) disc swelling can be mistaken for papilledema or ischemic neuropathy. A mild decrease in visual acuity is frequently reduced to the 20/50 level (at worst), and a pupillary defect is mild if present. Mild central scotoma and peripheral field constrictions, without any altitudinal loss, have been described with the papillopathy.[36] Resolution of the swelling occurs within 90 days, but the patient may be have a residual field defect despite vision recovery. Anterior ischemic optic neuropathy (AION) can also be encountered in diabetics, but the clinical course and associated visual sequella differ from those of diabetic papillopathy. Diabetes and hypertension are seen at a higher frequency in AION patients than in age-matched ION patients.[37] The presence of AION on a diabetic patient should suggest associated vascular disease (carotid artery disease), particularly in patients older than age 50.

Anterior segment involvement from diabetes is commonly encountered. The most common corneal se-

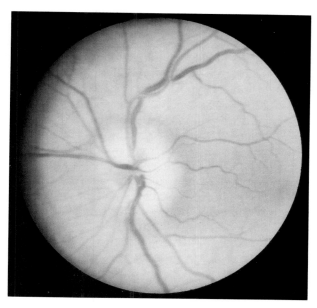

Fig. 9-2. Unilateral diabetic papillopathy in 34-year-old type I diabetic patient. The patient had 20/30 best corrected vision without associated APD. Mild red desaturation without visual field defect resolved over a 3-month period. Note the indistinct nerve head margins and lack of microinfarction or significant hemorrhages. No diabetic retinopathy was associated with neuropathy. (See also Plate 9-1.)

quella is poor healing following corneal insult, either ineffective or mechanical. The degree of impaired corneal healing correlates well with proliferative retinopathy.[37] This phenomenon is not caused by decreased epithelial mitosis but appears related to thickened basement membrane; axonal degeneration, and altered corneal sensation.[38] These changes appear to decrease the ability of the epithelium to adhere to the underlying stroma, predisposing diabetics to a protracted course when epithelial loss results from corneal erosion or abrasion. Minimal insult to the cornea can cause significant areas of epithelium to slough off with portions of basement membrane attached to them. Ineffective keratitis, which may or may not be related to contact lens wear, has prolonged healing times despite appropriate therapy and management.

Diabetes is one risk factor for the development of glaucoma. Primary open-angle glaucoma is seen more frequently in diabetic patients than in nondiabetics. Diabetic patients may have a higher average intraocular pressure (IOP) with nonproliferative retinopathy and manifest normotensive levels at the proliferative stages of retinopathy.[39,40] Small vessel disease associated with diabetes may play a role in perfusion of the optic nerve, placing the disc at risk of glaucomatous damage. Diabetics also manifest IOP elevations in response to topical steroids, and their IOP fluctuates with fluid intake more significantly than nondiabetics.[41–43] Diabetes-associated neovascular glaucoma is the second most frequent cause behind central retinal vein occlusion.[44] It is caused by diffuse ischemia from advanced retinopathy and may manifest bilaterally. Unilateral cases with grossly asymmetric retinopathy occur when significant carotid occlusion compromises ocular perfusion. Neovascular glaucoma is seen more frequently following intracapsular cataract extraction rather than extracapsular extraction. β-Blockers, epinephrine drugs, and carbonic anhydrase inhibitors must be used with caution to treat glaucoma in diabetic patients because of the propensity for developing significant systemic side effects. Hypoglycemic episodes, exacerbations of hyperglycemia, and increased systemic acidosis may be manifested without early warning signs; therefore, these patients should be monitored carefully for potential side effects.

Accumulation of sorbitol and fructose in the crystalline lens of the eye is implicated in cataract formation for diabetic patients. A two to four times higher incidence of cataract formation occurs in diabetic patients than nondiabetic patients and is related to the overall glycemic control of the patient. Cataracts are commonly seen in conjunction with some level of retinopathy. Cortical, posterior subcapsular, and nuclear opacities are most commonly seen in NIDDM patients. Cataract extraction is warranted when the patient's vision is impaired or if the opacity precludes the ability of the retinologist to effectively treat the retina when necessary. Snowflake cortical opacities are observed primarily in IDDM patients. They are of little visual significance and do not require extraction for most IDDM patients.

Refractive error shifts in diabetic patients most frequently occur toward increasing myopia, although increased hyperopia can occur. The shift in refractive error is acute and is related to the level of hyperglycemia. Accumulation of water in the lens from the hyperosmotic forces involved with sorbitol pathway byproducts alters the refractive indices of the eye. The amount of by-product accumulation in the lens is related to the level of hyperglycemia, which changes throughout the day. The stability of refractive error

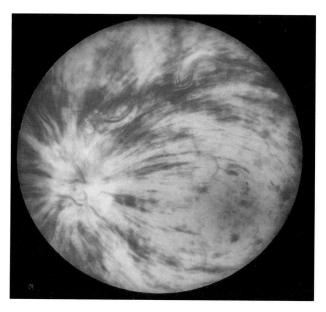

Fig. 9-3. CRVO in the left eye in a 53-year-old diabetic patient. Note the significant hemorrhage and lack of microinfarcts. Mild nonproliferative diabetic retinopathy was detected in the right eye. The occlusion resolved well with poor vision recovery that was due to the persistent edema. (See also Plate 9-2.)

is determined by the stability of the serum glucose. It is not only important for glucose levels to be in an acceptable range, but also the overall fluctuation of glucose levels are important for refractive error stabilization. A fluctuation of less than 80 to 100 mg/dl for the serum glucose levels over a 3- to 4-week period is recommended for stabilization of refractive error.

Retinal occlusive processes, particularly venous occlusion, occur more frequently than in nondiabetics (Fig. 9-3 and Plate 9-2). Up to 15 percent of patients with CRVO have diabetes, which may play a role in the development of the occlusion.[45] These may be seen without significant diabetic retinopathy. Other forms of retinal vascular disease are also observed in diabetic patients because of the extensive nature of vasculopathy in diabetes. Diabetic retinopathy can be complicated by retinal arteriosclerosis, ocular ischemic syndrome, and retinal plaques (from carotid artery disease), as well as other concurrent vasculopathies.

Patients with severe ketoacidosis are prone to infection. Orbital extension from inflammation in the surrounding paranasal air sinuses can cause an orbital cellulitis. Fungal infection, primarily mucormycosis, is characterized by inflammatory necrosis, which can involve the cavernous sinus rapidly following orbital extension. Because these patients are frequently in acute metabolic distress, hospitalization is required. Prompt treatment therefore can be rendered to preserve the patients' life.

Diabetic Retinopathy

The early vasculopathic changes associated with diabetic retinopathy have been well described, but the etiologic factors influencing their development remain elusive. The results of the collaborative Diabetic Retinopathy Study (DRS) and Early Treatment Diabetic Retinopathy Study (ETDRS) have provided ophthalmic practitioners with specific guidelines for intervention and treatment of diabetic retinopathy. Approaching diabetic retinopathy treatment from this perspective has maximized vision and minimized functional loss for many diabetics. No known cure is available for diabetes or diabetic retinopathy at this time; therefore, ophthalmic practitioners remain responsible in determining the proper classification, treatment, and management for each patient.

Specific changes in the retinal vasculature have been described with progression in diabetic retinopathy (Table 9-4). Pericytes participate in autoregulation of the retinal vasculature, and their death alters the normal vascular regulatory responses. Their dropout, caused directly by hyperglycemia, weakens the vessel wall structure, which precedes microaneurysmal formation. Endothelial cell dropout is influenced by increased blood flow rate in the retinal capillaries, which also weakens the vessel wall structure. Not all the etiologic factors influencing the development of microvascular changes of retinal vessels are known. Vessel wall disease results in the breakdown of the blood–retina barrier, causing intraretinal accumulation of blood products. These can be observed as hemorrhage, exudate, or retinal thickening and are seen

Table 9-4. Histopathologic Changes in Retinal Vessels Resulting From Diabetes

Vessel wall compromise resulting in a breakdown in the blood–retinal barrier
Capillary nonperfusion and closure resulting in ischemia
Neovascular growth of retinal and/or iris vessels

to varying degrees throughout the fundus. All retinal capillary beds are not affected uniformly; therefore, more or fewer vascular changes will be observed in each field of the retina. The extent to which these changes are seen throughout the fundus aids in the appropriate classification of diabetic retinopathy. Intraretinal accumulation of these products in the macular area is associated with vision loss and can occur at any stage of retinopathy.

Capillary nonperfusion (or dropout) and retinal ischemia are associated with impending vision loss. Capillary nonperfusion cannot be directly observed by ophthalmoscopy but requires the aid of fluorescein angiography to detect its presence and determine the extent of the capillary closure. Infarction of the overlying nerve fiber layer accompanies acute capillary closure; however, infarction resolves over a short period (i.e., a few weeks to 1 month). Resolution of the microinfarct does not imply reperfusion of that capillary bed but, rather some level of compensation by the surrounding beds. The ophthalmic practitioner cannot infer good capillary perfusion based solely on the absence of microinfarcts but should look for other signs associated severity of retinal vascular disease such as intraretinal microvascular abnormalities (IRMA), venous beading, and neovascularization. A fluorescein angiogram is needed to reveal the exact extent of capillary perfusion despite the presence or absence of these other findings. Microinfarcts are not observed with closure of the perifoveal capillary beds. There are insufficient nerve fibers in this area to manifest any observable microinfarct. Capillary closure in the perifoveal area would not be detected if microinfarcts were the only clue used to determine their presence in this area.

Progressive ischemia induces various retinal vascular changes that can be observed ophthalmoscopically. IRMA are engorged small retinal vessels that attempt to compensate for poor perfusion in the surrounding capillary beds. Progression in the number of areas of IRMA relates to increasing amounts of capillary disease and reflects the overall level of retinal schemia. The defined intraretinal course of these vessels helps differentiate them from neovascular vessel growth that has a random course and possible elevation. The fluorescein angiographic appearance of these vessels fails to reveal the significant leakage of dye commonly observed with neovascular vessels. Venous loops and beading are two large vessel responses to increasing levels of retinal ischemia. They serve as a poor prognostic indicator for long-term vision preservation because of their association with progressive diabetic retinal disease.

Neovascular vessels grow in response to capillary nonperfusion. Evidence supports an imbalance in stimulatory retinal growth factors and inhibitory retinal growth factors as the etiology for neovascular development.[46] Imbalance of the homeostatic mechanism in favor of excessive growth or insufficient inhibitory factors enhances the development of neovascular vessel growth. A number of growth factors are released by retinal tissue, which may be upset by tissue death from vascular disease. Neovascular vessel walls lack adequate structural support, predisposing the vessels to leakage and fibrous proliferation. Involvement of the vitreous cavity with associated fibrovascular tissue frequently leads to vitreous hemorrhage, tractional retinal detachment, and vision loss. This can occur despite aggressive laser or surgical intervention.

Classification of Diabetic Retinopathy

Diabetic retinopathy falls into two categories, either nonproliferative or proliferative retinopathy, based on the ophthalmoscopic and fluorescein angiographic characteristics. Each type of retinopathy can be divided into subcategories (Table 9-5), which has progressively higher risk for vision loss. The presence of clinically significant macular edema (CSME) associated with diabetes can occur at any stage of retinopathy, stressing the importance of critical evaluation of the macula at all stages of retinopathy. The modified Airlee House grading system for diabetic retinopathy[47] established standard photographs for grading retinal changes from diabetes. It serves as the standard for grading diabetic retinopathy. The appropriate classification need be determined only after critical evaluation of the retina and comparison to this system. A diabetic patient's risk of developing severe vision loss within a 5-year period is determined following proper classification.

Mild Nonproliferative Diabetic Retinopathy

Mild nonproliferative diabetic retinopathy (NPDR) is the earliest stage of retinopathy that can be observed. The presence of one hemorrhage or microaneurysm classifies the patient with this type of retinopathy (less severe than the Airlee House standard photograph 2A). No other hemorrhages, exudates, or microin-

Table 9-5. Characteristics of Diabetic Retinopathy

Mild NPDR
    One microaneurysm
    Criteria for moderate NPDR or higher not met
Moderate NPDR (one characteristic)
    Hemorrhage and/or microaneurysms in four retinal fields greater than standard photograph 2A with no fields of greater severity
    Retinal microinfarcts, venous beading, or IRMA found to a mild degree in one quadrant
    Criteria for severe NPDR not met
Severe NPDR (one characteristic)
    Severe hemorrhages and/or microaneurysms in four retinal quadrants
    Moderate venous beading in one quadrant (greater than or equal to standard photograph 6B)
    Moderate IRMA (greater than or equal to standard photograph 8A) in one quadrant without frank neovascularization
    Criteria for very severe NPDR not met
Very severe NPDR
    Two or more characteristics of severe NPDR present
    Criteria for PDR not met
Early proliferative retinopathy
    Neovascular vessels on or within 1 disc diameter of the optic nerve (NVD) whose size is a minimum of one-third to one-fourth disc diameter in size
High-risk proliferative retinopathy
    Neovascular vessels on or within 1 disc diameter whose size is less than one-third to one-fourth disc diameter if accompanied by a preretinal or vitreous hemorrhage
    NVE accompanied by a preretinal or vitreous hemorrhage
    Fibrovascular proliferation into vitreous
Nonspecific characteristics of proliferative disease
    NVD or NVE
    Preretinal or vitreous hemorrhage
    Fibrovascular proliferation

Abbreviations: IRMA, intraretinal microvascular abnormalites; NPDR, nonproliferative diabetic retinopathy; NVD, neovascularization of the disc; NVE, neovascularization elsewhere.
(Data from the Early Treatment Diabetic Retinopathy[47] and the Diabetic Retinopathy Study Research Group.[48])

farcts need be present. CSME may be present at this stage. This stage of retinopathy is associated with a 15 percent chance of developing into high-risk PDR within 5 years. Fluorescein angiography is not necessary as a diagnostic or therapeutic tool at this stage, because decisions regarding laser treatment need not be made at this stage. Efficacy in laser treatment at this stage has not been proved unless CSME is present. Evaluations should be performed every 6 months to monitor progression of this stage of retinopathy. Patients should be educated concerning visual symptoms related to macular edema at this stage. Patients should return for an evaluation whenever they experience symptoms of decreased vision.

Moderate Nonproliferative Diabetic Retinopathy

Moderate NPDR is associated with an increased number of retinal hemorrhages or microinfarcts in four retinal zones (as described in the modified Airlee House system). A patient with mild involvement in less than four zones cannot be classified at this level. Mild IRMA, minimal venous beading, or isolated microinfarction can be observed at this stage as long as less than four zones are involved. Approximately 17 percent of these patients progress to PDR within 1 year, and about 30 percent progress to high-risk PDR over a 5-year period. The macular area should be critically evaluated with a Goldmann-type fundus lens (for optimal view) or a clear slit lamp lens (90 D, 78 D or 60 D) for the presence of CSME. Laser treatment for CSME is necessary, with no proven efficacy for other laser treatment for this stage of retinopathy. These patients should be evaluated approximately every 6 months depending on the clinical presentation. Photographic documentation may be beneficial for this stage of retinopathy. Co-management with a retinologist may be considered if laser treatment for CSME is needed.

Severe Nonproliferative Diabetic Retinopathy

Severe NPDR is associated with increasing numbers of hemorrhages and microaneurysms in four or more zones and/or moderate venous beading in one or more zones. Moderate IRMA in one or more zones also places a patient in this category. No evidence of neovascularization is seen at this stage. Fluorescein angiography may be extremely helpful in differentiating between advancing IRMA and neovascularization. Macular edema may be present at this stage and be associated with decreased vision. These patients have about a 50 percent chance for progression to PDR within 1 year and a 60 percent chance of developing high-risk PDR within 5 years. Co-management with a retinologist should be considered because panretinal photocoagulation (PRP) may be necessary, considering the high risk of progression to high-risk PDR and vision loss. The guidelines for PRP are not well established for patients in this category, and the decisions concerning laser intervention are best determined on an individual basis. Regular evaluations should be performed every 3 months (at most) if laser treatment is deferred. Photographic documentation of the retinopathy is very beneficial at this stage.

An overlap of one or more of the clinical features of severe NPDR comprises the category of very severe NPDR (Fig. 9-4 and Plate 9-4). These patients are at high risk of suffering from vision loss and require laser treatment.

Proliferative Diabetic Retinopathy

If neovascularization is present, even to a small degree, the patient is considered to have early PDR. The

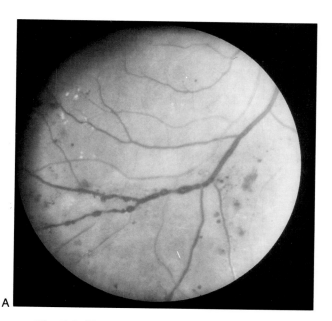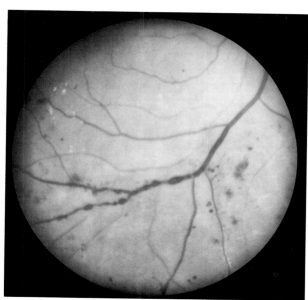

Fig. 9-4. Very severe nonproliferative diabetic retinopathy in a type II diabetic patient. **(A)** Severe venous beading present in three quadrants, which is more easily seen with **(B)** a red-free filter. (See also Plate 9-3.) The patient progressed to neovascularization of the disc within 6 months.

presence of neovascularization of the disc or neovascularization elsewhere still qualifies as PDR despite its location or small size. Some level of NPDR characteristics is observed at this stage in addition to the presence of neovascularization. All patients with PDR do not manifest extensive venous beading, IRMA, microinfarcts, microaneurysms, hemorrhages, and exudates throughout the entire fundus or posterior pole. Neovascularization may appear with observable retinal hemorrhages, exudates, microaneurysms, microinfarcts, IRMA, or venous beading to varying degrees. Extensive capillary closure may be associated with few microinfarcts, exudates or hemorrhages. Fluorescein angiography will reveal extensive areas of capillary closure despite the varying degrees of retinal hemorrhage or microinfarction. Patient with low-risk PDR will develop high-risk PDR 75 percent of the time within a 5-year period.[48]

These patients require PRP to minimize the risk of developing severe vision loss. The risk of severe vision loss is greatly diminished (approximately 50 percent) if PRP is performed. The efficacy of PRP for minimizing vision loss has been determined based on a full (1,500 to 1,800 spot) laser treatment, by the ETDRS guidelines. Partial treatment may help neovascularization regress in the acute post-laser treatment period; however, the same long-term response and visual preservation from a partial treatment has not been proved. Patients who have regression or stabilization of their proliferative disease still require routine care to monitor further progression. Follow-up every 2 to 3 months in coordination with a retinologist is recommended. Patients with retinopathy that does not meet the criterion for treatment by the DRS or ETDRS recommendations and still show multiple high-risk signs may be offered laser treatment at the discretion of the retinologist co-managing the patient's care.

Vitrectomy is beneficial for patients with recurrent or unresolving vitreous hemorrhage after 4 months. Some evidence supports early vitrectomy, but the long-term results do not appear significantly different. Endolaser or binocular indirect laser treatment at the time of vitrectomy has proven very beneficial for patients with proliferative retinopathy who could not be accessed for laser treatment before the vitrectomy. Retinal detachments associated with tractional vitreoretinopathy should be referred to a retinologist for evaluation and surgical intervention when detected.

Table 9-6. Characteristics of Clinically Significant Macular Edema

Retinal thickening at or within 500 μm of the center of the fovea
Hard exudates at or within 500 μm of the center of the fovea if there is thickening of the adjacent retina
Any area or retinal thickening equal to or larger than a disc diameter whose edge borders within 1 disc diameter of the center of the fovea

Diabetic Maculopathy

Diabetic maculopathy consists of both diabetic macular edema as well as ischemic maculopathy. Diabetic macular edema occurs at any stage of retinopathy, mild NPDR through high-risk PDR. It may be classified as either clinically significant or not clinically significant, depending on the presentation the size and proximity to the macula (Table 9-6).

Areas of leakage as evidenced by the presence of hemorrhage and/or exudation without retinal thickening are not considered to be CSME. These patients should be monitored bimonthly to monitor progression to CSME, and referral should be made to a retinologist for focal or grid laser treatment at the appropriate time. The ETDRS has shown a 50 percent progression to moderate vision loss for patients who have received focal laser treatment when compared with patients who have not. Patients with macular edema and high-risk retinopathy that requires PRP benefit from treatment of the maculopathy before PRP because the PRP may worsen the CSME. The sequencing of treatment should be determined by the retinologist.

Ischemic maculopathy has no observable signs by ophthalmoscopy. It results from capillary nonperfusion and closure at the edges of the Foveal avascular zone (FAZ). These vessels supply nutrition to the nerve fibers at the edge of the foveal pit. The unique retinal anatomy of the foveal and perifoveal areas do not allow for microinfarcts to manifest in this region; therefore, they will not be observed in the acute period of capillary closure at the edges of the foveal avascular zone (FAZ). The FAZ will appear irregular in shape or larger than normal, which is well demonstrated on fluorescein angiography (Figs. 9-5 and 9-6 and Plate 9-4). The ischemic maculopathy may represent a separate entity or be coincident with other areas of retinal ischemia.

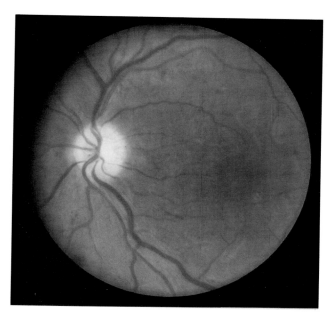

Fig. 9-5. Ischemic maculopathy in the left eye of a 32-year-old patient with type I diabetes. Note the lack of hemorrhage or microinfarction of the macular area despite a visual acuity of 20/100. The patient had early proliferative diabetic retinopathy in both eyes. Evaluation of the macula with a Goldmann contact lens revealed no evidence of retinal thickening. (See also Plate 9-4.)

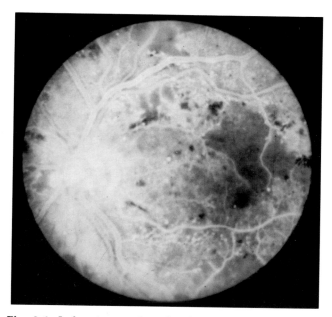

Fig. 9-6. Ischemic maculopathy demonstrated by fluorescein angiography. This is the fluorescein angiogram of the patient in Figure 9-5. Note the capillary nonperfusion of the perifoveal vascular network.

Ischemic maculopathy is seen in both IDDM and NIDDM patients after significant disease progression (i.e., after more than 20 years of well-controlled NIDDM). Ischemic maculopathy is related to diabetic retinopathy progression with the manifestation of ischemic foci involving the foveal area. Patients experience a gradual decrease of vision, which cannot be improved by refraction, yet the macular evaluation fails to reveal any macular edema. Mild decreased vision (20/30) in the early stages can progress to severe vision loss (20/200 or worse) with time. A central scotoma corresponding to the ischemic zone may be detected on Amsler grid evaluation. A pupillary defect is not associated with this entity because of the small amount of retina involved, but it can be indicative of extensive retinal ischemia. Laser treatment is ineffective and is therefore not a treatment option. No effective medical treatment for ischemic maculopathy is available at this time. Vision rehabilitative services should be considered for patients with significant vision loss from ischemic maculopathy.

DIABETIC TREATMENT AND EFFECTS ON RETINOPATHY

Clinical thought concerning treatment of the diabetic patient has changed since the results of the DCCT.[49] The results of this study have challenged traditional thinking concerning the "ideal" glucose levels in IDDM patients, with some implications for NIDDM patients. Despite the higher incidence of hypoglycemia, a direct relationship exists between strict glycemic control and decreased progression of diabetic retinopathy, neuropathy, and nephropathy.

A single glycosylated hemoglobin (HbA_{1C}) continues to be a valuable predictor of progression of mild-to-moderate retinopathy to more severe forms within 4 years.[26,27,50] Patients whose mean HbA_{1C} value was decreased from 9 to 7 percent had no beneficial effect on the retinopathy until after 3 years.[40,50] Stable HbA_{1C} values, reflecting long-term good glycemic control, appeared to have a positive effect on diabetic retinopathy that could not be reversed for approximately 4 years, despite poorer control during that period. The risk for progression to vision-threatening retinopathy from either macular edema or proliferative retinopathy was reduced by 48 to 54 percent in IDDM patients, whose mean serum glucose levels were reduced by 50 mg/dl (reflecting a decreased HbA_{1C} level from 9 to 7 percent). Patients with initiation of intensive therapy (as established by the DCCT) with no retinopathy at the onset of the treatment period, progressed to mild-to-moderate retinopathy in 76 percent of patients within 8- to 9-years.[49] This proved that a delay in the number of retinal microaneurysms will occur in patients undergoing intensive insulin therapy. The DCCT results also established similar beneficial effects on diabetic nephropathy and neuropathy. Because the cohort of IDDM patients in this study were young and had minimal macrovascular disease, a similar correlation between good glycemic control and macrovascular disease could not be established.

CONCLUSION

The treatment and management of diabetic retinopathy has been made easier with the guidelines established by the DRS, ETDRS, and Diabetic Retinopathy Vitrectomy Study (DRVS). Ophthalmic practitioners continue to be challenged by patients with diabetic retinopathy who cannot be easily classified or whose treatment may require an approach not well established by previous clinical trials. Patients with diabetic retinopathy can maintain vision and maximize their functional level with good glycemic control and laser treatment at the appropriate time. The classification of diabetic retinopathy, as determined by the ETDRS, has enhanced our understanding of diabetic retinopathy and the potential for vision loss, given each of these levels of retinopathy. It is important that the exact level of retinopathy be established for each patient and that evaluations be scheduled at regular intervals, depending on severity of diabetic retinopathy. Dilated eye examinations are crucial for diabetic patients with or without diabetic retinopathy, considering the lack of subjective symptoms in many diabetic patients despite the presence of high-risk retinopathy.

Eye care practitioners frequently detect ocular and systemic signs of uncontrolled or poorly controlled diabetes. Because many ocular manifestations are harbingers of inadequate systemic regulation of hyperglycemia, a critical evaluation of a patient's therapeutic regimen by the appropriate health-care provider is required. The sharing of information is necessary among health-care providers, so the ramifications of all clinical findings can be considered in the treatment and management plans for diabetics.

REFERENCES

1. Geiss LS, Herman WH, Goldschmid MG et al: Surveillance for diabetes mellitus—United States, 1980–1989. MMWR 42(SS-2): 1, 1993
2. Trends in diabetes mellitus mortality. MMWR 37(50), 1988
3. Lernmark A: Insulin-dependent diabetes mellitus. p. 35. In Davidson JK (ed): Clinical Diabetes Mellitus. A problem-oriented approach. 2nd Ed. Thieme Medical Publishers, New York, 1991
4. Lorenzi M: Diabetes mellitus. p. 463. In Fitzgerald PA (ed): Handbook of Clinical Endocrinology. Appleton & Lange, East Norwalk, CT, 1992
5. Gepts W: Pathologic anatomy of the pancreas in juvenile diabetes mellitus. Diabetes 14:619, 1965
6. MacCuish AC, Irvine WJ: Autoimmune aspects of diabetes mellitus. Clin Endocrinol Metab 4:435, 1975
7. Bottazzo GF, Dean BM, McNally JM, et al: In situ characterization of autoimmune phenomenon and expression of HLA molecules in the pancreas of diabetic insulitis. N Engl J Med 6:353, 1985
8. Friedlaender MH: Neurologic and endocrine diseases. p. 283. In: Allergy and Immunology of the Eye. 2nd Ed. Raven Press, New York, 1993
9. Davidson JK: Diabetic ketoacidosis and the hyperglycemic hyperosmolar state. p. 394. In Davidson JK (ed): Clinical Diabetes Mellitus. A Problem-Oriented Approach. 2nd Ed. Thieme Medical, New York, 1991
10. Salans LB, Cushman SW: Relationship of adiposity and diet to the abnormalities of carbohydrate metabolism in obesity. p. 267. In Katzen HL, Mahler RJ (eds): Advances in Modern Nutrition. Vol. 2. Diabetes, Obesity and Vascular Disease. John Wiley & Sons, New York, 1978
11. Feldt-Rasmussen B, Mathisen E, Deckert T: Effect of two years of strict metabolic control on progression of incipient nephropathy in IDDM. Lancet 2:1300, 1986
12. Grunwald JE, Brucker AJ, Schwartz SS et al: Diabetic glycemic control and retinal blood flow. Diabetes 39:602, 1990
13. Leicter SB: Association between glycemic control and degenerative complications of diabetes mellitus: a brief review of current concepts. p. 87. In Kerstein MD (ed): Diabetes and Vascular Disease. JB Lippincott, Philadelphia, 1990
14. Knatterud GL, Klimt CR, Goldner MG et al: Effects of hypoglycemic agents on vascular complications in patients with adult onset diabetes. VIII. Evaluation of insulin therapy: final report. Diabetes 31:1, 1982
15. Ambrus JL: Microvascular changes in diabetes. p. 9. In Kerstein MD (ed): Diabetes and Vascular Disease. JB Lippincott, Philadelphia, 1990
16. Pugliese G, Tiltion RG, Speedy A et al: Effects of very mild versus overt diabetes on vascular hemodynamics and barrier function in rats. Diabetologica 2:845, 1989
17. Beach KW, Brunzell JD, Conquest LL et al: The correlation of arteriosclerosis obliterans with lipoproteins in insulin-dependent and non-insulin dependent diabetes. Diabetes 28:836, 1979
18. De La Rubia G, Oliver FJ, Inoguchi T, King G: Induction of resistance to endothelin-1's biochemical actions by elevated glucose levels in retinal pericytes. Diabetes 41:1533, 1992
19. Pirart J: Diabetes mellitus and its degenerative complications: a prospective study of 4,400 patients observed between 1947 and 1973. Diabetes Care 1:168, 1978
20. West KM, Erdreich LJ, Stober JA: A detailed study of risk factors for retinopathy and nephropathy in diabetes. Diabetes 29: 501, 1980
21. Feldman JN, Hirsch SR, Beyer MM et al: Prevalence of diabetic nephropathy at the time of treatment for diabetic retinopathy. p. 9. In Friedman EA, L'Esperrance FA (eds): Diabetic Renal-Retinal Syndrome. Vol. 2. Grune & Stratton, Orlando, FL, 1982

22. Chronic disease reports: Deaths from diabetes—United States 1986. MMWR 38:543, 1989
23. Greene DA: Metabolic abnormalities in the diabetic peripheral nerve: relation to impaired function. Metabolism, suppl. 1. 32: 118, 1983
24. Greene DA, Lattimer SA, Sima AAF: Sorbitol, phosphoinositides and potassium-ATPase in the pathogenesis of diabetic complications. N Engl J Med 316:599, 1985
25. Clements RS Jr: Diabetic neuropathy—new concepts of its etiology. Diabetes 28:604, 1979
26. Klein R, Klein BEK, Moss SE et al: The Wisconsin eipdemiologic study of diabetic retinopathy: IX. Four year incidence and progression of diabetic retinopathy when age at diagnosis is less than 30 years. Arch Ophthalmol 107:237, 1989
27. Klein R, Klein BEK, Moss SE et al: The Wisconsin epidemiologic study of diabetic retinopathy: X. Four year incidence and progression of diabetic retinopathy when age at diagnosis is 30 years or more. Arch Ophthalmol 107:244, 1989
28. Miller N: Topical diagnosis of neuropathic ocular motility disorders. p. 652. In: Walsh and Hoyt's Clinical Neuro-Ophthalmology. 4th Ed. Vol. 2. Williams & Wilkins, Baltimore, 1985
29. Benson WE, Brown GC, Tasman W: Non-retinal ophthalmic abnormalities of diabetes. p. 110. In Benson WE, Broen GC, Tasman W (eds): Diabetes and Its Ocular Complications. WB Saunders, Philadelphia, 1988
30. Hayashim, Ishikawa S: Pharmacology of pupillary responses in diabetic—correlative study of the responses and grade of retinopathy. Jpn J Ophthalmol 23:65, 1979
31. Hreidarson AB: Pupil motility in long-term diabetes. Diabetologica 17:145, 1979
32. Appen RE, Chandra SR, Klein R, Myers FL: Diabetic papillopathy. Am J Ophthalmol 90:203, 1980
33. Lubow M, Makely TA: Pseudopapilledema of juvenile diabetes mellitus. Arch Ophthalmol 85:417, 1971
34. Glaser JS: Topical diagnosis: prechiasmal visual pathway. p. 1. In Tasman W, Jaeger EA (eds): Duane's Clinical Ophthalmology. Vol. 2. JB Lippincott, Philadelphia, 1993
35. Barr CC, Glaser JS, Blankenship G: Acute disc swelling in juvenile diabetes. Clinical profile and natural history of 12 cases. Arch Ophthalmol 98:2185, 1980
36. Skillern PG, Lockhart G: Optic neuritis and uncontrolled diabetes mellitus in 14 patients. Ann Intern Med 51:468, 1959
37. Rogell GD: Corneal hypaesthesia and retinopathy in diabetes mellitus. Ophthalmology 87:229, 1980
38. Ishida N, Rao GN, del Cerro M et al: Corneal nerve alterations in diabetes mellitus. Arch Ophthalmol 102:1380, 1984
39. Safir A, Paulsen EP, Klayman J et al: Ocular abnormalities in juvnile diabetics: frequent occurrence of abnormally high tension. Arch Ophthalmol 76:557, 1966
40. Blamksma LJ, Rouwe C, Drayer NJ: Retinopathy and intraocular pressure in diabetic children. Ophthalmologica 187:137, 1983
41. Becker B, Bresnik G, Chevrette L et al: Intraocular pressure and its response to topical corticosteroids in diabetes. Arch Ophthalmol 76:477, 1966
42. Becker B: Diabetes and primary open-angle glaucoma. Am J Ophthalmol 71:1, 1971
43. Hetherington J, Schaffer RN: Glaucoma research conference. Am J Ophthalmol 58:1065, 1964
44. Brown GC, Magargal LE, Schachat A et al: Neovascular glaucoma, etiologic considerations. Ophthalmology 91:315, 1984
45. Brown GC: Central retinal vein obstruction. p. 65. In Reineke RD (ed): Ophthalmology Annual. Vol. 1. Appleton-Century-Crofts, East Norwalk, CT, 1985
46. Widemann P: Growth factors in retinal diseases: proliferative vitreoretinopathy, proliferative diabetic retinopathy and retinal degeneration. Surv Ophthalmol 36(5):373, 1992
47. The Early Treatment Diabetic Retinopathy Study Research Group: Grading diabetic retinopathy from stereoscopic color fundus photographs—an extension of the modified Airlie House classification. ETDRS report number 10. Ophthalmology 98:786, 1991
48. The Diabetic Retinopathy Study Research Group: Two year course of visual acuity in severe proliferative diabetic retinopathy with conventional management. Diabetic retinopathy study report number 1. Ophthalmology 92:492, 1985
49. The Diabetes Control and Complications Trial (DCCT): N Engl J Med 329:683, 1993
50. Santiago JV: Lessons from the diabetes control and complications trial. Diabetes 42:1549, 1993

10 Hematologic Disease

HELENE M. KAISER

INTRODUCTION

Hematologic disorders include a wide range of conditions as a result of the many components of blood. The major blood components consist of erythrocytes, leukocytes, plasma cells, platelets, and coagulation factors.[1] Each, in an abnormal concentration, can disrupt hematopoiesis. Because of the highly vascularized nature of the eye, hematologic disorders cause many different ocular signs. This chapter outlines the major hematologic disorders and their ocular manifestations.

CASE REPORT

A 43-year-old black man presented with complaints of reduced vision in the left eye for 3 days. His medical history was remarkable for sickle cell trait. His ocular history was negative, and he was taking no medications.

Best visual acuities were OD 20/20, OS 20/400. Pupil responses were normal, with no afferent defects, and extraocular muscles were intact. Biomicroscopy revealed deep and quiet anterior chambers. Intraocular pressure was 18 mmHg OU by applanation. Dilated fundus examination of the right eye revealed areas of sea-fan-like neovascularization, superotemporal in the retinal periphery. Examination of the left eye was obscured by the presence of a vitreal hemorrhage.

The patient underwent scatter photocoagulation treatment of the sea-fans in the right eye. The vitreal hemorrhage in the left eye resolved over the next 2 months and subsequently revealed the presence of sea-fan neovascularization as the cause of vitreal hemorrhage. Laser treatment was also performed to the scattered sea-fan areas to promote regression of the neovascularization.

ERYTHROCYTE DISORDERS

Anemia

Anemia is one of the most common manifestations of disease in the world.[1] *Anemia* is defined as a reduction in the number of erythrocytes or a reduction in hemoglobin below a physiologic need set by tissue oxygen demand.[2] Anemia is not a disease but a symptom of a number of different diseases or disorders.[3] Anemia may be classified according to pathophysiologic mechanism, etiology, or morphologic appearance of the red blood cells (RBCs).[4] Pathophysiologic mechanisms of anemia are classified either by decreased erythrocyte production or increased erythrocyte loss.[5] One of the most common causes of anemia (25 percent) of the hospitalized population in the United States is iron deficiency, resulting in decreased hemoglobin and RBC production. Acute blood loss represents another 25 percent of cases hospitalized. Chronic inflammatory diseases that cause anemia also represent 25 percent of cases. All other causes of anemia represent the remaining percentage.[4]

The morphologic appearance of the erythrocyte can be classified by size (macrocytic, normocytic, or microcytic) and coloration (normochromic or hypochromic).[4] Laboratory evaluation of anemia includes the complete blood count: hemoglobin, hematocrit, white blood cell (WBC) count, differential, platelet count, RBC indices, and the peripheral blood smear[2] (see Ch. 1).

Macrocytic Anemia

In macrocytic anemia, the number of erythrocytes is greatly reduced, and the RBCs are much larger than normal.[6] Causes of macrocytic anemia include vitamin B_{12} (pernicious anemia) deficiency, folic acid deficiency, diseases of the stomach or small bowel, pregnancy, alcoholism, chemotherapy,[2] liver disease, hypothyroidism,[1] or "primary" marrow disorders.[7]

Ocular signs are more frequent with macrocytic anemia because the thrombocytopenia often associated with it enhances the hemorrhagic findings.[6,8] Ocular manifestations include white-centered hemorrhages (Roth spot), cotton-wool patches, a pale fundus, generalized retinal edema,[6] bilateral optic neuropathy, bilateral central or cecocentral scotomas[9,10] flame-shaped hemorrhages, venous tortuosity,[11,12] and eventual optic nerve atrophy.[10,13]

Normocytic Anemia

Normocytic anemia occurs when the absolute number of erythrocytes decreases and/or the quantity of blood in the body decreases. Common causes of normocytic anemia include blood loss, decreased production of blood elements (e.g., in aplastic anemia, anemia of chronic disease, liver disease, renal failure, "primary" bone marrow disorders, or endocrine disorders), or increased destruction of blood cells (found in extrinsic or intrinsic hemolytic anemia).[1,2,4,6,7]

The severity of the ocular signs is associated with the severity of the anemia. Ocular manifestations include retinal hemorrhages with or without central pallor; generalized edema; flame-shaped hemorrhages; pale veins; thread-like arterioles; numerous cotton-wool patches; anterior ischemic optic neuropathy;[5] eventual optic atrophy; visual field loss of arcuate, quadratic, or hemispheric patterns;[6,14] bilateral loss of vision usually within 48 hours of severe blood loss;[15] and blindness.[6]

Microcytic Anemia

Microcytic anemia is characterized by a decrease in the size of the erythrocytes with a decrease in hemoglobin (hypochromic).[3,6] The three major causes of microcytic anemia are iron deficiency, anemia of chronic disease, and thalassemia.[1,7] The most common cause of anemia throughout the world is iron deficiency.[7] The causative factors of iron deficiency include deficient diet, malabsorption, chronic blood loss (gastrointestinal, menstrual, blood donation), increased requirements (pregnancy, lactation), hemoglobinuria, or pulmonary hemosiderosis.[6,7]

Ocular signs are present only in unusually severe microcytic anemia.[6] They include flame hemorrhages with or without pale centers, round blot hemorrhages, exudates, generalized retinal edema, papilledema, cotton-wool patches, and venous tortuosity.[1,6,12,16]

Correct treatment of the specific anemia usually results in reversal of the ocular signs with good visual prognosis unless severe retinal or optic nerve infarction has occurred.[13,14]

Hemoglobinopathies

The most common inherited disorders in humans are hemoglobinopathies.[1] In patients with hemoglobinopathies, the abnormal clinical signs are the result of altered structure, function, or production of hemoglobin, the oxygen transportation protein of the blood.[1]

The five major classifications of hemoglobinopathies follow:

1. Structural hemoglobinopathies are the result of mutations that alter the amino acid sequence, and thus, the physical and chemical properties of the globin, such as solubility or oxygen affinity. Examples of structural alteration include sickle cell anemia.
2. Thalassemia syndromes are the result of defective and imbalanced globin-chain synthesis and precipitation of the unpaired chains.
3. Thalassemic-hemoglobin syndromes demonstrate features of both thalassemia and structural hemoglobinopathies.
4. Persistence of fetal hemoglobin occurs when production of fetal hemoglobin continues after the perinatal period.
5. Acquired hemoglobinopathies are the result of toxins or other disease processes.[1]

Hemoglobin is the major protein in the erythrocyte. It binds oxygen for transportation to the tissues. Each hemoglobin molecule consists of two pairs of globin-polypeptide chains.[2] Six different globin chains occur in normal hemoglobin: α, β, γ, δ, ϵ, and ζ.[17] Normal adult hemoglobin is made up of mainly (97 percent) hemoglobin A; the molecule of which consists of two α-globin chains and two β-globin chains ($\alpha_2\beta_2$). A very small portion (3 percent) comprises a pair of α-globin chains and a pair of δ-globin chains. A hemoglobin found in trace amounts after birth is fetal hemoglobin.[17] Fetal hemoglobin (HbF) contains a pair of α-globin chains and a pair of γ-globin chains.

Erythrocytes containing normal hemoglobin resemble a biconcave disc that is pliable and flexible and easily flows through capillaries. An alteration in the amino acid sequence in the globin chain, such as a single substitution of an amino acid, results in an abnormally functioning molecule.[2] This single substitution can cause changes in shape, oxygen affinity, pliability, solubility, electrophoretic movement, and life span of the hemoglobin molecule. The mutations are recorded according to the geographic location in the amino acid chain where the substitution occurred. When valine is substituted for glutamic acid in the sixth position of the β-globin chain, it is designated as $\alpha_2\beta_2^{6Glu\rightarrow Val}$ and is known as sickle hemoglobin (HbS). When lysine is substituted for glutamic acid, hemoglobin C (HbC) is recorded as $\alpha_2\beta_2^{6Glu\rightarrow Lys}$.[17] Erythrocytes containing HbS have an elongated or crescent shape, especially under conditions of hypoxia. The "sickled" cells are more rigid and tend to restrict blood flow in small blood vessels, and thus cause further tissue hypoxia.[18]

Thalassemia results in the presence of a genetic defect in the rate of synthesis of a protein chain.[19] Thalassemia and sickle hemoglobin can be inherited together and result in a condition called *sickle cell thalassemia*.[18]

Inheritance of the sickle hemoglobinopathies is autosomal co-dominant; each parent provides one gene for the hemoglobin. The distribution for sickle cell syndromes can be seen in Table 10-1. A hemoglobin electrophoresis is required for definitive diagnosis of the hemoglobin types.

The incidence of this condition follows: Of American blacks, 8 percent have sickle cell trait (AS), 0.4% have sickle cell anemia (SS), 0.2% have sickle cell disease (SC), and 0.1% have sickle cell thalassemia (SThal).[7,20,21]

SS has the most severe systemic symptomatology, with an unrelenting hemolytic anemia, periodic acute episodes of pain and fever, and a high mortality rate in early childhood.[7] The ocular complications of SS, however, are usually mild and asymptomatic.[10] SC and SThal have mild systemic symptoms but the most severe ocular complications.[22-24] AS is the mildest form, in terms of both systemic and ocular manifestations. Symptoms occur only in extreme circumstances of severe hypoxia.[1]

Ocular Complications

Ocular complications of the sickling hemoglobinopathies can be related directly or indirectly to vascular occlusion.[18] These complications can be grouped into three categories: nonretinal, nonproliferative retinopathy, and proliferative retinopathy.[10]

Nonretinal

Nonretinal ocular manifestations of sickling hemoglobinopathies can be seen in the conjunctiva. Short, comma-shaped vascular segments[17,21] in the lower bulbar conjunctiva[25] can most commonly be found in patients with SS and SC.[17] These conjunctival changes are asymptomatic. Rarely, the iris may demonstrate ischemia, atrophy, and occasionally neovascularization from the pupillary border to the collarette.[21,25]

Nonproliferative

Nonproliferative sickle retinopathy changes that are asymptomatic are listed in Table 10-2. Venous tortuosity is a common characteristic of sickling retinopathy.

Table 10-1. Sickle Cell Syndromes

Parents	Genotype	Diagnosis	Hemoglobin Distribution
HbA + HbA = AA	Normal	97% HbA
HbA + HbS = AS	Sickle cell trait	60% HbA, 40% HbS
HbS + HbS = SS	Sickle cell anemia	92% HbS, 8% HbF
HbS + HbC = SC	Sickle cell disease	50% HbS, 50% HbC
HbS + Thal = SThal	Sickle cell thalassemia	80% HbS, 20% HbF

(Data from Wyngaarden et al.,[1] Andreoli et al.,[2] and Schroeder et al.[7])

Table 10-2. Non-proliferative Sickle Cell Retinopathy

Asymptomatic lesions
  Venous tortuosity
  Black sunbursts
  Refractile deposits
  Silver-wire arterioles
  Salmon-patch hemorrhages
  Retinal holes
Symptomatic lesions
  Central retinal artery occlusion
  Macular artery occlusion
  Retinal venous occlusion
  Choroidal vascular occlusion
  Angioid streaks

In one study it was found in 47 percent of patients with SS and in 32 percent of patients with SC.[24] Venous tortuosity is associated with many other diseases and is not pathognomonic of sickle cell hemoglobinopathies.[18]

Black sunbursts are described as peripheral, black, ovoid, circumscribed fundus lesions that are approximately 0.5 to 2 DD in size with spiculate or stellate borders.[24] These lesions are likely the result of an acute vascular occlusion of the retina, causing deep retinal hemorrhage near the retinal pigment epithelium (RPE). The reparative process of the retina then produces RPE hypertrophy and hemosiderin deposition.[25–29] In a selected series, these lesions were observed in 71 percent of SThal patients, 43 percent of SS patients, and in 18 percent of SC patients.[24,30] In an unselected series, black sunbursts occurred in 41 percent of SC patients and 18 percent of SS patients.[26]

Glistening, refractile deposits in the retinal periphery occur as a result of hemosiderin-laden macrophages after they resorb the intraretinal blood.[31] These iridescent yellow spots can occur in retinal schisis cavities or in pigmented lesions or can be scattered in the retina.[26] In a unselected study, they were present in 25 percent of SC patients and 15 percent of SS patients.[26]

Silver wire arterioles in the hemoglobinopathies are the result of peripheral arteriolar occlusions.[18] The appearance of the silver wire arterioles can be a prognostic sign for the subsequent development of neovascular proliferation.[18,25]

A salmon-patch hemorrhage occurs when collecting sickled erythrocytes suddenly occlude an arteriole, causing a subsequent blow-out hemorrhage just distal to the occlusion.[31,32] These small, oval hemorrhages initially appear red, then change to pink, then orange, then yellow-white in color,[18] and often disappear. The hemosiderin may give rise to refractile deposits. The hemorrhage may also result in pigmented black sunbursts.[33] Because in the initial stages the hemorrhage may resemble a retinal hole, indirect ophthalmoscopy and scleral indentation are necessary to differentiate them.[23]

Retinal holes may develop in equatorial or pre-equatorial locations and are usually asymptomatic until they cause vitreous hemorrhages or retinal detachment.[18,23]

Symptomatic nonproliferative retinal lesions in sickling hemoglobinopathies (Table 10-2) can have devastating visual consequences. Fortunately, these complications are infrequent.[18] Central retinal artery occlusions have been reported in patients with SA and SS.[24,34–37] Macular arteriole occlusions in sickling hemoglobinopathies can produce significant visual defects. Cases have been reported in SS and SThal.[36,38] Unlike the peripheral location, vasoproliferation rarely occurs in the posterior pole of sickling patients.[18] Retinal venous occlusions are rare, but central retinal vein occlusions (CRVOs) have occurred in SS patients,[27,39] and branch retinal vein occlusions (BRVOs) have occurred in SC[40] and SS patients.[27] Choroidal vascular or posterior ciliary vessel occlusions have been reported in SA,[35] SC, and SThal patients.[41] Angioid streaks are an infrequent complication described in each of the sickling hemoglobinopathies.[42,43] Chronic hemolysis presumably results in deposition of iron in Bruch's membrane, rendering it more brittle.[29,42]

Proliferative

Proliferative sickle retinopathy is usually broken down into five different stages, based on fluorescein angiography and indirect ophthalmoscopy.[44] Stage 1 is characterized by peripheral retinal arteriolar occlusions. Sickled erythrocytes may act as microemboli[18] closing capillary beds. The interface area from perfused to nonperfused retina is obvious with fluorescein and appears as a grayish-brown discoloration of the anterior fundus with indirect ophthalmoscopy. The ischemic zone presents as a more blurred image with silver-wire or chalky white arterioles within the ischemic zone.[18,25]

Stage 2 consists of peripheral arteriolar-venular anastomoses. Blood is shunted from the occluded arterioles to the nearest venules at the interface of the nonperfused retina.[18,25] This represents enlargement of the pre-existing capillaries rather than new vessel growth.

Stage 3 of proliferative sickle retinopathy is characterized by sprouting of neovascular capillary buds toward the anterior nonperfused retina in an attempt to revascularize ischemic retina.[18] The new vessels sprout in a fan-shaped configuration, or a "sea-fan," with one major feeding arteriole and one major venule.[25] With time, additional vessels are incorporated and ultimately form a complex neovascular patch of vessels.[18]

Sea-fans are most common in patients with SC (59 percent) and SThal (33 percent).[24,45] The most common location for these lesions is superotemporal (46 percent), inferotemporal (29 percent), superonasal (18 percent), and finally, inferonasal (7 percent).[44]

Initially, the sea-fans are formed on the surface of the retina, but with time, they adhere to the cortical vitreous.[18] Through syneresis or degeneration of the vitreous, the sea-fans are pulled anteriorly into the vitreous toward the center of the globe. Occasionally, sea-fans undergo spontaneous regression and disappear.[18] Most commonly, however, neovascular sea-fans develop in the second to fourth decade of life, which places patients at risk of chronically progressive retinopathy (stages IV and V lesions) for the remainder of their lives.[18]

Stage 4, vitreous hemorrhage, occurs as a result of minor ocular trauma, vitreal collapse, or traction on adherent neovascular tissue.[18] In one selected study, it was the most common cause of visual loss in eyes affected with proliferative sickle retinopathy (44 percent) in SC patients.[46] It is relatively infrequent in SS or AS. The hemorrhage can be small and localized or massive. Clotted hemorrhage eventually organizes into white fibrous tissue. The patient usually remains asymptomatic unless the hemorrhage is massive or a retinal detachment occurs.[18,25] Risk factors for vitreal hemorrhage include the SC genotype, 60 degrees or more of the retinal circumference with proliferative sickle retinopathy, and a previous vitreal hemorrhage.[47]

Stage 5 is characterized by vitreous traction and retinal detachment.[18,37,40,45,48] Vitreous traction bands result from vitreal hemorrhages from the neovascular tissue. In one selected study, a tractional retinal detachment caused vision loss in 31 percent of SC patients.[46] Most tractional retinal detachments (85 percent) occur in cases with a pre-existing vitreous hemorrhage.[46] Most detachments are associated with retinal holes.[18] Most cases occur in patients with SC, although they have been reported in patients with AS[49] and SS.[27,50]

Causes of visual loss in untreated sickle cell retinopathy can occur secondary to nonproliferative and proliferative manifestations. The most common causes of acuity loss in nonproliferative cases are angioid streaks with disciform degeneration (57 percent).[46] The common proliferative causes are vitreal hemorrhage (44 percent) and tractional retinal detachment (31 percent) and epiretinal membranes (18 percent).[46]

Treatment

The treatment goal in sickle cell retinopathy is elimination of neovascular lesions to reduce the potential for vitreal hemorrhage and subsequent retinal detachment.[25] Thus, treatment options should be started at stage III of proliferative retinopathy.[18] Retinal neovascularization in sickling conditions can be eradicated by many methods, but Xenon or argon laser photocoagulation are the most typically used techniques.[25] According to Jampol et al.,[51] photocoagulation with a scatter technique should be the first treatment approach. This involves surrounding the neovascular lesion with laser burns without attempting to directly treat the sea-fan or the feeding vessels. Most sea-fans (83 percent) should show complete or partial regression. Scatter photocoagulation is currently the most effective and safest treatment for patients with sickle neovascularization.[52] A 360-degree peripheral circumferential technique of scatter photocoagulation has been suggested for patients who are extremely unreliable for follow-up.[51]

If scatter treatment does not produce regression of the neovascular lesions, then a direct feeder vessel photocoagulation should be considered.[51] Feeder vessel coagulation consists of high-intensity burns that stimulate pigmentary reactions and closure of the feeder arteriole and draining venule of the sea-fan.[53] Complications of this difficult procedure include choroidal neovascularization and increased risk of retinal detachment (with argon laser).[52] In addition, this technique requires the use of retrobulbar anesthesia, which can infrequently produce devastating complications such as blindness from retrobulbar hemorrhage occluding the central retinal artery.[54]

The surgical repair of retinal detachments is complicated by several factors: preretinal fibrovascular tissue frequently obscures retinal breaks, pronounced vitreal traction requires extensive buckles, and the rate of postoperative anterior segment necrosis is high.[18,45] A variety of preoperative and intraoperative prophylactic techniques can be used to increase the success of the surgery.

Polycythemia

Polycythemia, or erythrocytosis, is an abnormal elevation of the RBC count, hematocrit, and hemoglobin concentration.[1] Similar to anemia, it is not a disease but a sign of an underlying condition.[4]

Two distinct forms of this condition occur. Primary polycythemia, or polycythemia rubra vera, is characterized by increased RBC production for unknown reasons.[3] Hyperplasia of erythrocytic elements of the bone marrow result in elevation of the RBC count, elevated hemoglobin concentration, and an increase in the number of leukocytes and platelets.[3,6] Polycythemia is a disorder of middle-aged and older persons and is more frequent in men.[1,6] A routine blood count demonstrates an elevated RBC, an increased hematocrit, and increased hemoglobin level.

In the secondary polycythemias, a decreased oxygen supply to the tissues results in normal bone marrow stimulation to produce increased numbers of RBCs.[1,3] Living at high altitudes, congenital heart disease, chronic obstructive pulmonary disease, and abnormal hemoglobins that have an increased oxygen affinity can produce polycythemia.[1,4]

Symptoms of polycythemia result from expanded blood volume, increased blood viscosity, and an increased tendency toward clotting.[1,3] The elevated viscosity of the blood limits its ability to circulate and thus impairs the blood supply to the brain and other vital tissues. Decreased cerebral blood flow contributes to headaches, tinnitus, light-headedness, vertigo, dizziness, fainting, a feeling of fullness in the head, and visual irregularities.[1,3,4] Common visual complaints include blurred vision, scotomas, photophobia, entopic phenomena, and transient loss of vision.[6] Bleeding or thrombotic complications can also occur secondary to abnormal platelet function.

Ocular manifestations of polycythemia include venous engorgement and increased tortuosity of the vessels in the conjunctiva and retinal veins as a result of the hyperviscosity of the blood.[1,6,10,14] In cases of extreme venous stasis, retinal hemorrhages (deep and superficial), microaneurysms, cotton-wool spots, and retinal edema occur. This can progress to thrombosis of the central retinal veins with optic disc swelling.[5,6,10,14,17] Increased venous pressure or increased intracranial pressure may result in papilledema.[6] These findings can be found in both eyes and result in severe vision loss.[14]

Initial treatment of polycythemia is phlebotomy, or blood-letting, which reduces the RBC count and the blood volume.[1,3] In secondary polycythemias, treatment of the causative condition will relieve the polycythemia. If retinal venous occlusion has not yet oc-

curred, the visual outlook is good. Once venous occlusion has occurred, management of the retina is the same as for other cases of central vein occlusion.[14]

LEUKOCYTE DISORDERS

The leukocytes, or WBCs, that are normally present in the blood are polymorphonuclear leukocytes of the neutrophilic, basophilic, and eosinophilic types as well as lymphocytes and monocytes. The function of leukocytes is to protect the body against microorganisms that cause disease.[3] Changes in leukocyte quantity are more important than changes in their appearance in disease states. Also, it is clinically important to determine the specific type of leukocyte responsible for the quantitative change.[4]

Leukemia

Leukemia is a neoplastic blood disorder characterized by an abnormal proliferation of leukocytes.[6,55] Normal leukocytes mature, perform their function, die, and are removed from the circulation. Leukemic cells give rise to progeny that fail to differentiate, remain immature, and instead continue to proliferate in an uncontrolled fashion, overgrowing the normal cells. As the condition progresses, the leukemic cells rapidly accumulate and progressively replace the bone marrow. The loss of normal marrow function leads to a decreased production of normal RBCs, WBCs, and platelets. Thus, the common clinical complications of leukemia are anemia, infection, and bleeding. With time, the leukemic cells also infiltrate the lymph nodes, spleen, liver, and other tissues.[1,10,55]

Leukemia is classified clinically according to the duration and presentation as either acute or chronic. Acute leukemia is characterized by a swift, advancing downhill clinical course with accumulating immature cells incapable of combating infection in the peripheral blood.[6] The presentation at diagnosis usually includes evidence of anemia, hemorrhage, and infection as well as enlargement of the lymph nodes, spleen, and liver.[10,56] Typically, the acute leukemias occur more commonly in children and young adults and show no sexual preference.[6] If left untreated, death will occur within months after diagnosis.[56]

Chronic leukemias usually affect middle-aged and older persons with a typical presentation that is more vague and gradual. Often, many asymptomatic patients are diagnosed in routine physical examinations in an evaluation of other illnesses with routine hematologic studies.[1,6,10] A slight preponderance of affected men exists.[6] The typical symptoms are secondary to anemia, enlargement of the spleen, and an increase of the basal metabolic rate.[1] They include fatigue, lethargy, loss of appetite, weight loss, fever, and documented infections. The median survival of patients with chronic leukemia ranges from 5 to 8 years.[1]

Leukemia is also classified by the two predominant cell lines involved. The first is the myeloid (myelogenous) cell line in which the granular polymorphonuclear leukocytes predominate. The second type is the lymphoid (lymphogenous) cell line, in which the lymphocytes are the dominate cells. Thus, most leukemias fall into one of four types[1]:

Acute myelogenous leukemia (AML), 46 percent
Chronic lymphocytic leukemia (CLL), 29 percent
Chronic myelogenous leukemia (CML), 14 percent
Acute lymphocytic leukemia (ALL), 11 percent

In the United States, the leukemias account for about 3 percent of all cancers.[1]

The exact cause of leukemia is unknown. Ionizing radiation, such as from radiation treatments or survivors of the atomic bomb, increases the incidence of ALL, AML, and CML. The dosage of radiation, its distribution over time, and the age of the individual affect the magnitude of the risk.[1]

Two rare forms of leukemia, adult T-cell leukemia and hairy cell leukemia, have been linked to retroviruses. A genetic predisposition exists in congenital disorders such as Down syndrome, and risk is greater in a person who has an identical twin with leukemia.[1,3] A tendency to develop acute leukemia also exists after marrow hypoplasia secondary to heavy occupational exposure to benzene.[1]

Diagnosis of leukemia can be achieved by a variety of techniques. Bone marrow aspiration and biopsy with a peripheral blood smear evaluation is the typical method. The initial WBC count is usually over 100,000/mm^3 but can be depressed. The platelet count is always depressed in acute leukemia.[55] Classification of the leukemia can be achieved by using monoclonal antibodies reactive with cell-surface antigens.[1] Other methods include biopsy of lymph nodes, radiography, and computed tomographic scanning.[55]

Ocular signs are observed in both the acute and chronic forms of leukemia but are more common in the acute forms.[14,56] Any ocular structure may be involved.[10] Ocular manifestations are so common that perhaps 50 percent of leukemic patients will have an ocular sign at any given time, and nearly 100 percent will have ocular involvement at some point during the course of their disease.[57,58] Direct invasion by neoplastic cells causes most of the ocular involvement in leukemia.[59] Secondary ophthalmic findings are related to associated hematologic abnormalities of leukemia such as hyperviscosity and anemia or thrombocytopenia.[59,60]

Retinal involvement is the most frequent visible ocular manifestation of leukemia.[55,56] Retinal involvement can occur in many different forms. Tortuous dilated retinal veins is a common finding. The arteries and veins become more "yellowish" secondary to the decreased RBC count and increased WBC count. Posterior pole retinal hemorrhages can be seen at all levels of the retina and are most commonly round or flame-shaped.[56,59] Intraretinal hemorrhage may have a "white center," which represents cellular debris, capillary emboli, or an accumulation of leukemic cells.[56,58,61,62] Extensive hemorrhaging in the macular or peripapillary region, vitreal hemorrhage, or hemorrhagic retinal detachments may lead to blindness.[6] Less commonly, peripheral retinal microaneurysms are noted in cases of prolonged leukocytosis such as in cases of CML.[63] The resultant development of retinal neovascularization occurs in a sea-fan configuration and is most likely the result of secondary increased viscosity.[59]

Cotton-wool spots are a common finding secondary to ischemia from the anemia, hyperviscosity, or leukemic infiltration.[10,56] Localized retinal infarcts are more frequently found in adults than in children.[5] Generalized retinal edema can also occur.[6]

Leukemic infiltration of the retina resembles grayish-white preretinal masses. They are a rare finding and are associated with localized destruction, hemorrhage, and necrosis.[5,56,59]

Leukemic infiltration of the optic nerve occurs mainly in children with acute leukemia.[64] Infiltration of the prelaminar portion of the optic nerve head produces the clinical appearance of papillitis. Visual acuity usually remains good unless edema and hemorrhage of the infiltrate extend into the macular area.[56,59] Retrolaminar optic nerve infiltration by leukemic cells leads to profound vision loss.[55] Optic disc edema, elevation, and hemorrhage are usually present.[59] In addition, the optic nerve may indirectly be involved by an increase of intracranial pressure causing papilledema.[55] Furthermore, these manifestations can occur simultaneously, making differential diagnosis essential. A lumbar puncture is vital in every case for the differential. Orbital radiation therapy is the treatment of choice for leukemic infiltration of the optic nerve, and it should be performed on an emergency basis to avoid irreversible vision loss.[59]

Leukemic infiltration of the choroid is common histopathologically, but clinical changes are almost never apparent. The perivascular infiltration results in a thickening of the choroid with an overlying retinal pigment epithelial degeneration and clumping disturbances.[56] Secondary sequlae include drusen formation and serous detachments.

Anterior segment manifestations of leukemia are relatively infrequent.[59] Involvement can be unilateral or bilateral.[65] The clinical picture can include conjunctival injection,[11,59] spontaneous subconjunctival hemorrhage,[56] acute iridocyclitis, pseudohypopyon, spontaneous hyphema, elevated intraocular pressure, and a change in iris color.[66,67] Infiltration of the trabecular meshwork can presumably cause the elevated intraocular pressure.[68] Heterochromia iridis results from the presence of a diffuse involvement of the iris beginning at the root of the iris.[56,59,65] Nodular involvement of the iris can also occur.[59] Paracentesis of the aqueous humor can confirm the diagnosis. Low-dose anterior segment irradiation often leads to complete resolution of the iris infiltration.[66,67,69,70]

The avascular nature of the cornea protects it from direct invasion by leukemic cells.[56] Compromised vascular perfusion and limbic infiltration can lead to the formation of peripheral corneal infiltrates, corneal edema, and sterile corneal ring ulcers.[56,59,71]

Leukemia accounts for approximately 2 to 6 percent of the orbital tumors of childhood.[59,72,73] Orbital involvement is more common in acute than in chronic leukemia and more frequently in the lymphoid than in the myeloid cell type.[74,75] Leukemic involvement of the orbit can be the result of infiltration or hemorrhage. Infiltration can include the lid, orbit, lacrimal gland,[59] and rarely, the extraocular muscles.[56] An orbital focus of leukemic cells in myelogenous leukemia

has been called a *granulocytic sarcoma*, or *chloroma*.[56] These tumors may have a greenish color caused by the pigmented enzyme myeloperoxidase.[56,59] The appearance of a granulocytic sarcoma may occur at any time in the course of the myelogenous leukemia.[59] Most of these tumors occur in the first decade of life and indicate a poor prognosis for longevity.[59] Immunosuppression secondary to the leukemic process and secondary to chemotherapy makes leukemic patients susceptible to opportunistic infections.[56,76] Ocular disease can also occur secondary to bone marrow transplantation,[77] in the form of graft-versus-host disease.[77,78] Conjunctival lesions are used to correlate the severity of the graft-versus-host disease.[5]

PLATELET DISORDERS/ COAGULATION DISORDERS

Normal hemostasis is required to prevent pathologic bleeding. Hemostatic disorders usually indicate a defect in either the cellular component (platelet) or the humoral component (coagulation) of hemostasis.[7] Platelets, or thrombocytes, are the cell fragments that are derived from the bone marrow.[79] Normal platelet function and peripheral platelet blood counts greater than $100,000/\mu l$ are needed for normal hemostasis.[2] Platelets perform three main events in primary hemostasis. Platelets adhere to injured blood vessel walls with the help of coagulation factor VIII, the von Willebrand factor. Platelets then are activated and release endogenous substances that stimulate other surrounding platelets to clump together. Finally, the platelets form cellular aggregates, or the primary hemostatic plug.[79]

Secondary hemostasis then occurs through the humoral components of hemostasis. The surface of activated platelets initiates thrombin formation by a cascade reaction of coagulation factors in the intrinsic and extrinsic pathways. Thrombin then facilitates the conversion of fibrogen to fibrin, stimulates further platelet activation, and activates fibrin-stabilizing factors. Fibrin consolidates the platelet plug and captures erythrocytes to add strength to the permanent clot.[2] The proper interaction of all these components results in normal hemostasis.

Laboratory evaluation of hemostasis can be achieved with the following tests: prothrombin time, partial thromboplastin, platelet count, and bleeding time. Any abnormalities indicate that further investigation is necessary.[2]

Thrombocytosis

Thrombocytosis occurs when the platelet count exceeds 500,000/μl.[2] The causes of thrombocytosis can be divided into three major categories: (1) transitory thrombocytosis represents a physiologic mobilization of platelets following stress or exercise; (2) reactive thrombocytosis results from increased platelet production secondary to hemolysis, infection, hemorrhage, inflammatory disease, or malignancy; or (3) autonomous thrombocytosis occurs when production of platelets is independent of the normal regulatory processes. This last category may indicate a manifestation of a myeloproliferative disorder.[2,4]

The clinical findings of thrombocytosis are usually related to the expanded blood volume and increased blood viscosity, similar to polycythemia.[1,4] Thrombotic and hemorrhagic complications can also occur secondary to abnormal platelet function. Ocular manifestations would be similar to those encountered in hyperviscosity syndromes. Treatment involves treating the underlying disorder.

Thrombocytopenia

Thrombocytopenia occurs when there is a subnormal count of platelets, usually below 100,000/μl.[4] The principal manifestation of thrombocytopenia is bleeding. Platelet counts below 20,000/μl are frequently associated with spontaneous bleeding, which can be life-threatening.[4] Bleeding symptoms typically involve mucocutaneous lesions of petechiae and purpura and prolonged post-traumatic bleeding. Similar to anemia, thrombocytopenia should be considered a symptom to an underlying cause. Clinically, the causes of thrombocytopenia can be divided into four classes: decreased production, increased destruction, abnormal distribution, and intravascular dilution.[2,4]

Decreased platelet production can occur as a result of a decrease in the total number of megakaryocytes in the bone marrow secondary to drugs or radiation, ineffective thrombopoiesis secondary to nutritional disorders, or systemic infections. The ocular manifestations of thrombocytopenia include hemorrhages, especially preretinal hemorrhages in the macular area.[6]

Increased platelet destruction may be induced by commonly used drugs, such as digitalis, quinidine, thiazides, certain antibiotics, and gold salts.[2] Ocular manifestations of drug-induced thrombocytopenia can include vitreal and subconjunctival hemorrhages, hyphema, postsurgical hemorrhage,[80] and rarely, bilateral serous retinal detachments and disc edema.[81]

Increased platelet destruction can also result from an immune mechanism such that antibodies are directed against antigens on the platelet surface for unknown reasons, termed *idiopathic thrombocytopenic purpura* (ITP).[4] ITP occurs in two major patterns: an acute and a chronic form. In children, the acute form typically occurs as a self-limiting condition following a viral infection. The chronic form is usually found in young to middle-aged women. Symptoms include petechiae, easy bruising, ecchymoses, minor bleeding, epistaxis, and purpura. Ocular manifestations of ITP include flame-shaped retinal hemorrhages and, rarely, round macular hemorrhages.[8]

Thrombotic thrombocytopenic purpura (TTP), also known as Moschcowitz syndrome, is a condition of nonimmunologic accelerated destruction of platelets. This disorder is characterized by five clinical manifestations: thrombocytopenia, microangiopathic hemolytic anemia, neurologic abnormalities, renal dysfunction, and fever.[2,4] In TTP, spontaneous platelet activation and aggregation apparently occurs.[4] Ocular manifestations include retinal hemorrhage, papilledema, visual field loss, diplopia, and serous or exudative retinal detachment.[82,83] Treatment of TTP usually involves plasma transfusion and plasmapheresis.[4]

Abnormal distribution of platelets occurs in hypersplenism. In this condition, the total number of platelets is normal, but the vast majority of the platelets are pooled in the spleen, resulting in moderate thrombocytopenia. Typically, no severe hemorrhaging occurs.[2,4]

Intravascular dilutional thrombocytopenia occurs following massive transfusions. The need for platelet transfusions should be monitored if the patient's bone marrow is depressed or hemorrhaging occurs.[2,4]

Congenital Platelet Disorders

Inherited defects that result in platelet dysfunction include thrombasthenia, von Willebrand's disease, and thrombocytopathy. Thrombasthenia (Glanzmann syndrome) is characterized by prolonged bleeding time, absent platelet aggregation, and episodes of mucosal bleeding. It is inherited by an autosomal recessive gene.[2] Ocular manifestations include spontaneous preretinal and vitreal hemorrhages.[84] Treatment involves transfusions of normal platelets.

A common bleeding disorder that is also transmitted as an autosomal recessive trait is von Willebrand's disease. In this disorder, platelets are normal in number and structure but lack a plasma factor that is necessary to adhere to the vessel wall, called the von Willebrand factor. Signs of von Willebrand's disease include prolonged bleeding time, poor platelet adhesion, normal platelet aggregation, but absent platelet agglutination. Clinical findings include menorrhagia, mucosal bleeding, and bruising.[2] Ocular manifestations are included later in the discussion of hemophilia. Treatment consists of administering the von Willebrand factor.

Thrombocytopathy is a condition defined by the impaired expression of platelet procoagulant activity; it produces a mild bleeding tendency.[2] Familial exudative vitreoretinopathy, a retinal vascular disorder similar to retinopathy of prematurity, has been documented in two families in conjunction with familial thrombocytopathy.[85]

Acquired Platelet Disorders

Acquired platelet dysfunction occurs most commonly secondary to the ingestion of aspirin or other nonsteroidal anti-inflammatory drugs. These drugs cause platelets to exhibit impaired aggregation and release; thus, the bleeding time becomes prolonged and the amount of microaggregates of platelets is reduced. The duration of the platelet effects varies depending on the drug ingested.[2] Aspirin inhibits platelet function for up to 1 week,[86] while the inhibitory effect of other nonsteroidal anti-inflammatory drugs lasts less than 24 hours.[2] Ocular manifestations of aspirin-induced platelet dysfunction include large subretinal hemorrhages and vitreal hemorrhage in age-related macular degeneration.[87] Aspirin may make patients with choroidal neovascularization prone to bleeding and those with hyphema prone to rebleed; it may also cause bleeding problems in surgery.[88,89]

Hemophilia

Hemophilia is a hereditary disorder of coagulation that is transmitted by an X-linked gene. A deficiency of coagulation factor VIII results in hemophilia A; a deficiency of coagulation factor IX results in hemophilia B. Both factors VIII and IX are vital coagulation factors in the intrinsic pathway. Clinically, hemophilia is characterized by the insidious onset of hemorrhage occurring hours to days after trauma.[2] The extent of the deficiency determines the correlated severity of the hemorrhaging. A deficiency of less than 1 percent of normal activity results in severe hemorrhagic disease. Patients with activity greater than 5 percent have a milder clinical course, excluding trauma victims or patients undergoing surgery.[2] Clinical presentations include hemarthrosis, chronic synovitis, intramuscular hematomas, and central nervous system bleeding.[90]

Ocular manifestations of hemophilia include spontaneous and post-traumatic subconjunctival hemorrhage, orbital and periorbital hemorrhages, and postoperative bleeding.[91] Minor injuries can lead to significant hemorrhaging into ocular and orbital tissues and lead to secondary glaucoma and vision loss.[6] Ocular signs resulting from central nervous system hemorrhage include pupillary abnormalities, cranial nerve palsies, visual blurring, and papilledema.[90,91] Treatment requires replacement therapy of factor VIII.[2]

Anticoagulation Therapy

Anticoagulation therapy is used therapeutically to inhibit thrombosis in clinical conditions such as cardiac disease, pulmonary embolism, ischemic cerebrovascular disease, venous thromboembolism, and postoperative immobility.[5] The four main types of therapy used are antiplatelet agents, heparin, vitamin K antagonists, and thrombolytic agents. Each disrupts clotting at a different site in the coagulation pathway.[2] Heparin, coumarin, and warfarin are examples of anticoagulation agents.

Anticoagulation agents have been related to a number of hemorrhagic ocular conditions. Isolated vitreal hemorrhage and spontaneous hyphema have been reported. Massive subretinal and vitreal hemorrhage have also been described in age-related macular degeneration patients.[92–96]

PLASMA CELL DISORDERS

Plasma cells normally secrete immunoglobulins and maintain the immune system. The five subgroups of antibodies or immunoglobulins are immunoglobulin

γ (IgG), μ (IgM), α (IgA), δ (IgD), and ϵ (IgE). In the plasma cell disorders, neoplasms arise from a clone of immunoglobulin-secreting cells and produce a monoclonal immunoglobulin. If the amount of IgM and its plasma-producing cells is abnormally increased, the condition is termed Waldenström's macroglobulinemia. If the monoclonal immunoglobulin is IgG, IgA, IgD, or IgE, the disease is a multiple myeloma.[2]

Multiple Myeloma

Malignant proliferation of plasma cells results in a large number of identical abnormal plasma cells (myeloma cells). These myeloma cells tend to collect in the bone marrow and in the outer bone (osteolytic bone lesions). In most cases, the myeloma cells collect in many bones, hence multiple myeloma. Typically, a monoclonal antibody, usually IgG, is overproduced, which can cause osteoporosis, bone pain, hypercalcemia, anemia, renal disease, elevated sedimentation rate, and infection.[2] The symptoms may include bone pain, broken bones, weakness, fatigue, weight loss, and repeated infections.[2]

Ocular involvement can affect the cornea, causing stromal crystalline deposits.[97] Retinal manifestations can include microaneurysms, flame hemorrhages, infarcts, and exudative retinal detachments. Neuro-ophthalmic signs could include proptosis, diplopia, cranial nerve palsies, and optic nerve involvement.[98,99] The hyperviscosity syndrome is uncommon in multiple myeloma.

Waldenström's Macroglobulinemia

Waldenström's macroglobulinemia is due to overproduction of the antibody IgM by the plasmacytoid lymphocytes. This chronic disorder usually affects older individuals. Symptoms arise secondary to anemia and other physical properties of the elevated, large molecule monoclonal IgM. When the IgM level becomes elevated, plasma viscosity also becomes elevated. Clinical presentations include nosebleeds, mental confusion, and congestive heart failure of the hyperviscosity syndrome.[2]

Ocular manifestations are primarily the result of the hyperviscosity syndrome. Venous dilation, retinal hemorrhages, retinal edema, and exudative detachments occur in severe cases.[100] Disc edema, serous retinal detachments, and central retinal vein occlusion have also been reported.[101–104]

REFERENCES

1. Wyngaarden JB, Smith LH, Bennett JC: Cecil Textbook of Medicine. 19th Ed. WB Saunders, Philadelphia, 1992
2. Andreoli TE, Carpenter CC, Plum F, Smith LH: Cecil Essentials of Medicine. 2nd Ed. WB Saunders, Philadelphia, 1990
3. Miller BF, Keane CB: Encyclopedia and Dictionary of Medicine and Nursing. WB Saunders, Philadelphia, 1972
4. Greene HL, Glassock RJ, Kelley MA: Introduction to Clinical Medicine. BC Decker, Philadelphia, 1991
5. Williams GA: Ocular manifestations of hematologic diseases. p. 1. In Tasman W, Jaeger EA (eds): Duane's Clinical Ophthalmology. Vol. 5. JB Lippincott, Philadelphia, 1992
6. Cunningham RD: Retinopathy of blood dyscrasias. p. 1. In Tasman W, Jaeger EA (eds): Duane's Clinical Ophthalmology. Vol. 3. Lippincott, Philadelphia, 1992
7. Schroeder SA, Tierney LM, McPhee SJ, et al: Current Medical Diagnosis and Treatment. Appleton & Lange, E. Norwalk, CT, 1992
8. Rubenstein RA, Yanoff M, Albert DM: Thrombocytopenia, anemia and retinal hemorrhage. Am J Ophthalmol 65:435, 1968
9. Lerman S, Feldmahn AL: Centrocecal scotomata as the presenting sign in pernicious anemia. Arch Ophthalmol 65:381, 1961
10. Kanski JJ, James TE: The eye in Systemic Disease. 2nd Ed. Butterworth-Heinemann, Boston, 1990
11. Kanski JJ, James TE: Case Presentations in Medical Ophthalmology. Butterworth-Heinemann, Boston, 1991
12. Aisen ML, Bacon BR, Goodman AM, Chester EM: Retinal abnormalities associated with anemia. Arch Ophthalmol 101:1049, 1983
13. Foulds WS, Chisholm IA, Stewart JB et al: The optic neuropathy of pernicious anemia. Arch Ophthalmol 82:427, 1969
14. Grey RH: Vascular Disorders of the Ocular Fundus. Butterworth, Boston, 1991
15. Klewin KM, Appen RE, Kaufman PL: Amaurosis and blood loss. Am J Ophthalmol 86:669, 1978
16. Merin S, Freund M: Retinopathy in severe anemia. Am J Ophthalmol 66:1102, 1968
17. Newell FW. Ophthalmology—Principles and Concepts. 7th Ed. Mosby-Year Book, Philadelphia, 1992
18. Goldberg MF: Sickle cell retinopathy. p. 1. In Tasman W, Jaeger EA (eds): Duane's Clinical Ophthalmology. Vol. 3. JB Lippincott, Philadelphia, 1992
19. Weatherall DJ: The genetics of the thalassemias. Br Med Bull 25:24, 1969
20. Pearson HA: Hemoglobin S-thalassemia syndrome in Negro children. Ann NY Acad Sci 165:83, 1969
21. Kanski JJ: Clinical Ophthalmology—A Systematic Approach. Butterworth, Boston, 1989
22. Hannon J: Vitreous hemorrhage associated with sickle cell-hemoglobin C disease. Am J Ophthalmol 42:707, 1956
23. Munro S, Walker C: Ocular complications in sickle-cell haemoglobin C disease. Br J Ophthalmol 44:1, 1960
24. Welch RB, Goldberg MF: Sickle-cell hemoglobin and its relation to fundus abnormality. Arch Ophthalmol 75:353, 1966
25. Siegel D: Diagnosis and treatment of sickle cell retinopathy. J Am Optom Assoc 59:11, 1988
26. Bonanomi MT, Cunha SL, Targino de Araujo J: Funduscopic alterations in SS and SC hemoglobinopathies. Ophthalmologica 197:26, 1988
27. Condon PI, Sergeant GR: Ocular findings in homozygous sickle-cell anemia in Jamaica. Am J Ophthalmol 73:533, 1972

28. Okun E: Development of sickle cell retinopathy. Doc Ophthalmol 26:574, 1969
29. Romayananda N, Goldberg MF, Green WR: Histopathology of sickle cell retinopathy. Trans Am Acad Ophthalmol Otolaryngol 77:652, 1973
30. Goldberg MF, Charache S, Acacio I: Ophthalmologic manifestations of sickle cell thalassemia. Arch Intern Med 128:33, 1971
31. Condon PI, Serjeant GR: Ocular findings in sickle cell thalassemia in Jamaica. Am J Ophthalmol 74:1105, 1972
32. Jampol LM, Condon PI, Dizon-Moore R, et al: Salmon-patch hemorrhages after central retinal occlusion in sickle cell disease. Arch Ophthalmol 99:237, 1981
33. Luxenberg MN: The evolution of salmon-patch hemorrhages in sickle cell retinopathy. Arch Ophthalmol 107:1814, 1989
34. Kabakow B, van Weimokly SS, Lyons HA: Bilateral central retinal artery occlusion: occurrence in a patient with cortisone-treated systemic lupus erythematosus, sickle cell trait, and active pulmonary tuberculosis. Arch Ophthalmol 54:670, 1955
35. Stein MR, Gay AJ: Acute chorioretinal infarction in sickle cell trait: report of a case. Arch Ophthalmol 84:485, 1970
36. Acacio I, Goldberg MF: Peripapillary and macular vessel occlusions in sickle-cell anemia. Am J Ophthalmol 75:861, 1973
37. Goodman G, von Sallmann L, Holland MG: Ocular manifestations of sickle-cell disease. Arch Ophthalmol 58:655, 1957
38. Knapp JW: Isolated macular infarction in sickle-cell (SS) disease. Am J Ophthalmol 73:857, 1972
39. Lieb WA, Geeraets WJ, Guerry D III: Sickle-cell retinopathy. Acta Ophthalmol, suppl. 58:5, 1959
40. Polychronakos DJ, Theodossiadis G: Netzhautablosung bei Sichelzellenanamie. Klin Monatsbl Augenheilkd 153:203, 1968
41. Davies TG, Bansal NC: Bilateral endophthalmitis associated with sickle-cell haemoglobin C disease. Br J Ophthalmol 48:692, 1964
42. Paton D: The Relation of Angioid Streaks to Systemic Disease. Charles C Thomas, Springfield, IL, 1972
43. Geeraets WJ, Guerry D III: Angioid streaks and sickle-cell disease. Am J Ophthalmol 49:450, 1960
44. Goldberg MF: Natural history of untreated proliferative sickle retinopathy. Arch Ophthalmol 85:428, 1971
45. Goldberg MF: Retinal detachment associated with proliferative retinopathies. Ophthalmic Surg 2:222, 1971
46. Moriarty BJ, Acheson RW, Condon PI, Serjeant GR: Patterns of visual loss in untreated sickle cell retinopathy. Eye 2:330, 1988
47. Condon PI, Jampol LM, Farber MD et al: A randomized clinical trial of feeder vessel photocoagulation of proliferative sickle cell retinopathy. II. Update and analysis of risk factors. Ophthalmology 91:1496, 1984
48. Ryan SJ, Goldberg MF: Anterior segment ischemia following scleral buckling in sickle-cell hemoglobinopathy. Am J Ophthalmol 72:35, 1971
49. Isbey EK, Clifford GO, Tanaka KR: Vitreous hemorrhage associated with sickle-cell trait and sickle-cell hemoglobin C disease. Am J Ophthalmol 45:870, 1958
50. Kearney WF: Sickle-cell ophthalmopathy. NY State J Med 65:2677, 1965
51. Jampol LM, Farber M, Rabb MF, Serjeant G: An update on techniques of photocoagulation treatment of proliferative sickle cell retinopathy. Eye 5:260, 1991
52. Farber MD, Jampol LM, Fox P et al: A randomized clinical trial of scatter photocoagulation of proliferative sickle cell retinopathy. Arch Ophthalmol 109:363, 1991
53. Jacobson MS, Gagliano DA, Cohen SB et al: A randomized clinical trial of feeder vessel photocoagulation of sickle cell retinopathy: a long-term follow-up. Ophthalmology 98:581, 1991
54. Roth SE, Margaral LE, Kimmel AS et al: Central retinal-artery occlusion in proliferative sickle-cell retinopathy after retrobulbar injection. Ann Ophthalmol 20:221, 1988
55. Kincaid MC: Leukemia. In Gold DH, Weingeist TA (eds): The Eye in Systemic Disease. JB Lippincott, Philadelphia, 1990
56. Kincaid MC, Green WR: Ocular and orbital involvement in leukemia. Surv Ophthalmol 27:211, 1983
57. Duke-Elder S: System of Ophthalmology. Retina. Vol 10. CV Mosby, St Louis, 1967
58. Allan RA, Straatsma BR: Ocular involvement in leukaemia and allied disorders. Arch Ophthalmol 66:490–508, 1961
59. Rosenthal AR: Ocular manifestations of leukemia: a review. Ophthalmology 90:889, 1983
60. Schachat AP, Markowitz JA, Guyer DR et al: Ocular manifestations of leukemia. Arch Ophthalmol 107:697, 1989
61. Holt JM, Gordon-Smith EL: Retinal abnormalities in diseases of the blood. Br J Ophthalmol 53:245, 1969
62. Guyer DR, Schachat AP, Vitale S et al: Leukemic retinopathy: relationship between fundus lesions and hematologic profiles at diagnosis. Ophthalmology 96:860, 1989
63. Duke JR, Wilkinson CP, Sigelman S: Retinal microaneurysms in leukaemia. Ophthalmology 52:368, 1968
64. Ellis W, Little HL: Leukemic infiltration of the optic nerve head. Am J Ophthalmol 75:867, 1973
65. Johnston SS, Ware CF: Iris involvement in leukaemia. Br J Ophthalmol 57:320, 1973
66. Masera G, Carnelli V, Uderzo C et al: Leukaemic hypopyon in acute lymphoblastic leukaemia after interruption of treatment. Arch Dis Child 54:73, 1979
67. Zakka KA, Yee RD, Shorr N et al: Leukemic iris infiltration. Am J Ophthalmol 89:204, 1980
68. Rowan PJ, Sloan JB: Iris and anterior chamber involvement in Leukemia. Ann Ophthalmol 8:1081, 1976
69. Ninane J, Taylor D, Day S: The eye as a sanctuary in acute lymphoblastic leukaemia. Lancet 1:452, 1980
70. Abramson DH, Wachtel A, Watson CW et al: Leukemic hypopyon. J Pediatr Ophthalmol Strabismus 18:42, 1981
71. Wood Wj, Nicholson DH: Corneal ring ulcer as presenting manifestation of acute monocytic leukemia. Am J Ophthalmol 7:69, 1973
72. Nicholson DH, Green WR: Tumors of the eye, lids and orbit in children. p. 923. In Harley RD (ed): Pediatric Ophthalmology. WB Saunders, Philadelphia, 1975
73. Porterfield JF: Orbital tumors in children: a report of 214 cases. Int Ophthalmol Clin 2:319, 1962
74. Jakobiec FA, Jones IS: Lymphomatous plasmacytic, histiocytic, and hematopoietic tumors. p. 345. In Jones IS, Jakobiec FA (eds): Diseases of the Orbit. Harper & Row, Hagerstown MD, 1979
75. Reese AB, Guy L: Exophthalmos in leukemia. Am J Ophthalmol 16:718, 1933
76. Cogan DG: Immunosuppression and eye disease. Am J Ophthalmol 83:777, 1977
77. Hirst LW, Jabs DA, Tutschka PJ et al: The eye in bone marrow transplantation. Part 1. Clinical study. Arch Ophthalmol 101:580, 1983
78. Jabs DA, Wingard J, Green WR et al: The eye in bone marrow transplantation. Part III. Conjunctival graft-vs-host disease. Arch Ophthalmol 107:1343, 1988
79. Rybak ME: Disorders of hemostasis. In Nobel J (ed): Textbook of General Medicine and Primary Care. Little, Brown, Boston, 1987
80. Ackerman J, Goldstein M, Kanarek I: Spontaneous massive vitreous hemorrhage secondary to thrombocytopenia. Ophthalmic Surg 11:636, 1980
81. Klepach GL, Wray SH: Bilateral serous retinal detachment with thrombocytopenia during pencillamine therapy. Ann Ophthalmol 13:201, 1981
82. Percival SPB: Ocular findings in thrombotic thrombocytopenic purpura. Br J Ophthalmol 54:73, 1970
83. Lambert SR, High KA, Cotlier R et al: Serous retinal detach-

ments in thrombotic thrombcytopenic purpura. Arch Ophthalmol 103:1172, 1985

84. Vaiser A, Hutton WL, Marengo-Rowe AJ et al: Retinal hemorrhage associated with thrombasthenia. Am J Ophthalmol 80:258, 1975

85. Chaudhuri PR, Rosenthal AR, Goulstine DB et al: Familial exudative vitreoretinopathy associated with familial thrombocytopathy. Br J Ophthalmol 67:755, 1983

86. Burch JW, Stanford N, Majerus PW: Inhibition of platelet prostaglandin synthetase by oral aspirin. J Clin Invest 61:314, 1978

87. Mortada A, Abboud I: Retinal hemorrhage after prolonged use of salicylates. Br J Ophthalmol 57:199, 1973

88. Crawford JS, Lewandowski RL, Chan W: The effect of aspirin on rebleeding in traumatic hyphema. Am J Ophthalmol 80:543, 1975

89. Paris GL, Waltuch GF: Salicylate-induced bleeding problems in ophthalmic plastic surgery. Ophthalmic Surg 13:627, 1982

90. Eyster ME, Bill FM, Blaff PM: Central nervous system bleeding in hemophiliacs. Blood 51:1179, 1978

91. Rubenstein RA, Albert DM, Scheie HG: Ocular complications of hemophilia. Arch Ophthalmol 76:230, 1966

92. Butner RW, McPherson AR: Spontaneous vitreous hemorrhage. Ann Ophthalmol 14:268, 1982

93. Oyakawa RT, Michels RG, Blase WP: Vitrectomy for nondiabetic vitreous hemorrhage. Am J Ophthalmol 96:517, 1983

94. Koehler MP, Sholiton DB: Spontaneous hyphema resulting from warfarin. Ann Ophthalmol 15:858, 1983

95. Baba FE, Jarrett WH II, Harbin TS et al: Massive hemorrhage complicating age-related macular degeneration: clinicopathologic correlation and role of anticoagulants. Ophthalmology 93:1581, 1986

96. Kingham JD, Chen MC, Levy MH: Macular hemorrhage in the aging eye: the effect of anticoagulants. N Engl J Med 318:1126, 1988

97. Pinkerton RMH, Robertson DM: Corneal and conjunctival changes in dysproteinemia. Invest Ophthalmol 8:357, 1969

98. Clarke E: Plasma cell myeloma of the orbit. Br J Ophthalmol 37:543, 1953

99. Knaspp AJ, Gartner S, Henkind P: Multiple myeloma and its ocular manifestations. Surv Ophthalmol 31:343, 1987

100. Murphy RP: Treatment of hyperviscosity retinopathy. p. 247. In Ryan SJ, Dawson AK, Littel HL (eds): Retinal Diseases. Grune & Stratton, New York, 1985

101. Avashia JH, Fath DF: Bilateral central retinal vein occlusion in Waldenström's macroglobulinemia. J Am Optom Assoc 60:657, 1989

102. Feman SS, Stein RS: Waldenström's macroglobulinemia: a hyperviscosity manifestation of venous stasis retinopathy. Int Ophthalmol 4:107, 1981

103. Friedman AH, Marchevsky A, Odel JG et al: Immunofluorescent studies of the eye in Waldenström's macroglobulinemia. Arch Ophthalmol 98:743, 1980

104. Hayreh SS, Van Heuven WAJ, Hayreh MS: Experimental retinal vascular occlusion. Part 1. Pathogenesis of central retinal vein occlusion. Arch Ophthalmol 96:311, 1978

11 Pregnancy

MARK SAWAMURA

INTRODUCTION

The creation of life from the union of genetic information from two human beings is a truly remarkable phenomenon. In the months that constitute gestation, many impressive alterations occur within the expectant mother. Considering the myriad events transpiring during this period, it is understandable how gestation may influence the course of an underlying disease process or activate a latent form of pathology. In this chapter, many physiologic changes, including disease entities, are presented as they relate to the structure and function of the visual system and the surrounding adnexa during pregnancy.

The mother's body must undergo a variety of physiologic and metabolic alterations to support the burgeoning zygote. Endogenous hormones such as human chorionic gonadotropin, human placental lactogen, estrogens, and progesterone attain peak levels during this 40-week period. Additionally, other important hormones such as angiotensin II, aldosterone, renin, and cortisol will also attain elevated concentrations. Thyroid function escalates, and glucose metabolism is altered, increasing the requirements of insulin. Cardiac output is raised 30 to 50 percent, peaking between weeks 16 and 28.[1] Blood volume, particularly the plasma volume, increases up to 50 percent.[1] Blood pressure generally decreases and reaches a minimum at the junction of the second and third trimesters.[1] Glomerular filtration rate increases in the percentage of volume, at a rate very similar to that of cardiac output. Respiratory rate and oxygen consumption are also noted to increase. Finally, the body attains a state of relative immunosuppression, allowing acceptance of the fetal allograft.

CASE REPORT

A 22-year-old black woman presented to our clinic with an initial complaint of contact lens intolerance and slightly blurred vision for the past month. She had a history of soft contact lens wear for 5 years, and her medical history revealed that she was in the sixth month of her first pregnancy. She also disclosed a history of juvenile-onset diabetes of 11 years' duration, which was treated with insulin. In addition, the patient reported weight gain and noticeable facial edema in recent weeks. Further questioning divulged poor compliance keeping scheduled appointments with other medical professionals.

Best corrected visual acuity through the contact lenses measured 20/25⁻ OD, OS. Evaluation of the lenses revealed a slightly snug fit with accumulated protein deposition. Best corrected visual acuity through spectacle lenses was 20/20⁻ OD, OS. Ocular motilities, pupillary reactivity, color vision, and confrontation fields were all normal. External ocular examination revealed slight lid edema and focal constrictions in the vessels of the bulbar conjunctiva. Significant corneal edema was not appreciated. Tonometry by applanation measured 16 mmHg OU. Blood pressure measurements on the right arm and left arm were 150/95 and 150/100, respectively. Screening ophthalmoscopy revealed the presence of retinal hemorrhages; thus, the patient was dilated. A binocular fundus examination exposed the presence of scattered soft and hard exudates and retinal hemorrhages in both eyes. The

---

optic nerves had well-demarcated borders and healthy rim tissue. The retinal vasculature demonstrated points of focal constriction. Both maculae and peripheral retinae were clear in each eye. Our tentative diagnosis was retinopathy secondary to pregnancy-induced hypertension and diabetes. The patient was instructed not to wear contact lenses for the remainder of the pregnancy and immediately referred back to her obstetrician for further care. She was later diagnosed and treated for mild pre-eclampsia. Her diabetes was also placed under better control.

In the subsequent months, the patient was closely monitored for changes in retinal findings. Retinopathy in both eyes remained stable until after an uncomplicated delivery, when mild regression occurred. She then resumed wearing contact lenses without further problems.

VISUAL FUNCTION

Refractive error in the normal pregnant woman has been demonstrated to remain significantly constant through the gestational period.[2] Nonetheless, a small number of individuals have exhibited fluctuations exceeding 1.00 diopter.[3] These changes may or may not be solely associated with pregnancy. Additional reports attribute refractive error shifts to intracapsular lens swelling and corneal curvature changes.[4] No studies, however, have observed changes in refraction in patients with sufficient gestational edema. Such findings have been documented in other cases of systemic edema, such as renal and vascular disease.[5]

In addition, a decrease in amplitude of accommodation of greater than 1.00 diopter often appears in the second half of pregnancy.[3] Alterations in the permeability of the crystalline lens by estrogen and progestins is believed to be the mechanism.[2] Prepresbyopic patients may experience blur at near vision, but full recovery is expected in most individuals. Visual acuity, heterophoria measurements, accommodative convergence/accommodation (AC/A) ratios, and fusional ranges tend to remain relatively stable.[2] Hilton,[3] however, noticed significant fluctuation in calculated AC/A ratios in 49 percent of subjects. Proximal convergence was not measured and may have had a negative influence on his findings. Permanent changes in refractive status are not expected; therefore, refractions should be performed following delivery.

Electrophysiologic changes in the optic pathways have been noted during pregnancy. In a recent study, significant reductions were demonstrated in the early waves of visual-evoked potentials of gravid females.[6] This led the authors to believe that neural excitation and conduction improved during pregnancy.

CONTACT LENS WEAR

The majority of women who elect to wear contact lenses do so within the childbearing years. With metabolic and physiologic changes occurring during pregnancy, many women become intolerant or experience transient disturbances with lens wear. Imifadon et al.[7] found that 30 percent of pregnant women wearing soft or rigid contact lenses experienced symptoms, with nonspecific discomfort associated with rigid lens wear as the most common complaint.

Hormonal influences during pregnancy and normal lens wear, independently, increase tissue hydration in the corneal stroma. When these two factors compound during gestation, however, they can produce modifications in corneal topography and consequently lead to tight-fitting lenses. In addition, rigid lenses have been documented in situ, exhibiting loss of peripheral clearance during gestation.[8] Blackstone[9] reported a case of a young woman who experienced corneal flattening in the second trimester and subsequent steepening in the final trimester of gestation. Finally, Westerhout[10] reported two rigid-lens patients who experienced gross corneal edema and decompensation of the epithelium before unfortunate spontaneous abortions.

Many women combat increased intolerance to hard lenses in the first trimester and those suffering from pregnancy-induced hypertension are more likely to have overall difficulty.[8] Similarly, soft lens wear is complicated by altered tear volume, corneal changes, and increased deposition of proteins and mucous.[11]

Therefore, pregnancy is an ill-advised time to initiate contact lens fitting, especially in the presence of positive anterior segment findings. Management of the pregnant patient is problem oriented, whether it be lens modification, alteration of wearing time, or discontinuation of lens wear. Although a number of women may not experience symptoms, those patients who continue to wear lenses should be followed periodically.

ANTERIOR SEGMENT

Cornea

Weinreb et al.[12] measured central corneal thickness in pregnant subjects in comparison to a nongravid and postpartum control population. Data revealed a 3 percent increase in corneal thickness with insignificant fluctuation through each trimester of pregnancy. The return to baseline thickness shortly after delivery may suggest a hormonal influence on corneal fluid retention. In addition, Kiely et al.[13] observed thickness changes that were concurrent with fluctuating systemic estrogen levels in the menstrual cycle.

Corneal hydration produces a reduction in corneal sensitivity; however, the amount of edema is unrelated to the increase in corneal touch threshold values.[14] Decrease in corneal sensitivity during pregnancy has been demonstrated in several studies, with reversion to normal in the weeks following delivery.[14,15] Riss and Riss[15] did not find a correlation between the duration of pregnancy and the degree of abated corneal sensitivity.

Krukenberg spindles have been observed far more often in pregnant women than in the general population.[16] In four reported cases, each woman was black, possessed minimal refractive error, and exhibited mild signs of pigment dispersion syndrome. Hormonal influence on melanin-producing cell types in the anterior segment is believed to result in increased pigmentation. Spindle formations were noted to dissipate in late pregnancy via increased outflow also induced by hormones.[16] Finally, Thomas[17] noted the exacerbation of parenchymatous and marginal keratitis and the recurrence of an epithelial dystrophy during pregnancy.

Orbit

Vascular anomalies may present during pregnancy or postpartum in the form of orbit-related signs. Hormonal and maternal blood volume changes during gestation or labor can induce alterations in the vasculature in the periorbital tissues. Spontaneous carotidcavernous fistulas appear more frequently in women than men, and 25 to 30 percent of all cases in women occur in the latter stages of pregnancy or during delivery.[18] Signs such as bulbar conjunctival injection, proptosis, marked edema, and audible orbital bruit should point toward the diagnosis of a fistula. Patients should be referred for further vascular evaluation. Spontaneous resolution has been reported to occur in the months following delivery.[19]

Intermittent diplopia associated with pain and exophthalmos has transpired during labor caused by acute orbital hematoma.[20,21] Valsalva maneuver applied in the second stage of labor can greatly increase the pressure in the orbital veins, resulting in retrobulbar hemorrhage. Recovery is spontaneous in the weeks following delivery. Finally, growth of an orbital hemangioma has been described as progressive proptosis during the course of pregnancy.[22] Associated findings include retinal striae, posterior pole edema, and a mild ipsilateral abduction deficit. Some vascular tumors such as hemangiomas may grow under the influence of hormonal changes in the gravid women. In such a case, the encapsulated tumor was excised and the patient fully recovered.

Miscellaneous Changes

Blood flow through the bulbar conjunctival vascular bed has been noted to undergo alterations during uncomplicated pregnancies.[23,24] Entering the second half of gestation, blood flow gradually decreases, which continues through the first postpartum week. Biomicroscopic examination reveals granularity of the blood columns within the capillary beds. In a large study, Landesman et al.[24] reported these findings in 95 percent of their subjects with normal pregnancies. Additionally, in the second trimester, the number of functioning capillaries progressively reduces, which continues through the first postpartum week.[23] The tortuosity of the vessels remains unchanged. Idiopathic subconjunctival hemorrhages can present during gestation or labor. In such instances, one should rule out the presence of underlying vascular disease.

Morphologic changes have been documented in the conjunctival epithelium that correlate well with fluctuations in estrogen level.[25] As estrogen reaches peak levels, the maturation index of the stratified cuboidal epithelium is at its maximum. Studies, however, have been performed in menstruating women and not in pregnant subjects.

Schirmer strip evaluation has demonstrated a steady decline in lacrimal volume, with the most notable changes occurring in the third trimester.[26] Changes in the composition of the tear film is evident by the increased deposition of mucous and protein on contact lenses and reported intolerance to lens wear. In addition, tear lysozyme levels are also noted to elevate.[11,14]

Intraocular pressure measurements and corneal indentation pulse amplitudes are reduced during pregnancy.[27,28] Reduction in ocular rigidity,[29] decreased episcleral venous pressure,[30] increased outflow facility,[31] and reduced peripheral vascular resistance[28] have all been demonstrated and implicated as possible causes. Intraocular pressure decreases throughout gestation, reaching its lowest point at the end of the third trimester.[28] In another report, acute angle closure glaucoma was precipitated by labor in a patient with narrow anterior chamber angles.[32] It is well accepted that periods of physical and emotional stress may incite angle closure in predisposed individuals.

Ptosis has also been reported as a complication of pregnancy.[33] The reporting physicians hypothesized that increasing estrogen levels resulted in the infiltration of water molecules into the ground substance of the levator tendon. When evaluating patients with ptosis, the eye care practitioner must rule out the presence of additional neurologic deficits such as an unreactive pupil or cranial nerve involvement. Such signs may indicate a pathologic cause. Examination of old photographs can aid in determining the time of onset.

DERMATOLOGIC PROBLEMS

The facial and periorbital skin, like many organs, changes during pregnancy. Melasma, most commonly referred to as "the mask of pregnancy," may develop in 50 to 70 percent of pregnant women.[34,35] The clinical picture consists of sharply demarcated tan-to-brown patches, which resolve following delivery. This may present in a small variety of distribution patterns but is most common in the centrofacial region. Sunlight is believed to be a necessary component in its development. Pre-existing nevi may increase in size and should be monitored for signs of malignancy. Freckles, nevi, and scars also increase in pigmentation. The most dramatic changes relate to the vascular system of the dermis. Facial and eyelid edema may accompany generalized systemic edema. Small telangiectatic vessels, known as spider angiomas, may appear in a large majority of women, most

often during the first and second trimesters.[35] Subcutaneous capillary hemangioepitheliomas within the facial area may also first appear. Pre-existing hemangiomas tend to enlarge but recede in the postpartum period. Other facial and ocular dermatologic conditions associated with pregnancy include papular dermatitis of pregnancy,[36] hereditary angioedema,[36] acrodermatitis enteropathica,[37] and erythema multiforme.[34,36]

NEUROLOGIC MANIFESTATIONS

Cranial Nerves

Idiopathic facial palsy is observed in an increased incidence of threefold during pregnancy, with over 75 percent of cases occurring in the third trimester and first 2 weeks postpartum.[38] Hypotheses for the underlying mechanism have suggested a vascular-mechanical compression,[39] viral infection,[39] and a possible association with toxemia.[40–42] Spontaneous recovery may occur shortly after delivery. Prognosis is regarded as less favorable if loss of taste is experienced.

Trigeminal neuropathy may present in pregnancy, but a solid association has not been fully documented. In such instances, patients may develop sensory deprivation, often in a single branch of cranial nerve V. Latent demyelinating disease in pregnant women may activate trigeminal neuralgia.[38]

The cranial nerves responsible for visual transmission, pupillary function, and extraocular muscle movements are vulnerable to many pathologic states during pregnancy. Optic neuritis may appear during lactation shortly following delivery. Immunosuppressive activity in conjunction with underlying demyelinating disease may contribute to the onset of this disorder.[43] The frequency of such attacks is similar to the age-matched population and thus may not be a significant finding. One case, however, has presented during the second trimester without evidence of multiple sclerosis.[44] Additionally, cerebral complications such as infarction, tumorous growths, and increased intracranial pressure can manifest as cranial nerve deficits.

Jacobson[45] reported the manifestation of a superior oblique palsy during the uncomplicated pregnancies of three women. No systemic disease or focal neurologic signs were present at the time of diagnosis. Extrafoveal fixation and large vertical fusion ranges in these patients led the author to believe that the new-found diplopia resulted from decompensation of fusion ability.

Two cases of Adie's tonic pupil that presented during pregnancy have been reported.[46] A causal relationship was not established and may signify a coincidental finding. Transient neurologic deficits such as sixth nerve palsy[47] and Horner syndrome[48,49] have been noted as iatrogenic complications in spinal analgesia during labor. The sixth nerve is the most common cranial nerve affected and may present 7 to 21 days following anesthesia.[47] Recovery may take up to 3 months. Horner syndrome begins 1 hour after the administration of lumbar epidural anesthesia with an incidence up to 75 percent.[49] Complete and spontaneous resolution occurs 5 hours after cessation of the analgesic.

Cerebrovascular Complications

Pregnancy increases the risk of focal ischemic cerebrovascular events approximately 13-fold relative to an age-matched nonpregnant population.[50] Although 60 to 80 percent of all occlusive events occur in the arterial circulation, venous thrombosis must also be considered in the differential diagnosis.[50] Arterial occlusions are most often observed in the second and third trimesters and first week postpartum, whereas venous occlusions are generally seen in the first month postpartum.

Strokes can be caused by a wide variety of pathophysiologic entities (Table 11-1). In addition to ischemic-vascular events, pregnant women may suffer from hemorrhagic and arteritic disease. Intracranial hemorrhage from pre-existing aneurysms and arteriovenous malformations (AVM) accounts for 5 to 12 percent of all maternal deaths in pregnancy.[51,52] The risk of aneurysm rupture increases with each passing trimester, unlike for AVMs, which tend to bleed in the second trimester and during delivery.[53,54] Conscious patients suffering from a spontaneous subarachnoid hemorrhage note a severe occipital headache. The manifestations of ocular symptoms and signs are based on the location of the occlusive or hemorrhagic event. Cranial nerve deficit, visual field loss, transient ischemic attacks, and papilledema are some of the re-

Table 11-1. Causes of Cerebrovascular Complications and Associated Visual Signs

Cause	Mechanism	Reported Ocular Signs and Symptoms
Aneurysms	Hemorrhage	Cranial nerve palsy, visual field loss, disc edema, blurred vision
Atherosclerosis/hypertension	Hemorrhage Ischemia	Cortical blindness
Arteriovenous malformations	Hemorrhage	Stroke
Atrial fibrillation	Embolism	Stroke
Choriocarcinoma	Arterial occlusion Hemorrhage	Stroke
Hypercoagulation syndromes	Venous thrombosis	Cranial nerve palsy, papilledema, visual field loss, photophobia, transient loss of vision
Abrupt hypotension	Ischemia	Infarction of the chiasm
Mitral valve prolapse	Embolism	Transient ischemic attacks, stroke
Nephritis (acute)	Ischemic	Eyelid edema, papilledema, transient amblyopia, blur
Peripartum cardiomyopathy	Embolism	Stroke
Pregnancy-induced hypertension	Hemorrhage Ischemia	Transient vision loss, photopsia Hemianopsia
Sickle cell crisis	Thrombosis Arterial occlusion	Stroke
Systemic lupus erythematosus	Arteritis	Cranial nerve palsy
Subacute bacterial endocarditis	Embolism Subarachnoid Heme	Transient ischemia attacks Stroke
Takayasu's disease	Arteritis	Visual disturbances
Thrombotic thrombocytopenic purpura	Arterial thrombosis	Transient ischemic attacks

(Data from Weibers,[50] Donaldson,[54] Fehr,[55] King,[56] Rand,[57] Simolke et al.,[162] and Srinivisan.[163])

ported symptoms and signs.[55–57] In Table 11-1, the work *stroke* refers to cases of cerebrovascular accidents with no mention of specific ocular signs. Depending on their location, however, these vascular events can cause visual disturbance or field loss in conjunction with other neurologic deficits. These patients are best managed by neurovascular specialists.

When evaluating the patient suspected of suffering a cerebrovascular event, the following tests should be performed: blood pressure measurements for both arms, carotid and ocular bruits, and ophthalmoscopy to rule out the presence of emboli. A cardiac examination, blood testing, and noninvasive tests such as echocardiography and computed tomography (CT) scans should be performed by a physician. Within the first 6 weeks following a stroke, about 80 percent of the recoverable function will return.[54]

Intracranial Neoplasms

Although the incidence of brain tumors during pregnancy is not statistically different from that found in the age-matched general population, the effects of gestation on tumors are well documented.[58,59] The hormonal influences of pregnancy may incite tumor growth, with subsequent diminution in size postpartum. Those tumors that most often involve the visual pathways include pituitary adenomas, meningiomas, and gliomas.

Pituitary adenomas present with a peak incidence within the childbearing years and are the most common of all intrasellar mass lesions. Routine postmortem studies have documented the incidence of chromophobe adenomas as high as 13 to 25 percent in asymptomatic women.[60] In many instances, adenomas produce hormonal changes that may result in infertility. However, tumors may be present in the pregnant patient, especially if the patient is undergoing bromocryptine or gonadotropin therapy. Functional tumors such as prolactin-secreting adenomas are generally diagnosed on the basis of endocrinopathy, whereas nonfunctioning tumors are more often larger and compress adjacent structures such as the chiasm. Rapid expansion of pre-existing pituitary adenomas occurs primarily in the second and third trimesters; macroadenomas are affected more than microadenomas. However, it is also well documented that the pituitary gland undergoes normal physiologic enlargement as a consequence of hyperplasia of prolactin-secreting cells that occurs in pregnancy.[61] Ap-

proximately 40 percent of these patients develop symptoms around the junction of the first and second trimester, with headaches preceding the onset of visual disturbances by an average of 4.2 weeks.[60] If the adenoma reaches significant size, approximately 1 cm or more, compression of the optic chiasm can produce bitemporal hemianopsia of varying degree. Patients who remain stable over the course of pregnancy can postpone surgical or radiation treatment until after delivery. Visual fields should be closely monitored during pregnancy.

Lymphocytic adenohypophysitis is a rare autoimmune-related cause of pituitary gland enlargement and must be included in the differential diagnosis of pituitary adenoma. When diffuse lymphocytic infiltration of the pituitary gland occurs, a clinical picture of hypopituitarism is observed and may lead to death, if left untreated. Ninety-six percent of all reported cases have occurred in women, with virtually all cases associated with pregnancy.[61] Symptoms of headache and visual changes may present at any time but usually manifest in the third trimester. On diagnosis with laboratory tests, formal visual fields, and CT, treatment should include a trial of medical therapy followed by surgical resection by a neurosurgeon.

Meningiomas are benign, slow-growing, fibrous tumors that most often arise from the arachnoid mater or the middle layer of the meninges. They constitute 10 to 15 percent of all intracranial tumors.[62] During pregnancy, growth may be accelerated and then abate on delivery of the fetus. Enlargement may reoccur with breast-feeding and subsequent pregnancies.[63] Although the underlying mechanism of the altered growth pattern is not completely understood, recent studies tend to implicate hormonal effects on the tumor's progesterone and estrogen receptors.[64] Diagnostically, ophthalmologic and neurologic signs may aid in determining the location of a meningioma. These may include proptosis, optic atrophy, optociliary shunt vessels, afferent pupillary defect, cranial nerve palsies, papilledema, visual field loss, and decreased acuity. Symptoms may include headache, nausea, and dizziness, which unfortunately, from a diagnostic point of view, occur during a normal pregnancy. After the meningioma is confirmed by radiologic studies, surgical excision is the treatment of choice. Consideration of the degree of vision loss, prognosis for improvement, location of the tumor, and stage of pregnancy is required in determining the urgency of action. The patient is best monitored by a team of specialists: a neurosurgeon, obstetrician, and pediatrician.[65]

Glial tumors such as astrocytomas and oligodendrogliomas may undergo expansion as a result of the hormonal influences of pregnancy. This, however, has not yet been confirmed by experimental means.[66] Edema of the tissue surrounding the growing tumor tends to be greater during gestation because of the retention of body water, thus producing more severe symptoms. Patients may demonstrate signs such as papilledema, cranial nerve deficits, and sensory or motor dysfunction. Co-management with a specialist team is the best treatment. Corticosteroids may be used to postpone surgery.

Other tumors that have been reported in pregnancy include the rapid enlargement of a craniopharyngioma,[67] neurofibromas,[59] acoustic neuromas,[58,59] hemangiomas,[59] angiomas,[58,68] and cerebellar astrocytomas.[58,59] Each can potentially present with visual signs and symptoms. As previously mentioned, management is best handled with a team approach.

Benign Intracranial Hypertension

Similar to many other pathologic conditions, benign intracranial hypertension (BIH), otherwise known as pseudotumor cerebri, has a predisposition for women during the childbearing years. Epidemiologic studies, however, have determined that the incidence of this entity is not significantly greater than that among an age-matched nonpregnant population.[69] BIH most often appears in the first half of gestation, and is a diagnosis of exclusion. Recurrence in subsequent pregnancies has been reported, but a valid association has not yet been proven.[70] Symptoms may include intermittent headache, diplopia, nausea, vomiting, transient obscuration of vision, and tinnitus. Objective examination reveals the presence of optic disc edema and, possibly, involvement of cranial nerve VI (Fig. 11-1 and Plate 11-1). Following delivery or induced or spontaneous abortion, amelioration of symptoms occurs.

Patient management includes a thorough case history, blood pressure to rule out hypertensive disease, binocular ophthalmoscopic examination, and visual fields. An immediate referral should be made for neuroimaging and lumbar puncture to rule out other causes of increased intracranial pressure seen in pregnancy. Although the disease is usually self-limiting,

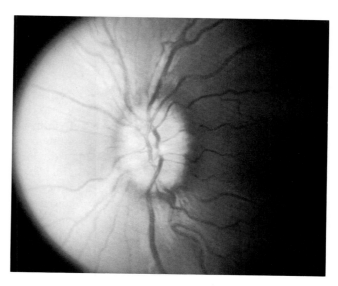

Fig. 11-1. Fundus photograph of disc edema in a patient diagnosed with benign intracranial hypertension. (See also Plate 11-1.)

medical intervention is sometimes required to preserve vision. This may include serial lumbar puncture, carbonic anhydrase inhibitors, and glucocorticoids.[71] In cases of persistent severe headaches or progressive optic nerve damage, surgical intervention may be indicated. Monitoring for changes in acuity and visual fields should be performed frequently. Termination of pregnancy is reserved only as a last resort. Subsequent follow-up is best performed with a team approach: obstetrician, neurosurgeon, and eye care professional.

Migraine Headaches

Migraine headaches are recurrent attacks of unilateral head pain, which may or may not be associated with visual and gastrointestinal disturbances. They tend to occur more often in females and peak in incidence in the childbearing years. Improvement in migrainous symptoms is reported to be as high as 60 to 87 percent of affected women during pregnancy.[72–74] Of the remaining migraine sufferers, two-thirds remain stable, while one-third worsen. Remission may occur in the second trimester, with the return of symptoms following delivery or during menses 2 or 3 months postpartum. Migraine headaches that first appear during gestation usually do so in the first trimester.[75,76] The best form of management is the least management. Traditional treatments of ergot alkaloids should be avoided, and analgesics such as acetaminophen used only when necessary.[74]

Wernicke's Encephalopathy

Wernicke's encephalopathy is an acute or subacute disorder resulting from thiamine deficiency and is usually associated with malnutrition and alcoholism. During the course of pregnancy, however, some individuals with hyperemesis gravidarum may develop this somewhat rare condition. *Hyperemesis gravidarum* refers to malignant vomiting and nausea in the pregnant mother, which results in dehydration and acidosis. In contrast to women with "morning sickness," affected women are more likely to lose rather than gain weight.

Histopathologically, vascular deformation and degeneration occur within the periventricular gray matter, resulting in impaired neurologic function. Classically, the encephalopathy presents as a triad of symptoms: ataxia, ophthalmoplegia, and impaired consciousness.[77] This triad, however, is not a constant finding. The ocularmotor and vestibular nuclei are often involved and may present as nystagmus and gaze palsies of varying severity and direction. Lateral rectus (VI) palsy seems to be most frequently reported.[78–80]

Management includes hospitalization and intravenous infusion of thiamine, glucose, water, and electrolytes. Ancillary neurologic testing may be performed to rule out additional involvement. In most reported cases, the ocular signs resolve on treatment.[77,78,80]

SYSTEMIC DISEASE

A collection of systemic diseases is associated with ocular signs such as diabetes, myasthenia gravis, and thyrotoxicosis. Many of these entities may be influenced over the course of pregnancy in the form of aggravation or amelioration of signs. In some instances, the conclusion of pregnancy will reactivate the disease process, and again its associated ocular signs will be manifested.

Autoimmune Disease

Myasthenia gravis is a disorder of the neuromuscular junction that is primarily seen in young women. The influence of pregnancy is unpredictable, and many women may experience the first symptoms of the disorder during gestation. Ptosis and diplopia are the two most common ocular symptoms reported by patients. While one-third of the patients have aggravation of symptoms, one-third show no change, and the remaining third show some improvement.[81] Risk of exacerbation is also increased in the postpartum period.[82]

Pregnancy may provide physiologic immune suppression, which results in the clinical improvement of many autoimmune diseases with noted ocular signs. Multiple sclerosis tends to stabilize or even improve, but the risk of relapse in the postpartum period increases.[83] Only 10 percent of women may experience relapse during pregnancy.[84] Systemic lupus erythematosus is another autoimmune disease influenced by the course of pregnancy. Past reports suggest a threefold increase in risk of exacerbation in the first half of pregnancy and a sevenfold increase in the first 2 months postpartum.[82] Gestational influence on other autoimmune disorders such as rheumatoid arthritis,[82] juvenile rheumatoid arthritis,[85] sarcoidosis,[86] and Vogt-Koyanagi-Harada syndrome[87,88] is manifested as amelioration or remission of signs and symptoms. This may include uveitis. Risk for exacerbation of signs is increased in the postpartum period. One case of Behçet's disease has been reported in which ocular signs first appeared in the second trimester of a fourth pregnancy.[89] Past history indicated that the patient had previous bouts of systemic involvement.

Connective Tissue Disorders

Characterized by ectopia lentis, arachnodactyly, and cataracts, Marfan syndrome may be first diagnosed in the office of the primary care practitioner. Although there are no current reports of the influence of pregnancy on the ocular signs, the risk for dissection of aortic aneurysms in the last trimester is increased.[90] Referral to the appropriate physician should be made. Similarly, pseudoxanthoma elasticum, another elastic tissue disorder, may be diagnosed by the presence of retinal angioid streaks. Changes to these separations in Bruch's membrane have not been reported in pregnancy; however, the patient may be at higher risk for developing cardiovascular complications.[91]

Endocrine Disease

Many of the clinical signs of hyperthyroidism such as heat intolerance, anxiety, and tachycardia are seen in normal pregnancy. This may create added difficulty in making the correct diagnosis. To further complicate matters, the thyroid gland may undergo enlargement in the first trimester, which persists through gestation.[92] Graves disease, when influenced, may be aggravated in early pregnancy and postpartum.[93] The disease tends to enter clinical remission in the latter half of pregnancy. Because of this confusion, ocular findings such as lid lag or exophthalmos can help differentiate Graves disease from "normal" metabolic disturbances. Management of thyrotoxicosis presents many problems and should be handled by an endocrinologist.

Hypertensive Disorders of Pregnancy

When evaluating an individual for hypertension during pregnancy, one must determine the specific disorder that afflicts the patient. At one time, *toxemia* was an all-inclusive term referring to any hypertensive disorder and its accompanying signs. Currently, more descriptive terms are used to separate these different entities.

Gestational hypertension refers to the development of hypertension during pregnancy or the first 24 hours following the delivery. In these patients, the blood pressure returns to baseline levels within 10 days of parturition. Another disorder, chronic hypertension, implies the presence of hypertension before pregnancy, before the week 20 of pregnancy, or persistent after 6 weeks postpartum. By contrast, pregnancy-induced hypertension (PIH) specifically refers to a hypertensive disorder that has no underlying cause other than gestation and is accompanied by either generalized edema or increased protein excretion, or both. PIH may be further categorized into two stages: pre-eclampsia and eclampsia. Severity of the hypertensive disease is based on symptoms and objective findings (Table 11-2). Additionally, patients can develop PIH superimposed on chronic hypertensive disease.

Introduction of the fetal (paternal) allograft into the host mother induces many biochemical and physiologic changes in the first trimester. In the normotensive pregnancy, trophoblast cells migrate from the burgeoning embryo into the uteroplacental arteries to create a low-pressure, high-flow system. This is achieved through the breakdown of internal vascular musculature and the release of vasodilating prostaglandins. In PIH, immunologic maladaptation disrupts trophoblast migration and produces free radi-

Table 11-2. Criteria for the Diagnosis of Pregnancy-Induced Hypertension

Mild pre-eclampsia
    Blood pressure
        Rise in systolic of ≥30 mmHg
        Rise in diastolic of ≥15 mmHg
        ≥140/90 mmHg
    Proteinuria
        >300 mg/L in a 24-h collection period or 1–2+ on dipstick testing
    Generalized edema

Severe pre-eclampsia (one or more of the following signs or symptoms present)
    Blood pressure: ≥160/110 mmHg
    Proteinuria: >5 g/24-h period or 3–4+ on dipstick
    Oliguria or decreased urine output: <400 ml/24 h
    Cerebral or visual disturbances (headache, blurred vision, scotomata)
    Pulmonary edema
    Epigastric or right upper quadrant pain
    Unexplained hepatic dysfunction
    Thrombocytopenia

Eclampsia
    Convulsions
    Coma

(Modified from American College of Obstetricians and Gynecologists,[164] with permission.)

cals and chemicals that promote vasoconstriction, platelet aggregation, and impair endothelial (vascular) layer function.[94] Capillary hypoxia and generalized vasoconstriction ultimately lead to the development of systemic hypertension, proteinuria, and edema.

Pre-eclampsia develops in approximately 5 percent of all pregnancies in the United States.[94,95] Of these women, 5 percent will manifest signs of eclampsia. Typically, the onset of pre-eclampsia occurs after week 20 of gestation. Women predisposed for developing PIH are typically poorly nourished primigravidas and may report a family history of PIH (Table 11-3). Unfortunately, some patients may succumb to the

Table 11-3. Risk Factors for the Development of Pregnancy-Induced Hypertension

Primigravida (first pregnancy)
Family history of pregnancy-induced hypertension
Diabetes mellitus
Multiple gestation pregnancy (twins, etc.)
Extremes of age (early adolescence and women >35 years)
Malnutrition
Hydatidiform mole (trophoblastic neoplasm)
Chronic renal disease
Hydrops fetalis

(Data from Chelsey.[165])

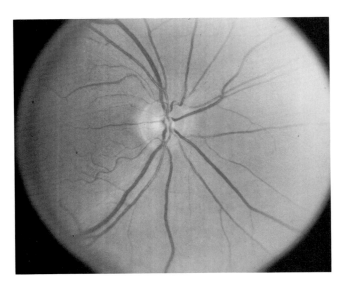

Fig. 11-2. Fundus photograph of generalized arteriolar attenuation. (Courtesy of Jane Stein, Philadelphia, PA.) (See also Plate 11-2.)

pathologic complications of this condition such as eclamptic encephalopathy.

The hallmark finding of retinal arteriolar angiospasm has been reported to occur in as high as 60 to 100 percent of patients diagnosed with PIH.[96] Initially, focal areas of arteriolar spasm predominate but tend to evolve into generalized vessel narrowing as the disease exacerbates (Fig. 11-2 and Plate 11-2). In addition, the incidence of retinal findings increases directly with blood pressure readings.[97] In a classic study, Jaffe and Schatz[98] examined mean arteriole/vein ratio and focal arteriolar constriction in a series of patients in various stages of pre-eclampsia. As the severity of the disease increased, the number of visible focal constrictions likewise increased, and the arteriole/vein ratio decreased. Involvement of the retinal capillary beds can result in areas of nonperfusion and associated edema. Other retinal signs such as hemorrhages, exudates, disc edema, and cotton-wool spots are almost exclusively observed in patients with additional systemic diseases.[98] Patients with superimposed hypertension develop retinal and choroidal vascular occlusion, whereas in those with pre-eclampsia, occlusions tend to be limited to the choroid.[99] In most cases, all vascular alterations are reversible with the delivery of the fetus.

Exudative retinal detachments are an infrequent finding in PIH. Studies report an incidence of 1 to 2 percent in patients with pre-eclampsia and up to 10 percent in those diagnosed with eclampsia.[96,100] Clinically, these detachments are most often bilateral and can present without frank hypertensive retinopathy[101] or PIH.[102] Choroidal hypoperfusion in conjunction with retinal pigment epithelium (RPE) dysfunction results in transudation of fluid into the subretinal space (Fig. 11-3 and Plate 11-3). Fluorescein angiography studies in patients with nonrhegmatogenous retinal detachments secondary to PIH have demonstrated areas of choroidal nonperfusion with leakage of dye through overlying areas of decompensated RPE.[103,104] Ophthalmoscopically, these points of leakage appear as yellowish-white opaque foci at the level of the RPE. Saito et al.[105] reported that the pattern of these foci may indicate their pathologic origins. Those arranged in a geographic pattern resulted from choroidal artery occlusion and ultimately led to areas of chorioretinal atrophy. A mosaic distribution was presumed to be associated with transient choroidal vascular insufficiency, and signs were not visible on examination shortly thereafter. Histopathologic studies noted thrombotic occlusion of choroidal vasculature and overlying necrosis of the stroma and RPE.[106] Patients may report blurred vision or photopsia as symptoms of an impending detachment. Following delivery, bullous detachments typically spontaneously resolve within the first 3 weeks postpartum, and vision returns to baseline.

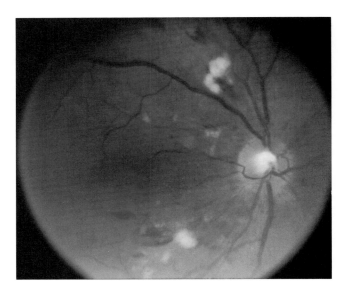

Fig. 11-3. Shallow inferior non-rhegmatogenous retinal detachment secondary to choroidal nonperfusion. (See also Plate 11-3.)

Focal alterations in the RPE may persist as yellow spots with pigmented centers, referred to as *Elschnig spots*. Gass and Pautler[107] described a series of cases of stable pigmentary changes in the pigment epithelium following reattachment of bullous retinal detachments. Each of these cases exhibited patterns bearing strong resemblance to tapetoretinal or heredomacular dystrophies. Finally, a case of bilateral peripheral neovascularization associated with PIH was reported with the likely pathogenesis of microvascular occlusion.[108]

The incidence of blindness in patients with diagnosed PIH is 1 to 5 percent and may be derived from a number of causes.[109,110] Aside from retinal findings such as vascular occlusion and retinal detachment, loss of vision may be of cortical origin. Patients who present with sudden visual loss in the presence of normal pupillary reactivity and fundus appearance may harbor cerebrovascular lesions. In PIH, the upper limit of autoregulation for cerebral blood flow by blood pressure may be exceeded, and subsequent disruption of the capillary endothelium ensues. Edema and ring hemorrhages appear in the cortical gray matter, with the parietal and occipital lobes most vulnerable.[111] Management includes an immediate cranial CT scan and medical therapy under the supervision of specialty care. Prognosis is usually excellent for the return of vision.

A summary of the signs and symptoms associated with PIH are listed in Table 11-4. The bulbar conjunctival vascular beds can experience changes in vessel caliber. Severe attenuation, tortuosity, and small areas of conjunctival hemorrhage have all been described in PIH.[23] Two cases of ischemic optic neuropathy have been reported in patients with pre-eclampsia with an episode of total transient blindness produced in one patient.[112] Recurrent episodes in the second patient resulted in permanent blindness.

During examination of a patient suspected to have pre-eclampsia, convulsions may be induced via photic stimulation.[113] Fundus evaluations however, should be performed because of the benefits of uncovering potential findings. Treatment of eclampsia involves antihypertensive agents, bed rest, and magnesium sulfate for seizure control. Frequent ophthalmoscopic examination should be performed by obstetric or ophthalmic professionals. When fetal maturity is reached, labor may be induced to reduce further risk to the mother.

Table 11-4. Ocular Signs and Symptoms of Pregnancy-Induced Hypertension

Amaurosis
Scintillation
Chromatopsia
Visual blur
Diplopia
Visual field loss (homonymous hemianopia, etc.)
Arteriolar constriction (retinal and conjunctival)
Facial and lid edema
Focal choridal infarcts (Elschnig spots)
Peripheral retinal neovascularization
Optic disc edema
Retinal edema
Retinal exudates
Retinal hemorrhages
Cotton-wool infarcts
Blindness secondary to
    Retinal ischemia following hemorrhage
    Exudative retinal detachment
    Central retinal artery or venous thrombosis
    Edema or hemorrhage in the occipital lobe
    Psychogenic disorder
    Optic nerve involvement
    Intracranial venous thrombosis
    Persistent spasm of retinal vessels

Effects of Pregnancy on Diabetes

Diabetic retinopathy is one of the leading causes of blindness in adults ranging in age between 24 and 64 in the United States.[114] It is well accepted that type I (insulin-dependent) diabetes mellitus of increasing duration heightens the incidence, severity, and progression of retinal vascular disease. Other factors that elevate severity of retinopathy are hypertension,[115] age of onset, and number of past pregnancies.[116] Pregnancy creates a state of insulin resistance, which requires close blood glucose monitoring. Therefore, young women with juvenile onset diabetes enter pregnancy at higher risk of developing retinopathy and suffering gestational complications. Because duration of the disease is such a critical component, it is recommended that women with juvenile-onset diabetes bear children at an early age.[117] Careful monitoring of retinopathy and blood glucose by eye care and obstetrics professionals, respectively, can help decrease blindness and fetal mortality.

Gestational diabetes mellitus is defined as carbohydrate intolerance that is first recognized during pregnancy[118]; it constitutes 90 percent of cases involving diabetes during gestation.[119] Proper diagnosis is important for this common disorder, because maternal and fetal morbidity rates are greatly enhanced. The best screening test is the 1-hour after 50-g oral glucose challenge.[118] Findings in the upper end of normal or those that seem suspicious should be further investigated because the test results are variable.[120] Furthermore, women developing gestational diabetes have a 50 to 60 percent chance of developing type II diabetes mellitus later in life.[121]

A number of reports indicate that women with diabetes mellitus without retinopathy have little risk of developing retinal changes during pregnancy. In a review of nine studies, Sunness et al.[122] discovered that 88 percent of the women did not develop retinopathy, 7 percent revealed mild background changes, and the remaining 5 percent demonstrated less subtle background retinopathy. One patient was noted to have preproliferative changes. Regression occurred in 57 percent of the subjects postpartum. With respect to gestational diabetes, the prevalence of retinal vascular tortuosity increases and has been shown to persist at least 5 months postpartum.[123] These patients, however, are not at increased risk of developing diabetic retinal changes.

Recent studies tend to indicate that many women experience exacerbation of background diabetic retinopathy (BDR), which regresses on delivery.[123–125] This waxing and waning of the state of retinopathy reaches its peak in the second trimester with gradual improvement through the postpartum period. Although progression to more severe states of background retinopathy is not believed to be significant, the small number of women who develop proliferative changes are considered to be at much higher risk. Additionally, patients with more severe BDR are at higher risk of developing proliferative changes. Studies show that 2 to 16 percent of women with background retinopathy at the onset of pregnancy will present with proliferative changes at some point during gestation.[123–130] These mounting changes are generally reported to occur between weeks 20 and 28. Sunness[131] noted the conversion of 43 percent of patients with initial BDR to the preproliferative stage in three studies. However, patients with less than 10 microaneurysms and dot hemorrhages per eye before gestation were studied and found not to exhibit significant change throughout pregnancy.[122]

Sinclair et al.[132] described several patients who developed diabetic macular edema in association with preproliferative and proliferative changes. Initially, each had minimal background changes but also possessed some form of nephropathy, including pregnancy-induced hypertension. Those individuals with the highest urine protein exhibited the greatest amount of retinal edema. In patients with macular edema, focal laser treatment is usually withheld due to the high rate of spontaneous recovery in the postpartum period. Treatment is indicated, however, in cases of long-standing edema with declining acuity or exudate material bearing down on the fovea.

The severity of proliferative retinopathy correlates well with the presence of angiopathy in other organs such as the kidney.[129] In addition, increased fetal morbidity has been associated with the presence of proliferative retinopathy in a number of studies.[126,133] In one review of many studies, exacerbation of pregestational proliferative retinopathy was exhibited in 46 percent of 122 total cases.[122] Progression of retinopathy was less likely in those women receiving scatter panretinal laser photocoagulation (26 percent) than those who did not (58 percent). Proliferative retinopathy, in the absence of panretinal laser, may spontaneously regress in the latter stages of pregnancy. However, involution of proliferative retinal changes following panretinal laser procedures transpires in 86 percent of the patients.[134]

Acute optic disc edema associated with juvenile-onset diabetes has been reported during pregnancy.[135] Although this pathologic change has a benign course, a full work-up is required to rule out more serious causes of disc edema. Misdiagnosis may often lead to unnecessary therapeutic abortion. Resolution of the edema to baseline levels occurs in the absence of any specific therapy.

Protocol for ophthalmologic examination in the diabetic woman during the childbearing years recommends a baseline dilated fundus examination within 12 months of a planned pregnancy (Table 11-5). Once pregnant, the diabetic mother should be examined once in the first trimester to assess the presence or severity of retinopathy. The frequency of subsequent examinations is determined by the severity of retinal and systemic disease. A follow-up within the first 3 months postpartum is also suggested. Color fundus photography is a useful tool to document and monitor retinal changes. Scatter panretinal laser photocoagulation by an experienced retinologist is recommended in the presence of proliferative disease with high-risk characteristics as defined by the Diabetic Retinopathy

Table 11-5. Recommendations for the Ophthalmologic Management of Pregnant Diabetics

1. Previously diagnosed diabetics	Baseline dilated fundus examination within 12 months of a planned pregnancy; comprehensive eye examination in the first trimester; frequency of follow-up examinations based on severity of retinopathy; patients should be counseled on the risk of development or progression of diabetic retinopathy
2. Women with insulin-dependent diabetes <5 years, no retinopathy, nephropathy, or hypertension	Perform ophthalmoscopy at least once between weeks 20 and 30 of gestation
3. Women with insulin-dependent diabetes >5 years, no retinopathy, nephropathy, or hypertension	Dilated fundus examination at least once per trimester
4. Women with mild nonproliferative retinopathy, nephropathy, or hypertension	Dilated fundus examination at least once per month
5. Women with moderate or severe nonproliferative retinopathy, significant nephropathy, and proteinuria	Patient to be educated before or early in pregnancy regarding the potential risk to the eyes; dilated fundus examinations at least monthly
6. Women with active proliferative retinopathy, especially with high risk characteristics as defined by the Diabetic Retinopathy Study	Panretinal scatter photocoagulation
7. Women who develop severe optic disc neovascularization in the first trimester that responds very poorly to aggressive laser photocoagulation	Therapeutic abortion may be recommended
8. Women who develop gestational diabetes mellitus	No increased risk of the development of diabetic retinopathy; previous guidelines for monitoring do not apply in such cases

(Data from Sinclair et al.[166] American Diabetes Association,[167])

Study.[136] The presence of one of the following is indicative of high-risk proliferative retinopathy: (1) neovascularization on the optic disc or within 1 diameter of the nerve head that is greater than one-quarter to one-third of the disc area; (2) neovascularization of the optic disc or within 1 diameter of the nerve head that is less than one-quarter to one-third of the disc area, if a fresh vitreous or preretinal hemorrhage is present; or (3) neovascularization elsewhere in the retina, if a fresh preretinal or vitreous hemorrhage is present. Persistent neovascularization of the optic disc may be a sign of increased fetal and maternal mortality due to diffuse systemic vascular disease (Fig. 11-4 and Plate 11-4). Therapeutic abortion may be recommended in such instances.

Coagulopathies

Myriad hematologic complications can occur during pregnancy and the puerperium. In many instances, the disease process may be fatal, requiring aggressive intensive care as the only means to preserve the life of the expectant mother.

Disseminated intravascular coagulation is an acquired syndrome characterized by the disturbance in homeo-

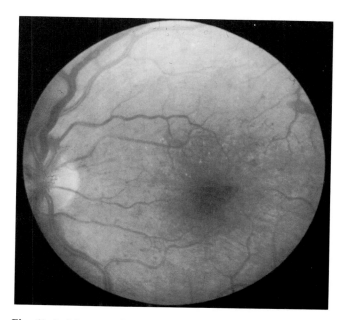

Fig. 11-4. Neovascularization of the optic disc with diabetic macular edema. (See also Plate 11-4.)

stasis of the body's clotting cascade. It develops during pregnancy secondary to an underlying disease entity and may present in acute or chronic forms. PIH is well established as one predisposing factor.[137] The primary disease process induces clot formation in the microvasculature, resulting in localized fibrin deposition. The subsequent fibrinolytic response reduces the body's platelet and coagulation factors. Thrombus formation may then become widespread within the smaller vessels of the body. Within the eye, fibrin-platelet clots may form at the level of the submacular and peripapillary choriocapillaris. In most instances, these changes are not visible but in severe cases can manifest as signs of occlusive disease such as choroidal hemorrhage, cystoid macular edema, and serous retinal detachment.[138,139] Symptoms reported include xanthopsia (shimmering of vision) and visual blur. Treatment is targeted at the underlying disease.

Thrombotic thrombocytopenia purpura is a rare, acute hematologic syndrome that can occur during pregnancy and may possess a genetic predisposition.[140] Although is not well understood at this time, the classic features include the aggregation of platelets or thrombosis in small vessels, thrombocytopenia, and hemolysis. Neurologic manifestations appear in one-half of cases and include paresis, headache, and visual disturbances.[137] Ocular symptoms are reported in approximately 10 percent of cases.[131] Documented signs include yellow subretinal infiltrates, disc edema, arteriolar constriction, vitreous hemorrhage, and serous retinal detachment.[131,141,142] These patients should be placed under the care of obstetricians for appropriate blood testing and treatment.

Amniotic fluid embolism is a rare but very serious complication in the intrapartum or early postpartum period. Mortality is reported in the 86 percent range.[143] Embolic material within the amniotic fluid deposits in the microvasculature of the heart, lung, brain, and eye. Within the eye, ischemic retinopathy is the manifestation of retinal arteriolar occlusions. Localized branch and complete artery occlusions have been documented.[143,144] Large areas of pigmentary disruption have been attributed to underlying choroidal ischemia.[144] Ophthalmoscopic examinations should be performed on all patients suspected of having amniotic fluid embolism.

POSTERIOR SEGMENT

The posterior segment of the eye is a highly vascularized structure that exhibits signs of systemic alterations, of which pregnancy is no exception. Pregnant women may develop complications secondary to pregnancy, or pregnancy may aggravate a pre-existing disease process. The retina and underlying choroid may often be used as a gauge to monitor the health of the expectant mother in such diseases as diabetes and PIH.

Choroidal Malignant Melanoma

Malignant melanoma of the choroid is a potential lethal entity rarely documented in pregnancy. Many of the cases reported, unfortunately, have a grim outcome.[145–147] Shields et al.[146] ascertained the transformation of suspicious choroidal lesions to active uveal melanomas in seven patients during gestation. Subretinal fluid and adjacent detachments were noted in all cases. Tumor analysis indicated that no histopathologic differences were evident when compared with melanomas from nonpregnant women. Accelerated growth attributed solely to the physiologic and hormonal changes of pregnancy could not be definitively determined. In a recent large case-control study, Holly et al.[148] reported a decrease in relative risk for the development of uveal melanoma with the increase in the number of live births. Women with suspicious posterior segment lesions should be watched throughout pregnancy. Referral to an ocular oncologist is recommended as the best form of management. Treatment options include observation, radiotherapy, or enucleation.

Idiopathic Central Serous Chorioretinopathy

Idiopathic central serous chorioretinopathy (ICSC) is a posterior segment disorder that presents with a frequency 10 times greater in men than in women.[149] Although usually associated with periods of stress in young or middle-aged men, ICSC can also present during pregnancy. During gestation, a number of physiologic, vascular, and hormonal changes transpire and may predispose pregnant women to the development of ICSC.

ICSC has been reported to occur in each trimester and even recur in subsequent pregnancies.[150] Patients may complain of reduced acuity followed by metamorphopsia, micropsia, dyschromatopsia, and may demonstrate a refractive shift toward hyperopia. Binocular funduscopic examination reveals a circumscribed area of elevation in the posterior pole with alterations to the normal light reflex of the foveal zone

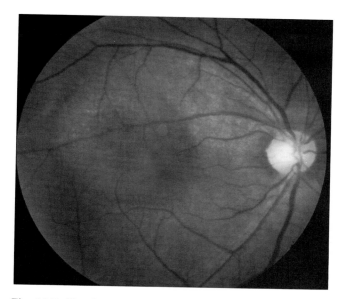

Fig. 11-5. Fundus photograph of central serous chorioretinopathy. (See also Plate 11-5.)

(Fig. 11-5 and Plate 11-5). Such findings represent a serous detachment of the neurosensory retina and/or the underlying RPE. Additionally, a high percentage of pregnant patients with ICSC present with white, fibrous, subretinal exudate around a focalized areas of RPE detachment.[151] Gass[152] noted that the appearance of exudate with ICSC was much greater among pregnant patients than nonpregnant patients and may indicate a new clinical entity. Management should include avoiding the diagnostic use of fluorescein angiography and assuring the patient about the gradual return of vision in the following months. Usually, vision returns to baseline postpartum. Periodic ophthalmologic examinations are highly recommended.

Retinal Occlusive Disorders

Retinal vascular occlusions in late pregnancy and following labor have been associated with embolism and thrombosis. A rare ophthalmoscopic picture resembling Purtscher's retinopathy has been reported in several women complaining of visual loss immediately following delivery.[153] Observed white areas of ischemic retina and flame hemorrhages translated into areas of nonperfusion, leakage, and arterial obstruction on fluorescein angiography. The pathophysiology of occlusion is poorly understood but may be attributed to complement-induced leukoemboli.[154] In

addition, vascular occlusions in pregnancy have also been reported in conjunction with primary antiphospholipid antibody syndrome[154] and protein S deficiency.[155]

Miscellaneous Posterior Segment Disorders

Hemorrhagic retinitis, in the form of retinal and subhyaloid hemorrhages, has been documented as a finding in hyperemesis gravidarum.[156] When such observations are made, they are regarded as signs of grave prognosis. It is imperative that patients undergo frequent ophthalmologic examinations to monitor for retinal changes. If hemorrhaging is discovered, the pregnancy should be terminated immediately.[1]

Additional reports of retinal disease include pericentral retinal degeneration,[157] idiopathic retinal phlebitis,[158] and toxoplasmic retinochoroiditis.[159] In the case of pericentral retinal degeneration, the patient reported progressive deterioration of bilateral ring scotomas during consecutive pregnancies.[157] Fundus examination revealed a depigmented zone around both maculae. Pregnancy has also been implicated as a factor in the reactivation of latent toxoplasmosis.[159] It is recommended that such patients undergo antibody titers for toxoplasmosis once each trimester. Similar to their orbital counterpart, choroidal hemangiomas may enlarge and subsequently regress during pregnancy.[160] Finally, one case of choroidal osteoma presenting during gestation has been documented.[161]

REFERENCES

1. Berkow R (ed): Normal pregnancy, labor, and delivery. p. 1744. In Berkow R (ed): The Merck Manual. 15th Ed. Merck, Rahway, NJ, 1987
2. Manges TD, Banaitis DA, Roth N et al: Changes in optometric findings during pregnancy. Am J Optom Physiol Optics 64: 159, 1987
3. Hilton GF: Some effects of pregnancy on the eye. Am J Optom Arch Am Acad Optom 35:117, 1958
4. Curtin BJ: Pseudomyopia. p. 455. In: The Myopias. Harper & Row, New York, 1985
5. Rosenwasser HM: Aetiology of systemic oedema and its effect on contact lens wearing. Optician 163:8, 1972
6. Tandon OP, Bhatia S: Visual evoked potential responses in pregnant women. Indian J Physiol Pharmacol 35:263, 1991
7. Imafidon CO, Imafidon JE, Akingbade OA, Onwudiegwu U: Symptomatology of contact lens wear in pregnancy. Optom Vis Sci, suppl. 12, 68:111, 1991
8. Phillips AJ, Stone J: Contact Lens: A Textbook for Practitioner and Student. 3rd Ed. Butterworth, Boston, 1989
9. Blackstone D: Wearing difficulties during pregnancy. Optician 149:12, 1965
10. Westerhout D: Pregnancy and contact lens problems. Optician 154:27, 1967

11. Imafidon CO, Imafidon JE: Contact lens wear in pregnancy. J Br Contact Lens Assoc 14:75, 1991
12. Weinreb RN, Lu A, Beerson C: Maternal corneal thickness during pregnancy. Am J Ophthalmol 105:258, 1988
13. Kiely PM, Carney LG, Smith G: Menstrual cycle variations of corneal topography and thickness. Am J Optom Physiol Optics 60:822, 1983
14. Millodot M: The influence of pregnancy on the sensitivity of the cornea. Br J Ophthalmol 61:646, 1977
15. Riss B, Riss P: Corneal sensitivity in pregnancy. Ophthalmologica 183:157, 1981
16. Duncan TE: Krukenberg spindles in pregnancy. Arch Ophthalmol 91:355, 1974
17. Thomas CI: Corneal lesions from generalized metabolic disturbances. p. 678. In: The Cornea. Charles C Thomas, Springfield, IL, 1955
18. Raskind R, Johnson N, Hance D: Carotid cavernous fistula in pregnancy. Angiology 28:671, 1977
19. Toya S, Shiobara R, Izumi J: Spontaneous carotid cavernous fistula during pregnancy or in the post-partum state. J Neurosurg 54:252, 1981
20. Jacobson DM, Itani K, Digre KB et al: Maternal orbital hemangioma associated with labor. Am J Ophthalmol 105:547, 1988
21. Nucci P, Bianchi S, Pierro L, Brancato R: Diplopia after labour. Br J Obstet Gynecol 98:227, 1991
22. Zauberman H, Feinsod M: Orbital hemangioma growth during pregnancy. Acta Ophthalmol 48:929, 1970
23. Landesman R: Retinal and conjunctival vascular changes in normal and toxemic pregnancy. Bull NY Acad Med 31:376, 1955
24. Landesman R, Douglas RG, Holze E: The bulbar conjunctival vascular bed in the toxemia of pregnancy. Am J Obstet Gynecol 68:170, 1954
25. Kramer P, Lubkin V, Potter W, et al: Cyclic changes in conjunctival smears from menstruating females. Ophthalmology 97:303, 1990
26. Imafidon JE, Imafidon CO: Influence of gestation on lacrimal liquid production. Optom Vis Sci, suppl. 12, 68:35, 1991
27. Horven I, Gjonnaess H: Corneal indentation pulse and intraocular pressure in pregnancy. Arch Ophthalmol 91:92, 1974
28. Horven I, Gjonnaess H, Kroese A: Blood circulation changes in the eye and limbs: with relation to pregnancy and female sex hormones. Acta Ophthalmol 54:203, 1976
29. Phillips CI, Gore SM: Ocular hypotensive effect of late pregnancy with and without high blood pressure. Br J Ophthalmol 69:117, 1985
30. Wilke L: Episcleral venous pressure and pregnancy. Acta Ophthalmol, suppl. 125:40, 1975
31. Green K, Phillips CI, Cheeks L et al: Aqueous humor flow rate and intraocular pressure during and after pregnancy. Ophthalmol Res 20:353, 1988
32. Kearns PP, Dhillon BJ: Angle closure glaucoma precipitated by labour. Acta Ophthalmologica 68:225, 1990
33. Sanke RF: Blepharoptosis as a complication of pregnancy. Ann Ophthalmol 16:720, 1984
34. Eudy SF, Baker GF: Dermatopathology for the obstetrician. Clin Obstet Gynecol 33:728, 1990
35. Parmley T, O'Brien T: Skin changes during pregnancy. Clin Obstet Gynecol 33:713, 1990
36. Dotz W, Berman B: Dermatologic problems of pregnancy. p. 452. In Cherry SH, Berkowitz RL, Kase NG (eds): Rovinsky and Guttmacher's Medical, Surgical, and Gynecologic Complications of Pregnancy. 3rd Ed. Williams & Wilkins, Baltimore, 1985
37. Cameron JD, McClain CJ, Doughman DJ: Acrodermatitis enteropathica. p. 630. In Gold DH, Weingeist TA (eds): The Eye in Systemic Disease. JB Lippincott, Philadelphia, 1990
38. Massey EW: Mononeuropathies in pregnancy. Semin Neurol 8:193, 1988
39. Korcyzn AD: Bell's palsy and pregnancy. Acta Neurol Scand 47:603, 1971
40. Hilsinger RL, Adour KKA, Doty HE: Idiopathic facial paralysis, pregnancy, and the menstrual cycle. Ann Otolaryngol 84:433, 1975
41. Pope TH, Kenan PD: Bell's palsy in pregnancy. Arch Otolaryngol 89:52, 1969
42. Robinson JR, Pou JW: Bell's palsy: a predisposition of pregnant women. Arch Otolaryngol 95:125, 1972
43. Erkkila H, Raitta C, Iivanainen M et al: Optic neuritis during lactation. Graefes Arch Clin Exp Ophthalmol 222:134, 1985
44. Trautman JC: Optic neuritis during lactation: comment. Surv Ophthalmol 30:273, 1985
45. Jacobson DM: Superior oblique palsy manifested during pregnancy. Ophthalmology 98:1874, 1991
46. Gnadt GR: Two cases of Adie's tonic pupil which occurred during pregnancy. South J Optom 9:37, 1991
47. Bryce-Smith R, Macintosh RR: Sixth nerve palsy after lumbar puncture and spinal analgesia. Br Med J 1:275, 1951
48. Carrie LES: Horner's syndrome following obstetric extradural block. Br J Anaesth 48:611, 1976
49. Schachner SM, Reynolds AC: Horner syndrome during epidural analgesia for obstetrics. Obstet Gynecol, suppl. 59:31S, 1982
50. Wiebers DO: Ischemic cerebrovascular complications of pregnancy. Arch Neurol 42:1106, 1985
51. Wiebers DO: Subarachnoid hemorrhage in pregnancy. Semin Neurol 8:226, 1988
52. Hunt HG, Schifrin BS, Suzuki K: Ruptured berry aneurysms and pregnancy. Obstet Gynecol 43:827, 1974
53. Holcomb WL, Petrie RH: Cerebrovascular emergencies in pregnancy. Clin Obstet Gynecol 33:467, 1990
54. Donaldson JO: Cerebrovascular disease. p. 137. In: Neurology of Pregnancy. 2nd Ed. WB Saunders, Philadelphia, 1989
55. Fehr PE: Sagittal sinus thrombosis in early pregnancy. Obstet Gynecol, suppl. 59:7S, 1982
56. King A: Neurologic conditions occurring as complications of pregnancy. Part I. Arch Neurol Psychiatry 63:471, 1950
57. Rand CW: Two cerebral complications of pregnancy: brain tumor and spontaneous subarachnoid hemorrhage. Clin Neurosurg 3:104, 1957
58. Haas JF, Janisch W, Staneczek W: Newly diagnosed primary intracranial neoplasms in pregnant women: a population based assessment. J Neurol Neurosurg Psychiatry 49:874, 1980
59. Roelvink NCA, Kamphorst W, Van Alphen HAM et al: Pregnancy-related primary brain and spinal tumors. Arch Neurol 44:209, 1987
60. Magyar DM, Marshall JR: Pituitary tumors and pregnancy. Am J Obstet Gynecol 132:739, 1978
61. Fiegenbaum SL, Martin MC, Wilson CB et al: Lymphocytic adenohypophysitis: a pituitary mass lesion occurring in pregnancy. Proposal for medical treatment. Am J Obstet Gynecol 164:1549, 1991
62. Wilson WB: Meningiomas of the anterior visual system. Surv Ophthalmol 26:109, 1981
63. Bickerstaff ER, Small JM, Guest IA: The relapsing course of certain meningiomas in relation to pregnancy and menstruation. J Neurol Neurosurg Psychiatry 21:89, 1958
64. Wan WL, Geller JL, Feldon SE et al: Visual loss caused by rapidly progressive intracranial meningiomas during pregnancy. Ophthalmology 97:18, 1990
65. Goldberg M, Rappaport ZH: Neurosurgical, obstetric, and endocrine aspects of meningioma during pregnancy. Isr J Med Sci 23:825, 1987
66. Olivi A, Brem RF, McPherson R, Brem H: Brain tumors in pregnancy. p. 85. In Goldstein PJ, Stern BJ (eds): Neurological Disorders of Pregnancy. 2nd Ed. Futura, Mount Kisco, NY, 1992

67. Sachs BP, Smith SK, Cassar J: Rapid enlargement of a craniopharyngioma in pregnancy. Br J Obstet Gynecol 85:557, 1978

68. Rubin SM, Jackson GM, Cohen AW: Management of the pregnant patient with a cerebral venous angioma: a report of two cases. Obstet Gynecol 78:929, 1991

69. Powell JL: Pseudotumor cerebri and pregnancy. Obstet Gynecol 40:713, 1972

70. Elian M, Ben-Tovim N, Bechar M, Bornstein B: Recurrent benign intracranial hypertension during pregnancy. Obstet Gynecol 31:685, 1986

71. Kassam SH, Hadi HA, Fadel HE et al: Benign intracranial hypertension in pregnancy: current diagnostic and therapeutic approach. Obstet Gynecol Surv 38:314, 1983

72. Lance JW, Anthony M: Some clinical aspects of migraine. Arch Neurol 15:356, 1966

73. Massey EW: Migraine during pregnancy. Obstet Gynecol Surv 32:693, 1977

74. Reik L: Headaches in pregnancy. Semin Neurol 8:187, 1988

75. Callaghan N: The migraine syndrome in pregnancy. Neurology 18:197, 1968

76. Sommerville BW: A study of migraine in pregnancy. Neurology 22:824, 1972

77. Nightingale S, Bates D, Heath PD, Barron SL: Wernicke's encephalopathy in hyperemesis gravidarum. Postgrad Med J 58:558, 1982

78. Chaturachinda K, McGregor EM: Wernicke's encephalopathy and pregnancy. J Obstet Gynecol Br Comm 75:969, 1968

79. Jollife N, Wortis H, Fein HD: The Wernicke syndrome. Arch Neurol Psychiatry 46:569, 1941

80. Wood P, Murray A, Sinha B et al: Wernicke's encephalopathy induced by hyperemesis gravidarum: case reports. Br J Obstet Gynecol 90:583, 1983

81. Parry GJ, Heiman-Patterson TD: Pregnancy and autoimmune neuromuscular disease. Semin Neurol 8:197, 1988

82. Pitkin RM: Autoimmune diseases in pregnancy. Semin Perinatol 1:161, 1977

83. Nelson LM, Franklin GM, Jones MC et al: Risk of multiple sclerosis exacerbation during pregnancy and breast feeding. JAMA 259:3441, 1988

84. Birk K, Smeltzer SC, Rudick R: Pregnancy and multiple sclerosis. Semin Neurol 8:205, 1988

85. Ostensen M: Pregnancy in patients with a history of juvenile rheumatoid arthritis. Arthritis Rheum 34:881, 1991

86. Mayock RL, Sullivan RD, Greening RR: Sarcoidosis and pregnancy. JAMA 164:158, 1957

87. Friedman Z, Granat M, Neumann E: The syndrome of Vogt-Koyanagi-Harada syndrome and pregnancy. Metabol Pediatr Syst Ophthalmol 4:147, 1980

88. Steahly LP: Vogt-Koyanagi-Harada syndrome and pregnancy. Ann Ophthalmol 22:59, 1990

89. Hurt WG, Cooke CL, Jordan WP et al: Behçet's syndrome associated with pregnancy. Obstet Gynecol, suppl. 53:31S, 1979

90. Elias S, Berkowitz RL: The Marfan syndrome and pregnancy. Obstet Gynecol 47:358, 1976

91. Berde C, Willis DC, Sandberg EC: Pregnancy in women with pseudoxanthoma elasticum. Obstet Gynecol Surv 38:339, 1983

92. Halme JK: Endocrine system changes. p. 43. In Bishop EH, Cefalo RC (eds): Signs and Symptoms in Disorders of Pregnancy. JB Lippincott, Philadelphia, 1983

93. Amino T, Tanizawa O, Mori H: Aggravation of thyrotoxicosis in early pregnancy and after delivery in Grave's disease. J Clin Endocrinol Metabol 55:108, 1982

94. Zeeman GG, Dekker GA: Pathogenesis of pre-eclampsia: a hypothesis. Clin Obstet Gynecol 35:317, 1992

95. Knuppel RA, Drukker RA: Hypertension in pregnancy. In Knuppel RA, Drukker JE (eds): High-Risk Pregnancy: A Team Approach. WB Saunders, Philadelphia, 1986

96. Hallum AV: Eye changes in hypertensive toxemia of pregnancy. JAMA 106:1649, 1936

97. Mussey RD, Mundell BJ: Retinal examinations: a guide in the management of the toxic hypertensive syndrome of pregnancy. Am J Obstet Gynecol 37:30, 1939

98. Jaffe G, Schatz H: Ocular manifestations of preeclampsia. Am J Ophthalmol 103:309, 1987

99. Saito Y, Omoto T, Kidoguchi K et al: The relationship between ophthalmoscopic changes and classification of toxemia in toxemia of pregnancy. Acta Soc Ophthalmol Jpn 94:870, 1990

100. Fry WE: Extensive bilateral retinal detachment in eclampsia, with complete reattachment. Arch Ophthalmol 1:609, 1929

101. Oliver M, Uchenik D: Bilateral exudative retinal detachment in eclampsia without hypertensive retinopathy. Am J Ophthalmol 90:792, 1980

102. Brismar G, Schimmelpfennig W: Bilateral exudative retinal detachment in pregnancy. Acta Ophthalmologica 67:699, 1989

103. Fastenberg DM, Fetkenhour CL, Choromokos E et al: Choroidal vascular changes in toxemia of pregnancy. Am J Ophthalmol 89:362, 1980

104. Mabie WC, Ober RR: Fluorescein angiography in toxaemia of pregnancy. Br J Ophthalmol 64:666, 1980

105. Saito Y, Omoto T, Fukuda M: Lobular pattern of choriocapillaris in pre-eclampsia with aldosteronism. Br J Ophthalmol 74:702, 1990

106. Klein BA: Ischemic infarcts of the choroid: a cause of retinal separation in hypertensive disease with renal insufficiency: a clinical and histopathological study. Am J Ophthalmol 66:1069, 1968

107. Gass JDM, Pautler SE: Toxemia of pregnancy pigment epitheliopathy masquerading as a heredomacular dystrophy. Trans Am Ophthalmol Soc 83:114, 1985

108. Brancato R, Menchini U, Bandello F: Proliferative retinopathy and toxemia of pregnancy. Ann Ophthalmol 19:182, 1987

109. Beeson JH, Duda EE: Computed axial tomography scan demonstration of cerebral edema in eclampsia preceded by blindness. Obstet Gynecol 60:529, 1982

110. Will AD, Lewis KL, Hinshaw DB et al: Cerebral vasoconstriction in toxemia. Neurology 37:1555, 1987

111. Donaldson JO: Eclampsia. p. 269. In: Neurology of Pregnancy. 2nd Ed. WB Saunders, Philadelphia, 1989

112. Beck RW, Gamel JW, Willcourt RJ et al: Acute ischemic optic neuropathy in severe eclampsia. Am J Ophthalmol 90:342, 1980

113. Folk JC, Weingeist TA: Fundus changes in toxemia. Ophthalmology 88:1173, 1981

114. Elman KD, Welch RA, Frank RN et al: Diabetic retinopathy in pregnancy: a review. Obstet Gynecol 75:119, 1990

115. Jovanovic-Peterson L, Peterson CM: Diabetic retinopathy. Clin Obstet Gynecol 34:516, 1991

116. Klein BEK, Klein R: Gravidity and diabetic retinopathy. Am J Epidemiol 119:564, 1984

117. Johnston GP: Pregnancy and diabetic retinopathy. Am J Ophthalmol 90:519, 1980

118. Cousins L, Baxi L, Chez R et al: Screening recommendations for gestational diabetes mellitus. Am J Obstet Gynecol 165:493, 1991

119. Berry JL, Gabbe SG: Diabetes mellitus in pregnancy. p. 399. In Knuppel RA, Drukker JE (eds): High-Risk Pregnancy: A Team Approach. WB Saunders, Philadelphia, 1986

120. Harlass FE, Brady K, Read JA: Reproducibility of the oral glucose tolerance test in pregnancy. Am J Obstet Gynecol 164:564, 1991

121. Boone MI, Farber ME, Jovanovic-Peterson L, Peterson CM: Increased retinal vascular tortuosity in gestational diabetes mellitus. Ophthalmology 96:251, 1989

122. Sunness JS, Gass JDM, Singerman LJ et al: Retinal and choroidal changes in pregnancy. p. 262. In Singerman LJ, Jampol

LM (eds): Retinal and Choroidal Manifestations of Systemic Disease. Williams & Wilkins, Baltimore, 1991

123. Laatikainen L, Larinkarl J, Teramo K, Raivio KO: Occurrence and prognostic significance of retinopathy in diabetic pregnancy. Metab Pediatr Ophthalmol 4:191, 1980

124. Moloney JBM, Drury MI: Effect of pregnancy on the natural course of diabetic retinopathy. Am J Ophthalmol 93:745, 1982

125. Ohrt V: The influence of pregnancy on diabetic retinopathy with special regard to the reversible changes shown in 100 pregnancies. Acta Ophthalmol 62:603, 1984

126. Beetham WP: Diabetic retinopathy in pregnancy. Trans Am Ophthal Soc 48:205, 1950

127. Cassar J, Kohner EM, Hamilton AM et al: Diabetic retinopathy and pregnancy. Diabetologia 15:105, 1978

128. Dibble CM, Kochenour NK, Worley RJ et al: Effect of pregnancy on diabetic retinopathy. Obstet Gynecol 59:699, 1982

129. Horvat M, MacLean H, Goldberg L, Crock GW: Diabetic retinopathy in pregnancy: a 12 year prospective study. Br J Ophthalmol 64:398, 1980

130. Phelps RL, Sakol P, Metzger BE et al: Changes in diabetic retinopathy during pregnancy: correlations with regulation of hyperglycemia. Arch Ophthalmol 104:1806, 1986

131. Sunness JS: Pregnancy and the eye. Ophthalmol Clin North Am 5:623, 1992

132. Sinclair SH, Nesler C, Foxman B et al: Macular edema and pregnancy in insulin-dependent diabetes. Am J Ophthalmol 97:154, 1984

133. Klein BEK, Klein R, Meuer SM et al: Does the severity of diabetic retinopathy predict pregnancy outcome? J Diab Complications 2:179, 1988

134. Sunness JS: The pregnant woman's eye. Surv Ophthalmol 32:219, 1988

135. Ward SC, Woods DR, Gilstrap LC, Hauth JC: Pregnancy and optic disc edema of juvenile-onset diabetes. Obstet Gynecol 64:816, 1984

136. The Diabetic Retinopathy Study Research Group: Preliminary report on effects of photocoagulations therapy. Am J Ophthalmol 81:383, 1976

137. Laros RK: Acquired coagulation disorders. p. 178. In Laros RK (ed): Blood Disorders in Pregnancy. Lea & Febiger, Philadelphia, 1986

138. Cogan DG: Ocular involvement in disseminated intravascular coagulopathy. Arch Ophthalmol 93:1, 1975

139. Cogan DG: Disseminated intravascular coagulopathy and related vasculopathies. p. 497. In Ryan SJ (ed): Retina. Vol. 2. CV Mosby, St. Louis, 1989

140. Wiznitzer A, Mazor M, Leiberman JR et al: Familial occurrence of thrombotic thrombocytopenic purpura in two sisters during pregnancy. Am J Obstet Gynecol 166:20, 1992

141. Hemmeter W: Presumed thrombotic thrombocytopenic purpura associated with bilateral serous retinal detachments. Am J Ophthalmol 105:421, 1988

142. Leff SR, Yarian DL, Masciulli L et al: Vitreous hemorrhage as a complication of HELLP syndrome. Br J Ophthalmol 74:498, 1990

143. Chang M, Herbert WNP: Retinal arterial occlusion following amniotic fluid embolism. Ophthalmology 91:1634, 1984

144. Fischbein FI: Ischemic retinopathy following amniotic fluid embolization. Am J Ophthalmol 67:351, 1969

145. Seddon JH, MacLaughlin DT, Albert DM et al: Uveal melanomas presenting during pregnancy and the investigation of oestrogen receptors in melanomas. Br J Ophthalmol 66:695, 1982

146. Shields CL, Shields JA, Eagle RC et al: Uveal melanoma and pregnancy: a report of 16 cases. Ophthalmology 98:1667, 1991

147. Siegal R, Ainslie WH: Malignant ocular melanoma during pregnancy. JAMA 185:542, 1963

148. Holly EA, Aston DA, Ahn DK et al: Uveal melanoma, hormonal and reproductive factors in women. Cancer Res 51:1370, 1991

149. Cruysberg JR, Deutman AF: Visual disturbances during pregnancy caused by central serous choroidopathy. Br J Ophthalmol 66:240, 1982

150. Chumbley LC, Frank RN: Central serous retinopathy and pregnancy. Am J Ophthalmol 77:158, 1974

151. Fastenberg DM, Ober RR: Central serous choroidopathy in pregnancy. Arch Ophthalmol 101:1055, 1983

152. Gass JDM: Central serous chorioretinopathy and white subretinal exudation during pregnancy. Arch Ophthalmol 109:677, 1991

153. Blodi BA, Johnson MW, Gass JD et al: Purtscher's-like retinopathy after childbirth. Ophthalmology 97:1654, 1990

154. Acheson JF, Gregson RMC, Merry P, Schulenberg WE: Vaso-occlusive retinopathy in the primary anti-phospholipid antibody syndrome. Eye 5:48, 1991

155. Greven CM, Weaver RG, Owen J, Slusher MM: Protein S deficiency and bilateral branch retinal artery occlusion. Ophthalmology 98:33, 1991

156. Stander HJ: Haemorrhagic retinitis in vomiting of pregnancy. Surg Gynecol Obstet 54:129, 1932

157. Hayakasa S, Ugomori S, Kanamori M, Setogawa T: Pericentral retinal degeneration deteriorates during pregnancies. Ophthalmologica 200:72, 1990

158. Spitzberg DH: Retinal phlebitis associated with pregnancy. Ann Ophthalmol 14:101, 1982

159. ONiki S: Prognosis of pregnancy in patients with toxoplasmic retinochoroiditis. Jpn J Ophthalmol 27:166, 1983

160. Pitta C, Bergen R, Littwin S: Spontaneous regression of a choroidal hemangioma following pregnancy. Ann Ophthalmol 11:772, 1979

161. McLeod BK: Choroidal osteoma presenting in pregnancy. Br J Ophthalmol 72:612, 1988

162. Simolke GA, Cox SM, Cunningham FG: Cerebrovascular accidents complicating pregnancy and the puerperium. Obstet Gynecol 78:37, 1991

163. Srinivisan K: Puerperal cerebral venous and arterial thrombosis. Semin Neurol 8:222, 1988

164. American College of Obstetricians and Gynecologists: Management of Pre-eclampsia. ACOG Technical Bulletin No. 91. February 1986

165. Chelsey LC: Epidemiology of preeclampsia-eclampsia. p. 35. In: Hypertensive Disorders in Pregnancy. Appleton-Century-Crofts, E. Norwalk, CT, 1978

166. Sinclair SH, Nesler CL, Schwartz SS: Retinopathy in the pregnant diabetic. Clin Obstet Gynecol 28:536, 1985

167. American Diabetes Association: Eyecare guidelines for patients with diabetes mellitus. Diabetes Care 11:745, 1988

168. American College of Physicians, American Diabetes Association, American Academy of Ophthalmology: Screening guidelines for diabetic retinopathy. Ophthalmology 99:1626, 1992

12 Dermatologic Disease

GEORGE E. WHITE

INTRODUCTION

Identification and Terminology

A patient with a dermatologic (skin) disorder requires a comprehensive history. This should include duration of lesion, onset, other locations, symptoms, family history, associated allergies, and previous treatment. The physical examination should evaluate the extent of the lesions as well as the extent of the condition. This requires the patient to completely disrobe. A careful assessment of the primary lesion is completed, together with review of secondary lesions and distribution of disease. The differential diagnosis is based on physical examination, blood test, skin biopsy, Gram stain, and Wood's light examination.[1]

The primary lesion should be identified. Most skin disorders begin with a primary lesion. Once cutaneous disease has been diagnosed and a differential diagnosis is made, treatment can be initiated. The clinical entities include macule, papule, plaque, nodule, wheal, pustule, vesicle, and bullae.[1-3]

A secondary lesion seen during physical examination is one that has developed during the course of the skin disorder. These include scales, crusts, erosions, ulcers, fissure, atrophy, scar, excoriation, comedone, milia, cyst, burrow, lichenification, telangiectasia, petechiae, and purpura.[1-5] (See the Appendix for examples of primary and secondary lesions.)

Skin Anatomy

The skin is divided into three layers: epidermis, dermis, and subcutaneous layer. The epidermis is the outermost layer, which is very thin. It ranges from 1.5 mm on the palms of the hands and soles of the feet to 0.05 mm on the eyelids. The dermis varies in thickness from 3.0 mm on the back to 0.3 mm on the eyelid. It consists of collagen fibers and vascular structures. The cutaneous layer is the innermost layer, which consists of most of the nerve endings. This provides the sensations of temperature, pain, and touch. The sebaceous glands and hair follicles have their base in the cutaneous layer.

Treatment

The skin's function is to protect. Any disruption that removes water, lipids, or protein from the surface epithelium will compromise function. Restoration of the normal function of the epithelium is accomplished therapeutically with mild detergent soaps, emollients, and lotions. These are most often lubricants, antibiotics, or steroids.[5-7] Regarding the categories of dermatites, the old adage applies—"If it's wet, dry it; if it's dry, wet it."

Dry cutaneous diseases demonstrate lost water and lipids from the epithelium. They require emollient creams and ointments in their remediation. Wet diseases are noted by exudative inflammation. Treatment consists of wet compresses that suppress the inflammation and remove the crust. Once the wet phase of the disease is controlled, emollient creams and ointment may be initiated.[1-3,5-7]

Vehicle

The vehicle, or base, is the substance in which the active ingredient is dispensed. The base determines the rate at which the active ingredient is absorbed through the skin. These include creams, ointments, gels, solutions or lotions, and aerosols.[1,6,7]

A cream mixture of an oily organic base, water, and preservatives. Creams are versatile in treatment and are therefore the most frequently prescribed base.

197

They are usually white and greasy but are acceptable cosmetically. They cause a drying effect with extended use and are recommended with acute exudative inflammation.

An ointment consists of a petroleum base with little or no water. They are usually preservative free. They are usually clear, very greasy, and provide greater lubrication. They are recommended for dryer lesions. They provide greater penetration.[1,7,8]

The gels are mixtures of propylene glycol and water or alcohol. They have a jelly-like consistency and are very sticky. They feel unpleasant and are not prescribed frequently. They are very useful in acute exudative inflammation such as poison ivy.

The solutions or lotions contain water and alcohol as the major ingredients. They appear clear or milky and are most useful on treatment of hair-covered skin because they penetrate the hair easily.

The aerosols are in a base that is suspended under pressure of isobutane or a propane propellant. They are a useful vehicle for treating the hairy areas or moist lesions such as lesions caused by poison ivy.[1,4,6]

They are also useful in patients who lack mobility and cannot reach certain body areas. Emollient creams and lotions restore water and lipids. Creams are thicker than lotions. These greasy lubricants should not be applied to wet lesions, because they promote secondary infection.[1–3]

Topical Corticosteroids

Topical corticosteroids are valuable treatment tools in the management of dermatologic disease. Understanding the preparations and their proper use is easier if they are categorized by potency. Potency is determined by the drug's ability to cause vasoconstriction of the small vessels in the dermis. Topical corticosteroids have been categorized in seven groups—from group 1, the strongest, to group 7, the weakest. The best results are obtained when the correct group is administered for a specified time. Use of more potent steroids or excessive periods can cause atrophy of the tissue or adrenal suppression.[9,10] Ocular side effects include elevation in intraocular pressures and posterior subcapsular cataracts.[1–3,9,10] Patients should be monitored carefully. Many skin diseases can be chronic or recur. Extensive use of steroids can cause significant side effects and must be monitored carefully.

CASE REPORT

A 52-year-old white Irish man presented for eye examination with complaints of irritated eyes. He stated that his eyes had been red and irritated intermittently for months and that the symptoms had recently become almost constant. In addition, the eyes were sore and sensitive to light. He claimed that this had affected his vision slightly; however, he was tearing frequently, which made it difficult for him to keep his eyes open.

He claimed to be in good health. He was currently being treated for essential hypertension with enalapril maleate (Vasotec) and for rheumatoid arthritis with raudawia and naproxen (Naprosyn). He saw his family doctor about every 3 to 4 months for regular follow-up care. He claimed that his hypertension was well controlled.

He claimed to have had a previous excision of two chalazions from his eyelids. He had had three metallic foreign bodies removed from his corneas. No sequelae were noted. He had a history of recurring red eye and many minor eye infections since adolescence. He had been treated by many different eye care practitioners for many years for what was called *chronic conjunctivitis*.

He stated that his maternal grandmother had cataract surgery of both eyes. His father had cataract surgery in his right eye and early macular degeneration in both eyes. The patient had a few relatives who had skin eruptions and ruddy complexions similar to his.

The patient's vision with spectacles was 20/40 OU. Multiple pinholes showed an improvement to 20/25 OU. The pupils were examined and were found to respond normally to light and accommodation. The extraocular muscles were full and smooth in all fields of gaze.

A slight hyperopic astigmatic correction ($+1.00 - 0.75 \times 90 + 1.25 - 0.50 \times 90$) at distance and an add appropriate for his age ($+1.75$) corrected his vision to 20/20 OU at distance and near.

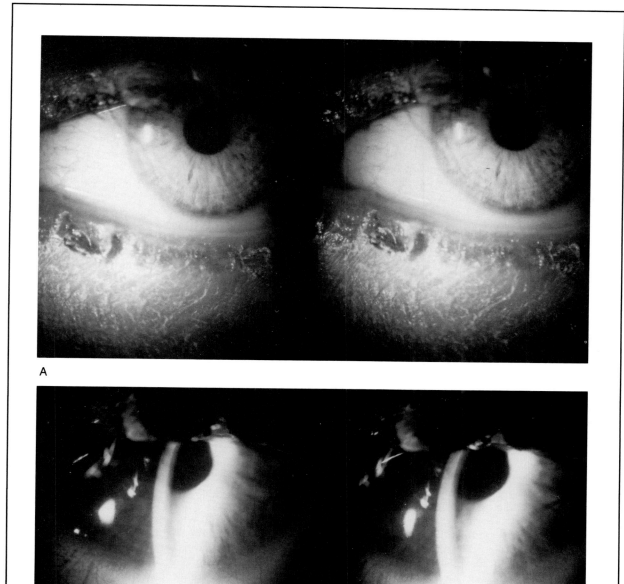

Fig. 12-1. (A&B) Ulcerative staphylococcal blepharitis, secondary blepharoconjunctivitis, and secondary uveitis. (See also Plate 12-1.)

Careful examination of the anterior segment of the eye with the biomicroscope showed the following findings: The eyelids were hyperemic, with many flaky and greasy deposits at the base of the lashes (Fig. 12-1 and Plate 12-1). The pattern of the lashes indicated that some of the lashes were missing. Small ulcers were present in the lashes in both eyes. A small chalazion was noted on the right upper lid. Generalized edema was present in all four lids. The areas of contact between the inflamed lids and the globe showed corneal involvement. The corneas showed inflammation and heavy areas of stippling. The conjunctiva was red; some redness was noted in the episcleral vessels. A seromucous discharge was present in the tear film. The eyes were very watery and constantly tearing. Evaluation of the anterior chamber showed a mild amount of white blood cells.

Applanation tonometry with Goldmann was deferred but was completed with a noncontact air puff tonometer. It measured 15 mmHg OU.

A dilated examination was completed. The media was clear. The cup/disc ratios were measured at 0.2 × 0.2 OU. The retinal vasculature showed some compressions demonstrating long-standing hypertension. The macular reflexes were noted in both eyes. The peripheral retinas were examined, and paving stone degeneration was seen in both eyes.

The diagnosis was acute ulcerative blepharitis, chalazion of the right upper lid, acne rosacea, secondary keratoconjunctivitis, and secondary iritis.

The patients was started on 5 percent homatropine ophthalmic drops in each eye, three times daily. He was given tobradex ointment (an antibiotic steroid combination) to be placed on all four lids, three times per day, and tobradex suspension to be used topically in the eye, three times per day in each eye.

On 2-day follow-up, a significant reduction in symptoms was seen. The lids were still red, and ulcers were still present, but the inflammation was reduced about 50 percent. The corneas still had moderate staining with fluoroscein. The anterior chamber was quiet with no white blood cells noted. The conjunctival injection was still present but was reduced about 50 percent. The patient was instructed to continue all medications. He was also given lids scrubs to be done with baby shampoo morning and night.

On 1-week follow-up, almost no symptoms were present. The conjunctivas were white and quiet. The anterior chamber was quiet. Minimal staining of the corneas was noted. The lids were still inflamed, but the ulcerations were healed. Lids and lashes were very clean, with no deposits, flakes, or greasy deposits noted. The patient was told to discontinue the homatropine and tobradex drops to the eyes. He was to continue the tobradex ointment to the lids. He was also asked to continue the lid scrubs with the baby shampoo. He was asked to use warm compresses to the right eyelid to aid in reduction of the chalazion. At this time, his lids were under reasonable control. He was told about the acne rosacea; the ruddy complexion and inflammation of the skin of the lids, cheek, and nose need to be kept in check to avoid flare-up of inflammation of the blepharitis. He was administered erythromycin tablets, 250 mg orally, three times daily.

On 2-week follow-up, minimal redness in the lid margins was seen. The chalazion in the upper right lid had resorbed almost completely. The conjunctiva and corneas were both clear. The acne rosacea on the face and nose showed a significant reduction in redness and inflammation. The patient was told that a telephone consultation with his primary care doctor was made, and long-term erythromycin therapy was prescribed. All other medications were discontinued. He was told of the recurrent nature of blepharitis, especially in patients with acne rosacea. He was asked to continue the oral medication and lid scrubs with baby shampoo and was scheduled for reevaluation in 3 months.

CHRONIC STAPHYLOCOCCAL BLEPHAROCONJUNCTIVITIS

Etiology

A bacterial infection of the lid and secondarily infecting the closely located conjunctiva is referred to as blepharoconjunctivitis. The infection is caused most commonly by Staphylococcus aureus and Staphylococcus epidermidis. Cultures of eyelids and conjunctiva were compared for microbial growth in staphylococcal blepharoconjunctivitis. The results of the eyelid cultures showed 50 percent growth of S. aureus and 92 percent growth of S. epidermidis.[11–14] The results of the conjunctival cultures showed 23 percent growth of S. aureus and 85 percent growth of S. epidermidis.[12–16] Other microbial growth included Propionibacterium spp.

Clinical Presentation

Blepharoconjunctivitis is one of the most commonly occurring diseases seen in a general eye care practice. The chronic form of blepharitis has symptoms that range from asymptomatic to itching, burning, foreign body sensation, and mild discharge. The symptoms wax and wane over the history of the disease. The eyelids have a characteristic scaly or crusty deposition at the base of the lashes at the lid margins (Fig. 12-2 and Plate 12-2). Scales are hard and brittle and are less greasy than those found in seborrheic blepharitis. In most cases, a characteristic redness or erythema is seen on the lid margin (tylosis). Edema is also found occasionally on the lid margin. Madarosis, or loss of lashes, is frequently seen. Long-term, poorly managed cases often result in loss of many lashes and thickened, leathery-appearing lids. Signs and symptoms of chronic cases are almost always bilateral. Unilateral disease should caution the optometrist to verify patency of the lacrimal drainage system and to investigate the cause of the lid disease to determine whether it is secondary to staphylococcus dacryoadenitis.[17-19]

The crustiness of the lashes occurs with associated collarettes surrounding each cilia. Ten to fifteen percent of these chronic cases are seen to have associated hordeolum and chalazia.[11,12,15,16] The chronically infected lid is in close apposition with the globe, and often the conjunctiva and cornea are secondarily infected. Bulbar, tarsal conjunctival hyperemia and papillary hypertrophy occur. Inferior superficial punctate keratitis, will also be found which is due to the pooling of the tears. The pooling of staphylococcal antigens during sleep can lead to an excess amount of *Staphylococcus* spp. on the lid margin, leading to marginal infiltrative keratitis and subsequent marginal corneal ulceration.[13,14,16,18,20,21] These cause inferior punctate staining on the lower half of the cornea. Staining will be seen directly adjacent to the affected patients' lids and their association with the globe.

Marginal stromal infiltration begins with a hypersensitivity reaction caused by a release of potent exotoxins from the *Staphylococcus* bacterium.[17-19,21] These tend to occur clinically at 2-, 4-, 8-, and 10-o'clock positions on the corneal limbus in close apposition of the lid to the globe. Without proper treatment, this may progress to micropannus and neovascularization of the affected cornea. With progression, a central in-

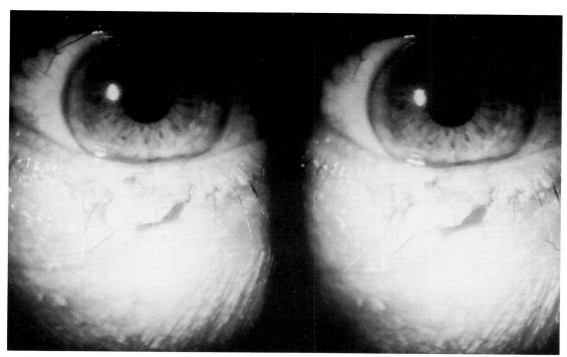

Fig. 12-2. Staphylococcal blepharitis. Heavy deposition and crustiness are seen in the lash margin. Also note the irregular number and consistency of lashes in the bottom lid compared to the top lid. (See also Plate 12-2.)

fected staphylococcal corneal ulcer may develop. This appears as a dense white or yellowish stromal infiltrate with an overlying epithelial defect. On instillation of sodium fluorescein, this epithelial defect will show pooling, followed by a subsequent diffuse seepage into the anterior stroma. The surrounding area will take on a whitish gray haze as stromal edema occurs. Striate keratitis or folds in Descemet's membrane may develop as the edema progresses posteriorly. These cause inferior punctate staining on the lower half of the cornea. Staining will be seen directly adjacent to the affected patients' lids and their physical position against the globe.

Many patients diagnosed with blepharitis also have keratoconjunctivitis sicca. The symptoms are similar, and it is difficult to differentiate the two diseases until the blepharitis is controlled. The blepharitis patients, however, have altered meibomian gland function, which is one of the components of the tear film.[11,13,22-24] This causes the resultant ocular surface disease and unstable tear film. One study indicated that as many as 20 to 25 percent of blepharitis patients have concomitant dry eyes.[11,22-24] Therefore, it is imperative to carefully evaluate patients for dry eye syndrome after signs of blepharitis are well controlled.[11,22-25]

Patients with staphylococcal blepharitis should be instructed not to wear contact lenses until healed or the disease is under excellent control. Lenses will become heavily deposited, and secondary ulceration of the cornea is a strong possibility. Furthermore, contact lenses require healthy levels of tear exchange for proper movement and centration, which may be compromised.

Management

The most important component to curing staphylococcal blepharoconjunctivitis is a clear understanding of the treatment that the patient must accomplish. Warm compresses are used with a facecloth on both the upper and lower lids. This should be done for 5 to 10 minutes, three to four times per day. The facecloth should be kept very warm.[20,21] This treatment will loosen the crusty scaly debris, which clings to the base of the lashes. It also loosens the meibomian secretions that may be hardened or stuck in the meibomian orifices.

The second part of the treatment is lid scrubs.[20,21] The lid margins should be scrubbed with baby shampoo or any of the commercially available lid scrub kits. This can be accomplished with a facecloth or cotton-tipped applicators. Care must be taken not to irritate the globe. This treatment reduces the bacterial count on the lids and removes debris on the lids or lashes. The shampoo or cleansing chemicals need to be rinsed off the lids at the end of the treatment.

The third part of the treatment is use of an antibiotic ointment, which is placed on the lids and carefully rubbed into the surface.[20,21] The antibiotic of first choice is bacitracin.[20] It is bactericidal, and most staphylococcal spp. are sensitive to it. Erythromycin is the second drug of choice and is used if the patient is allergic to bacitracin.[20] The aminoglycosides such as tobramycin or gentamycin should be reserved for more serious or resistant infections. Either of these ointments is rubbed into the surface after the warm compresses and the lid scrubs. This allows for maximum absorption. If significant infection is present or if corneal infection or ulceration is suspected, an aminoglycoside may be chosen.[20] In addition to being more potent, the aminoglycosides are also available in both ointment and solution. They can be applied topically in drop form to the globe as well as topically to the lids in the form of ointment. If hypersensitivity reactions occur, such as infiltrates or exotoxins, topical steroids may be used.[17,23,24] The use of steroids is controversial, however. If steroids are used, therapy should be short-term. Steroid use is associated with many risks. Steroids are designed to suppress the immune system and can further exeracerbate bacterial infection and promote fungal infection.

Patients diagnosed with keratoconjunctivitis sicca should be treated with topical artificial tear therapy.

Occasionally, patients need to be treated with systemic antibiotics. Erythromycin, tetramycin, cephalosporins, or penicillinase-resistant penicillin may be used in these patients.[20-23] Sulfonamides are not recommended, because sensitivity testing has shown significant resistance for many staphylococcal spp.[20-23]

ACUTE ULCERATIVE BLEPHAROCONJUNCTIVITIS
Etiology

Acute ulcerative blepharoconjunctivitis is caused by *S. aureus* or *S. epidermidis*. The clinical picture differs significantly from chronic staphylococcal blepharoconjunctivitis.

Clinical Presentation

The symptoms of acute ulcerative blepharoconjunctivitis are very different from those of chronic blepharitis. The patient experiences a great deal of discomfort, which is due to the ulcerative formations present on the lids. Significant inflammation is present, and the patient is obviously uncomfortable. With the lids heavily inflamed and ulcerated, association of the conjunctiva and cornea is frequent (Fig. 12-3 and Plate 12-3). In the presence of secondary involvement—infection and/or inflammation of the conjunctiva—the patient must be treated accordingly. If the cornea is involved with infection or inflammation, the clinical picture may change drastically. The cornea may be involved with secondary punctate epitheliopathy, usually in the inferior half or third.[18–21,26] More involvement of the cornea may result in sterile infiltrates on the peripheral or marginal limbus of the cornea. As these inflammatory changes advance, micropannus formations and eventual neovascularization of the cornea occur. Ultimately, the cornea may develop an infectious corneal ulcer, which can result in inflammation of the uvea.[18,20,21] Secondary uveitis of the entire anterior segment of the eye may result, causing more significant symptoms.

Management

The treatment for ulcerative blepharitis involving only the eyelids is steroid antibiotic ointment, three to four times daily. Once the inflammation is controlled, the conventional treatment for blepharitis may be initiated. Steroids should be used carefully and discontinued when inflammation has resolved.[6,10,20]

Other treatment may be needed, depending on the associated findings with the ulcerative lids. If the disease is advanced and involves the entire anterior segment, as in uveitis, a powerful cycloplegic agent such as 5 percent homatropine every 6 hours and topical steroids to reduce the inflammatory response should be administered.[10] These should be tapered as soon as the inflammation is controlled. If the cornea is involved with a corneal ulcer, a powerful cycloplegic drop such as 5 percent homatropine should be used every 6 hours with powerful topical antibiotics such as norfloxacin (Chibroxin) every 1 to 2 hours. Very careful monitoring of the cornea and close follow-up are needed in managing corneal ulcers. Ulcers of the cornea should be cultured during treatment. This will aid in making a differential diagnosis. It is especially helpful in those recalcitrant cases that show limited

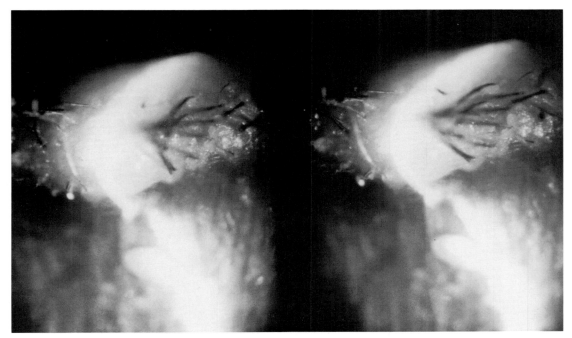

Fig. 12-3. Ulcerative staphylococcal blepharitis. This slide shows 3^{++} inflammation in the lid margin. Tremendous ulceration of the lid margin is seen. (See also Plate 12-3.)

improvement in the first 2 to 3 days. Confirmation of the exact diagnosis will then be available for reevaluation of antibiotic therapy.

SEBORRHEIC BLEPHAROCONJUNCTIVITIS

Etiology

Seborrheic blepharitis is a localized form of classic seborrheic dermatitis. This is a common, chronic inflammatory disease that affects different age groups. A yeast, *Pityrosporum ovale,* is thought to be the causative agent. When seborrheic dermatitis affects infants, it is referred to as *cradle cap.*[1,2] In young children, it is called *tinea amiantacea,* and in adolescents and adults, it is referred to as *classic seborrheic dermatitis.*[27]

Clinical Presentation

Seborrheic blepharitis has been classified into three different categories: pure seborrheic blepharitis, mixed staphylococcal/seborrheic blepharitis, and seborrheic blepharitis with secondary meibomianitis. Seborrheic blepharitis is most commonly seen in patients older than the age of 50.[1,2,16,19,21,27] The symptoms include burning, tearing, and minor discharge. Patients frequently complain of foreign body sensation. These symptoms wax and wane as they do in staphylococcal blepharitis but not nearly as much. The eyelids are much less inflamed, but the debris or crusty deposition on the lid margin is very greasy (Fig. 12-4 and Plate 12-4). This greasy crusty deposition in seborrheic blepharitis is called a *scurf* (Fig. 12-5 and Plate 12-5).[1,2,12,15,16] Seborrheic blepharitis is marked by frequent exacerbations and remission of patient symptoms (discussed previously in the section on staphylococcal blepharitis). Seborrheic blepharitis with secondary meibomianitis results in significant symptoms of burning and foreign body sensation, especially in the morning.[13,23,27] The clinical signs are a foamy tear film and retained material within the meibomian glands. These glands are easily palpated or massaged and opened, and the retained meibum is easily expressed. These glands show a mild inflammation on the palpebral conjunctival surface.

These patients frequently have associated keratoconjunctivitis sicca, which is due to the tear film instability caused by the retention of meibum in the meibomian glands.[11,13,20] The symptoms of sicca may not be noted until the seborrheic blepharitis is well controlled.

Patients with significant seborrheic blepharitis should be cautioned about contact lens wear. This condition is usually chronic and may create heavy deposits on contact lenses as well as secondary infections. Contact

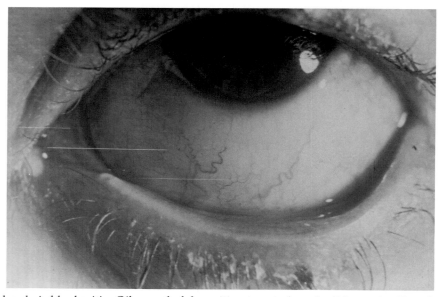

Fig. 12-4. Seborrheic blepharitis. Oily scruf of deposition is noted on the lid margin. (See also Plate 12-4.)

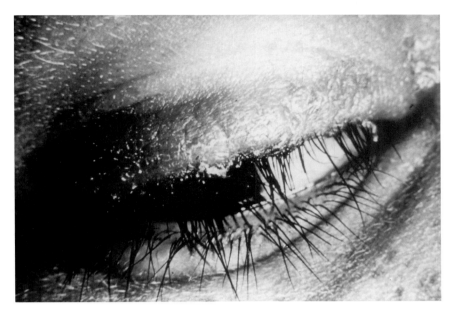

Fig. 12-5. Seborrheic blepharitis. Oily scruf of deposition is noted on lid margin. (See also Plate 12-5.)

lens wear may be considered in patients with mild seborrheic blepharitis that is well controlled and who are compliant and well supervised; caution should be exercised in these patients.

Management

The most significant factor in treating seborrheic blepharitis is understanding that this disease is chronic. There no cure; the goal of treatment therefore is control of this disease. Frequent exacerbations and remissions are very common. This is a dermatitis affecting other areas of the body as well as the eyelids.[11,12,14,20,24]

The patient must be taught lid hygiene. Cleaning the lid margins will reduce the amount of scruf formation and restore normal meibomian excretion. Warm compresses should be used for 5 to 10 minutes in a massaging motion. This accomplishes two tasks. First, it loosens all the debris on the lid margins and forces any retained meibum out of the meibomian glands. Second, it warms the lids, melting any of the meibum that may be hardened and retained within the gland orifices. The lid margins should be cleaned with baby shampoo or commercially available lid preparations, morning and night, and the shampoo should be thoroughly cleansed off the lids. Topical antibiotics are recommended for patients with the mixed form of seborrheic/staphylococcal blepharitis and seborrheic blepharitis with secondary meibomianitis.[21,23,24] These agents have little effect on patients with pure seborrheic blepharitis.

Systemic antibiotics are indicates in patients with secondary meibomianitis.[11,13,23] The recommended therapy is 250 mg of tetracycline, four times per day. In patients with meibomianitis without rosacea, the dosage of tetracycline may be tapered or discontinued after about 3 months of therapy.[11,15,16,23] Patients with rosacea, secondary keratoconjunctivitis sicca, and meibomianitis may require low-dose long-term therapy of about 250 mg/day to control the disease.[11,15,16,23] It is important to note that patients who require systemic tetracycline therapy need to take precautions. Ingestion of this drug is usually recommended on an empty stomach or about 2 hours after meals. This causes significant stomach upset in patients and may not be tolerated. It may be necessary to switch the patient to erythromycin, 250 mg, four times per day, or doxycycline, 100 mg, two times per day.[21–24] Neither tetracycline nor doxycycline should be administered to children, because these antibiotic can affect dental enamel. They are also contraindicated in pregnant and lactating mothers.[21–23,24]

It is imperative to remember that seborrheic blepharitis is part of systemic dermatitis, which is most probably affecting other parts of the skin. The involvement varies among patients. Those patients with significant associated seborrhea should be co-managed with a dermatologist.

CHALAZION

Etiology

Chalazions are characterized by chronic granulomas of the meibomian glands. They may also result in inflammation of these glands.

Clinical Presentation

Characteristic swelling in the adjoining tissue usually is seen. The swelling or edema is caused by retention of secretions and formation of granulation material and inflammatory products. The tumor-like growth may continue to a size of 8 to 10 mm in diameter. If it breaks through the tarsal plate anteriorly (toward the skin side), it is called a *fistula*.[28–31] If it continues to grow and extends through the lid from the conjunctiva to the skin surface, it is referred to as an *abscess*.[28–31] In addition to the meibomian glands, the Zeis or Moll's glands can be the site of a chalazion. The most common location is a marginal chalazion of the meibomian gland at the lid margin. These tend to be small and resolve quickly and easily, because they are very superficial and close to the surface. Therefore, they open very quickly. The amount of discomfort associated with the chalazion depends directly on their location. For example, the deeper they are in the lid tissue, the more nerve roots are disturbed and therefore the more symptoms are felt by the patient. Chalazions are more commonly found in patients with chronic blepharitis, certain dermatites such as acne rosacea, and seborrhea.[11,23,24,27,28]

Management

In cases of small chalazions of the lid margins with little to no symptoms, no specific treatment may be needed. In most cases, however, the patient is started on warm compresses for 15 minutes, three times per day, to the affected lids and topical antibiotic ointments. If inflammation is noted in the area of the chalazion, either on the skin side or the conjunctival surface, topical corticosteroids may be used. Systemic or oral antibiotics are not usually helpful.

If the patient has a chalazion that is soft and palpable to the touch, indicating that it is fairly recent in origin and not calcified, local injection with a corticosteroid may be beneficial.[28,30,32–35] A small volume of about 0.2 to 2.0 ml of triamcinolone acetate (Kenalog), 5 mg/ml, is usually used.[28,30,32–35] A 23-gauge needle or larger is required because of the molecular size of triamcinolone.[28,30,32–35] One or more intralesional injections are made. The patient is seen in 1 week. Repeat injections may be necessary. This treatment is particularly helpful if the patient has multiple lesions or if they are located near the lacrimal drainage system.

If surgical excision is the treatment chosen, excision on the conjunctival surface is preferred. Local infiltration anesthesia is used near the base of the chalazion.[28–30,34,35] If the lesion is large, the block is applied to both sides of the lesion. A chalazion clamp is applied, and a vertical incision is made in the lesion. Curettage and excision of the granuloma and sac are accomplished. Careful inspection of the remaining tissue and removal of any remaining granuloma are completed.[28,29,31] Care should be exercised not to remove any normal tissue, if possible. Electrocautery can be used to prevent bleeding. An antibiotic ointment is placed at the site. The clamp is removed, and a pressure bandage is applied. Antibiotic ointments can be given topically for 3 to 4 days but are usually not necessary.

If an external excision is needed, a horizontal incision is made about 3 mm from the lid margin.[28,29] These are usually made in the normal folds of the lid skin. After removal of the granuloma and the sac, the wound is closed with 6–0 silk or similar suture material.

Cautions

Care must be taken when treating chalazions near the lid margins to prevent notching of the lid.[28,29] This is unsightly and may cause exposure keratitis. Intralesional steroid injections may cause hypopigmentation in dark-complexioned patients.[28,32–35] To minimize this complication, the injection should be made through the conjunctival surface; insoluble aqueous steroid preparations are preferred to the crystalline suspensions.[28,32–35]

DEMODEX

Etiology

Demodex is caused by an infestation of the eyelid by two different mites. *Demodex folliculorum* is found in the eyelash follicles and hair, *D. brevis* infests the meibomian and sebaceous glands.[36–40] They usually affect adults and affect the eyelids, eyebrow, and nasal regions of the body.

Clinical Presentation

D. folliculorum infest the hair follicles of the eyelid. The mite pierces and destroys epithelial cells and deposits a characteristic cuffing on the surface of the lid[36,39–41] (Figs. 12-6 and 12-7 and Plates 12-6 and 12-7).

D. brevis destroys the glands of the eyelid, both meibomian and sebaceous.[36–40] This subsequently causes instability of the lipid layer of the tear film.

Patients experience symptoms of itching and burning and often notice a crusty deposition on the lid margin. The appearance of this disease is very similar to staphylococcal blepharitis and is frequently misdiagnosed

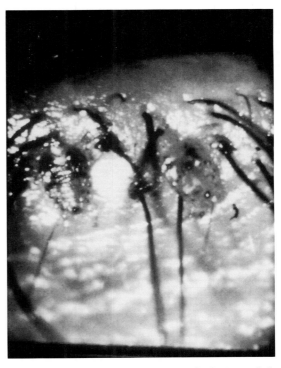

Fig. 12-7. *Demodex folliculorum.* Magnified view of the deposits in the lid. (See also Plate 12-7.)

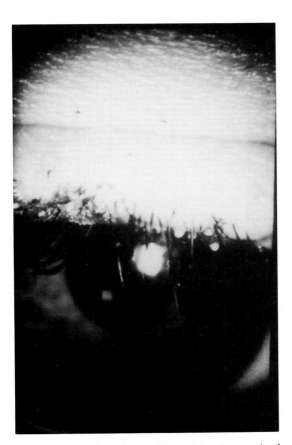

Fig. 12-6. *Demodex folliculorum.* Deposition is seen in the lid margin. (See also Plate 12-6.)

initially. Careful examination of the lid with the light microscope will show the exoskeletons of these parasites.

Any patient who contracts a *Demodex* infestation should discontinue lens wear until complete eradication is confirmed by the eye care practitioner.

Management

Determining the extent of the infestation is imperative. The experienced viewer will note the mites within the orifices of the glands on slit lamp examination. Most diagnoses are made with the light microscope and by epilating a cilia.

The treatment of choice is to topically anesthetize the lids and carefully clean the infested lid with saline. A cotton-tipped applicator is used to cleanse between each eyelash, and the cuffing or deposition must be completely cleaned.[37,39–41] For many years, ether was recommended for cleansing of the lids.[37,40,41] Ether is dangerous and highly toxic to the cornea. Antibiotic ointment is placed on the lid margins at bedtime for a few weeks. The recommended antibiotics include sulfacetamide or neosporin/bacteracin/polymixin B.[36-41] This reduces bacterial overgrowth and slows down the migration of the mites. It must be stressed that all members of the household should be examined. This is a difficult infestation to control because of recalcitrant cases and recontamination.

ACNE ROSACEA

Etiology

The cause of acne rosacea is unknown.[42-45] It affects patients after the age of 30 and seems to be seen mostly in people of Celtic origin.[42-45] The erythema is exacerbated by sunlight, extreme cold, and alcohol, and it was once thought to be caused by coffee.[42,44,46] It is the heat of the coffee and not the caffeine that causes the erythema. Therefore, hot drinks of any kind should be avoided.

Clinical Presentation

Patients with this skin disorder usually have ocular manifestations. Symptoms include burning, conjunctival hyperemia, grittiness or conjunctivitis with soreness, telangiectasia of the lid, staphylococcal blepharitis, hordeolum, chalazion, superficial corneal punctate staining, and corneal vascularization.[42-45, 47,48] Abnormal tear production is common.

The characteristic clinical signs include erythema of the lid tissues, edema, telangiectasic vessels, papules, and pustules (Figs. 12-8 and 12-9 and Plates 12-8 and 12-9). These affect the cheeks, nose, and eyelids. Most of these patients have very oily skin. This disease is chronic and usually worsens in appearance with age. The deep inflammation seen on the nose results in hypertrophy of the tissue and extreme disfigurement, called rhinophyma.[42,45,49,50]

Patients with acne rosacea are not good candidates for contact lens wear and are not recommended for contact lens wear.[42,43,45,49] Occasionally, a patient may present already wearing lenses. This presents a more difficult management decision. Extreme caution should be exercised when monitoring these patients with contact lenses, because a low-grade inflammation usually is present in the lids. Contact lens intolerance is usually experienced by the patient.

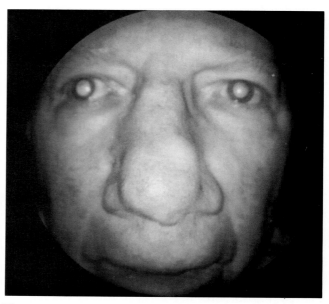

Fig. 12-8. Acne rosacea. Telangiectacic vessels are seen in the cheek and the rhinophyma (distorted nose). (See also Plate 12-8.)

Management

The skin and the eyes must be treated with oral antibiotics and isotretinoin (Accutane).[43,45,49,51-55] The antibiotic of choice is tetracycline or erythromycin. The recommended dosage is 250 mg orally, four times per day. Recalcitrant or resistant cases may be treated with 200 mg of metronidazole, twice daily.[51,53,54,56] The medication is continued until the pustule formation and inflammation have cleared. Patients have a variable response to treatment. Pustule formation and inflammation may clear in 2 to 4 weeks or flare up and require long-term management with a minimal dosage. Isotretinoin, 0.5 percent mg/kg/day for 20 weeks, has been found to be very effective.[51,54,54,56] Recent studies have shown that combination treatment of severe refractory rosacea resulted in no relapses in 85 percent of cases by the end of the first year of treatment.[51,53,54,56]

Topical treatment with metronidazole is not as effective but may be used for initial treatment in mild cases or for maintenance dosage after cessation of systemic antibiotics.[43,51,54-56] Patients with rhinophyma may benefit from localized electrocautery treatment to reduce unsightly telangiectasic vessels.[46,49-51,54-56]

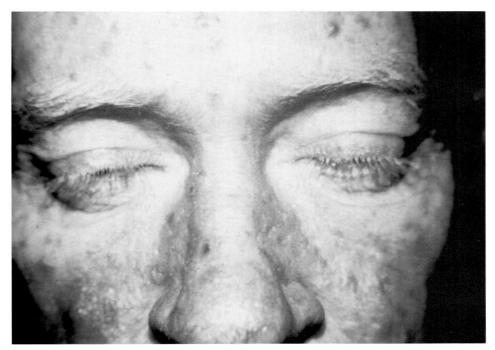

Fig. 12-9. Acne rosacea. Typical rosacea appearance on the facial areas as well as on the lids. Note the papules and pustules in this typical case of acne rosacea. (See also Plate 12-9.)

ACNE

Etiology

Acne is a disease of the pilosebaceous glands.[57,58] It is most commonly seen in puberty-aged children and adolescents. The duration and the intensity of its reaction varies tremendously with the individual patient. Acne begins when sebum production increases.[57,58] A bacteria, *Propionibacterium acnes*, proliferates in the sebum. Follicular epithelial linings become altered and form plugs called *comedones*.[2,57,58]

Clinical Presentation

Sebaceous glands are located in many places on the body. They are concentrated on the facial region. The glands produce an oily material called *sebum*. Blockage of the canal is referred to as a *comedone*. The opening to this comedone may be very thin in a closed comedone or white head or papule.[2,57,58] An open comedone, or blackhead, occurs if the opening of the gland is dilated or open. The closed comedone is the precursor to inflammatory acne papules, pustules, or cysts.[2,57,58] The normal flora include the bacteria *P. acnes*.[2,57,58] This organism becomes trapped inside the comedone and helps to cause the inflammation. It is very sensitive to several antibiotics such as tetracycline.[27,57,59,60]

Management

Most cases are managed by a combination of vitamin A acid, benzoyl peroxide, and antibiotics.

Vitamin A acid, or tretinoin (Retin-A), is the drug of choice in noninflamed acne.[27,52,59,61] The tretinoin solution is topically applied to the skin and causes drying of oily skin. Tretinoin cream is used for lubricating and is therefore used for dry skin.[27,52,59,62] Tretinoin causes fragmentation of the microplug and expulsion of comedone. During the active treatment, the stratum corneum is thinned making the patient more susceptible to sunburn.[27,59,61] Astringents and strong acne soaps should be avoided.[27,59,61] This treatment should be continued and monitored over 6 to 12 weeks.

Benzoyl peroxide is antibacterial and is therefore very helpful in treating inflammatory acne.[52,59,62] This preparation is available in a water-based gel, an alcohol-based gel, and an acetone-based gel. Water-based gels are less irritating and are therefore more easily tolerated. The alcohol-based gels, however, are usually more effective.[63,64] The treatment produces drying and desquamation to scaliness, peeling, and cracking of the affected skin.[27,52,57,59,61] It reduces the size of the sebaceous gland. Caution should be exercised, because this is a bleaching agent and can ruin clothing. It has been found to be easily tolerated by patients, and very few allergic reactions have been reported.

Oral antibiotics have been used safely and have been found to be effective in many cases.[27,63,64] The desired effect is to reduce the amount of the bacteria, *P. acnes*. Antibiotics are prescribed in divided doses. The most common prescribed is tetracycline. Precautions in prescribing have been previously discussed. Other antibiotics used include erythromycin, minocycline, clindamycin, ampicillin, cephalosporins, and trimethoprim.[27,63,64]

Isotretinoin (10-, 20-, and 40-mg capsules) is an oral retinoid related to vitamin A.[54,56,58] It has been found to be very effective in the treatment of acne and is given for patients resistant to conventional treatments. Isotretinoin is given in individual doses of 1 mg/kg/day for a 20-week course.[56] The result of this treatment is a significant reduction in sebaceous gland size. Significant side effects are noted with this drug. For example, it causes significant birth defects and should not be given to pregnant women.[56,63,64] It also causes significant elevations in serum triglyceride levels, and raises the sedimentation rate.

Acne is not a contraindication for wearing contact lenses. Some of the treatments used in management of the disease, however, can cause problems in contact lens management. The drying agents, such as benzyol peroxide, can create some difficulty on the lids if they prevent normal function of secretion of the sebaceous glands.[56,61,63,64] The skin of the eyelid can become cracked and dried and make lens insertion and removal difficult and uncomfortable. Treatment of acne with isotretoin causes almost complete reduction in all oil gland production during the 20-week treatments.[56,63,64] This reduces the normal amount of lubrication needed for contact lens movement and positioning. Therefore, during treatment with isotretinoin, contact lens wear should be discontinued. Contact lens wear should not resume until tear film is evaluated by the optometrist.

REFERENCES

1. Ebling FJ: The normal skin. In Rock A (ed): Textbook of Dermatology. 4th Ed. Blackwell Scientific Publications, Oxford, England, 1986.
2. Habif TP: Clinical Dermatology. 2nd Ed. CV Mosby, St. Louis, 1990.
3. Holbrook D, Wolff K: p. 64. Structure and development of the skin. In Fitzpatrick TB (ed): Dermatology in General Medicine. McGraw-Hill, New York, 1987
4. Fisher AA, Pascher F, Kanof N: Allergic contact dermatitis due to ingredients of vehicles. Arch Dermatol 104:286, 1971
5. Soll DB, Winslow R: Surgery of the eyelids. Clin Ophthalmol 5:6, 1982.
6. McKenzie AW: Percutaneous absorption of steroids. Arch Dermatol 86:911, 1972
7. Trevor-Roper PD: Diseases of the eyelids. Int Ophthalmol Clin 14:362, 1974
8. Stoughton RB: Are topical glucocorticoids equivalent to the brand name? J Am Acad Dermatol 18:138, 1988.
9. Brubaker RF, Halpin JA: Open angle glaucoma associated with topical administration of flurandrenolide to the eye. Mayo Clin Proc 50:320, 1975
10. Burry J: Topical drug addiction: adverse effects of fluorinated corticosteroid creams and ointment. Med J Aust 1:393, 1973.
11. Bowman RW, Dougherty JM, McCulley JP: Chronic blepharitis, and dry eyes. Int Ophthalmol Clin 27:27, 1987
12. Dougherty JM, McCulley JP: Comparative bacteriology of chronic blepharitis. Br J Ophthalmol 68:524, 1984
13. McCulley JP, Scallis GF: Meibomian keratoconjunctivitis. Am J Ophthalmol 84:788, 1988
14. McCulley JP: Blepharoconjunctivitis. Int Ophthalmol Clin 24:65, 1984
15. Dougherty JM, McCulley JP: Analysis of free fatty acid component of meibomian secretions in chronic blepharitis. Invest Ophthalmol Vis Sci 27:52, 1986
16. Dougherty JM, McCulley JP: Bacterial lipases and chronic blepharitis. Invest Ophthalmol Vis Sci 27:486, 1986
17. Thygeson P: Bacterial factors in chronic catarrhal conjunctivitis: role of toxin-forming staphylococci. Arch Ophthalmol 18:373, 1937
18. Thygeson P: Complications of Staphylococcus blepharitis. Am J Ophthalmol 68:446, 1969
19. Valenton M, Okumoto M: Toxin producing strains of Staphylococcus epidermidis. Arch Ophthalmol 89:186, 1973
20. Leibowitz HM, Capino D: Treatment of chronic blepharitis. Arch Ophthalmol 106:720, 1988
21. Smolin G, Okumoto M: Staphylococcal blepharitis. Arch Ophthalmol 95:812, 1977
22. McCulley JP, Dougherty JM: Bacterial aspects of chronic blepharitis. Trans Ophthalmol Soc UK 105:314, 1986
23. McCulley JP, Sciallis GF: Meibomian keratoconjunctivitis. Am J Ophthalmol 84:778, 1977
24. McCulley JP, Dougherty JM, Deneau DG: Classification of chronic blepharitis. Ophthalmology 189:1173, 1983
25. Leyden JJ, Thew M, Kligman AM: Steroid rosacea. Arch Dermatol 110:619, 1974
26. Leyden JJ, Kligman AM: The case for topical antibiotics. Prog Dermatol 10:3, 1976
27. Burton JL, Shuster S: The relation between seborrhea and acne vulgaris. Br J Dermatol 85:197, 1971
28. Epstein GA, Allen MP: Combined excision and drainage with intralesional corticosteroid injection in the treatment of chronic chalazia. Arch Ophthalmol 106:514, 1988
29. Gershen HJ: Chalazion excision. Ophthalmic Surg 5:75, 1975
30. King RA, Ellis PP: Treatment of chalazia with corticosteroid injections. Ophthalmic Surg 17:351, 1986
31. Perry HD, Seriuk RA: Conservative treatment of chalazia. Ophthalmology 87:218, 1980

32. Pizzarello LD: Intralesional corticosteroid therapy of chalazia. Am J Ophthalmol 85:818, 1978
33. Dua HS, Nilawar DV: Nonsurgical therapy of chalazion. Am J Ophthalmol 94:424, 1982
34. Sloas HA, Jr: Treatment of chalazia with injectable triamcinolone. Ann Ophthalmol 15:78, 1983
35. Vidaurri LJ, Jacob P: Intralesional corticosteroid treatment of chalazia. Ann Ophthalmol 18:339, 1986
36. English FP, Iwamoto T, Darrell RW: The vector potential of Demodex folliculorum. Arch Ophthamol 84:83, 1970
37. English FP, Nutting WB: Demodicosis of ophthalmic concern. Am J Ophthalmol 91:362, 1981
38. English FP, Cohn D, Groeneveld ER: Demodectic mites and chalazion. Am J Ophthalmol 100:482, 1985
39. Coston TO: Demodex folliculorum blepharitis. Trans Am Ophthalmol Soc 65:361, 1967
40. Roth AM: Demodex folliculorum in hair follicles of the eyelid skin. Ann Ophthalmol 11:37, 1979
41. Heacock CE: Clinical manifestation of demodicosis. J Am Optom Assoc 57:914, 1986
42. Browning DJ, Proia AD: Ocular rosacea. Surv Ophthalmol 31:145, 1986
43. Brown SI, Shahinian L: Diagnosis and treatment of ocular rosacea. Am Acad Ophthalmol Otolaryngol 85:779, 1978
44. Dupont C: The role of sunshine in rosacea. J Am Acad Dermatol 15:713, 1986
45. Jenkins MS, Brown SI, Lempert SL, Weinberg RJ: Ocular rosacea. Am J Ophthalmol 88:618, 1979
46. Wilkin JK: Oral thermal-induced flushing in erythematotelaniectatic rosacea. J Invest Dermatol 76:15, 1981
47. McCulley JP: Blepharitis associated with acne rosacea and seborrheic blepharitis. Trans Ophthalmol 17:53, 1985
48. Sneddon IB: The treatment of steroid-induced rosacea and perioral dermatitis. Dermatologica, suppl. 1, 152:231, 1976
49. Dolezal R, Schultz RC: Early treatment of rhinophyma: a neglected entity? Ann Plast Surg 11:393, 1983
50. Verde SF: How we treat rhinophyma. J Dermatol Surg Oncol 6:560, 1980
51. Bleicher PA, Charles JH, Sober AJ: topical metronidazole therapy for rosacea. Arch Dermatol 123:609, 1987
52. Gomez EC, Kaminester L, Frost P: Topical halcinonide cream and betamethasone valerate: effects on plasma cortisol. Arch Dermatol 113:1196, 1977
53. Hoting E, Paul E, Plewig G: Treatment of rosacea with isotretinoin. Int J Dermatol 25:660, 1986
54. Nielson PG: Metronidazole treatment in rosacea. Int J Dermatol 27:1, 1988
55. Polack FM, Goodman DF: Experience with a new detergent lid scrub in the management of chronic blepharitis. Arch Ophthalmol 106:719, 1988
56. Turjanmaa K, Reunala T: Isotretinoin treatment of rosacea. Acta Derm Venereol (Stockh) 67:89, 1987
57. Katz HI, Hien NT, Prawer SE: Superpotent topical treatment of psoriasis vulgaris: clinical efficacy and adrenal function. J Am Acad Dermatol 16;804, 1987
58. Kligman AM: An overview of acne. J Invest Dermatol 62:268, 1974
59. Frankel RK, Strauss JS, Yim Yip S: Effect of tetracycline on the composition of sebum in acne vulgaris. N Engl J Med 273:850, 1965
60. Resh W, Stoughton RB: Topically applied antibiotics in acne vulgaris. Arch Dermatol 112:182, 1976
61. Fisher AA: Problems associated with "generic" topical medications. Cutis 41:313, 1988
62. May P, Stein EJ, Ryter RJ, Levy P: Cushing's syndrome from percutaneous absorption of triamcinolone cream. Arch Intern Med 136:612, 1976
63. Rasmussen JE: The case against topical antibiotics. Prog Dermatol 11:21, 1977
64. Rasmussen JE: Percutaneous absorption of topically applied triamcinolone acetonide in children. Arch Dermatol 114:1165, 1978

SUGGESTED READINGS

Allansmith MR, Ross RN: Phlyctenular keratoconjunctivitis. Clin Ophthalmol 4:1, 1986
Stoughton RB: Bioassay systems for formulation of topically applied glucocorticoids. Arch Dermatol 106:825, 1972
Zaidman GW, Brown SI: Orally administered tetracycline for phylctenular keratoconjunctivitis. Am J Ophthalmol 92:173, 1981

Appendix 12-1
Examples of Primary and Secondary Skin Lesions

Primary Lesions

Macule: A circumscribed, flat discoloration. It can appear brown, red, or blue or may be hypopigmented.[1-3]
Examples: brown—café-au-lait sports, freckle; blue—ink (tattoo), mongolian spot; red—drug eruptions, juvenile rheumatoid arthritis (Still's disease), secondary syphilis; hypopigmented—piebaldism, postinflammatory psoriasis, tuberous sclerosis, vertiligo.

Papule: Elevated solid lesions up to 0.5 cm in diameter. The color can vary. They can become confluent to form plaques.[1-3]
Examples: Flesh colored—basal cell epithelioma, closed comedone (acne), milia, molluscum contagiosum; red—acne, atopic dermatitis, insect bites, urticaria; brown—keratitis follicularis, melanoma, warts; blue—blue nevus, lymphoma, Kaposi sarcoma, melanoma.

Plaque: A circumscribed, elevated, superficial solid lesion more than 0.5 cm in diameter, often formed by the confluence of papules.[1-3]
Examples: Eczema, discoid lupus erythematosis, seborrheic dermatitis, psoriasis.

Nodule: A circumscribed, elevated, solid lesion more than 0.5 cm in diameter. A large nodule is referred to as a tumor.[1-3]
Examples: Basal cell carcinoma, furuncle, hemangioma, Kaposi sarcoma, lymphoma, melanoma, neurofibromatosis, squamous cell carcinoma.

Wheal: A firm edematous plaque resulting from infiltration of the dermis. These are transient and last only a short time.[1-3]
Examples: Angioedema, hives, urticaria, insect bites.

Pustule: A circumscribed collection of leukocytes and free fluid that varies in size.[1-3]
Examples: Acne, candidiasis, herpes simplex, herpes zoster, impetigo, psoriasis, rosacea, varicella.

Vesicle: A circumscribed collection of free fluid up to 0.5 cm in diameter.[1-3]
Examples: Pemphigus vulgaris, bullous pemphigoid, diabetes.

Bulla: A circumscribed collection of free fluid more than 0.5 cm in diameter.[1-3]
Examples: Pemphigus vulgaris, bullous pemphigoid, diabetes.

Secondary Lesions

Scales: Excess dead epidermal cells that are produced by abnormal keratinization and shedding.[1-3]
Examples: Erythema craquele, pityriasis rosacea, secondary syphilis, tinea versicolor, xerosis.

Crusts: Collection of dried sebum and cellular debris, scab.[1-3]
Examples: Acute eczematous inflammation, impetigo, tinea capitus.

Erosions: A focal loss of epidermis, erosions do not penetrate below the dermoepidermal junction and therefore heal without scarring.[1-3]
Examples: Candidiasis, ezcematous diseases, senile skin.

Ulcers: A focal loss of epidermis and dermis.[1-3]
Examples: Chancre, decubitus, ischemia, neoplasms, pyoderma gangrenosum, stasis ulcers.

Fissure: A linear loss of epidermis and dermis, sharply defined.[1-3]

Examples: Chapped hands, eczema of fingertips.

Atrophy: A depression in the skin resulting from thinning of the epidermis or dermia.
Examples: Aging, discoid lupus erythematosus, topical or intralesional steroids.

Scar: An abnormal formation of connective tissue implying dermal damage. After damage, they become thickened and pink but flatten and blanch with time.[1-3]
Examples: Acne, burns, herpes zoster, varicella.

Color Plates

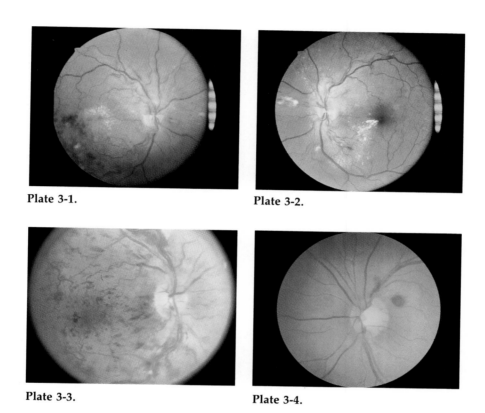

Plate 3-1.

Plate 3-2.

Plate 3-3.

Plate 3-4.

Plate 3-1. Moderate hypertensive retinopathy in the right eye, with scattered intraretinal hemorrhages and macular star formation. The optic disc appears edematous. (Photograph courtesy of Drs. Leonard V. Messner and Stephanie S. Messner.)

Plate 3-2. Moderate hypertensive retinopathy in the left eye, with scattered intraretinal hemorrhages, cotton-wool spots, and optic disc edema. A partial macular star is present. (Photograph courtesy of Drs. Leonard V. Messner and Stephanie S. Messner.)

Plate 3-3. Nonischemic central retinal vein occlusion in the right eye. Intraretinal hemorrhage, retinal edema, and retinal vein engorgement are evident. (Photograph courtesy of Dr. Leonard V. Messner.)

Plate 3-4. White-centered hemorrhage in the left eye, temporal to the optic nerve disc. Additional nerve fiber hemorrhage is located directly superior to the optic disc. The patient has a history of transient vision loss and a mitral valve prolapse.

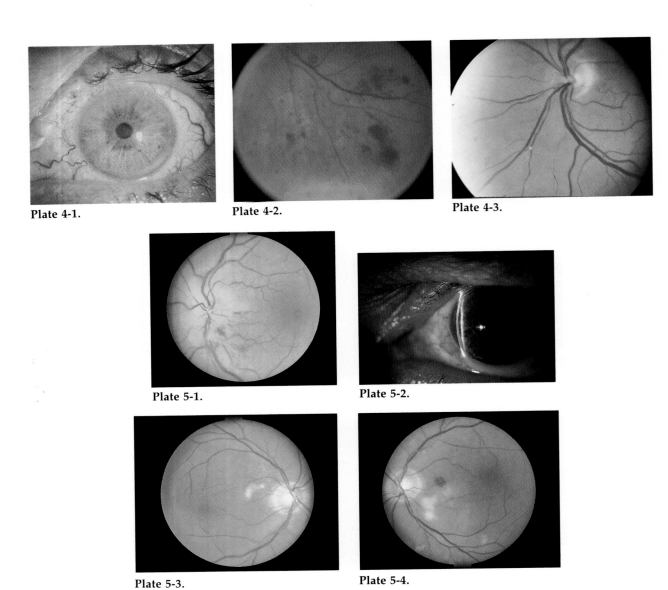

Plate 4-1.

Plate 4-2.

Plate 4-3.

Plate 5-1.

Plate 5-2.

Plate 5-3.

Plate 5-4.

Plate 4-1. Dilated, tortuous epibulbar vessels characterize ischemia to the anterior segment.

Plate 4-2. Venous stasis retinopathy. Note the mid-peripheral blot and dot hemorrhages as well as the dilated veins.

Plate 4-3. Hollenhorst plaque lodged in the branch of a retinal arteriole. These bright, glistening particles represent cholesterol emboli from carotid atheromas.

Plate 5-1. Anterior ischemic optic neuropathy in the left eye of a patient with systemic lupus erythematosus.

Plate 5-2. Peripheral corneal furrowing in the same patient in Fig. 5-2. Note the thinning of the biomicroscope beam inside the limbal area, which was present in a 360-degree area. No progression to corneal ulceration has occurred during the 8 years of the follow-up care.

Plate 5-3. Large microinfarct in the superior papillomacular bundle of the right eye in a patient with systemic lupus erythematosus. There was no drop in vision associated with the presence of the microinfarct. No evidence of diffuse vaso-occlusive retinopathy was appreciated.

Plate 5-4. Multiple microinfarcts were seen in the left eye of the same patient in Plate 5-3. Note the blossom hemorrhage off the 2:30 o'clock area of the disc. The retinopathy in both eyes cleared within 3 weeks after the patient was treated with oral steroids.

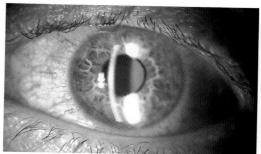

Plate 5-5.

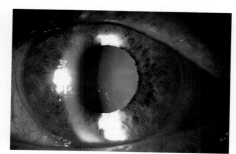

Plate 5-6.

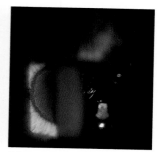

Plate 5-7.

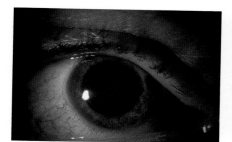

Plate 5-8A.

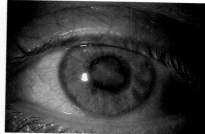

Plate 5-8B.

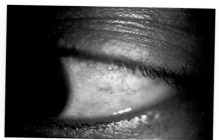

Plate 5-9.

Plate 5-5. Ankylosing spondylitis patient with active iridocyclitis in the left eye. Recurrences involved both eyes with a predilection for the left eye. Patient was successfully treated with topical medications without developing cataracts, glaucoma, or macular edema. Posterior synechia did develop.

Plate 5-6. Same patient as in Fig. 5-9, with evidence of broken posterior synechia following treatment with topical steroids and cycloplegics.

Plate 5-7. Fixed posterior synechia in a patient with ankylosing spondylitis after recurrent episodes of iridocyclitis. Note the posterior synechia with fibrosis at the pupil border, which extended from 7:00 to 1:00 o'clock. No medical regimen was successful in breaking the synechia.

Plate 5-8. Patient with Reiter syndrome. **(A)** Recurrent uveitis in the right eye. Patient has steroid-responding glaucoma, which complicated the treatment and management of the inflammation. This eye went on to develop macular edema, poorly controlled glaucoma, and vision loss. **(B)** Left eye. Fixed posterior synechia between 1:00 and 3:30 o'clock distorted the pupil but the decreased vision of "count fingers" was caused by cataract formation and glaucoma. These findings were evident at initial presentation years after the initial diagnosis.

Plate 5-9. Episcleritis of the left eye in a patient with Crohn's disease. Note the sectoral injection in a triangular shape pointing toward the limbus. The recurrent episodes occurred prior to the onset of colitis four times over a 2-year period. Topical steroids were necessary to control the episcleritis and the colitis responded very well to systemic steroid therapy.

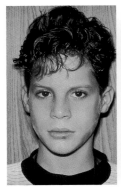

Plate 7-1.

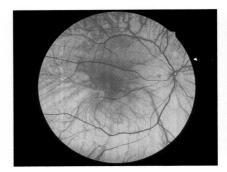

Plate 7-2.

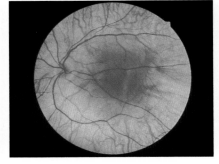

Plate 7-3A.

Plate 7-3B.

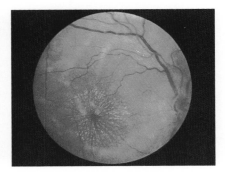

Plate 8-1.

Plate 7-1. Healthy 11-year-old boy with dark hair but somewhat lighter cutaneous pigmentation than his mother.

Plate 7-2. Pigmented irides with transillumination defects and severe photophobia.

Plate 7-3. Albinotic fundus with prominent choroidal vessels. **(A)** Right eye, **(B)** left eye.

Plate 8-1. Circinate background diabetic maculopathy.

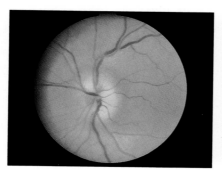

Plate 9-1.

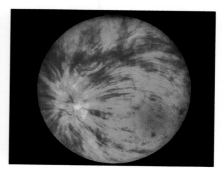

Plate 9-2.

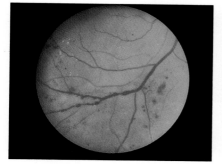

Plate 9-3A.

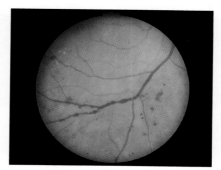

Plate 9-3B.

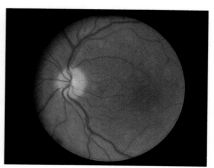

Plate 9-4.

Plate 9-1. Unilateral diabetic papillopathy in 34-year-old type I diabetic patient. The patient had 20/30 best corrected vision without associated APD. Mild red desaturation without visual field defect resolved over a 3-month period. Note the indistinct nerve head margins and lack of microinfarction or significant hemorrhages. No diabetic retinopathy was associated with neuropathy.

Plate 9-2. CRVO in the left eye in a 53-year-old diabetic patient. Note the significant hemorrhage and lack of microinfarcts. Mild nonproliferative diabetic retinopathy was detected in the right eye. The occlusion resolved well with poor vision recovery that was due to the persistent edema.

Plate 9-3. Severe nonproliferative diabetic retinopathy in a type II diabetic patient. **(A)** Severe venous beading present in three quadrants, which is more easily seen with **(B)** a red-free filter. The patient progressed to neovascularization of the disc within 6 months.

Plate 9-4. Ischemic maculopathy in a 32-year-old patient with type I diabetes. Note the lack of hemorrhage or microinfarction in the macular area despite a visual acuity of 20/100. The patient had early proliferative diabetic retinopathy in both eyes. Evaluation of the macula with a Goldmann contact lens revealed no evidence of retinal thickening.

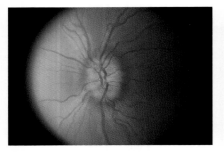

Plate 11-1.

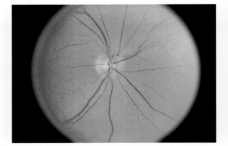

Plate 11-2.

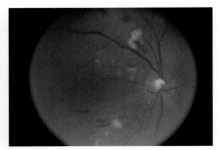

Plate 11-3.

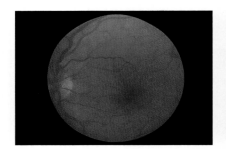

Plate 11-4.

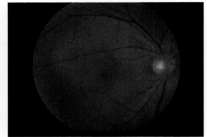

Plate 11-5.

Plate 11-1. Fundus photograph of disc edema in a patient diagnosed with benign intracranial hypertension.

Plate 11-2. Fundus photograph of generalized arteriolar attenuation. (Courtesy of Jane Stein, Philadelphia.)

Plate 11-3. Shallow inferior non-rhegmatogenous retinal detachment secondary to choroidal nonperfusion.

Plate 11-4. Neovascularization of the optic disc with diabetic macular edema.

Plate 11-5. Fundus photograph of central serous chorioretinopathy.

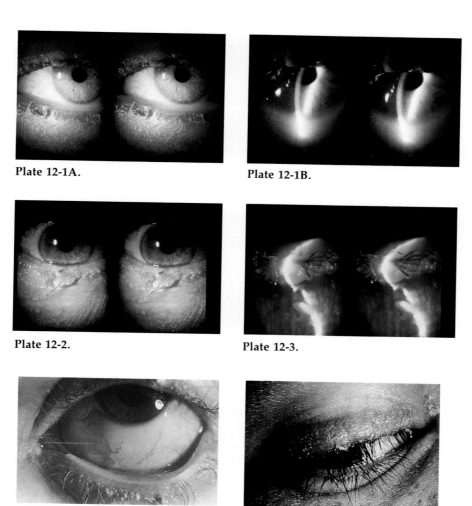

Plate 12-1A.

Plate 12-1B.

Plate 12-2.

Plate 12-3.

Plate 12-4.

Plate 12-5.

Plate 12-1. (A & B) Ulcerative staphylococcal blepharitis, secondary blepharoconjunctivitis, and secondary uveitis.

Plate 12-2. Staphylococcal blepharitis. Heavy deposition and crustiness are seen in the lash margin. Also note the irregular number and consistency of lashes in the bottom lid compared to the top lid.

Plate 12-3. Ulcerative staphylococcal blepharitis. This slide shows 3^{++} inflammation in the lid margin. Tremendous ulceration of the lid margin is seen.

Plate 12-4. Seborrheic blepharitis. Oily scruf of deposition is noted on the lid margin.

Plate 12-5. Seborrheic blepharitis. Oily scruf of deposition is noted on lid margin.

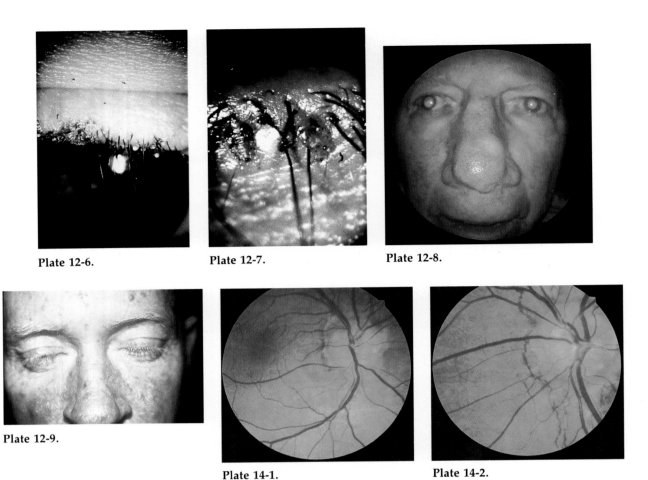

Plate 12-6.

Plate 12-7.

Plate 12-8.

Plate 12-9.

Plate 14-1.

Plate 14-2.

Plate 12-6. *Demodex folliculorum.* Deposition is seen in the lid margin.

Plate 12-7. *Demodex folliculorum.* Magnified view of the deposits in the lid.

Plate 12-8. Acne rosacea. Telangiectacic vessels are seen in the cheek and the rhinophyma (distorted nose).

Plate 12-9. Acne rosacea. Typical rosacea appearance on the facial areas as well as on the lids. Note the papules and pustules in this typical case of acne rosacea.

Plate 14-1. View of a right posterior pole with a mild presentation of angioid streaks. The angioid streaks are primarily limited to the optic nerve head with several extensions. The streaks themselves appear as red-orange crags deep in the retina. The optic nerve head appears elevated due to buried drusen and also present are several observable drusen bodies.

Plate 14-2. A more magnified view of the angioid streaks in the left posterior pole with a moderate degree of presentation. Note the expanded width of the streaks, which indicates a higher degree of risk of the development of subretinal neovascular changes.

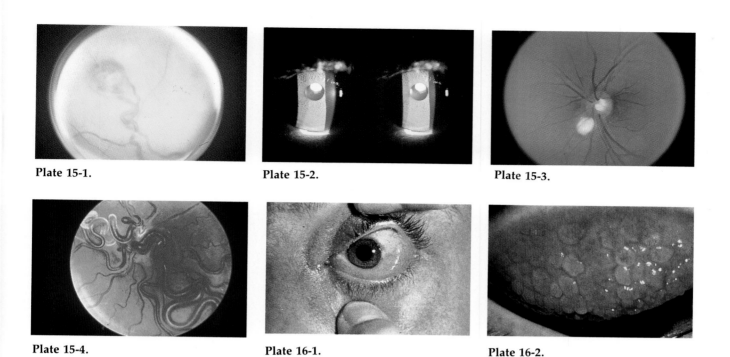

Plate 15-1.

Plate 15-2.

Plate 15-3.

Plate 15-4.

Plate 16-1.

Plate 16-2.

Plate 15-1. Retinal hemangioma with dilated afferent and efferent vessels. (Photograph courtesy of Dr. Edward Deglin.)

Plate 15-2. Iris nodules in a patient with neurofibromatosis. (Photograph courtesy of Jane Stein.)

Plate 15-3. Astrocytic hamartoma. (Photograph courtesy of Jane Stein.)

Plate 15-4. Arteriovenous malformation. (Photograph courtesy of Dr. Edward Deglin.)

Plate 16-1. Limbal vernal conjunctivitis. Note the limbal papilla.

Plate 16-2. Palpebral vernal conjunctivitis. Note the cobblestone appearance of the papillae on this everted upper lid.

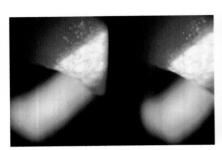

Plate 16-3.

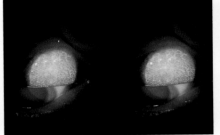

Plate 16-4.

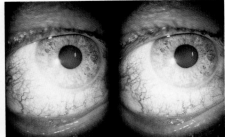

Plate 16-5.

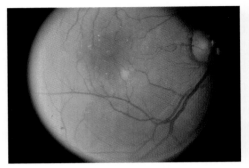

Plate 17-1.

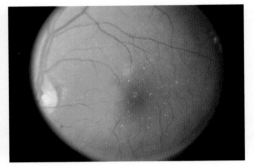

Plate 17-2.

Plate 16-3. Giant papillary conjunctivitis. Note the rounded papillary hypertrophy as contrasted to the flattened papillae of vernal as seen in Plate 16-2.

Plate 16-4. Giant papillary conjunctivitis. Fluorescein helps delineate the papillae by pooling around the bases. Note also the staining of the apices.

Plate 16-5. Toxic conjunctivitis secondary to topical antibiotic administration.

Plate 17-1. Right eye. Note the small, refractile particles in the perimacular area.

Plate 17-2. Left eye. Note the talc particles trapped by the small arterioles in the parimacular area.

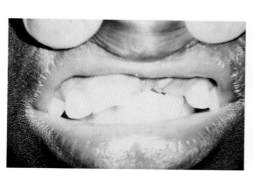

Plate 18-1.

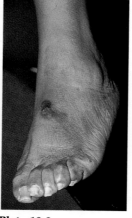

Plate 18-2.

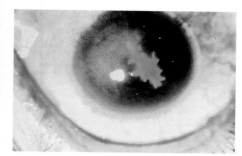

Plate 18-3.

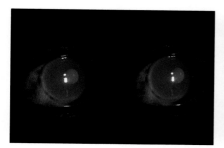

Plate 19-1.

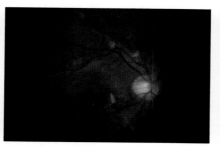

Plate 19-2.

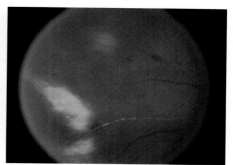

Plate 19-3.

Plate 18-1. Malformed "notched" teeth in Hutchinson's triad. (Photograph courtesy of Jane Stein.)

Plate 18-2. Bony abnormalities of foot secondary to congenital syphilis. (Photograph courtesy of Jane Stein.)

Plate 18-3. Herpetic corneal ulcer. (Courtesy of Dr. Andrew Gurwood.)

Plate 19-1. The patient from the case report: a premenopausal women infected with HIV. She presented with a reduced break-up time, debris in the tear film, and a reduced tear meniscus. She had symptomatology of dry eye secondary to HIV infection. (Photograph courtesy of Jane Stein.)

Plate 19-2. Cotton-wool spots and retinal microvascular changes. (Photograph courtesy of Jane Stein.)

Plate 19-3. Early CMV exhibited in the superior nasal quadrant of the retina. (Photograph courtesy of Jane Stein.)

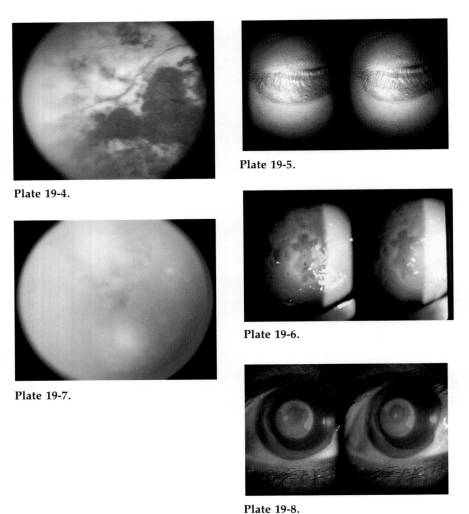

Plate 19-4.

Plate 19-5.

Plate 19-6.

Plate 19-7.

Plate 19-8.

Plate 19-4. Advanced CMV. Note the white granular retinal necrosis. exudate, and hemorrhaging that are characteristic of CMV retinitis. (Photograph courtesy of Jane Stein.)

Plate 19-5. Kaposi's sarcoma on the lower lid. (Photograph courtesy of Jane Stein.)

Plate 19-6. Herpes simplex corneal dendrite. (Photograph courtesy of Jane Stein.)

Plate 19-7. Active toxoplasmosis adjacent to a scar due to toxoplasmosis. (Photograph courtesy of Jane Stein.)

Plate 19-8. Corneal chemical burn or "tattoo" secondary to a wet alcohol disinfected tonometer tip. (Photograph courtesy of Jane Stein.)

13 Oncologic Disease

MARK A. SHUST

INTRODUCTION

In its 1987 Annual Cancer Statistics Review, the National Cancer Institute estimates the death rate from cancer in the United States to be about 483,000 cases per year.[1] In one study of eyes from patients who died from systemic carcinoma a 9 percent incidence of cancer metastatic to the uvea was noted.[2] Based on these figures, one can expect approximately 50,000 new cases of systemic cancer metastatic to the uvea each year. Compared to an estimated 1,900 new cases of primary intraocular cancer per year, it becomes clear that carcinoma metastatic to the uvea is the most common type of intraocular malignancy.[1]

Uveal metastatic disease may be the earliest sign of a systemic malignancy in almost 50 percent of patients with choroidal metastases.[3] Thus, the optometrist may often be the first health care professional to diagnose systemic metastatic disease in a patient with or without any previous history of malignancy. This chapter reviews the ocular manifestations of systemic oncologic disease, including metastatic lesions of the eye and orbit.

CASE REPORT

A 68-year-old black woman presented for an eye examination with complaints of mild blurring and distortion of the vision in the left eye for the past month. She underwent a mastectomy 2 years ago because of breast cancer.

Best corrected visual acuities were OD 20/20, OS 20/30. External examination was unremarkable, and pupil responses were normal with no afferent defects. Slit lamp examination revealed no anterior segment abnormalities, and intraocular pressures were 18 mmHg OU by applanation. Dilated fundus examination revealed a round, slightly elevated yellow and white subretinal lesion in the posterior pole of the left eye extending superiorly from the inferotemporal retinal vascular arcade up to and including the macula. B-scan ultrasound revealed a curvilinear echo, which bowed forward from the posterior ocular wall with moderate internal reflectivity.

No significant changes were noted in the size of the lesion during the next 2 years, after which the patient died of widespread systemic metastatic disease. Postmortem histologic examination of the ocular lesion confirmed it to be a metastasis from the primary tumor in the breast.

OCULAR AND ORBITAL METASTATIC DISEASE

Metastasis of cancer to the eye and orbit occurs almost exclusively by hematogenous dissemination because there are no intraocular lymphatic channels. Tumor cells are carried through the internal carotid artery to the ophthalmic artery, by which they reach the ocular region. The uvea is the most common location of ocular metastases, presumably because of its extensive vascularity and relatively slow blood flow.[3,4]

A predilection for left-sided involvement has frequently been reported.[5-12] The usual explanation for this left-sided predilection is based on anatomic differences in the carotid systems on the two sides. Blood

215

flows directly into the left common carotid from the aorta, whereas a more tortuous route must be taken to reach the right common carotid artery through the innominate artery. Therefore, it was postulated that fewer tumor cells were likely to reach the right internal carotid circulation and ultimately the right ophthalmic artery. Several other studies, however, have failed to confirm this asymmetric distribution of metastasis between the two eyes.[13–16] Involvement of both eyes at time of initial examination may occur in almost 30 percent of patients with metastasis of cancer to intraocular structures.[17]

Site of Primary Tumor

Tumors that metastasize to the eye or orbit are carcinomas in almost all cases except those in children, in whom embryonal tumors and sarcomas occur with greater frequency.[18,19] The most common site of primary malignancy metastatic to the eye and orbit in women is the breast, accounting for 62 to 77 percent of patients in this group. In men, the most common primary tumor site is the lung, accounting for approximately 26 to 49 percent of cases in this group and 14 to 30 percent overall. In about 8 to 18 percent of total cases, the site of primary malignancy could not be identified with certainty.[3,13,20] Other documented primary tumor locations include the kidney, testicle, prostate, pancreas, colon, rectum, stomach, thyroid, ileum, skin, esophagus, bladder, uterus, ovary, oral squamous cell, undifferentiated sarcoma, submandibular adenocystic carcinoma, glomus jugulare chemodectoma, neuroblastoma, bronchial carcinoid, Ewing sarcoma and Wilm tumor.[3,13,18,20,21]

Location of Metastasis to Eye and Orbit

Cancer metastatic to the eye and orbit most often involves the uveal tract.[21] Because of its rich blood supply, the posterior choroid is the most common location of intraocular metastasis and is affected 10 to 20 times more often than the iris or ciliary body.[19] Metastasis of breast cancer occurs with equal frequency to the uvea and orbit, whereas lung tumors preferentially invade the choroid rather than the orbit.[13] Isolated metastasis to the uvea occurs six to nine times more often than the orbit in adults. In children, however, intraocular metastasis of cancer is known to be exceedingly rare in comparison to orbital metastasis.[16,22]

Choroid

Approximately 40 percent of choroidal metastases occur deep to the macula and rarely are found anterior to the equator.[13] About 40 percent of the lesions are at least partially located between the superotemporal and inferotemporal retinal vascular arcades.[17] Choroidal metastases from the breast and lung may occur as multifocal lesions in about one-third of cases.[21] A choroidal metastasis typically appears as a creamy yellow placoid or dome-shaped lesion during ophthalmoscopic examination that may vary in size and elevation.[4,21] Metastatic tumors have no intrinsic pigment, but changes in the overlying retinal pigment epithelium may occur, causing an appearance of pigment clumping on the surface of the tumor.[23] A nonrhegmatogenous retinal detachment is associated with the lesion in 72 percent of eyes.[21] Patients with choroidal metastases may be asymptomatic but will usually report a painless blurring of vision and, in some cases, may complain of pain or photopsia.[4,19,21]

Ultrasonography is sometimes useful in evaluating patients with suspected choroidal metastases. B-scan ultrasound of metastatic tumors will usually reveal a curvilinear echo that bows forward from the posterior ocular wall with moderate-to-high internal reflectivity and no choroidal excavation or orbital shadowing, unlike that seen with a primary choroidal melanoma. In some cases multiple tumors may be found. Secondary overlying retinal detachment may often be detected as a moderately high-intensity linear echo associated with the mass, which may be seen to shift with changes in position of the patient's head. A-scan ultrasonography will show a sharp initial spike and moderate-to-high internal reflectivity, whereas malignant melanomas will usually show a low reflectivity. The back portion of the A-scan pattern will often climb as it approaches the region of the sclera, a phenomenon known as "negative-angle κ."[4,19,23]

The differential diagnosis of a metastatic choroidal tumor includes amelanotic malignant choroidal melanoma, amelanotic choroidal nevus, choroidal hemangioma, choroidal osteoma, uveal effusion syndrome, central serous choroidopathy, Harada's disease, posterior scleritis, and rhegmatogenous retinal detachment.[4,17,24]

Anterior Uvea

Metastases to the iris and ciliary body are much less common than those to the choroid and account for approximately 4 to 11 percent of intraocular metastases.[17,23,25,26] An iris metastasis is almost always amelanotic and typically presents as a single or multiple yellow-white gelatinous mass within the iris stroma that may have numerous surface vessels.[4,21,23] In some cases, the tumor cells will be loosely cohesive and may settle in the anterior chamber, forming a pseudohypopyon. Unlike primary melanomas, which are most often located in the inferior half of the iris, metastatic tumors involve the superior and inferior portions of the iris with equal frequency. Another distinction is that metastatic iris tumors tend to grow much more rapidly than do primary malignancies. Most patients with iris metastases are asymptomatic or have mild visual disturbances in the affected eye. A metastatic tumor of the ciliary body may appear similar to an amelanotic melanoma, although ciliary body metastases are often difficult to detect clinically.[4] Injected epibulbar vessels and signs suggestive of anterior uveitis may be seen in association with metastasis to the ciliary body and angle structures, as well as a shallow anterior chamber, subluxated lens, and cataract.[4,17,25,26] Other clinical signs associated with metastatic disease to the anterior uvea include elevated intraocular pressure, hyphema, ocular inflammation, iris neovascularization, and infiltration of the cornea and adjacent angle structures.[17,21,25,26] The differential diagnosis of a metastatic tumor to the anterior uvea includes amelanotic melanoma of the iris and ciliary body, iris cysts, granulomatous anterior uveitis, retained intraocular foreign body, and retinoblastoma.[4,21]

Retina and Vitreous

Metastatic disease of the retina is relatively uncommon, accounting for less than 1 percent of metastases to the eye and orbit.[4,20,27,28] Retinal metastases tend to be rather friable, and tumor cells may seed into the vitreous cavity, simulating a retinitis. The tumor cells may also cause a retinal vascular obstruction in which a patchy yellow lesion may be seen associated with hemorrhage or exudate.[4,21] Certain lymphoproliferative disorders such as large cell lymphoma may also disseminate into the vitreous.[4]

Optic Nerve and Optic Disc

Metastasis of cancer to the optic disc is uncommon. In some cases direct extension of a juxtapapillary choroidal metastasis to the optic disc may occur, but on rare occasions a malignancy can metastasize to the disc alone.[4,17,21,29] Metastases of the optic disc may be associated with decreased visual acuity and visual field defects.[19] Edema of the optic disc, dilation and

tortuosity of retinal vessels, an afferent pupillary defect, and retinal hemorrhage, vein occlusion, or artery occlusion can be seen in these patients. Edema, hyperemia, or atrophy of the disc may be noted in patients with meningeal carcinomatosis of the optic nerve sheath.[4,17,21,29]

Conjunctiva and Sclera

Conjunctival and scleral metastasis occurs in association with intraocular metastasis in approximately 2 percent of eyes. Scleral involvement occurs in up to 11 percent of patients with uveal metastasis, usually by direct extension of the tumor.[17,21] Conjunctival metastases typically resemble fleshy vascularized tumors.[21] Involvement of the conjunctiva may also occur in patients with lymphoproliferative disorders such as leukemia and lymphoma.[30]

Orbit

Metastatic disease to the eye appears to occur with significantly greater frequency than to the orbit. A series of studies have estimated that 2 to 9 percent of orbital tumors are metastatic and that 11 to 32% of metastases to the ocular region involve the orbit.[5,20,23,31–35] There are some important differences in the types of orbital metastases between adults and children. In adults, most orbital metastatic tumors are carcinomas, whereas in children metastases are more likely to originate from embryonal neuronal tumors or sarcomas.[19,34,36]

The most common primary cancer sites metastatic to the orbit in adults are the breast in women and the lung in men, similarly to the case of uveal metastatic disease.[3,32] Most metastases of cancer to the orbit are unilateral, although bilateral cases have been reported.[32,37] Common findings during clinical examination include noncomitant strabismus with diplopia, a palpable mass, reduced visual acuity, edema and chemosis of the lids and conjunctiva, and ptosis.[19,21,34] In cases of selective metastasis to the lacrimal gland, optic nerve, or extraocular muscles, variations in the clinical presentation may be observed and can often lead to misdiagnosis. An interesting variation that may occur in patients with scirrhous breast carcinoma is the presence of enophthalmus instead of exophthalmos. This phenomenon occurs as a result of sclerosis induced by the invading tumor cells, which causes retraction of the globe.[38–41] Ophthalmoplegia and orbital pain can also occur and may be more marked early in the course of orbital metastases than in primary orbital tumor.[31] A rapid onset of any of these signs or symptoms should alert the optometrist to the possibility of an orbital metastasis, or perhaps a very aggressive primary orbital malignancy, as a rapid clinical course is not characteristic of benign orbital tumors.[34]

Noteworthy are studies that have suggested that most women with metastasis of breast carcinoma to the orbit will report a prior history of treatment for breast cancer.[33,34] The average interval of time between the diagnosis of the primary tumor in the breast and metastasis to the orbit is 2 to 5 years, although an interval of up to 27 years has been documented.[32,35] By contrast, orbital metastasis of lung cancer frequently appears before or simultaneously with diagnosis of the primary lesion in the lung.[3,32,42–44]

The most common orbital metastatic tumor in children is neuroblastoma. Ewing sarcoma and Wilm tumor are also of diagnostic importance, but both occur with lesser frequency.[23,34,45,46] Neuroblastoma is one of the most prevalent childhood tumors, accounting for approximately 10 to 15 percent of pediatric malignancies.[47–50] A neuroblastoma is most commonly described as a malignant neoplasm of embryonic neuroblastic tissues, which under normal circumstances, would form the sympathetic nervous system and ganglia.[34] The primary tumor site is the adrenal medulla in up to 50 percent of cases, other retroperitoneal areas in 25 percent, the head and neck in 2 to 5 percent, and the mediastinum in another 10 percent of cases. Neuroblastomas metastasize to the orbit rather than to the globe, unlike metastatic tumors in adults.[23,51–53] Most patients are younger than 4 years, with one-half younger than 2 years.[19] Orbital metastasis is believed to occur in approximately 11 to 38 percent of patients having primary neuroblastoma, with abdominal tumors showing the greatest tendency for orbital metastasis.[34,37] Neuroblastomas may occur as a primary tumor within the orbit, but only in extremely rare instances.[36] Clinically, the child with orbital metastasis of neuroblastoma typically presents with an abrupt onset of proptosis and displacement of the globe.[51,52,54,55] Ecchymosis of the eyelids is common as a result of hemorrhage, which occurs when the tumor expands rapidly and outgrows its blood supply.[19] Bilateral involvement may occur in 20 to 55 percent of cases.[56–58] The metastasis tends to lodge in the zygomatic bone, such that a mass in the cheek or temple area may sometimes coexist with the proptosis.[19] Fundus examination may reveal optic nerve head edema and dilation of retinal veins.[34] A prior diagnosis of primary neuroblastoma will have been made in 97 percent of patients with orbital symptoms.[16] Most patients with orbital metastases from a previously undetected abdominal tumor will have a palpable abdominal mass, which should not be overmanipulated because dissemination of tumor cells into the bloodstream may occur.[19] Affected children often have signs of systemic illness such as skin pallor, weakness, fever, and malaise.[34]

A number of ophthalmic signs may be seen in patients with primary neuroblastoma of the cervical sympathetic chain, even in the absence of orbital metastasis, including Horner syndrome and opsoclonus. The presence of heterochromia suggests that the tumor is congenital.[16,19,34,59,60]

The prognosis is generally poor for patients with metastasis of neuroblastoma to the orbit. The 3-year survival rate is approximately 11 percent. For patients having Horner syndrome but no orbital involvement, however, the 3-year survival rate is 79 percent.[34,54]

Ewing sarcoma is a primary malignant neoplasm of the bone usually seen in individuals between 10 and 25 years of age. The tumor usually originates in the long limb bones or the trunk bones and has a strong predisposition to metastasize to other bones and to the lung.[19,34,62] Studies have reported an 11 to 42 percent incidence of orbital metastasis among patients with systemic Ewing sarcoma.[16,57] In rare cases, this tumor has also been recognized to occur as a primary lesion of the bones in the orbit.[62]

Orbital metastasis of Ewing sarcoma presents clinically as a unilateral, rapidly progressive proptosis, usually on the same side as the primary lesion. Bilateral involvement is rare, unlike that seen with neuroblastoma.[16,19,34] Conjunctival and palpebral hemorrhages may also be seen in association with the proptosis. Patients with ocular signs almost always present with a prior history of malignancy of the bones.[34] The treatment of Ewing sarcoma is not particularly effective because of its early dissemination, and most patients with widespread metastasis have a fatal course.[19,34]

Wilms tumor, also known as nephroblastoma, is a neoplasm of embryonic kidney cells and accounts for approximately 20 percent of childhood cancers.[34,57] It usually occurs in children between the ages of 1 and

5 years, but may sometimes be seen in newborns and young infants.[34,37] As with neuroblastoma and Ewing sarcoma, the orbital metastasis almost always occurs after the abdominal Wilms tumor has been diagnosed. The clinical presentation is that of a rapidly progressive unilateral proptosis and displacement of the globe commonly associated with ecchymosis of the eyelids and conjunctiva. In some cases, the metastatic tumor may even create a deformity of the head.[34,46] The occasional association of Wilms tumor with aniridia is a condition known as Miller syndrome.[58] Most patients with orbital metastasis of Wilms tumor have widespread systemic involvement and usually survive for only a few months.[34]

Eyelids

Metastasis of cancer to the eyelids is rare and accounts for less than 1 percent of eyelid malignancies.[63–66] Metastasic lid lesions may present as recurrent chalazia, ulcerated lesions, diffuse swelling, multicentric nodules, or chronic blepharoconjunctivitis. The lesion usually appears on the dermis or less commonly on the palpebral conjunctiva. The most common primary tumor site is the breast, accounting for 35 percent of eyelid metastases, followed by the skin (16 percent), and the gastrointestinal and urogenital tracts (10 percent each). Metastatic eyelid disease may be detected before diagnosis of the primary tumor in up to 45 percent of cases. In one case, signs of eyelid metastasis occurred 10 years after radical mastectomy for breast carcinoma.[63]

Cancer-Associated Retinopathy

Cancer-associated retinopathy, or paraneoplastic retinopathy, is a condition characterized by progressive photoreceptor degeneration with subsequent visual deterioration.[67–70] This entity is believed to occur as a remote, nonmetastatic effect of the primary tumor as a result of either a tumor cell product that is toxic to the retina or a tumor antigen that stimulates an autoimmune response within certain retinal cells. Symptoms typically include reduced visual acuity, visual obscurations, nyctalopia, and photopsia. Associated visual field defects may include a ring scotoma, central scotoma, or generalized field constriction. Ophthalmoscopic examination will reveal attenuated or sheathed retinal arterioles and a normal optic nerve head. A delay in the transit time is seen with fluorescein angiography along with areas of hypofluorescence corresponding to areas of retinal pigment

epithelial atrophy. The electroretinogram and electrooculogram are both reduced or extinguished altogether in these patients. Paraneoplastic retinopathy has been associated with cancers of the breast, lung, and cervix.[21,70,71]

Prognosis

The prognosis for patients with metastasis of cancer to the eye and orbit depends on the type of primary lesion as well as the stage and extent of systemic metastatic disease. In general, however, the long-term prognosis for patients with any metastatic disease is poor. Various sources have reported an overall average survival of 7.4 to 10.5 months from the time of ocular diagnosis in patients with metastasis of systemic cancer to the eye and orbit.[3,13,17]

LYMPHOID TUMORS

Lymphoid tumors can involve almost any part of the eye or ocular adenxa. Unfortunately, the clinical behavior and histopathologic characteristics of lymphoid tumors are not clearly understood. There is also some confusion regarding the relationship of ocular lymphoid lesions to systemic disease. To further complicate matters, the classification systems used to organize these disorders are continuously undergoing change and modification. A comprehensive review of lymphoproliferative disease is beyond the scope of this chapter, but the following is a brief discussion of the more common associated ocular manifestations. A description of ocular findings in patients with leukemias and plasma cell tumors can be found in Chapter 10.

Lymphomas

Lymphomas are a group of malignant neoplasms that primarily affect the lymphatic system and account for about 3 percent of all cancers. They are usually found in the lymph nodes but may sometimes develop in extranodal sites such as the skin, gut, bone marrow, and oropharyngeal region as well as the ocular structures. Lymphomas are broadly divided into Hodgkin's disease and non-Hodgkin's lymphoma, based on histologic and clinical characteristics.[72] Non-Hodgkin's lymphoma occurs three times more commonly than Hodgkin's disease and accounts for the vast majority of orbital lymphoid tumors.[72,73] Intraocular involvement of lymphomas is extremely rare except with large cell lymphoma, previously known as reticulum cell sarcoma, which is a highly malignant type of non-Hodgkin's lymphoma but is discussed here as a separate entity.[74]

Non-Hodgkin's Lymphoma

Orbital lymphoid lesions account for approximately 7.5 to 11 percent of all orbital tumors.[75–77] However, the incidence of orbital involvement in patients with systemic lymphomas is only about 1 percent.[78] Most cases occur in adults, and the eye care practitioner should suspect leukemia as the primary systemic disease in any child diagnosed with an orbital lymphoid tumor.[73,79]

Orbital lymphoid tumors related to non-Hodgkin's lymphoma most often present clinically as a proptosis or displacement of the globe in a patient between the age of 45 and 65.[73] Visual acuity and ocular motility is minimally impaired, except in advanced cases.[73,80] The tumor tends to involve the superior and anterior regions of the orbit and exhibits a predilection for involvement of the lacrimal gland. Thus, most orbital lymphoid tumors cause a downward displacement of the eye, and a firm mass can often be palpated through the upper eyelid. In cases with involvement of the anterior orbit, subconjunctival extension may sometimes be noted as a pink "salmon-patch"-type lesion in the conjunctival fornix.[73] Most cases occur unilaterally, and simultaneous bilateral presentation or recurrence after excision is suggestive of a malignant tumor.[81]

Large Cell Lymphoma

Also known as histiocytic lymphoma or reticulum cell sarcoma, large cell lymphoma is divided into a systemic type and a less common central nervous system (CNS) type. The primary sites of involvement with the systemic type are the lymph nodes, visceral organs, and infrequently, the uveal tract. The CNS type primarily affects the CNS and produces ocular manifestations more often. Ocular changes may precede CNS or systemic involvement by many months or sometimes even years.[74,82,83] Large cell lymphoma is a disease of older persons and generally affects individuals older than 50 years of age. Ocular manifestations often begin unilaterally, but bilateral involvement eventually occurs in 80 percent of cases.[74]

Affected patients typically complain of a painless blurring of vision. Slit lamp examination frequently re-

veals keratic precipitates along with vitreous cells resembling that of intermediate uveitis. Fundus examination may reveal multifocal yellow infiltrative subretinal lesions with areas of hyperpigmentation.[74,84] Vitreous cells are believed to occur secondary to the retinal lesions, although histologic studies have sometimes been unable to reveal the presence of tumor cells in the retina.[85,86] Exudative retinal detachment occurs rarely as a late complication.[74] Many patients are often misdiagnosed as having uveitis, and any individual older than age 50 with signs of bilateral diffuse uveitis should be suspected of having large cell lymphoma.[87]

Orbital involvement with large cell lymphoma is quite infrequent and usually consists of swelling of the eyelids, which may be associated with proptosis and orbital discomfort.[84]

Hodgkin's Disease

Orbital involvement in Hodgkin's disease occurs much less often than in non-Hodgkin's lymphoma. Almost all patients with orbital manifestations of Hodgkin's disease have had a prior diagnosis of systemic disease, unlike those with non-Hodgkin's lymphoma, which may sometimes even occur as a primary tumor. Hodgkin's disease typically occurs in individuals between the ages of 35 and 55. Ocular findings present clinically as a progressively enlarging unilateral or bilateral orbital mass with no preference for specific areas of the orbit.[84]

Burkitt's Lymphoma

Burkitt's lymphoma is a distinct type of malignant lymphoma that was originally described as a solid, rapidly progressive lymphoma occurring most often in the jaw and abdomen of African children. Burkitt's lymphoma accounts for almost one-half of all childhood malignancies in East Africa.[88,89] More recently, however, an American (non-African) and an acquired immunodeficiency syndrome (AIDS) form have also been recognized.[90] Orbital involvement in the American and AIDS-related forms occurs significantly less often than in the African form.[73]

The various forms of Burkitt's lymphoma differ in clinical appearance.[90] The African form typically involves the jaw bones, orbit, and viscera. Orbital involvement occurs in 50 percent of cases, usually by erosion of the tumor from the primary site in an adjacent maxillary bone. Rapidly progressive proptosis and upward displacement of the globe is usually observed and may ultimately result in severe visual loss.[73,91,92]

The American form usually involves the lymph nodes, bone marrow, and abdominal viscera. A rapidly progressive unilateral proptosis as a result of direct extension to the orbit from a primary ethmoid sinus tumor occurs most often.[93] In some cases, however, a bilateral proptosis may be seen in patients with involvement limited to the orbital soft tissues.[73,94]

The AIDS-related form is similar in many ways to the American form except that initial involvement of the CNS occurs much more frequently. It usually occurs in immunosuppressed homosexual men with clinical signs of AIDS.[90] Orbital findings are typically unilateral and may involve the anterior orbital soft tissues in the absence of bone involvement.[73]

As with all lymphomas other than large cell lymphoma, intraocular involvement with Burkitt's lymphoma is extremely rare.

EVALUATION

The evaluation of all patients with suspected metastatic or secondary ocular tumors should include an extensive history inquiring into previous malignancies as well as a thorough physical examination with specific emphasis on the detection of systemic oncologic disease. It is worth repeating that most patients with metastatic breast cancer will report a prior history of treatment for malignancy, whereas patients with metastatic lung cancer will frequently develop ocular findings simultaneously with or before detection of the primary tumor in the lungs.[32–34,42–44] Ancillary studies that are sometimes useful in the diagnostic work-up of patients include ultrasound, computed tomographic scan, magnetic resonance imaging, fluorescein angiography, and fine-needle aspiration biopsy in some cases.[4,21,34,71]

MANAGEMENT

Treatment of ocular and orbital metastatic disease is essentially palliative. In cases of ocular metastasis, intervention is generally indicated with involvement or impending involvement of the fovea by tumor or subretinal fluid, anterior uveitis, glaucoma, or pain. Orbital metastases usually require therapy when pain, diplopia, or optic neuropathy are evident.[21] External beam irradiation therapy to the tumor is the usual course of treatment when necessary.[17,33,95,96] However, a metastatic tumor of the eye or orbit that is undergoing regression with chemotherapy alone should require no specific ocular therapy. The potential side effects as well as benefits of chemotherapy and radiotherapy must be evaluated when considering these options.

REFERENCES

1. 1987 Annual Cancer Statistics Review. p. 1.20. U.S. Department of Health and Human Services, Public Health Service, National Institutes of Health, National Cancer Institute, Bethesda, MD, 1987
2. Nelson CC, Hertzberg BS, Klintworth GK: A histopathologic study of 716 unselected eyes in patients with cancer at the time of death. Am J Ophthalmol 95:788, 1983
3. Ferry AP, Font RL: Carcinoma metastatic to the eye and orbit. I. A clinicopathologic study of 227 cases. Arch Ophthalmol 92:276, 1974
4. Shields JA: Diagnosis and Management of Intraocular Tumors. CV Mosby, St. Louis, 1983
5. Hart WM: Metastatic carcinoma to the eye and orbit. In Zimmerman LE (ed): Tumors of the eye and adnexa. Int Ophthalmol Clin 2:465, 1962
6. Hogan MJ, Zimmerman LE: Ophthalmic Pathology. 2nd Ed. WB Saunders, Philadelphia, 1962
7. Duke-Elder S, Perkins ES: Diseases of the uveal tract. p. 917. In Duke Elder S (ed): System of Ophthalmology. CV Mosby, St. Louis, 1966
8. Reese AB: Tumors of the Eye. 2nd Ed. Paul B. Hoeber, New York, 1963
9. Walsh FB, Hoyt WF: Clinical Neuro-ophthalmology. 3rd Ed. Williams & Wilkins, Baltimore, 1969
10. Data Analysis. Lifetime Learning Publications, Balmont, CA, 1980
11. Jenses OA: Metastatic tumors of the eye and orbit: a histopathological analysis of a Danish series. Acta Pathol Microbiol Immunol Scand 212:201, 1970
12. DeOcampo G, Espiritu R: Bronchogenic metastatic carcinoma of the choroid. Am J Ophthalmol 52:107, 1961
13. Freedman MI, Folk JC: Metastatic tumors to the eye and orbit: patient survival and clinical characteristics. Arch Ophthalmol 107:1215, 1987
14. Bloch RS, Gartner S: The incidence of ocular metastatic carcinoma. Arch Ophthalmol 85:673, 1971
15. Albert DM, Rubenstein RA, Scheie HG: Tumor metastasis to the eye. Part 1. Incidence in 213 adult patients with generalized malignancy. Am J Ophthalmol 63:723, 1967
16. Albert DM, Rubenstein RA, Scheie HG: Tumor metastasis to the eye. Part 2. Clinical study in infants and children. Am J Ophthalmol 63:727, 1967
17. Shakin EP, Shields JA, Augsburger JJ: Metastatic carcinoma to the eye: an analysis of 200 patients. Paper presented at the Wills Eye Hospital Annual Clinical Conference, 1985
18. Ferry AP: Metastatic carcinoma of the eye and ocular adnexa. Int Ophthalmol Clin 7:615, 1967
19. Basic and Clinical Science Course. Section 4: Ophthalmic pathology and intraocular tumors. American Academy of Ophthalmology, San Francisco, 1991
20. Hutchison DS, Smith TR: Ocular and orbital metastatic carcinoma. Ann Ophthalmol June 869, 1979
21. Shakin EP, Shields JA: The eye and ocular adnexa in systemic malignancy. In Duane's Clinical Ophthalmology. Vol. 5. JB Lippincott, Philadelphia, 1991

22. Feman SS, Apt L: Eye findings associated with pediatric malignancy. J Pediatr Ophthalmol 9:224, 1972
23. Devron CH: Clinical Ocular Oncology. Churchill Livingstone, New York, 1989
24. Michelson JB, Stephens RF, Shields JA: Clinical conditions mistaken for metastatic cancer to the choroid. Ann Ophthalmol 11:149, 1979
25. Sierocki J, Charles N, Schafron KM et al: Carcinoma metastatic to the anterior ocular segment. Cancer 45:2521, 1980
26. Ferry AP, Font RL: Carcinoma metastatic to the eye and orbit: A clinicopathologic correlation study of 26 patients with carcinoma metastatic to the anterior segment of the eye.
27. Young SE, Cruciger N, Lukeman J: Metastatic cancer to the retina: a case report. Ophthalmology 86:1350, 1979
28. Robertson DM, Wilkerson CP, Murray JL et al: Metastatic tumors to the retina and vitreous cavity from primary melanoma of the skin. Ophthalmology 88:1296, 1981
29. Arnold A, Helper R, Foos R: Isolated metastasis to the optic nerve. Surv Ophthalmol 26:75, 1981
30. Kincaid MC, Green WR: Ocular and orbital involvement in leukemia. Surv Ophthalmol 27:211, 1983
31. Henderson JW: Orbital Tumors. WB Saunders, Philadelphia, 1973
32. Shields CL, Shields JA, Peggs M: Metastatic tumors to the orbit. Ophthalmic Plast Reconstr Surg 4:73, 1988
33. Font RL, Ferry AP: Carcinoma metastatic to the eye and orbit. III. A clinicopathologic study of 28 cases metastatic to the orbit. Cancer 38:1326, 1976
34. Shields JA: Diagnosis and Management of Orbital Tumors. WB Saunders, Philadelphia, 1989
35. Howard GM, Jakobiec FA, Trokel SL et al: Pulsating metastatic tumor of the orbit. Am J Ophthalmol 85:767, 1978
36. Jakobiec FA, Rootman J, Jones IS: Secondary and metastatic tumors of the orbit. p. 503. In Jones IS, Jakobiec FA (eds): Diseases of the Orbit. Harper & Row, Hagerstown, MD, 1979
37. Henderson JW, Farrow GM: Orbital Tumors. 2nd Ed. Brian C. Decker (Thieme-Stratton), New York, 1980
38. Cline RA, Rootman J: Enophthalmos: a clinical review. Ophthalmology 91:229, 1984
39. Manor RS: Enophthalmos caused by orbital metastasis of breast cancer. Acta Ophthalmol 52:881, 1974
40. Randot M, Varga M: Metastatic tumor of the orbit. Ann Ophthalmol 7:1465, 1975
41. Sacks JG, O'Grady RB: Painful ophthalmoplegia and enophthalmos due to metastatic carcinoma: simulation of essential facial hemiatrophy. Trans Am Acad Ophthalmol 75:351, 1971
42. Buys R, Abramson DH, Kitchin FD et al: Simultaneous ocular and orbital involvement from metastatic bronchogenic carcinoma. Ann Ophthalmol 14:1165, 1982
43. Divine RD, Anderson RL, Ossoinig KC: Metastatic small cell carcinoma masquerading as orbital myositis. Ophthalmic Surg 13:483, 1982
44. Ferry AP, Naghdi MR: Bronchogenic carcinoma metastatic to the orbit. Arch Ophthalmol 77:214, 1967
45. Porterfield J: Orbital tumors in children. Int Ophthalmol Clin 2:319, 1962
46. Apple DJ: Wilm's tumor metastatic to the orbit. Arch Ophthalmol 80:480, 1968
47. Gross RE, Farber S, Martin LW: Neuroblastoma sympatheticum: a study and report of 217 cases. Pediatrics 23:1179, 1959
48. Lingley J, Sagerman R, Santulli T, Wolff J: Neuroblastoma, management and survival. N Engl J Med 277:1227, 1967
49. DeLorimier AA, Bragg KU, Linden G: Neuroblastoma in childhood. Am J Dis Child 118:441, 1969
50. Neuroblastoma, editorial. Lancet 1:379, 1975
51. Mortada A: Clinical characteristics of early orbital metastatic neuroblastoma. Am J Ophthalmol 63:1787, 1967
52. Alfano JE: Ophthalmological aspects of neuroblastomatosis: a study of 53 verified cases. Trans Am Acad Ophthalmol Otolaryngol 72:830, 1968
53. Shubert EE, Oliver GL, Jaco NT: Metastatic neuroblastoma causing bilateral blindness. Can J Ophthalmol 4:100, 1969
54. Musarella M, Chan HSL, DeBoer G et al: Ocular involvement in neuroblastoma: prognostic implications. Ophthalmology 91: 936, 1984
55. Traboulsi EI, Shammas IV, Massad M et al: Ophthalmological aspects of metastatic neuroblastoma: report of 22 consecutive cases. Orbit 3:247, 1984
56. Coley B, Higinbotham N, Bowden L: Endothelioma of bone (Ewing's sarcoma). Ann Surg 128:533, 1948
57. Anderson WAD, Scotti TM: Synopsis of Pathology. CV Mosby, St. Louis, 1980
58. DiGeorge AM, Harley RD: The association of aniridia, Wilm's tumor and genital abnormalities. Trans Am Ophthalmol Soc 63:64, 1965
59. Sivaramasubramanian P: Solitary metastatic orbital tumor due to sympathetic neuroblastoma. Br J Ophthalmol 47:312, 1963
60. Apple DJ: Metastatic orbital neuroblastoma originating in the cervical sympathetic ganglion chain. Am J Ophthalmol 68:1093, 1969
61. Lichtenstein L: Bone Tumors. CV Mosby, St. Louis, 1972
62. Alvarez-Berdecia A, Schut L, Bruce DA: Localized primary intracranial Ewing's sarcoma of the orbital roof case report. J Neurosurg 50:811, 1979
63. Mansour AM, Hidayat AA: Metastatic eyelid disease. Ophthalmology 94:667, 1987
64. Aurora AL, Blodi FC: Lesions of the eyelids: a clinicopathologic study. Surv Ophthalmol 15:94, 1970
65. Weiner JM, Henderson PN, Roche J: Metastatic eyelid carcinoma. Am J Ophthalmol 101:252, 1986
66. Mansour AM: Metastatic lid disease. Orbit 4:247, 1985
67. Sawyer RA, Selhorst JB, Zimmerman LE et al: Blindness caused by photoreceptor degeneration as a remote effect of cancer. Am J Ophthalmol 81:606, 1976
68. Klingele TG, Burde RM, Rappazzo JA et al: Paraneoplastic retinopathy. J Clin Neuro Ophthalmol 4:239, 1984
69. Keltner JL, Roth AM, Chang RS: Photoreceptor degeneration: possible autoimmune disorder. Arch Ophthalmol 101:564, 1983
70. Grunwald GB, Klein R, Simmonds MA et al: Autoimmune basis for visual paraneoplastic syndrome in patients with small cell lung carcinoma. Lance 3:658, 1985
71. Augsburger JJ, Shields JA: Fine needle aspiration biopsy of solid intraocular tumors: techniques and instrumentation. Ophthalmic Surg 15:34, 1984
72. Jakobiec FA, Nelson D: Lymphomatous, plasmacytic, histiocytic, and hematopoietic tumors of the orbit. In Duane's Clinical Ophthalmology. Vol. 5. JB Lippincott, Philadelphia, 1991
73. Shields JA: Diagnosis and Management of Orbital Tumors. WB Saunders, Philadelphia, 1989
74. Kanski JJ, Thomas DJ: The Eye in Systemic Disease. Butterworth-Heinemann, Boston, 1990
75. Henderson JW, Farrow GM: Orbital Tumors. 2nd Ed. Brian C. Decker (Thieme-Stratton), New York, 1980
76. Kennedy RE: An evaluation of 820 orbital cases. Trans Am Ophthalmol Soc 82:134, 1984
77. Shields JA, Bakewell B, Augsburger JJ et al: Classification and incidence of space-occupying lesions of the orbit. A survey of 645 biopsies. Arch Ophthalmol 102:1606, 1984
78. Rosenberg SA, Diamond HD, Jalowitz B et al: Lymphosarcoma: a review of 1269 cases. Medicine 40:31, 1961
79. Shields JA, Bakewell B, Augsburger JJ et al: Space occupying orbital masses in children: a review of 250 consecutive biopsies. Ophthalmology 93:31, 1986
80. Yeo JH, Jakobiec FA, Abbott GF et al: Combined clinical and computed tomographic diagnosis of orbital lymphoid tumors. Am J Ophthalmol 94:235, 1982
81. Jakobiec FA, McLean I, Font R: Clinicopathologic characteris-

tics of orbital lymphoid hyperplasia. Ophthalmology 86:948, 1979

82. Appen RE: Posterior uveitis and primary cerebral reticulum cell sarcoma. Arch Ophthalmol 93:123, 1975

83. Neault RW, Van Scoy RE, Okazaki H, MacCarty CS: Uveitis associated with isolated reticulum cell sarcoma of the brain. Am J Ophthalmol 73:431, 1972

84. Shields JA: Diagnosis and Management of Intraocular Tumors. CV Mosby, St. Louis, 1983

85. Kennerdell JS, Johnson BL, Wizoteskey HM: Vitreous cellular reaction: association with reticulum cell sarcoma of the brain. Arch Ophthalmol 93:1341, 1975

86. Minckler DS, Font RL, Zimmerman LE: Uveitis and reticulum cell sarcoma of the brain and bilateral neoplastic seeding of vitreous without retinal or uveal involvement. Am J Ophthalmol 80:433, 1975

87. Char DH: Clinical Ocular Oncology. Churchill Livingstone, New York, 1989

88. Burkitt D, O'Conor GT: Malignant lymphoma in African children. I. A clinical syndrome. Cancer 14:258, 1961

89. Templeton AC: Orbital tumors in African children. Br J Ophthalmol 55:254, 1971

90. Brooks HL, Downing J, McClure JA et al: Orbital Burkitt's lymphoma in a homosexual man with acquired immune deficiency. Arch Ophthalmol 102:1533, 1984

91. Feman SS, Niwayana G, Hepler RS et al: "Burkitt tumor" with intraocular involvement. Surv Ophthalmol 14:106, 1969

92. Karp LA, Zimmerman LE, Payne T: Intraocular involvement in Burkitt's lymphoma. Arch Ophthalmol 85:296, 1971

93. Blakemore WS, Ehrenberg M, Fritz KJ et al: Rapidly progressive proptosis secondary to Burkitt's lymphoma. Origin in the ethmoid sinuses. Arch Ophthalmol 101:1741, 1983

94. Zak TA, Tisher JE, Afshani E: Infantile non-African Burkitt's lymphoma presenting as bilateral fulminant exophthalmos. J Pediatr Ophthalmol Strabismus 19:294, 1982

95. Mewis L, Young SE: Breast carcinoma metastatic to the choroid: analysis of 67 patients. Ophthalmology 89:147, 1982

96. Thatcher N, Thomas PRM: Choroidal metastasis from breast carcinoma. Clin Radiol 26:549, 1975

14 Connective Tissue Disorders

ANASTAS F. PASS

INTRODUCTION

Connective tissue is the tissue that supports the various structures within the body. Connective tissue is made up of fibroblasts, fibroglia, collagen fibrils, and elastic fibrils. Structures supported by the connective tissue include the collagenous, elastic, mucous, reticular, osseous, and cartilaginous tissues. Because all these tissues exist (at times) ambiguously throughout the body, disorders involving the connective tissue system can manifest diverse presentations. Connective tissue disorders have also been melded with the collagen and collagen-vascular disorders. Collagen is the main supporting protein component of bone, cartilage, connective tissue, skin, and tendons.

The definition of connective tissue disorders is indistinct, in that it has been classified inconsistently. The following disorders grouped in the collagen and collagen-vascular group have been synonymous with connective tissue disorders: ankylosing spondylitis, cranial arteritis, polyarteritis nodosa, polymyositis, Reiter syndrome, relapsing polychondritis, rheumatic fever, rheumatoid arthritis (adult or juvenile), scleroderma, Sjögren syndrome, systemic lupus erythematosus, Wegner's granulomatosis, Marfan syndrome, Weill-Marchesani syndrome, osteogenesis imperfecta, and Paget's disease. Although all these disorders can be associated with ocular findings (blue sclera, corneal defects, glaucoma and vision loss), they are primarily collagen and bone disorders (see Ch. 5). Specific to connective tissue disorders are Ehlers-Danlos syndrome and pseudoxanthoma elasticum (PXE). Ocular findings associated with these two connective tissue disorders are ocular fragility and retinal angioid streaks. Angioid streaks, however, are more of a hallmark of PXE. Excluding Paget's disease, the collagen and collagen-vascular disorders previously noted do not demonstrate this retinal artifact. Paget's disease (osteitis deformans), a skeletal disorder, can manifest angioid streaks in up to 15 percent of those affected.[1]

Angioid streaks are primarily breaks in Bruch's membrane. They can vary in presentation by extent of retinal involvement, color, and distribution. Angioid streaks are progressive and degenerative. They may be associated with vision loss and choroidal neovascularization, both of which may be prevented depending on the stage of presentation.

This chapter describes connective tissue disorders with regard to pathophysiology, systemic presentation, and ocular findings. Clinical presentation is discussed as well as appropriate ocular diagnostic procedures for differential assessment and systemic testing, which may also be necessary for the assessment. Because the eye care practitioner's responsibility does not stop at merely assessing an ocular presentation of a systemic disorder, additional testing procedures and treatment considerations are presented. Angioid streaks, which are demonstrated with both Ehlers-Danlos syndrome and (primarily) PXE, are discussed as a separate entity.

CASE REPORT

A 35-year-old white woman presented with a chief concern of a recent decrease in vision of the right eye, although she also noted a somewhat decreased left vision relative to what it has been. The acute vision loss in the right eye had been noted for the past 2 days. The overall vision decrease had been noted for several months.

On questioning, she reported no history of injury, ocular diseases, or ocular surgery. She did report a "dryness" that has existed for several years. She used ocular lubricants as needed to resolve the problem successfully. Her last visual/ocular examination was reported as approximately 8 years previous.

Inquiry into her medical history revealed the presence of systemic hypertension (for 8 years) and a duodenal ulcer (identified 8 months previously) for which she was hospitalized and treated. No history of diabetes, thyroid disorders, or severe cardiovascular disorders (the patient was diagnosed with a mitral valve prolapse at the time the hypertension was diagnosed) was given. She added anecdotally the existence of cramps in her lower extremities that have existed for several years. No family ocular and medical histories were noted because she was adopted.

Her current medications included chlorothiazide (Diuril) 250 mg (twice per day) and nizatidine (Axid) 150 mg taken at bedtime. She reported no known allergies to medication or the environment.

Entering unaided and best visual acuity were OD 20/100 and OS 20/30 with no improvement with pinhole. The best visual correction was determined to be OD $+.25/-.50 \times 020$ and OS $+.50/-.25 \times 165$. The pupillary reaction was brisk and equal to light. No afferent pupillary defect was noted. Ocular motility was unrestricted. Blood pressure was recorded at 130/85 mmHg (right arm, seated) at 2:10 PM. Keratometric assessment was noted to be OD $43.50/44.50 \times 175$ and OS $44.00/44.75 \times 005$ without any central distortion.

External assessment revealed minor inferior superficial punctate keratitis approximately equal between the two corneas. No associated blepharitis, meibomitis, or lagophthalmos was noted. The remaining external findings were unremarkable (adnexa, anterior chamber, iris, lens and anterior vitreous). Intraocular pressure measured by applanation tonometry was 14/16 mmHg at 2:35 PM.

Dilated fundus examination demonstrated clear media and a 20/20 fundus view. Pigmented mottling of the fundus was noted in both eyes throughout the posterior poles. Angioid streaks were present in both eyes; however, the presentation in the right eye was far more extensive (involving the macula). The angioid streaks in the right eye were noted around the optic nerve head (ONH) in a circumferential and radial pattern. Several of the streaks were noted in the macular area. It was difficult to assess the existence of any subretinal neovascular membrane (SRNM). There was the presence of an subretinal hemorrhage adjacent to the macula inferiorly. The angioid streaks in the left eye appeared to present only adjacent to the optic nerve head. Drusen-like lesions were noted throughout both fundi.

The optic nerve heads of both eyes presented with clear and distinct margin, were well perfused, and had no evidence of nerve head drusen. The angioid streaks appeared to emanate from the optic nerve head's; however, the right eye was significantly more involved.

On additional questioning at this point in the examination, the patient reported noticing an "excess of stretchy skin in the arm pits and inner elbow areas." Palpation and examination of the skin along the neck also revealed a thickening with some indication of hyperelasticity. The involved areas of the neck also appeared to have a peau d'orange presentation, although not to the degree of the antecubital areas.

The patient was tentatively diagnosed with PXE based on the clinical findings. Decreased vision was attributed to retinal degenerative changes associated with PXE. The acute vision loss of the right eye was attributed to the macular hemorrhage associated with the angioid streaks. The pigment mottling of the fundus was attributed to retinal peau d'orange also consistent with PXE.

After educating and counseling the patient with regard to the results of the examination, a retinal fluorescein angiogram was ordered to determine the extent of the degenerative Bruch's membrane involvement, investigate for neovascular nets associated within the retinal breaks, and determine the potential sites for treatment with laser therapy.

Table 14-1. Systemic Complications Seen
With Ehlers-Danlos Syndrome

Hyperextensibility of the joints and skin
Cutaneous pseudotumor
Subcutaneous nodules
Skin fragility
Vascular fragility, aneurysms, spontaneous rupture
Bruising
Poor wound healing

Table 14-3. Ocular Complications
Seen With Ehlers-Danlos Syndrome

Ocular fragility
Blue sclera
Epicanthal folds, lid laxity (Metenier's sign)
Corneal thinning, keratoconus, keratoglobus
Staphyloma
Myopia
Angioid streaks
Retinal hemorrhage
Hemorrhagic retinal detachment
Globe rupture

EHLERS-DANLOS SYNDROME

Ehlers-Danlos syndrome is a connective tissue disorder that involves both the collagen and elastic fibers with secondary calcification (Table 14-1). Typical systemic findings include hyperextensibility of the joints and skin, vascular and visceral fragility, fragile skin, cutaneous pseudotumor (usually seen on elbows and knees), and calcifications in the subcutaneous tissue.[2] Nine different subtypes of Ehlers-Danlos syndrome have been identified; the differentiation is determined by clinical presentation.[3] The most prominent expression of Ehlers-Danlos syndrome is through autosomal dominance, although it has been suggested that a recessive form also exists.[4] The most common subtype is type I, or Ehlers-Danlos syndrome (gravis), which manifests hyperextensibility of the joints and skin, cutaneous pseudotumor, subcutaneous calcifications, poor wound healing, bruising, and ocular fragility. Because of vascular fragility, hemorrhaging and spontaneous rupture can occur in the peripheral vasculature, although this is most often observed in the bowel and intestines.[5] Intracranial aneurysms, including vertebral involvement, have also been noted[6] (Table 14-2).

Type I (gravis) along with type VI (oculoscoliotic) are the two subtypes of Ehlers-Danlos syndrome that present with more significant retinopathy as demonstrated by angioid streaks. Type VI, however, is a much rarer form and, overall, angioid streaks are not considered a hallmark of the disease. More typical ocular findings are epicanthal folds, lid tissue redundancy, blue scleras, myopia, keratoconus retinal de-

Table 14-2. Neurologic Complications
Seen With Ehlers-Danlos Syndrome

Carotid-cavernous fistula
Intracranial aneurysms
Hemorrhage

tachment, and globe rupture. The tissue redundancy about the eye is associated with the epicanthal folds. Ehlers-Danlos patients with lid tissue involvement usually show an ease of lid eversion due to this redundancy (Metenier sign).[4] With the progression of the disease, scleral and corneal thinning become more manifest (Table 14-3). The exact mechanism of corneal thinning—keratoconus or keratoglobus—is still not well understood, but it has been postulated that it is due to abnormal mucopolysaccharide and collagen synthesis within the cornea.[7]

The ocular fragility of Ehlers-Danlos syndrome can also explain the increase in myopia with varying presentation of irregular astigmatism. As the globe itself becomes more fragile, the compromised scleral tissue thins. This causes a blue discoloration of the sclera (from the underlying uvea). As noted with keratoconus, with the progression of the corneal thinning in Ehlers-Danlos syndrome, breaks in Descemet's membrane can manifest an acute hydrops. Ectopia lentis can occur with Ehlers-Danlos syndrome, although this is not common. A concern, however, is that mild trauma can cause the compromised globe to rupture. Rupture sites occur at the weakened and thinned sclera, although the primary rupture site appears to be the cornea.[8]

PSEUDOXANTHOMA ELASTICUM

PXE is a connective tissue disorder that principally involves the elastic fibers with secondary calcification of the elastic fibers. The incidence in the general population is about 1:160,000.[9] PXE is primarily an autosomal recessive genetic disorder, although dominant forms have also been identified.[10,11] Etiologic investigation of the tissue involvement has demonstrated that the lesions associated with PXE comprise elastic fibers in the connective tissues and not collagen.[12]

Table 14-4. Systemic Complications Seen With Pseudoxanthoma Elasticum

Gastrointestinal bleeding
Ulcerative colitis
Hypertension
Kidney complications
Hemorrhage
Cramps
Paresthesia

Table 14-5. Neurologic Complications Seen With Pseudoxanthoma Elasticum

Progressive dementia
Mental disturbance
Hemorrhage
Paralytic cranial nerve palsy
Vision loss

The affected tissues include the skin, cardiovascular system, and eyes (Table 14-4). The primary involvement of proliferation of elastic fibers of the skin in PXE is generally a benign presentation. The redundancy of the tissue presents as a velvety thickened area with the appearance of an orange peel; this is typically described as peau d'orange. The skin areas most commonly involved with PXE are the neck, axilla, antecubital, and inguinal regions. These areas of redundant skin display hyperelasticity (Fig. 14-1). Yellow nodule-like lesions occur in these areas. These lesions are located in the elastic fibers of the middle and lower dermis and represent calcification of the elastic fibers.[13] The calcification can be easily identified with calcium stains after biopsy, which is helpful in the diagnosis of the disease.[14]

Changes in the elastic fibers of the cardiovascular system in a patient with PXE can present with far more serious clinical (systemic) findings. Because of the

fragility of the vascular wall, patients with PXE may exhibit hemorrhages and rupture in the peripheral vascular system. Gastrointestinal bleeding due to primary disease in the gastric vessel wall has been documented.[15] Hypertension is also a potential result of the peripheral vascular degeneration and is attributed, in part, to arterial degeneration in the kidney. Also associated with the peripheral vascular degeneration is the potential for cramps, paresthesias, and neurovascular deficits.[16] (Table 14-5).

The effects of PXE on the eye have been attributed to the phenotype.[10,11] The most common ocular presentations are degenerative changes of the (presumed) elastic tissue within Bruch's membrane[17] (Table 14-6). These breaks, or angioid streaks, form "cracks" reminiscent of broken glass. The presentation of angioid streaks is bilateral with asymmetry. Because of the presence of angioid streaks, which are breaks in Bruch's membrane, the potential for fibrovascular ingrowth and, hence, SRNMs can occur. When SRNMs occur beneath the foveal area, central vision is severely compromised.[18] With the development of the fibrovascular tissue, imminent vascular rupture and choroidal hemorrhage occur and therefore the development of hemorrhagic retinal detachment.

Also associated with PXE is the grainy retinal pigment epithelium (RPE), giving a mottled appearance. This mottling has also been termed a peau d'orange presentation. Drusen-like lesions may also present with

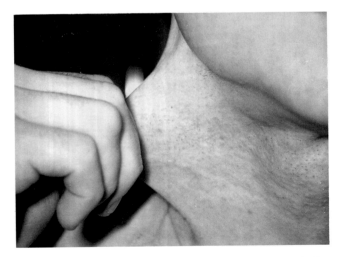

Fig. 14-1. Hyperelasticity and redundancy of the neck skin on a young adult male patient with PXE. Note the degree to which the skin can be manipulated.

Table 14-6. Ocular Complications Seen With Pseudoxanthoma Elasticum

Angioid streaks
Retinal pigment epithelium mottling (peau d'orange)
Retinal hemorrhage
Hemorrhagic retinal detachment
Drusen of retina and ONH
Blue sclera
Myopia

varying degrees of hyperpigmentation located through the fundus, particularly in the areas of the angioid streaks.[18]

Connective tissue degeneration within the sclera causes a bluish discoloration that can manifest due to the underlying uvea. With progressive fragility of the globe secondary to the degeneration of the scleral integrity, a myopic shift can be measured in conjunction with irregular astigmatism.

ANGIOID STREAKS

First described in 1889 by Doyne[19] and then later termed *angioid streaks* in 1892 by Knapp.[20] Angioid streaks present bilaterally as a rule and in the posterior aspects of the globe (Figs. 14-2 and 14-3). Rarely, they can be seen anterior to the equator. The configuration of angioid streaks is thought to be consistent with the global lines of force.[21] They are hypothesized to be due to the mechanical stresses induced by the extraocular muscles during eye movements over time. The color presentation of the angioid streak will vary depending on the overall pigmentation presentation of the retina. A darkly pigmented fundus may show

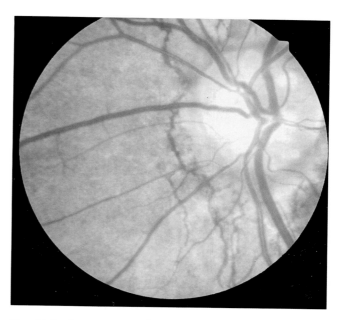

Fig. 14-3. A more magnified view of the angioid streaks in the left posterior pole with a moderate degree of presentation. Note the expanded width of the streaks, which indicates a higher degree of risk of the development of subretinal neovascular changes. (See also Plate 14-2.)

darker angioid streaks with liberated RPE pigment lining the border (and possibly within the break itself). Angioid streaks in the blonde fundus may present with a more red appearance and little RPE pigment associated with the retinal break.

Histopathologic studies of angioid streaks demonstrate the presence of basophilia and calcification.[22–24] Although the existence of localized deposition basophilia is consistent with the aging process,[1] a greater prevalence of basophilia occurs in the angioid streak. The presence of the calcification is consistent with the destructive process in the elastic tissue of connective tissue disorders previously discussed. The involvement of the choriocapillaris has been associated with the close proximity to the elastic component of Bruch's membrane. The overlying RPE is, in fact, present but thinned. Histologic studies show that the angioid streaks of PXE and Paget's disease demonstrate similar histopathologic profiles. Although PXE is the most common syndrome to present with angioid streaks, Paget's disease and sickle cell hemoglobulinopathies are also associated with angioid streaks.[18] Table 14-7 shows the systemic conditions associated with angioid streaks and their reported frequencies. The most common pathogenesis is due to

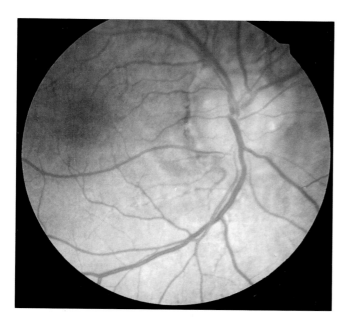

Fig. 14-2. View of a right posterior pole with a mild presentation of angioid streaks. The angioid streaks are primarily limited to the optic nerve head with several extensions. The streaks themselves appear as red-orange crags deep in the retina. The optic nerve head appears elevated due to buried drusen and also present with several observable drusen bodies. (See also Plate 14-1.)

Table 14-7. Systemic Conditions Associated With Angioid Streaks and Their Reported Frequencies

Condition, Comments	Possible Mechanism	Reported Frequency (%)
Pseudoxanthoma elasticum Autosomal recessive (two forms) Dominant (two forms)	Abnormal apatite (Ca^{2+}) formation in Bruch's membrane	55–87
Paget's disease (osteitis deformans)	Abnormal apatite (Ca^{2+}) formation in Bruch's membrane	8–20
Hemoglobin SS (sickle cell disease)	Abnormal apatite formation in Bruch's membrane	<Age 40, 1–6 >Age 40, 6–22
Other hemoglobinopathies	Abnormal apatite deposition in Bruch's membrane	Low, probably <6
Acquired hemolytic anemia	Fe^{11} deposition	Uncommon
Other connective tissue diseases Ehlers Danlos I, (dominant) Ehlers Danlos VI, (recessive, lytyl hydroxylase deficiency) Marfan (dominant)	Uncertain	Uncommon
Metabolic abnormalities Hyperparathyroidism Hyperphosphatemia Acromegaly Pituitary dwarfism Lead poisoning	Uncertain	Uncommon

(From Newsome,[18] with permission.)

the abnormal apatite of calcium formation in Bruch's membrane. This has not necessarily been demonstrated, however, with sickle cell hemoglobulinopathies. The latter do have abnormal mineralization processes within Bruch's membrane; however, the exact mechanism is not known. As can be seen in Table 14-7, the frequency of reported angioid streaks in PXE is 55 to 87 percent.

Fluorescein angiography is necessary to fully investigate the presence of the angioid streaks but, more importantly, to identify and locate the possible existence of SRNMs. Angioid streaks show early hyper-

fluoresence in the transit. This finding is due to the filling of the choriocapillaris that has "bunched" at the border of the angioid streak, delineating the defect in Bruch's membrane, which is easily seen through a thinned RPE. Because of leaking of the fluorescein into the intravascular space and the angioid streak, a hyperfluorescence persists and may coincide with the location of the early phase hyperfluoresence.[25] If serous leakage from the choroidal vessels occurs, serous detachment of the RPE may occur. Leakage of blood in the same area may cause the development of a disciform detachment of the RPE, a possible precursor to SRNM formation. Development of SRNMs, which may appear as a gray or greenish-gray discoloration of the retina, signifies a potential threat to vision, particularly if this occurs in the macular area.

Fluorescein angiography will localize the area needed for treatment as well as indicate the type of laser to be used depending on the proximity to the foveal area. If the SRNM exists outside the foveal avascular zone (FAZ) greater than 200 μm (extrafoveal), argon laser photocoagulation is indicated. If the SRNM exists within 1 to 199 μm from the FAZ (juxtafoveal), krypton red laser photocoagulation is indicated. If the SRNM exists at the FAZ, the patient may be watched or laser photocoagulation may be elected. The risks and benefits of photocoagulation need to be considered thoroughly.[26]

MANAGEMENT OF OCULAR COMPLICATIONS ASSOCIATED WITH CONNECTIVE TISSUE DISORDERS

Typically, a patient with PXE will manifest associated skin abnormalities, and the diagnosis of this particular connective tissue disorder is simplified. The appropriate retinal assessment can then be made in conjunction with a systemic assessment with internal medicine. A patient with angioid streaks as the sole observable manifestation represents an unknown and should undergo systemic laboratory testing to aid the eye care practitioner in the differential diagnosis. The Bascom Palmer Eye Institute has developed a scheduled array of testing to aid in diagnosis, and it includes the following: radiographs of the skull, abdomen, and lower extremities; a biochemical assay, including serum alkaline phosphatase, calcium, and phosphorous; hemoglobin electrophoresis; and skin biopsy. These tests will differentiate the presentation of angioid streaks as a possible cause of PXE, Paget's disease, or the sickle hemoglobulinopathies.[1]

The primary work-up for the observed ocular complication of angioid streaks is direct view of the fundus with appropriate lenses, although a contact fundus lens would provide the greatest degree of resolution and assessment. Visual field assessment may be considered to determine the status of the field as well as to provide a baseline for any overlying pathology that may also affect the visual field (i.e., glaucoma). The most important investigation involves fluorescein angiography to establish the actual extent of the damage to the retina (Bruch's membrane) and to identify the presence or absence of SRNMs. Identification of SRNMs is essential to appropriately determine the site of laser photocoagulation treatment.

Continued follow-up of the patient is an important aspect of patient care. In the absence of symptomology, intervals between follow-up visits should not exceed 6 months. When eye signs are visible, follow-up every 3 months is appropriate. Patients should be educated to present themselves immediately if visual symptomology (i.e., vision change, metamorphopsia, and/or scintillations) occurs.

SUMMARY

Patients with connective tissue disorders such as Ehlers-Danlos syndrome or PXE will manifest a myriad of systemic and ocular complications. The systemic effects of these disorders must not be dismissed by the eye care practitioner, because many of these patients may not be under the care of a physician. A thorough case history is important because it may bring to light systemic changes a patient may not have considered significant. Furthermore, as for all systemic disorders, it is also important to recognize the obvious or subtle skin changes that present with these disorders. Communication with the patient's physician is important when suspected changes arise; appropriate systemic and neurologic testing or imaging can best be coordinated with a joint effort.

The patients with connective tissue disorders should be followed closely to identify impending ocular changes that may result in the loss of vision or the globe itself. The time frame for evaluations will be dictated by the current presentation of the patient. Given a patient with minimal signs, however, intervals between visits should be no longer than 6 months. With severe ocular changes (i.e., SRNMs or imminent rupture), immediate assessment and treatment must be provided. Above all, patient education provides the best opportunity to maintain the integrity of vision and systemic health.

REFERENCES

1. Clarkson JG, Altman RD: Angioid streaks. Surv Ophthalmol 26:235, 1982
2. Pinnell SR, Murad S: Disorders of collagen. p. 1434. In Stanbury JB, Wyngaarden JB, Frederickson DS et al (eds): The Metabolic Basis of Inherited Disease. McGraw-Hill, New York, 1983
3. Renie WA: Goldberg's Genetic and Metabolic Eye Disease. 2nd Ed. Little, Brown, Boston, 1986
4. Beighton P: Serious ophthalmological complications in Ehlers-Danlos syndrome. Br J Ophthalmol 54:263, 1970
5. Lach B, Nair SG, Russell NA, Benoit BG: Spontaneous carotid-cavernous fistula and multiple arterial dissections in type IV Ehlers-Danlos syndrome: case report. J Neurosurg 66:462, 1987
6. de Paepe A, van Landegem W, de Keyser F, de Reuck J: Association of multiple of intracranial aneurysms and collagen type III deficiency. Clin Neurol Neurosurg 90:53, 1988
7. Maumanee IH: The cornea in connective tissue disease. Ophthalmology 85:1010, 1978
8. Kenyon KR, Fogle JA, Grayson M: Dysgeneses, dystrophies and degenerations of the cornea. p. 4. In Duane TD, Jaeger EA (eds): Clinical Ophthalmology. Vol. 4. Harper & Row, Philadelphia, 1981
9. Engelman MW, Fliegelman MT: Pseudoxanthoma elasticum. Cutis 21:837, 1978
10. Pope FM: Two types of autosomal recessive pseudoxanthoma elasticum. Arch Dermatol 110:209, 1974
11. Pope FM: Autosomal dominant pseudoxanthoma elasticum. J Med Genet 11:152, 1974
12. Findlay GH: On elastase and the elastic dystrophies of the skin. Br J Dermatol 66:16, 1954
13. Nerad JA, Whitaker DC: Pseudoxanthoma elasticum. p. 596. In Gold DH, Weingeist TA (eds): The Eye in Systemic Disease. JB Lippincott, Philadelphia, 1990
14. Fitzpatrick TB, Eisen AZ, Wolff K et al: Dermatology in General Medicine. 2nd Ed. McGraw-Hill, New York, 1979
15. Solomon LM, Esterly NB: The skin and the eye. p. 508. In: Goldberg's Genetic and Metabolic Eye Disease. Little, Brown, Boston, 1974
16. Miller NR: Aneurysms. p. 1982. In Walsh T (ed): Clinical NeuroOphthalmology. 4th Ed. Williams & Wilkins, Baltimore, 1991
17. Dryer R, Green WR: The pathology of angioid streaks: a study of 21 cases. Trans Pa Acad Ophthalmol Otolaryngol 31:158, 1978
18. Newsome DA: Angioid streaks and Bruch's membrane degenerations. p. 271. In Newsome DA (ed): Retinal Dystrophies and Degenerations. Raven Press, New York, 1988
19. Doyne RW: Choroidal and retinal changes: the result of blows to the eyes. Trans Ophthalmol Soc UK 9:128, 1889
20. Knapp H: On the formation of dark angioid streaks as an unusual metamorphosis of retinal hemorrhage. Arch Ophthalmol 21:289, 1892
21. Adelung JC: Zur genese der angioid Streaks. Klin Monatsbl Augenheilkd 119:241, 1951
22. Hagadorn A: Angioid streaks. Arch Ophthalmol 21:935, 1939
23. Verhoeff FH: Histopathologic findings in a case of angioid streaks. Br J Ophthalmol 32:431, 1948
24. Gass JDM, Clarkson JG: Angioid streaks and disciform macular detachment in Paget's disease (osteitis deformans). Am J Ophthalmol 75:576, 1973
25. Federman JL, Shields JA, Tomer TL: Angioid streaks: fluorescein angiographic features. Arch Ophthalmol 93:951, 1975
26. Macular Photocoagulation Study Group: Argon laser photocoagulation for neovascular maculopathy: five-year results from randomized clinical trials. Arch Ophthalmol 109:1109, 1991

15 The Phakomatoses

SARAH L. FOSTER

INTRODUCTION

The phakomatoses are a group of neuro-ophthalmico-cutaneous disorders with varied presentation. They are congenital, and for the most part have a dominant heredity. They are characterized by tumors and cysts that are spread throughout the body and give widespread symptomatology based on their location. The Dutch ophthalmologist van der Hoeve[1] first used the term *phakomatoses,* meaning "mother-spot," or birthmark, to describe these syndromes in 1932. He coined this term because skin involvement is a feature common to members of the group, and the conditions have a hereditary basis. Phakomatoses include (1) angiomatosis of the cerebellum and retina (von Hippel-Lindau syndrome, (2) neurofibromatosis (Recklinghausen's disease), (3) tuberous sclerosis (Bourne-ville's disease), and (4) encephalotrigeminal angiomatosis (Sturge-Weber syndrome). It has been suggested that ataxia-telangectasia (Louis-Barr), Wyburn-Mason syndrome, and Klippel-Trenaunay-Weber syndrome be included in the group; however, their inclusion has not been accepted traditionally.

All of the phakomatoses are caused by disseminated hamartomas. A hamartoma is a tumor composed of cells that are normally found in the involved tissue. Hamartomas are spread throughout the central nervous system, retina, and skin. Von Hippel-Lindau syndrome and Sturge-Weber syndrome arise from vascular anomalies that are of mesodermal origin. Tuberous sclerosis and neurofibromatosis are neuroectodermal dysplasias.

CASE REPORT

A 41-year-old white woman presented to the eye clinic complaining of a sudden decrease in vision in the right eye. This was of particular concern to the patient because her grandmother was blind before her death following intracranial surgery for a "brain tumor." Remaining ocular and systemic histories were noncontributory. Best corrected visual acuity was 20/70 OD and 20/20 OS. Pupils were round, equal in size, and normally reactive, with no afferent pupillary defect. Extraocular muscles were unrestricted. Slit lamp examination and applanation tonometry were entirely within normal limits. Dilated fundus examination was remarkable for the presence of a 4-disc-diameter yellow-red mass in the superior retinal midperiphery in the right eye. A tortuous dilated artery entered the mass, and an engorged vein drained it. The mass was surrounded by subretinal exudate, which extended inferiorly into the macular area. The entire macula was thickened. The left eye was within normal limits.

The diagnosis was made of retinal hemangioma (von Hippel's disease) in the right eye. Coats disease and racemose hemangiomatosis were considered but discounted because neither explained the presence of the yellow-red retinal mass. Immediate consultation was sought with a retina subspecialist, who performed fundus fluorescein angiography and subsequent cryotherapy of the hemangioma. Because the patient had a retinal hemangioma as well as a suspicious, possibly positive family history (blind family member with a "brain tumor"), consultation was also sought with an internist to rule-out the systemic manifestations of von Hippel-Lindau syndrome. A complete blood count and electrolytes were ordered as well as a magnetic resonance image of the brain, urine test, and abdominal computed tomography scan. The entire systemic work-up was negative.

At the 3-month follow-up, the visual acuity had improved to 20/25 OD, and the patient was asymptomatic. The primary eye care practitioner then meticulously examined the patient's three children and her 66-year-old mother, none of whom were symptomatic. The patient's mother exhibited two small (1 disc diameter) retinal hemangiomas, one in the retinal periphery of each eye. These were both treated with photocoagulation. She adamantly refused a systemic work-up. The children's ocular and systemic examinations were within normal limits. Regular follow-up was recommended for all family members at 6-month intervals for the patient's mother and yearly intervals for her children.

ANGIOMATOSIS OF THE RETINA AND CEREBELLUM (VON HIPPEL-LINDAU SYNDROME

Eugen von Hippel first described angiomatosis retinae at the Heidleberg Congress in 1904.[2] Because of its autosomal dominant heredity, von Hippel's disease affects many members of the same family, but reports of affected families are very rare. In 1926, Avrid Lindau, the Swedish neurologist, correlated angiomatosis retinae with angiomatous cysts in the cerebellum and established the entity von Hippel-Lindau syndrome.[3,4]

Von Hippel's disease initially presents with a small (2 to 3 disc diameter) round, yellowish red retinal tumor or plexus of capillaries with large dilated afferent and efferent feeder vessels. The initial appearance is usually during childhood or adolescence. The tumor is often located in the peripheral retina, although it can also be present in the posterior pole. Progression is variable, but the tumor usually enlarges gradually and begins to leak exudate because of changes in the permeability of the vessel walls. Slowly enlarging capillary and precapillary arteriovenous shunts develop. The lesion may not change for months or years, but it can eventually grow to form a raised globular growth fed by a dilated arteriole and drained by a dilated tortuous vein (Fig. 15-1 and Plate 15-1). With time, the hemangioma becomes a rounded, reddish mass. The gray-white exudate surrounding the tumor can often obscure the view of the hemangioma completely. In many long-standing cases, massive exudation can resemble Coats disease and confound the diagnosis. Often, retinal detachment, massive gliosis, retinal edema, macular star, papilledema, and recurrent hemorrhage are observed in the late stages. Secondary glaucoma with narrowing of the anterior chamber can result. Affected eyes can become phthisical or at least functionally useless.

Histologically, the growth is composed of a plexus of thin-walled capillaries with areas of cystic degeneration and neovascularization. Fibrous tissue is present in and around the hemangioma. Glial tissue is pronounced during the late stages. Exudation is demonstrated by fluorescein angiography of the angioma, which shows massive leaking of dye.

The differential diagnosis includes multiple congenital aneurysms, Coats disease, racemose arteriovenous aneurysm, and choroidal melanoma. Multiple congenital aneurysms are localized dilations occurring in the veins or arteries, or both. Angiomatosis retinae must have dilation of the feeder arteriole and companion venule. When multiple congenital aneurysms present with dilation of both the artery and vein, they can be difficult to differentiate from von Hippel's disease in its late stages. Racemose arteriovenous aneurysm—a congenital anomalous communication be-

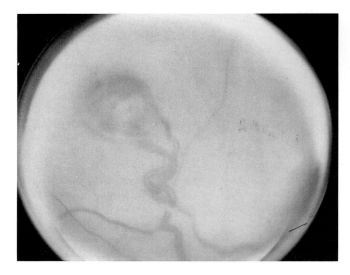

Fig. 15-1. Retinal hemangioma with dilated afferent and efferent vessels. (Photograph courtesy of Dr. Edward Deglin.) (See also Plate 15-1.)

tween the artery and the vein (see the section, *Wyburn-Mason syndrome*)—also has enlarged and tortuous afferent and efferent vessels, but it has no exudation or gliosis, as is present in angiomatosis retinae. A visual field test can be used to rule out a choroidal melanoma. Angiomatosis retinae will show a sector defect, especially if the hemangioma is located near the optic nerve. The melanoma will show a scotoma correlating exactly to its size and position.

Signs and symptoms of angiomatosis retinae depend on the location and extent of the lesion. Few symptoms are present when the early lesion is in the retinal periphery. If an early lesion is found near the macula, Amsler anomalies can be demonstrated. Treatment also depends on the location and extent of the lesion. Photocoagulation is the method of choice for retinal lesions. A single application is usually effective when the lesion is in the early stages. If exudative areas are present, cryotherapy is the treatment of choice. If a retinal detachment and exudate are present, all forms of treatment are usually unsuccessful.

The role of the eye care practitioner in managing patients with von Hippel's disease cannot be overemphasized. Because von Hippel's disease usually occurs in many members of a family as a result of its autosomal dominant heredity, it is extremely important to carefully examine all members of the family of an affected patient at regular intervals with the binocular indirect ophthalmoscope. Successful photocoagulation of an existing hemangioma does not cure the disease; other retinal hemangiomas are quite likely to appear. It is imperative that the eye care practitioner not allow an asymptomatic patient to become complacent. Routine examination and diligent follow-up can prevent eventual blindness in patients affected with von Hippel's disease.

As previously mentioned, Lindau recognized retinal angiomatosis as part of a symptom complex involving the central nervous system. Angiomatosis can also be present in the cerebellum, medulla, spinal cord, kidney, and pancreas. The symptoms experienced by the patient with Lindau's disease are those produced by the brain tumor. Increased intracranial pressure can cause headache, nausea, vomiting, and papilledema. The resulting cerebellar disturbances may include staggering gait and inability to walk a straight line, positive Romberg sign, nystagmus, ataxia, adiadokinesis (neck stiffness), and dizziness. The eye care practitioner may note decreased corneal reflex on the side of the tumor or a visual field defect caused by the increased intracranial pressure. Treatment involves surgical removal of the tumor.

The most important role of the eye care practitioner in the management of Lindau's disease is diagnosis of asymptomatic von Hippel-Lindau syndrome in family members of patients with known von Hippel-Lindau syndrome. Lindau suggested that 25 percent of patients with retinal angiomas have central nervous system involvement. The diagnosis is most easily confirmed by location of incipient retinal lesions. The detection of incipient nervous system or visceral lesions requires complicated and costly radiologic techniques. The eye care practitioner is responsible for monitoring asymptomatic family members. If a retinal lesion is located, it should be treated as previously mentioned, and arrangements should be made for neurologic work-up for Lindau's disease. Because von Hippel-Lindau syndrome has autosomal dominant heredity, patients should be counseled as to the likelihood of passing on the disease to their offspring.

NEUROFIBROMATOSIS

Neurofibromatosis (Recklinghausen's disease) was first described in 1882 by Frederick Daniel von Recklinghausen.[5] Neurofibromatosis is a congenital disease characterized by multiple tumors of the skin and cutaneous pigmentation. The tumors arise from the sheaths of cranial, spinal, peripheral, and sympathetic nerves. Abnormalities most commonly involve the brain, bone, and optic nerve. Incomplete forms of the disease are commonly observed. Signs and symptoms may not be evident until early adulthood and may be activated by puberty, pregnancy, and menopause. Neurofibromatosis affects 1 person in 3000.[6]

Neurofibromatosis is characterized by dermal pigmentation and multiple tumors that arise from the Schwann cells of the peripheral nerves. Two types of tumors occur: plexiform neuromas and fibroma molluscum. Plexiform neuromas are subcutaneous tumors that protrude from beneath the skin. They are soft to the touch and contain many tortuous knotty cords that give them the consistency of a "bag of worms." They arise from superficial peripheral nerves. Plexiform neuromas often involve the upper lid and adjacent temple and can be associated with a bony defect in the temporal region. Often, generalized enlargement of the orbit on the affected side occurs, or a bony defect in the sphenoid with complete absence of the orbital roof is seen[7] (Fig. 15-2). The eye care practitioner is likely to be faced with problematic plexiform neuroma of the lids. This is quite difficult to treat surgically and is often best left alone. I have had surprising success in treating these large, ptotic lids with a crutch device attached to the patient's spectacles. This lifts the heavy lid off the visual axis, allowing the patient an adequate visual field. Fibroma molluscum are solitary pedunculated cutaneous neurofibromas that may be scattered over the entire body (Fig. 15-3). The surface of these tumors is easily invaginated. They arise from cutaneous nerves, either from the sheath of a Schwann cell or from perineural connective tissue.[9,10] If the tumor arises from a Schwann cell, it is called a *schwannoma*. Fibroma molluscum can also involve the eyelids.

Neurofibromatosis can result in enlargement of a particular part of the body. When this is extreme, it is termed *elephantiasis neuromatosis* and can result in grotesque deformities.

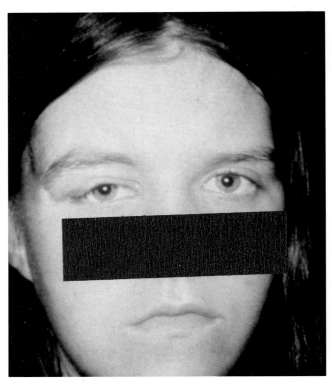

Fig. 15-3. Fibroma molluscum of the right upper lid. (Photograph courtesy of Dr. Edward Deglin.)

Café-au-lait spots are brown lesions ranging in shade from pale to very dark and ranging in size from 1 mm to many centimeters. They can occur anywhere in the body and are found in 10 percent of the population in general. A patient with six or more café-au-lait spots greater than 1.5 cm in diameter invariably has Recklinghausen's disease.[11,12] Axillary freckling and pigmentation are also pathognomonic of the disease.

Ocular Findings

Allende considered the ocular involvement in neurofibromatosis in order of frequency as follows: lids, optic nerves, orbit, retina, iris, cornea, and conjunctiva.[13] Neurofibromatosis of the lids is described above.

Neurofibromatosis can be associated with glaucoma. Anderson[14] believed that congenital glaucoma occurs only in the presence of upper lid involvement, but exceptions to this generalization have been reported.[15] The cause of glaucoma in patients with neurofibromatosis is unclear. The presence of congenital

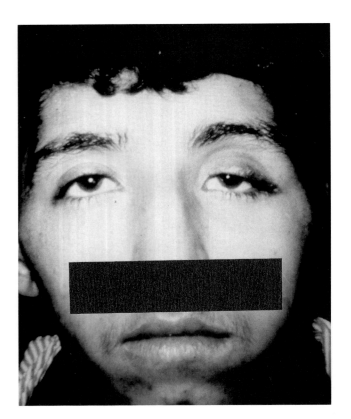

Fig. 15-2. Plexiform neuroma of the left orbit and temporal region. (Photograph courtesy of Dr. Edward Deglin.)

defects of the angle or disturbed metabolism has been suggested because of involvement of the ciliary nerves. Anterior displacement of the iris root may cause it to contact the posterior cornea, yielding angle closure.[16] Grant and Walton[17] have described some generalizations. They note that, usually, glaucoma occurs in neurofibromatosis in the presence of palpable and visible neurofibromas in the lid as well as facial hemihypertrophy on the involved side. They also note that 50 percent of cases of plexiform neuroma are associated with congenital glaucoma of the ipsilateral eye. They drew three conclusions regarding the mechanism. First, neurofibroma infiltrate the angle and obstruct the outflow of aqueous, a mechanism that occurs early in life (before age 2 years). Second, thickening of the choroid and the ciliary body pushes the iris forward, which causes stretching and enlargement of the cornea from the increased intraocular pressure; this mechanism also occurs early in life. Third, fibrovascular formation within the angle results in peripheral anterior synechiae and neovascular glaucoma; this mechanism occurs later in life.

Orbital neurofibroma can result in proptosis.[18] Orbital tumors can be fibroma molluscum or plexiform neuromas. Both can result in proptosis and displacement of the globe or extraocular muscle palsies, or both. Tumors of the optic nerve can result in a globe that protrudes straight forward and can be associated with optic atrophy and an enlarged optic canal. Posterior orbital encephalocele may occur and cause pulsating exophthalmos.[19] Also reported are pulsation of the globe,[19] pulsating enophthalmos,[20] and intermittent exophthalmos.[21] The mechanisms of these phenomena are unclear.

Retinal tumors resemble those of tuberous sclerosis (see the section, *Tuberous Sclerosis*). Medullated nerve fibers have been described in patients with neurofibromatosis.[22] Shapland and Greenfield[23] described glial proliferation around the disc and in the peripheral retina. They postulated the presence of a metabolic agent derived from the tumor cells that stimulated this glial reaction.

Neurofibromatosis of the iris presents as multiple small brown raised nodules on the anterior stroma[24] (see Fig. 15-4 and Plate 15-2). These nodules, called *lisch nodules,* are histopathologically identical to the iris nodules often seen in patients without neurofibromatosis. Usually, the iris lesions are identified after the diagnosis of neurofibromatosis. The iris may be-

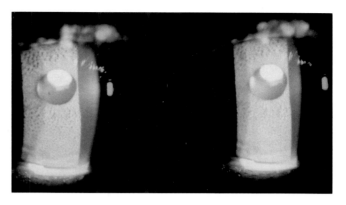

Fig. 15-4. Iris nodules in a patient with neurofibromatosis. (Photograph courtesy of Jane Stein.) (See also Plate 15-2.)

come atrophic, and the pupil may be decentered, possibly secondary to sympathetic nerve damage.[16] Heterochromia can result.

Optic atrophy can occur in patients with neurofibromatosis. This can result from papilledema secondary to increased intracranial pressure from an intracranial neurofibroma, or from an intraneural or intraorbital fibroma. Marshall[25] reports an increased frequency of glioma of the optic nerve and optic chiasm in individuals with neurofibromatosis.

Patient symptoms depend on the location and severity of the tumors. Treatment can include local excision when necessary, but the results are not good, and the prognosis is variable. Surgery should be avoided if possible.

TUBEROUS SCLEROSIS

Desir Maglore Bourneville,[26] a physician whose interest was in mentally retarded and epileptic children, first described tuberous sclerosis (Bourneville's disease) in 1880. The name arises from the multiple potato-like tumors in the cerebrum and other organs.[26] Tuberous sclerosis is a heredofamilial disease composed of a triad of signs: mental deficiency, epilepsy, and adenoma sebaceum. Psychiatrists call this triad *epiloia.* Males are most commonly affected.[27]

The diagnosis is usually made in this country in mental hospitals. According to Golden[28] tuberous sclerosis affects 1 in 30,000 persons. Thirty percent die by age 5, and 75 percent die by age 20.

Cutaneous lesions are usually the earliest sign of the disease. Adenoma sebaceum, the principle cutaneous lesion, presents as small reddish brown papules, 1 to 4 mm in diameter that form a butterfly pattern over the nose, cheeks, and nasolabial folds. A shagreen patch is usually seen on the back as a slightly elevated pigskin texture or "orange-peel" textured area. White macules, termed *ash leaf* lesions, are pathognomonic of tuberous sclerosis and are often the first sign of the disease.[29–31] The term *ash leaf* arises from the linear oval shape of the lesions, which have one rounded end and one pointed end. They are found on the trunk and limbs of 86 percent of patients with tuberous sclerosis. They can range in size from 1 mm to several centimeters and can range in number from very few to 75.[32] Nevi, moles, fibromas, and café-au-lait spots can also be evident on the skin. Small fibromas, Coeren's tumors, can be localized to the sides of the nails on the fingers and toes.

Systemic findings include rhabdomyosarcoma of the heart, tumors of the thyroid, kidney, uterus, and intestines, as well as congenital defects such as spinabifida, ectopic testes, and horseshoe kidney.[31]

Ocular Findings

The most common ocular finding is the astrocytic hamartoma, which presents in the retina, usually in the posterior pole, although it can be anywhere. The astrocytic hamartoma is a gray-white lesion with mulberry-like nodules (Fig. 15-5 and Plate 15-3). It is usually about 1 disc diameter in size and is composed of hyaline material, which may have areas of calcification. If calcification is present, the astrocytic hamartoma will be visible radiologically. The lesion originates in the nerve fiber layer and can extend to the ganglion cell layer but not below. There is no effect on surrounding vasculature and no retinal reaction. Growth, if any, is slow. The astrocytic hamartoma may metastasize within the eye by seeding. A piece may pinch off and travel in the vitreous to another area of the retina, where it triggers new growth. Salom, in Messinger and Clarke,[33] listed four other types of retinal changes seen in tuberous sclerosis: (1) yellowish red spots, (2) blurred pigmented spots, (3) clearly outlined nevoid spots and nevi, and (4) pigmented changes identical to those occurring in other types of retinitis. Additional retinal tumors have been described as oval circular white or gray areas in the retinal periphery that resemble medullated nerve fibers but are rather dull in appearance.

Other ocular findings include optic nerve head drusen and vitreous clouding, as well as white pedunculated tumors of the palpebral conjunctiva and yellowish red thickenings of the bulbar conjunctiva.

ENCEPHALOTRIGEMINAL ANGIOMATOSIS

The complete form of encephalotrigeminal angiomatosis (Sturge-Weber syndrome)—a triad of skin, eye, and brain involvements—was first described by Sturge[34] in 1879 and then by Weber[35] in 1922. The syndrome is characterized by a cutaneous nevus (venous angioma) along the distribution of the branches of the cranial nerve V, hemangiomas of the ipsilateral meninges and choroid, and unilateral, congenital glaucoma. In some cases epilepsy, hemiplegia, and areas of intracranial calcification may be present. Many incomplete forms of the syndrome also occur: (1) Schirmer syndrome, oculocutaneous angiomatosis with late glaucoma; (2) Lawford syndrome, oculocutaneous angiomatosis with glaucoma; (3) Milles syndrome, oculocutaneous angiomatosis with choroidal angiomatosis without glaucoma; (4) Krabbe syndrome, encephalotrigeminal angiomatosis; and (5) Jahnke syndrome, neuro-oculocutaneous angiomatosis without glaucoma.[36] In contrast to the other phakomatoses, the mode of inheritance is not clear.

The most striking feature of Sturge-Weber syndrome

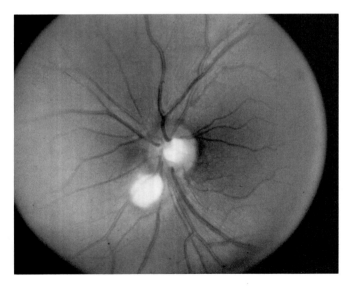

Fig. 15-5. Astrocytic hamartoma. (Photograph courtesy of Jane Stein.) (See also Plate 15-3.)

is the skin lesion: a flat, venous hemangioma often called *nevus flammeus* or *port-wine stain* because of its brilliant deep red or purple color. The lesion is usually unilateral and most often lies over the distribution of the first branch of the trigeminal nerve. Often the eyelid is involved. Occasionally, the nevus will overlay the distribution of the first and second branches of the trigeminal nerve, but only rarely does it involve all three branches. The lesion usually does not cross the midline. It can be pale in color, rendering it harder to recognize, but the affected skin has a raised and uneven texture, which aids in detection. The nevus is often present at birth but can become more apparent during early childhood. The lesion may affect the nasal mucosa, buccal mucosa, and/or conjunctiva. Occasionally, localized hemihypertrophy of the involved tissues is present. Forty percent of affected patients have vascular hyperplasia of the cheeks and lips. Less common cutaneous manifestations are (1) disseminated angiomas and nevi, (2) varices of the legs and arms, and (3) café-au-lait spots.[31]

The most prominent encephalogic feature of Sturge-Weber syndrome is angiomas of the meninges, which are present on the same side as the facial nevus. The angiomas may cause convulsions, usually occurring on the contralateral side to the lesion. The convulsions may cause recurrent hemiplegia or hemiparesis. Mental retardation may be present, ranging from mild deficiency to complete amentia. Treatment is aimed at controlling the seizures.

Ocular Findings

Glaucoma is the most notable ocular manifestation of Sturge-Weber syndrome. Facial nevi coexist with glaucoma, and both may be associated with intracranial lesions, although any of these may occur independently.[37] Authors have suggested that angiomas of the lids or conjunctiva are most likely associated with glaucoma.[38] Glaucoma may be present from birth, but the precise pathogenesis is not known. Berkow[39] describes an abnormal anterior chamber angle with the longitudinal muscle of the ciliary body inserted anterior to the scleral spur in a Sturge-Weber patient. Other theories suggest abnormal sympathetic innervation to the eye or increased episcleral venous pressure. Choroidal hemangioma has been exhibited in many patients with facial nevi and glaucoma whose eyes were enucleated for glaucoma.[37] Choroidal hemiangioma presents as a yellowish, elevated circular area that disappears or diminishes with scleral

depression. This can be difficult to see clinically, which is why they are often detected only after enucleation; fundus fluorescein angiography, however, can be helpful in identifying them. Other ocular findings include telangectasia of the iris, conjunctiva, and episclera. Telangectasias of the iris may result in heterochromia, with the affected side having more pigmentation than the nonaffected side. Hebold[40] reports two instances in which the pupil was larger on the side opposite the cutaneous lesion. Retinal vessels can show tortuocity and dilation. Visual field defects, mainly homonymous hemianopsia contralateral to the facial nevus, have been reported.[41]

Treatment is aimed at controlling the glaucoma, although the results are usually disappointing. Medical or surgical treatment is usually necessary to control the neurologic involvement. The prognosis for most patients with Sturge-Weber syndrome is poor; most die in the second or third decade of life.

WYBURN-MASON SYNDROME

Wyburn-Mason syndrome is not traditionally considered a phakomatosis. The syndrome is characterized by retinal and central nervous system involvement with arteriovenous malformations, also termed *racemose hemangiomas* and *cirsoid aneurysms*. In 1874, Magnus[42] first reported involvement of the retinal vessels. The vessels appear dilated and tortuous and bulge forward from the retina. In 1943, Wyburn-Mason[43] reported a series of cases from which he concluded that arteriovenous malformations of the retina were likely to be paired with intracranial arteriovenous malformations. These associated arteriovenous malformations all involve the retina as well as the following: (1) the orbit and optic nerve, causing proptosis, bruits, and dilation of conjunctival vessels; (2) the ipsilateral maxilla, pterygoid fossa, and mandible, causing severe epistaxis and oral hemorrhage; (3) the ipsilateral basifrontal area and sylvian fissure, causing epilepsy, intracranial hemorrhage, hemiplegia, and hemianopsia; and (4) the posterior fossa, causing cranial nerve or brainstem involvement.[19]

Retinal arteriovenous malformations are usually monocular. The vessels become enlarged and tortuous, such that differentiating the artery from the vein is difficult (Fig. 15-6 and Plate 15-4). The malformations are most often located in the midperiphery and are surrounded by creamy white fibrous glial tissue that engulfs the vessels. Vision can range from normal to

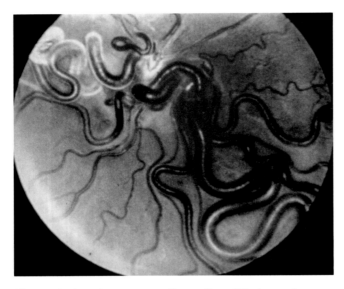

Fig. 15-6. Arteriovenous malformation. (Photograph courtesy of Dr. Edward Deglin.) (See also Plate 15-4.)

very poor, although the visual capacity of the eye is usually unchanged. The lesions are not associated with glaucoma and almost never bleed. Histologically, the affected vessels become so large that they occupy the entire thickness of the retina and protrude anteriorly into the vitreous. The retina shows cystic degeneration between the vessel walls.

The differential diagnosis include Sturge-Weber syndrome and angiomatosis retinae. Sturge-Weber syndrome exhibits choroidal changes that could be confused with arteriovenous anastomoses. Wyburn-Mason syndrome does not, however, include glaucoma or skin lesions, which are found in Sturge-Weber syndrome. Early angiomatosis retinae could be confused with arteriovenous malformations, but angiomatosis retinae will eventually bleed and exude, whereas arteriovenous malformations do not change over time.

Because arteriovenous malformations usually do not deteriorate, no ocular treatment is necessary once a definitive diagnosis has been made.

REFERENCES

1. Van der Hoeve J: The Doyne memorial lecture: eye symptoms in phakomatoses. Trans Ophthalmol Soc UK 52:380, 1932
2. von Hippel E: Uber eine sehr Erkrankung der Netzhaut. Arch Ophthalmol 59:83, 1904
3. Lindau A: Studien uber Kleinhirncysten. Bau, Pathogenese und Beziehungen zur Angiomatosis Retinae. Acta Pathol Microbiol Scand, suppl. 1:1, 1926
4. Lindau A: Zur Frage der Angiomatosis retinae und ihrer Hirnkomplikationen. Acta Ophthalmol 4:196, 1927
5. von Recklinghausen FD: Ueber die multiplen Fibrome der Haut und ihre Beziehung zu den multiplen Neuromen. Hirschwald, Berlin, 1882
6. Brain WR: Diseases of the Nervous System. Oxford University Press, London, 1933
7. Rosendal T: Some cranial changes in Recklinghausen's neurofibromatosis. Acta Radiol 19:373, 1938
8. Kulvin MM: Surgical repair of neurofibromatosis of eyelid. Am J Ophthalmol 32:1231, 1949
9. Heard G: Nerve sheath tumors and von Recklinghausen's disease of the nervous system. Ann R Coll Surg Engl 31:229, 1962
10. Weber FP, Perdrau JR: Periosteal neurofibromatosis with a short consideration of the whole subject of neurofibromatosis. Q J Med 23:151, 1930
11. Crowe FW, Schull WJ: Diagnostic importance of cafe-au-lait spots in neurofibromatosis. Arch Intern Med 91:758, 1953
12. Adams RD, Reed WB: Neurocutaneous diseases. p. 1393. In Fitzpatrick TB et al (eds): Dermatology in General Medicine. McGraw-Hill, New York, 1971
13. Allende FP: Diffuse neurofibromatosis involving the bulbar conjunctiva. Arch Ophthalmol 33:110, 1945
14. Anderson JR: Hydrophthalmia or Congenital Glaucoma: Its Causes, Treatment and Outlook. Cambridge University Press, London, 1939
15. MacMillan JA, Cone WV: Solitary neurofibroma of the orbit. Arch Ophthalmol 10:51, 1933
16. Davis FA: Plexiform neurofibromatosis (Recklinghausen's disease) of the orbit and globe with associated glioma of the optic nerve. Report of a case. Arch Ophthalmol 22:761, 1939
17. Grant WM, Walton DS: Distinctive findings in glaucoma due to neurofibromatosis. Arch Ophthalmol 79:127, 1968
18. Moore JG: Neonatal neurofibromatosis. Br J Ophthalmol 46:682, 1962
19. Walsh FB, Hoyt WF: Clinical Neuro-ophthalmology. 3rd Ed. Williams & Wilkins, Baltimore, 1969
20. Dabezies OH, Walsh FB: Pulsating enophthalmos in association with neurofibromas of the eyelid. Trans Am Acad Ophthalmol Otolaryngol 3:885, 1961
21. Mayfield FH, Wilson CB: The pathological basis for postural (intermittent) exophthalmos: case report. J Neurosurg 26:619, 1967
22. Moore AE: Neurofibromatosis associated with proptosis and defect of orbital wall. Aust N Z J Surg 5:314, 1936
23. Shapland CD, Greenfield JG: A case of neurofibromatosis with meningeal tumor involving the left optic nerve. Trans Ophthalmol Soc UK 55:257, 1935
24. Goldstein I, Wexler D: Melanosis uveae and melanoma of the iris in neurofibromatosis (Recklinghausen). Arch Ophthalmol 3:288, 1930
25. Marshall D: Glioma of the optic nerve. Am J Ophthalmol 37:15, 1954
26. Bourneville DM: Sclerose tubereuse des circonvolutions serebrales: idiote et epilepsie hemiplegique. Arch Neurol 1:81, 1880
27. Cockayne EA: Inherited Abnormalities of the Skin and Its Appendages. Oxford University Press, London, 1933
28. Golden, GS: Tuberous sclerosis. Minn Med 47:881, 1964
29. Gold AP, Freeman JM: Depigmented nevi, the earliest sign of tuberous sclerosis. Pediatrics 35:1003, 1965
30. Fitzpatrick TB, Szabo G, Hori Y, et al: White leaf-shaped macules: earliest sign of tuberous sclerosis. Arch Dermatol 98:1, 1968
31. Tasman W, Tager E: Duane's Clinical Ophthalmology. Revised. JB Lippincott, Philadelphia, 1992
32. Critchley M, Earl CJC: Tuberose sclerosis and allied conditions. Brain 55:311, 1932

33. Messinger HS, Clarke BE: Retinal tumors in tuberous sclerosis; review of the literature and report of a case with special attention to microscopic structure. Arch Ophthalmol 18:1, 1937
34. Sturge WA: A case of partial epilepsy, apparently due to a lesion of one of the vaso-motor centers of the brain. Trans Clin Soc Lond 12:162, 1879
35. Weber FP: Right-sided hemi-hypotrophy resulting from right-sided congenital spastic hemiplegia with morbid condition of left side of brain, revealed to radiograms. J Neurol Psychopathol 3:134 (Aug), 1922
36. Francois J: Heredity in Ophthalmology. CV Mosby, St. Louis, 1961
37. Dunphy EB: Glaucoma accompanying nevus flammeus. Am J Ophthalmol 18:709, 1935
38. Anderson JR: Hydrophthalmia or Congenital Glaucoma, Its Causes, Treatment, and Outlook. Cambridge University Press, London, 1939
39. Berkow JW: Retinitis pigmentosa associated with Sturge-Weber syndrome. Arch Ophthalmol 75:72, 1966
40. Hebold O: Haemangiom der weichen Hirnhaut bei Naevus vasculosus des Gesichts. Arch Psychiatr Nervenkr 51:445, 1913
41. Tyson HH: Nevus flammeus of face and globe associated with glaucoma, vascular changes in the iris, and calcified vascular growth in the left occipital lobe of the brain, with right homonymous hemianopsia. Arch Ophthalmol 8:265, 1932
42. Magnus H: Aneurysma arterioso-venosum retinate. Virchows Arch A Pathol Anat Histopathol 60:38, 1874
43. Wyburn-Mason R: Arteriovenous aneurysm of midbrain and retina, facial naevi and mental changes. Brain 66:163, 1943

16 Allergy

SUSAN E. MARREN

CASE REPORT

A 25-year-old white woman presented complaining of itchy eyes that watered slightly. When asked, she admitted to a runny nose and sinus congestion. The nasal symptoms had not disturbed her as much as the ocular symptoms, however. She had discontinued soft contact lens wear 2 weeks before, which brought some relief, but she was still somewhat uncomfortable.

She reported similar occurrences in past springs but she had not been so uncomfortable as to seek care. She had a mildly atopic history; some lotions and cosmetics had caused itching and redness in the past. She had not been able to trace her present problems to any new product and had stopped using eye makeup at the same time that she stopped wearing contact lenses. We ruled out common allergens: new carpet, new pets, and new detergent or fabric softener. With the pollen count at its highest in years and a history of mild seasonal recurrences, the diagnosis seemed most likely to be seasonal allergic conjunctivitis.

As is often the case, slit lamp examination provided very little corroborating evidence. Her tear film appeared trashy but of a normal volume. No blepharitic flakes were seen. The meibomian glands were free flowing, and the expressant was clear and free of particles. A mild papillary hypertrophy of the upper and lower tarsal conjunctiva was noted. Grade 1[+] hyperemia of the bulbar and tarsal conjunctiva was present with no hyperemia or scaling of the skin of the adnexa.

These findings ruled out dry-eye syndrome, contact dermatitis, and blepharitis, all of which can confuse the diagnosis of seasonal allergic conjunctivitis.

She rated the itching at 7 on a scale of 1 to 10 and confessed to some vigorous eye rubbing at night when she removed her spectacles. We explained to her that the eye rubbing causes mast cell release, which only intensifies the itch[1] and recommended cold compresses instead, along with a mild topical decongestant–antihistamine combination. Because some relief can be obtained for ocular symptoms by oral treatment, and because she clearly had a concomitant allergic rhinitis, we recommended an over-the-counter oral antihistamine–decongestant combination to relieve symptoms. She was to refrain from contact lens wear and use of eye cosmetics until she showed significant improvement.

At follow-up our patient was much happier. Our slit lamp findings were almost unchanged, but she reported significantly less itching and tearing. We suggested she continue with the topical decongestant–antihistamine four times per day, cold compresses as needed for itching, and the oral medication until she noticed the symptoms abating. I wanted to see her again before she resumed contact lens wear. I allowed her to resume use of hypoallergenic cosmetics.

She came back in 1 month ready to resume contact lens wear. We explained that some care systems are more suitable for people with allergies and switched her to a peroxide system, emphasizing the importance of weekly enzymatic treatments. We also suggested she return in advance of the next year's hay fever season to initiate cromolyn treatment and hopefully forestall the discomfort she had suffered this year.

SEASONAL ALLERGIC CONJUNCTIVITIS

Seasonal allergic conjunctivitis (SAC) is typified in the preceding case report. It is usually mild, associated with mild-to-moderate itching and injection. Tearing or a minor amount of white mucus (or both) may be present. The patient may complain of some photophobia[2] and burning.[3] Patients with SAC are usually sensitive to pollens. Those sensitive to grass pollens tend to suffer in May and June, and those sensitive to ragweed are more likely to suffer in August and September.[3,4]

Pathophysiology

SAC is considered to be largely a type 1 hypersensitivity, which is known by several names: immediate, humoral, anaphylactic, or immunoglobulin E (IgE)-mediated. The classic type 1 hypersensitivity is the reaction to pollen seen in hay fever. Other classic examples are asthma, allergy to penicillin, and bee sting.

In type 1 sensitivity, the first exposure to an antigen causes manufacture of IgE antibodies that are specific for that antigen. The IgE antibodies bind to mast cells.[5] When the specific antigen or allergen is reintroduced, it binds with two adjacent IgE antibodies, bridging them. This causes the membrane of the mast cell to become more permeable to the influx of calcium ions. After several intervening steps, the cell releases vasoactive amines, including histamine, eosinophil chemotactic factor of anaphylaxis, and kinins.[6] In addition, the change in the membrane allows the formation of the precursors of prostaglandins, thromboxanes, and leukotrienes.[2] All of these are involved to some extent in the inflammatory reaction that follows. For example, eosinophil chemotactic factor causes an influx of eosinophils, which can, in turn, cause basophils to release histamine. A type 1 hypersensitivity reaction therefore can be muddied by a basophil-mediated reaction, which is more classically a type 4 hypersensitivity.

Differential Diagnosis

No clinical signs whatsoever may be noted in SAC, and the condition may be remarkably similar to a mild dry eye or blepharitis. The seasonal nature and lack of clinical evidence for dry eye or blepharitis are helpful in these cases. Any history of allergic rhinitis, eczema, or food allergies also contributes to the diagnosis of allergic conjunctivitis.[7] Viral conjunctivitis can be expected to show a more follicular than papillary reaction in the tarsal conjunctiva and should be accompanied by preauricular lymphadenopathy. The cardinal symptom of any allergic condition is itching, and often the differential diagnosis can be based on the degree of itching the patient reports.

Treatment

Because most treatment is centered around mast cells and histamine release, most of this discussion concerns these. It is important to understand, however, that allergy is a very complex arena and not fully understood.

Histamine release in the eye is known to cause itch, redness, tearing, and chemosis.[5] The mast cells that are known to release histamine are considered the "sentinel" cells of the body, being clustered around the natural openings of the body.[2] The external eye, except the cornea, is richly supplied with mast cells.

The first order of treatment for any allergic condition is to avoid the allergen that precipitated the attack. The allergen must be identified correctly and then eliminated from the environment. This cannot always be done, and, indeed, one of the setbacks in immunotherapy results from a failure to correctly identify all allergens. When the allergen is airborne, avoidance is often impossible. Immunotherapy is possible in many cases and is discussed later in this chapter; however, it is said to be less successful in treating ocular allergy than allergic rhinitis.[3,7,8]

Because SAC tends to be mild and is self-limited, treatment is primarily to alleviate symptoms. Drugs with potentially dangerous side effects are contraindicated. Irrigation with an artificial tear and cold compresses may bring relief. A topical vasoconstrictor such as naphazoline hydrochloride can be prescribed as often as five times per day. Because naphazoline can raise intraocular pressures slightly, it may not be advisable for some glaucoma patients.[5] A topical antihistamine may also block some of the effects of histamine that result in itching and vasodilation. One to two drops every 3 to 4 hours is recommended for the pyrilamine maleate, pheniramine maleate, and antazoline phosphate preparations commercially avail-

Table 16-1. Antihistamine–Decongestant Topicals Available by Prescription

Drug Name	Active Ingredient(s)	Concentration (%)
Albalon A	Antazoline phosphate,	0.5
	naphazoline hydrochloride	0.05
Naphcon A	Pheniramine maleate,	0.3
	naphazoline hydrochloride	0.025
Prefrin A	Pyrilamine maleate,	0.1
	phenylephrine hydrochloride	0.12
Vasocon A	Antazoline phosphate,	0.5
	naphazoline hydrochloride	0.05

able.[5] Some available preparations are listed in Tables 16-1 and 16-2.

Oral antihistamines bring some relief and are especially helpful in the presence of an accompanying rhinitis.[3,9] The drowsiness typically caused by antihistamines tends to be greatly reduced in two recently developed drugs, terfenadine (Seldane) and astemizole (Hismanal), both available by prescription. Both drugs have been shown to be of some benefit in allergic rhinoconjunctivitis.[10] Over-the-counter antihistamines may be helpful to the patient at nighttime, when drowsiness is a more tolerable side effect (Table 16-3).

Cromolyn sodium inhibits the release of the vasoactive amines from the mast cells as well as the formation of prostaglandins and leukotrienes. It is said to stabilize the mast cell.[2] Cromolyn has been used for many years for asthma,[11] and in recent years has been

Table 16-2. Over-the-Counter Topical Decongestants

Drug Name	Active Ingredient(s)	Concentration (%)
Allerest Eye Drops	Naphazoline hydrochloride	0.012
Allergy Drops	Naphazoline hydrochloride	0.012
	polyethylene glycol 300	0.2
Clear Eyes	Naphazoline hydrochloride	0.012
Comfort Eye Drops	Naphazoline hydrochloride	0.03
Degest 2	Naphazoline hydrochloride	0.012
Naphcon	Naphazoline hydrochloride	0.012
VasoClear	Naphazoline hydrochloride	0.02
VasoClear A	Naphazoline hydrochloride,	0.02
	zinc sulfate	0.25

Table 16-3. Oral Antihistamines Available Over-the-Counter

Drug Name	Ingredient(s)
Chlor-Trimeton	Chlorpheniramine maleate
Benadryl	Diphenhydramine (available under many brand names)
Dimetane	Brompheniramine maleate

successfully used in treating patients with seasonal and perennial allergic rhinitis.[12–14] Other mast cell stabilizers, nedocromil sodium 2 percent, and lodoxamide tromethamine, are being tested for ocular allergies[15,16] and vernal conjunctivitis.[17] Cromolyn is considered to be very safe,[18] and the minor adverse reactions are rare.[19] These consist of conjunctival injection, watery eyes, itchy eyes, dryness around the eye, puffy eyes, eye irritation, and stye formation.

Cromolyn takes time to have an effect and is best given in anticipation of a seasonal exacerbation. Even in an acute allergic episode, however, cromolyn 4 percent may be initiated four to six times daily in conjunction with or shortly after initiation of one of the vasoconstrictor–antihistamine combinations. Once the cromolyn begins to have an effect, the other drugs may be tapered off and discontinued.[3]

Steroids may be used concomitantly with cromolyn, and in fact, cromolyn use often allows the steroids to be tapered or discontinued.[20,21] Again, because of their severe side effects and because SAC is mild and self-limited, steroids are limited to only the "most severe and recalcitrant cases."[3] Steroids should not be permitted in the presence of contact lens wear.[22]

ALLERGIC RHINITIS

Allergic rhinitis is the most common form of atopic disease with estimates of prevalence ranging from 5 to 22 percent. The symptoms are sneezing, runny nose, nasal congestion, and itchy nose and eyes.[8] Because many patients suffering with allergic conjunctivitis also have allergic rhinitis, some notes about its treatment seem warranted. For the patient with seasonal allergic rhinitis, pharmacologic treatment makes the most sense. See Tables 16-3 and 16-4 for over-the-counter preparations. Patients who cannot tolerate the medications, however, might benefit from immunotherapy.

Table 16-4. Over-the-Counter Oral Antihistamine–Decongestant Combinations

Drug Name	Antihistamine	Decongestant
Actifed	Triprolidine hydrochloride	Pseudoephedrine hydrochloride
Allerest	Chlorpheniramine	Phenylpropanolamine maleate
Contac	Chlorpheniramine	Phenylpropanolamine maleate
Dimetapp	Brompheniramine	Phenylpropanolamine maleate
Drixoral	Dexbrompheniramine maleate	Pseudephedrine sulfate
Sudafed Plus	Chlorpheniramine maleate	Pseudephedrine hydrochloride

For those optometrists with little experience beyond ocular conditions, it is important to note the rising use of topical steroid sprays for the nose as a first line of treatment for ocular allergy. Unlike topical ocular steroids and systemic steroids, nasal steroids are almost completely free of side effects. The control offered is excellent, and the main reason they are not in greater use is that some patients are resistant to spraying the nose.[8]

PERENNIAL ALLERGIC CONJUNCTIVITIS

A condition that is very similar to SAC though somewhat milder is perennial allergic conjunctivitis (PAC). As the name implies, the condition is generally year-round, although there may be seasonal exacerbations.[23] In SAC, the causative allergens are usually pollens, and their seasonal release accounts for the seasonal nature of the disease. In PAC the sensitivities are more likely to be to molds, dust mites, animal dander, feathers,[3] and even foods.[6] Their ubiquitous nature explains the chronicity of the disease.[3] PAC is also more likely than SAC to be associated with perennial allergic rhinitis.[23]

Differential Diagnosis

The differential diagnosis again is generally based on a lack of evidence to support blepharitis or dry eye. Sometimes a patient will have both PAC and blepharitis. The blepharitis must be cleared up first; fortunately, this usually ameliorates the symptoms somewhat, even in PAC. Differentiating early dry eye and PAC may be largely based on the subjective evaluation of the itching.

I have treated one patient with a past history of severe vernal conjunctivitis whose case presented an especially puzzling differential diagnosis. The major clue that led me to believe he had a dry eye was the very mild degree of itching he reported. However, because he had been diagnosed with vernal conjunctivitis as a young man, I felt that his idea of what constituted "moderate" itching might have been colored by that experience. I recommended he alternate artificial tears and a new, mild over-the-counter topical decongestant weekly and report back on which one offered the most relief. When he returned, he said they were equal in relieving his symptoms, from which I concluded he had a mild dry eye and continued only the artificial tears.

Treatment

Treatment for PAC is the same as for SAC. Elimination of the antigen where possible is the first recommendation. This is more easily accomplished if the antigens are dust or animal dander.[3] Topical vasoconstrictors, antihistamines, and mast cell stabilizers often bring relief. Oral antihistamines may help, especially with concomitant rhinitis, as in approximately 75 percent of cases.[23] Experimental evidence supports the value of immunotherapy in treatment of allergy to mold.[24]

Allergen immunotherapy is a process in which the patient is tested for specifically which antigens cause an allergic reaction. Then, very small amounts of that antigen are injected under the skin in increasing doses over time, resulting in a reduced response of the body to natural exposure to the antigen. Success depends on exact identification of the antigens—no easy task. Sometimes symptoms return after immunotherapy is stopped.[25] Furthermore, patients make a significant investment of dollars and time, with no guarantees. Ocular allergy is less responsive than allergic rhinitis and asthma. However, many patients with multiple significant allergic involvements (e.g. allergic rhinitis and allergic conjunctivitis), are profoundly relieved by immunotherapy.[25] Patients who cannot be managed medically without inducing undesirable side effects should be referred for consultation and testing. Today there is some experimentation with and controversy about oral immunotherapy, as well.[26–28]

VERNAL CONJUNCTIVITIS

Vernal conjunctivitis is an uncommon, seasonally recurrent, bilateral allergic inflammation of the conjunctiva. It occurs more commonly in warm, dry climates such as Greece, Italy, Israel, parts of South Africa, and parts of the Southwestern U.S. The disease usually begins before the age of ten; twice as many sufferers are males as females.[29] The disease is most common in the spring, early summer, and fall[30] but some patients suffer year-round. The disease generally lasts 4 to 10 years. There is often a family history of atopy: infantile eczema, allergic rhinitis, or asthma.[2]

The symptoms of vernal conjunctivitis are severe itching that worsens as the day wears on,[2,29] burning, photophobia, and ropy discharge. In addition, some patients complain of foreign body sensation, ptosis, and matting of the lids. Sometimes the mucus is so thick and tenacious that it forms a pseudomembrane over the upper lid.[3]

There are two forms of vernal conjunctivitis: the limbal form and the palpebral form (Figs. 16-1 and 16-2 and Plates 16-1 and 16-2). Usually, features of both are present, but one or the other form predominates. In the limbal form, gelatinous swellings of the upper limbal conjunctiva occur; the swelling may form a sort of hood that overhangs the cornea by a couple of millimeters. The palpebral form is characterized by papil-

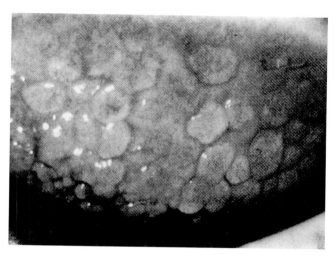

Fig. 16-2. Palpebral vernal conjunctivitis. Note the cobblestone appearance of the papillae on this everted upper lid. (See also Plate 16-2.)

lary hypertrophy, which may be mild at first but eventually forms huge cobblestones with tiny twigs of vessels in the center.[30] The papillae are usually greater than 1 mm in diameter and, in severe disease, fluorescein staining on the tips of the apices may occur. In chronic disease, white lines of scarring that run parallel to the lid margin, known as Arlt's lines, may be seen on the palpebral conjunctiva of the upper lid.

Horner-Trantas dots are associated with vernal conjunctivitis. These are chalky white concretions of eosinophils. They used to be considered pathognomonic for vernal conjunctivitis but have been reported in giant papillary conjunctivitis as well.[31] The Horner-Trantas dots generally last about 1 week.[32]

The feature of vernal conjunctivitis that causes the most discomfort is corneal involvement. The usual picture is a superficial punctate keratitis of the superior cornea. Small patches of necrotizing epithelium in the same area may be noted, however. This condition is known as *keratitis epithelialis vernalis of Togby.*[30] Small grayish white epithelial opacities in the same area are known as *farinaceous epithelial keratitis.*[32] Micropannus often results from vernal conjunctivitis; full pannus, rarely.

Less commonly, the cornea is involved to the extent of ulceration, a so-called shield ulcer, which is in the oval shape of a shield, is shallow, with grayish white

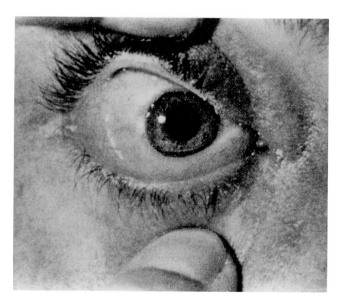

Fig. 16-1. Limbal vernal conjunctivitis. Note the limbal papilla. (See also Plate 16-1.)

Table 16-5. Numbers of Mast Cells in Conjunctiva of Normal and Vernal Conjunctivitis Patients

	Normals	Vernal
Number of mast cells in conjunctival substantia propria	5,000/mm^3	9,000/mm^3
Number of mast cells in upper tarsal conjunctiva	0	16,000/mm^3

borders and necrotic debris in the center. Stromal infiltrates are associated, and the ulcer may scar.[30]

Patients with vernal conjunctivitis often are sensitive to grass pollens, although desensitization has not proven beneficial as yet. Patients usually have a family history of atopy.[33] Vernal conjunctivitis in the younger patient may have some relationship with atopic keratoconjunctivitis (AKC) that develops as the patient ages.[34] Patients often have a personal history of infantile eczema, allergic rhinitis, or asthma, but vernal conjunctivitis can occur in the nonatopic patient as well.[2]

The number and distribution of mast cells in the conjunctiva of the patient with vernal conjunctivitis differ markedly from normal (Table 16-5). When it is remembered that mast cell degranulation is the precursor to itching, it is not remarkable that the itch of vernal conjunctivitis may be quite severe. In fact, vernal conjunctivitis is one of the diseases associated with eye rubbing implicated in the development of keratoconus.

Differential Diagnosis

The differential diagnosis of vernal conjunctivitis from AKC can be based on the location of the more severe involvement, which will be superior in vernal conjunctivitis and inferior in AKC. In addition, vernal conjunctivitis patients are usually younger and are more likely to report seasonal exacerbations. Differentiating vernal conjunctivitis from giant papillary conjunctivitis (GPC) can usually be based on the history of chronic use of a foreign body, such as a contact lens or ocular prosthesis, as the instigating factor for GPC. Table 16-6 provides a summary of the differential diagnosis of vernal conjunctivitis from GPC and AKC. Differentiating vernal conjunctivitis from SAC may be based on the greater severity of signs and symptoms in the former.[22]

Table 16-6. Differential Diagnosis of GPC, Vernal Conjunctivitis, and AKC

	GPC	Vernal	AKC
Itch	+	+ +	+ + +
Age of patient	Any; typically adolescence to 50s	3–20	20–50
History of contact lens wear	+	–	–
History of dermatitis	–	±	+ +
Papillary hypertrophy	+ + Upper lid	+ + Upper lid	+ Lower lid
Corneal involvement	±	+	+ + +

Abbreviations: AKC, atopic keratoconjunctivitis; GPC, giant papillary conjunctivitis.

Treatment

Treatment of vernal conjunctivitis consists of cold compresses or even ice packs if the swelling is very severe, topical vasoconstrictors–antihistamines, and mast cell stabilizers. In addition, moving to a cold, moist climate and use of air conditioning are generally beneficial if possible.[2] Topical or systemic steroids may be needed to stop the cycle of the itch and are usually necessary to control corneal involvement.[22,35]

Typically, severe disease is treated with steroids, such as 1 percent prednisolone every 2 hours, until the cornea clears. Then the steroid is tapered while the mast cell stabilizer and decongestant–antihistamine combination are continued. Moderate disease is treated with steroids as often as twice daily until the symptoms diminish; the steroid then is tapered, and the patient is controlled with the mast cell stabilizer and decongestant–antihistamine combination. When the disease seems to have remitted, many eye care practitioners continue to prescribe the mast cell stabilizer prophylactically for some time, depending on the patient's tendency to experience recurrences.[2,3]

The risks of using steroids must be weighed. We know topical steroids cause glaucoma and cataracts and permit secondary infection. Therefore, treatment depends mainly on the mast cell stabilizers and the decongestant–antihistamine combination with the steroids used in pulses only as needed.

Oral administration of aspirin for vernal conjunctivitis has been reported. The risks of Reye syndrome for young patients, gastritis, decreased platelet function, and exacerbation of asthma must be considered before recommending aspirin.[4,36,37] Topical cyclosporine, a nonsteroidal immunomodulating agent, has been used in patients with vernal conjunctivitis who were refractory to conventional treatment.[38] At the time of this writing, cyclosporine was considered too expensive to use in any but the most recalcitrant cases. An extreme form of treatment that has been successfully used on some refractory patients is surgical mucous membrane grafting. In this procedure, mucous membrane from the lower lip was grafted over the tarsus following removal of the diseased tissue.[39]

ATOPIC KERATOCONJUNCTIVITIS

AKC is a keratoconjunctivitis associated with atopic dermatitis. In fact, 25 percent of patients with atopic dermatitis develop AKC.[22] Patients are usually men, aged 29 to 47. The disease may begin in late adolescence and last through the 40s or 50s. Itching is moderate to severe and year-round, little affected by changes of season. Burning and tearing with a watery or mucopurulent discharge also occurs.[2] Some patients complain of photophobia and dryness.[22,29]

The lid margins are indurated and lichenified; the palpebral conjunctiva of the lower lid is more involved than the upper lid and shows a papillary hypertrophy. The bulbar and palpebral conjunctiva will be inflamed, chemotic, and thick. The papillae are generally not as large as those seen in vernal conjunctivitis. Follicles in the lower cul de sac may also be present.[29] The patient typically has a concurrent atopic dermatitis, often affecting the upper lids.[2] The bulbar conjunctiva is usually hyperemic and chemotic.[4]

AKC can be blinding due to the severe corneal involvement that is possible with this condition. This may range from a punctate epithelial keratitis, usually of the lower third of the cornea, to ulceration, scarring, and pannus with vascularization. AKC is associated with keratoconus and posterior and anterior subcapsular cataracts.[2,4] Trantas dots have been reported.[40] Conjunctival scarring can be so severe as to displace or stenose the puncta and induce ectropion or entropion and trichiasis.[22]

A secondary staphylococcal blepharitis is often present. Herpes simplex keratitis seems to be more prevalent in AKC patients. The tendency toward secondary infection is probably related to the disordered immunity thought to occur in AKC.

Pathophysiology

AKC is believed to be related to type I immediate hypersensitivity and type IV delayed hypersensitivity reactions.[3] It is probably less understood than vernal conjunctivitis or GPC, and the prognosis for improvement is much worse.[22] The cause of AKC is unknown. Foster et al.[41] describe AKC as a "complex immunoregulatory dysfunction at the local ocular level."

Mast cells are found in the epithelium of the conjunctiva and in the fibrovascular core of the papillae in the lower tarsal conjunctiva in AKC, whereas no mast cells are found in the conjunctival epithelium of control subjects.[42]

Differential Diagnosis

Differentiating AKC from blepharitis can be difficult because there is often a concomitant blepharitis with AKC. The itch of AKC is more severe than that expected in blepharitis. The indurated and macerated eyelids and any associated eczema suggest a diagnosis of AKC. Vernal conjunctivitis is associated with more involvement in the upper lid as opposed to the lower lid involvement of AKC; vernal conjunctivitis is found in younger patients than in AKC; and is more likely to be associated with warm, dry weather (Table 16-6).

Treatment

Treatment of AKC depends on steroids to alleviate symptoms and prevent blindness. Pulses of topical steroids in addition to antihistamines and mast cell stabilizers are the typical treatment. Cold compresses may help the severe itch. Sometimes systemic steroids are needed to control the disease.

The blepharitis must be controlled as best as possible with lid hygiene and bland antibiotic ointment.[3] Some cases may require the addition of low-dose systemic tetracycline.[43]

Ulcerative blepharitis can frequently accompany AKC. Compelling evidence suggests that this finding is symptomatic of candida infection, necessitating scrapings and cultures when ulcerative blepharitis fails to respond to treatment.[44]

GIANT PAPILLARY CONJUNCTIVITIS

GPC is very similar in appearance to the palpebral form of vernal conjunctivitis. GPC is chiefly characterized by the formation of papillae larger than 0.3 mm in diameter on the palpebral surface of the upper lid, with hyperemia, and mucus. These papillae usually form first in the zone nearest the fold. Later, papillae form in the zones closer to the lid margin (Fig. 16-3) and Plate 16-3). An exception to this formation pattern occurs when the irritant causing the papillary hypertrophy is a localized irritant (e.g., a suture) as opposed to a coated contact lens surface.[45] The conjunctiva is also hyperemic. One case has been reported of GPC that resembled the limbal form of vernal conjunctivitis with limbal inflammation and Trantas dots.[46] In later stages, mucus can be visualized between the papillae, and the tops of the larger papillae form craters and the apices stain with fluorescein.[47] White, scar-like heads may be noted on the papillae; these regress as the papillae regress. The conjunctival epithelium thickens initially, while still translucent. Later, it may become so densely infiltrated by inflammatory cells that it becomes opaque, and the underlying vasculature is no longer visible.[48]

GPC occurs in wearers of polymethylmethacrylate (PMMA) and rigid gas-permeable (RGP) lenses, as well. In PMMA wearers, GPC tends to resemble that seen with sutures and other localized foreign bodies. That is, scattered hyperemic giant papillae are interspersed with more normal-looking, smaller papillae. In RGP-associated GPC, the papillae are smaller and fewer in number than those seen with soft lens GPC, and they occur nearer the lid margin or in the central zone. The apices are more likely to be flattened and cratered in GPC associated with hard or rigid lenses than with soft lenses.

Symptoms are itching (especially on lens removal), mucus formation, increased lens awareness, excessive lens movement, and even dislocation. The doctor may note that the contact lens centers higher than when originally fitted, in severe cases even baring the inferior cornea. GPC is always associated with a foreign body in the eye,[47] usually a contact lens but also ocular prostheses or sutures. Therefore, it has been called an iatrogenic disease.[49]

The role of atopy in susceptibility to GPC is unclear. Some researchers find a relationship[42,46–48] whereas others do not. I believe that a patient with a history of atopy should be cautioned, at the very least, that contact lens wear may be uncomfortable or even impossible during allergic episodes, and that stringent care measures must be followed to avoid the development of GPC. Similarly, because I have seen focal GPC-type reactions to focal irritants such as nicks or large deposits, I urge replacement of such lenses, regardless of the degree of irritation. Clearly, some patients are more susceptible, and it is interesting to note that monkeys who had contact lenses from GPC patients sutured to their upper lids developed signs similar to GPC while those monkeys who similarly "wore" lenses from asymptomatic patients remained free of signs.[50]

Pathophysiology

The most well-known and widely accepted model for understanding GPC was developed by Allansmith.[48] This theory holds that the foreign body is not itself antigenic but that it becomes coated with tear proteins, which become altered and induce an allergic reaction of the cutaneous basophilic type (a variation of type 4 hypersensitivity). There are also arguments for GPC as a type 1 hypersensitivity based on the numbers of eosinophils, degranulated mast cells, and immunoglobulins seen. Clearly, however, GPC requires at least 3 weeks to develop, which indicates a more delayed hypersensitivity. The presence of eosinophils has been associated with both type 1 and type 4 hypersensitivities and can even be induced by trauma without immunologic challenge. Moreover, type 1 hy-

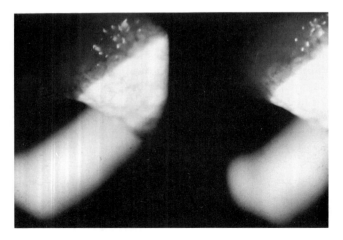

Fig. 16-3. Giant papillary conjunctivitis. Note the rounded papillary hypertrophy as contrasted to the flattened papillae of vernal as seen in Fig. 16-2. (See also Plate 16-3.)

persensitivity is associated with transient acute edema, which is not a feature of GPC.[47]

Type 4 hypersensitivity is also known as the tuberculin type, cellular, cell-mediated, or delayed hypersensitivity reaction. It differs from type 1 hypersensitivity in that no immunoglobulins are involved; the antigen reacts with sensitized T lymphocytes. The classic is the Mantoux tuberculin reaction, which is used to test for exposure to tuberculosis. Another classic example is contact dermatitis. A second type 4 hypersensitivity is cutaneous basophil hypersensitivity, also known as the Jones Mote reaction. This is not well understood but is believed to be a delayed hypersensitivity reaction with a primarily basophilic infiltrate occurring transiently 24 hours after cutaneous rechallenge with the sensitizing antigen.

Evidence also indicates that mechanical trauma contributes to GPC.[51,52] Greiner[53] reported on a patient with an epithelialized foreign body of 8 months' duration. The patient reported no symptoms of itching, mucus, or foreign body sensation. Papillae were formed on the part of the upper lid that would have been in contact with the epithelialized foreign body. The tissue between and surrounding the papillae was hyperemic. Because the foreign body was completely covered by epithelium, there was no antigenic challenge from a coated foreign body in contact with the lid. Within 1 month of removal of the foreign body, the papillary response had resolved.[53]

The contact lens may become coated with an antigen, the trauma of the coated contact lens against the conjunctiva may alert the immune system to the presence of the antigen, and so effects from both trauma and hypersensitivity are present.[22]

Differential Diagnosis

Of basic importance in diagnosing vernal conjunctivitis or GPC is the ability to differentiate between a papillae and a follicle. Follicles are usually found in the lower tarsus, with the exception of inclusion conjunctivitis. Papillae will usually have several blood vessels in their centers as well as around the base, whereas follicles have only the blood vessels around the base. The walls of follicles are more sloping as compared to the more columnar cobblestone appearance of the papillae.

Usually, differentiating vernal conjunctivitis from GPC is not a problem, because vernal conjunctivitis patients are young, usually male, and usually are not wearing contact lenses when the disease develops. GPC is always associated with some foreign body in the eye. In addition, the itch in vernal conjunctivitis is much more profound than the itch in GPC. Further, vernal conjunctivitis is more likely to be associated with a punctate keratitis than is GPC (Table 16-6).

Part of diagnosing GPC at an early stage and preventing it from becoming problematic is careful scrutiny of the upper tarsal conjunctiva. The best means to delineate papillary hypertrophy is by instillation of fluorescein and evaluation with a cobalt light. The fluorescein stains the mucus, if present, and pools around the base of the papillae, setting them in relief and making the number and size of the papillae much easier to judge (Fig. 16-4 and Plate 16-4). The tissue

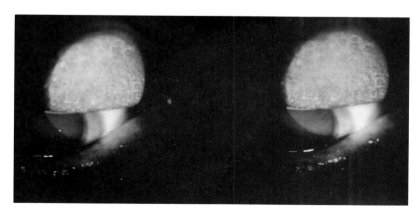

Fig. 16-4. Giant papillary conjunctivitis. Fluorescein helps delineate the papillae by pooling around the bases. Note also the staining of the apices. (See also Plate 16-4.)

should also be viewed with white light to look for infiltration and hyperemia.[22,54]

Treatment

The theories about pathology discussed above have a role in considering treatment. Mechanical trauma is assumed to be from two sources in contact lens wearers, both the lens edge and the surface of discrete deposits on the lens. Consequently, part of the recommendation for management includes changing the fit of the lenses and replacing lenses frequently enough to avoid excessive contact between discrete deposits and the eyelid. Different polymers are known to have different levels of attraction for coatings and deposits. Therefore, a polymer different from that which the patient was wearing when the GPC developed is often recommended. Furthermore, because mast cells are found in conjunction with GPC, mast cell stabilizers are used to help control the GPC in patients for whom the above changes are not sufficient.[55–57] GPC resolves without pharmacologic treatment when the offending agent is removed. This is easily accomplished with contact lenses, although it is not always the most welcome alternative to the patient, and indeed, in cases of extreme refractive error, is an understandably unwelcome solution.

Treatment depends on the stage at which the GPC is diagnosed. Stage 1 GPC is characterized on routine check-up by an elicited history of mild itch following lens removal but no mucus formation; the only sign is mild, small papillary hypertrophy. Probably the only treatment necessary is enhanced lens cleanliness with a more effective daily cleaner and weekly use of a protein-specific enzymatic cleaner. The patient should also be advised to watch for recurrence of the itching, excessive lens awareness, and mucous formation. If increased hygiene alone is not sufficient, or if the lenses are more than 6 months old, replace the lenses with identical clean lenses.

Stage 2 GPC features minor pain and discomfort with lens wear, sticky eyelids on waking, itching, increased lens awareness, and mild blurring after hours of wear. If the lenses are very old, simply replacing them with clean, new lenses and instituting the care regimen recommended below may suffice. Chances of success are increased, however, by refitting the patient in a different polymer and design.[3]

Stage 3 GPC adds an increase in the excessive move-

ment of the lens with the blink and accumulation of mucus during lens wear. In stage 4, the patient has grown intolerant of the lenses. Pain or severe foreign body sensation forces the patient to abandon lens wear. Sometimes the upper lid is so affected as to cause a pseudoptosis.

If the lens decenters on the blink, or if you see fluorescein staining of the apices of the papillae, heavy mucus on the conjunctiva, or significant tarsal hyperemia, the patient must discontinue lens wear.[3,4] Most symptoms will resolve after about 5 days. Allansmith[48] suggests refitting 3 to 5 days after symptoms have abated. Some authors recommend at least a month without contact lenses.[3,4] At the very least, the conjunctiva should be free of injection, and no corneal staining should be observed.[3] The papillary hypertrophy will remain unchanged for some time.

Some doctors recommend pharmacologic assistance during this period of withdrawal. Cromolyn may be used and then continued as maintenance after contact lens wear is reinstituted. No adverse effects of cromolyn use in the presence of contact lens wear have been reported.[58] The cromolyn may be initiated at four times per day and then tapered to the point that any further reduction results in an exacerbation of symptoms.[32] Allansmith[48] also points out that some patients are helped by irrigating the conjunctiva with sterile nonpreserved saline two or three times per day after contact lens wear is reinstituted.

Some authors have advocated a short course of mild steroids if the inflammation is severe; others warn that steroids are ineffective in GPC.[3,4,48,59]

Lens care following the refit should avoid further aggravation by any antigens. Most authors recommend hydrogen peroxide systems,[48] daily cleaning with an effective cleaner not preserved with thimerosal, and once- or twice-weekly enzymatic cleaning. Nonpreserved saline in aerosol spray cans is helpful. Chemical disinfection systems should be avoided because of the possibility that the preservative/disinfectant can become antigenic. Moreover, Allansmith[48] cautions that placing a contact lens soaked in chemicals on a compromised conjunctiva is "too great an insult." Heat is thought to bake on deposits, altering tear proteins, and making them more antigenic. Most authors agree that heat disinfection should be avoided.[48] Allansmith[48] recommends papain as the most effective and best tolerated of the enzymes. However, the subtilisin A enzyme, which acts in peroxide, is very convenient and is probably as effective.

Again, the patient may benefit from frequent replacement programs and should at least be watchful for the first tell-tale post-wear itch. Those in frequent replacement programs may safely avoid the enzyme cleaning step but must remain scrupulous in daily cleaning all the same. With extended wear, the antigenic-coated contact lens is in contact with the upper lid for too long a period of time. Therefore, extended wear is strictly contraindicated in GPC. Follow-up for GPC patients should be more often than for routine patients: Donshik and Ehlers[22] recommend every 3 months.

On occasion, GPC cannot be adequately controlled with the preceding measures. Sometimes, because of the decentering effect that the papillae exert on the lens, the patient cannot be adequately refitted with soft contact lenses. In these cases, an RGP lens may be tried. Care should be taken to minimize edge thickness, and the polymers that have a greater propensity to attract protein deposition should be avoided. A smaller lens diameter would be reasonably expected to carry less antigenic load. RGP lenses are easier to keep clean than soft lenses and are smaller in diameter. However, GPC does occur in RGP wearers and even PMMA wearers as well,[60] so scrupulous care must be taken. Donshik and Ehlers[22] recommend the

fluoropolymers for patients who develop GPC while wearing silicon acrylate.

Prosthetic eyes may be cleaned with the same cleaners used to clean rigid contact lenses, and some patients even use enzyme treatments on their prostheses. They can also be held against the sponge tool on a contact lens modification unit and polished clean. If hygiene improvement fails to control symptoms and a new plastic prosthesis does not bring relief, evidence indicates that glass prostheses are not associated with GPC, possibly because they do not last as long as plastic.[61]

CONTACT ALLERGY

Pathophysiology

Contact allergy is a type 4, or delayed, hypersensitivity. It is local and mediated by sensitized T lymphocytes, therefore requiring some time to develop. Sensitivity may develop as early as 5 to 10 days or may occur after years of exposure. When an allergic reaction takes place, it may become evident within 12 hours of the exposure or as long as 72 hours later, but usually it is between 24 and 48 hours.

The most common causes of contact allergy of the conjunctiva or eyelid are ingredients of ophthalmic preparations and cosmetics[62,63] (Fig. 16-5 and Plate

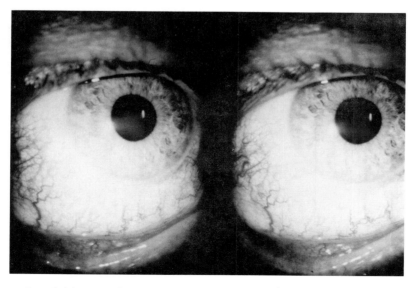

Fig. 16-5. Toxic conjunctivitis secondary to topical antibiotic administration. (See also Plate 16-5.)

16-5). Major offenders in ophthalmic drugs are neomycin, bacitracin, the sulfonamides, epinephrine, anticholinergics such as atropine, miotics such as pilocarpine, and antivirals. Papain, thimerosal, and chlorhexidine have been implicated in reports of allergic conjunctivitis.

Cosmetic ingredients that tend to be sensitizing are lanolin and lanolin derivatives, p-phenylenediamine, and propylene glycol, as well as many of the fragrances and preservatives. Allergic reactions can also occur to chemicals used in various sectors of industry; the classic cause of type 4 hypersensitivity, poison ivy, can also affect the eyes.[29]

The allergic reaction may be isolated to the conjunctiva, especially in contact lens solution allergies, or to the eyelid, as in cosmetic allergies. An allergic dermatoconjunctivitis with both conjunctival and eyelid involvement may occur. Sometimes keratitis is also noted. Patients complain of itching, which may be severe, burning, red swollen eyelids, and excessive tearing. With corneal involvement, patients will also report photophobia. Signs are redness, scaling, and edema of the eyelid skin. Papules or vesicles, crusting, or oozing may also be present. The conjunctiva may be injected and chemotic.[29] A follicular hypertrophy[3] or corneal infiltrates[64] may be noted.

Differential Diagnosis

If scaling and edema of the eyelids are observed, the diagnosis is usually evident. If lid involvement is only minimal, however, the condition may resemble SAC or PAC. In these cases, patient history of onset is more important. Toxic conjunctivitis can be similar; in this case the onset more closely follows exposure,[3] and the itching is usually less severe.

Treatment

Treatment depends on primarily identifying and removing the offending antigen. This requires a careful history. For conjunctival irritation, a topical lubricant and cold compresses will bring some relief. A topical antihistamine may help in more moderate cases,[29] for severe cases, a topical steroid may be indicated.[22] For lid involvement, oral antihistamines, cold compresses, and, if severe, a topical steroid in a cream base may be necessary.[29]

REFERENCES

1. Greiner JV, Peace DG, Baird RS, Allansmith MR: Effects of eye-rubbing on the conjunctiva as a model of ocular inflammation. Am J Ophthalmol 100:45, 1985
2. Allensmith MR, Ross RN: Ocular allergy and mast cell stabilizers. Surv Ophthalmol 30:229, 1986
3. Ehlers WH, Donshik PC: Allergic ocular disorders: a spectrum of diseases. CLAO J 18:117, 1992
4. Donshik PC: Allergic conjunctivitis. Int Ophthalmol Clin 28:294, 1988
5. Hegeman SL: Antihistaminic drugs. p. 299. In Bartlett JD, Jaanus SD (eds): Clinical Ocular Pharmacology. Butterworth, Boston, 1984
6. Stites DP: Basic and Clinical Immunology. Lange Medical Publications, Los Altos, CA, 1982
7. Kari O, Salo OP, Bjorksten F, Backman A: Allergic conjunctivitis total and specific IgE in the tear fluid. Acta Ophthalmol (Copenh) 63:97, 1985
8. Naclerio RM: Allergic rhinitis. N Engl J Med, 325:860, 1991
9. Juniper EF, Carier A, Trebilcock AL et al: Effects of oxatomide compared with chlorpheniramine in allergic rhinoconjunctivitis. Clin Allergy 11:61, 1981
10. Juniper EF, White J, Dolovich J: Efficacy of continuous treatment with astemizole (Hismanal) and terfenadine (Seldane) in ragweed pollen-induced rhinoconjunctivitis. J Allergy Clin Immunol 82:670, 1988
11. Berman BA, Ross RN: Cromolyn: a review. Clin Rev Allergy 1:6, 1983
12. Chandra RK: Double-blind controlled crossover trial of 4% intranasal sodium cromoglycate in patients with seasonal allergic rhinitis. Ann Allergy 49:131, 1982
13. Hasegawa M: The effect of sodium cromoglycate on the antigen-induced nasal reaction in allergic rhinitis as measured by rhinometry. Clin Allergy 6:359, 1976
14. Pelikan Z, Pelikan-Filipek M: The effects of disodium cromoglycate and beclomethasone dipropionate on the immediate response of the nasal mucosa to allergen challenge. Ann Allergy 49:283, 1982
15. Blumenthal M, Casale T, Dockhorn R et al: Efficacy and safety of nedocromil sodium ophthalmic solution in the treatment of seasonal allergic conjunctivitis. Am J Ophthalmol 113:56, 1992
16. Friedlaender MH: Immunologic aspects of diseases of the eye. JAMA 268:2869, 1992
17. Bonini S, Barney NP, Schiavone M et al: Effectiveness of nedocromil sodium 2% eyedrops on clinical symptoms and tear fluid cytology of patients with vernal conjunctivitis. Eye 6:648, 1992
18. Toogood JH: Multicenter surveillance of long-term safety of sodium cromoglycate. Acta Allergol, suppl. 13:S44, 1977
19. Ostler HB: Alpha-1-antitrypsin and ocular sensitivity to cromoglycate. Lancet 2:1287, 1982
20. Friday GA, Biglan AW, Hiles DA et al: Treatment of ragweed allergic conjunctivitis with cromolyn sodium 4% ophthalmic solution. Am J Ophthalmol 95:169, 1983
21. Ostler HB, Martin GR, Dawson CR: The use of disodium cromoglycate in the treatment of atopic ocular disease. p. 99. In Leopold IH, Burns RP (eds): Symposium on Ocular Therapy. Wiley, New York, 1977
22. Donshik PC, Ehlers WH: The contact lens patient and ocular allergies. Int Ophthalmol Clin 31:133, 1991
23. Dart JKG, Buckley RJ, Monnickenda M et al: Perennial allergic conjunctivitis: definition, clinical characteristics and prevalence. Trans Ophthalmol Soc UK 105:513, 1986
24. Karlsson R, Agrell B, Dreborg S et al: A double-blind, multicenter immunotherapy trial in children, using a purified and standardized Cladosporium herbarum preparation. Allergy 41:141, 1986
25. Creticos PS: Immunotherapy with allergens. JAMA 268:2834, 1992

26. Orbanek R, Burgelin KH, Kahle S et al: Oral immunotherapy with grass pollen in enterosoluble capsules: a prospective study of the clinical and immunological response. Eur J Pediatr 149: 545, 1990

27. Bjorksten B, Moller C, Broberger U et al: Clinical and immunological effects of oral immunotherapy with a standardized birch pollen extract. Allergy 41:290, 1986

28. Moller C, Dreborg S, Lanner A: Oral immunotherapy of children with rhinoconjunctivitis due to birch pollen allergy, a double blind study. Allergy 41:271, 1986

29. Jennings B: Mechanisms, diagnosis, and management of common ocular allergies. J Am Optom Assoc, suppl. 61:S32, 1990

30. Wallace W: Diseases of the conjunctiva. p. 583. In Barlett JD, Jaanus SD (eds): Clinical Ocular Pharmacology. Butterworth, Boston, 1984

31. Buckley RJ: Pathology and treatment of giant papillary conjunctivitis. II. The British perspective. Clin Ther 9:451, 1987

32. Goen TM, Siebolt K, Terry JE: Cromolyn sodium in ocular allergic diseases. J Am Optom Assoc 57:526, 1986

33. Duke-Elder S: Diseases of the Outer Eye: Conjunctiva. In Duke-Elder S (ed): System of Ophthalmology. Vol. 8. CV Mosby, St. Louis, 1965

34. Jay JL: Clinical features and diagnosis of adult atopic keratoconjunctivitis and the effect of treatment with sodium cromoglycate. Br J Ophthalmol 65:335, 1981

35. Rice NSC, Easty DL, Garner A et al: Vernal keratoconjunctivitis and its management. Trans Ophthalmol Soc UK 91:483, 1971

36. Abelson MD, Butrus SI, Weston J: Aspirin therapy in vernal conjunctivitis. Am J Ophthalmol 95:502, 1983

37. Meyer E, Kraus E, Zonis S: Efficacy of antiprostaglandin therapy in vernal conjunctivitis. Br J Ophthalmol 71:497, 1987

38. Bleik JH, Tabbara KF: Topical cyclosporine in vernal conjunctivitis. Ophthalmology 98:1679, 1991

39. Tse DT, Mandelbaum S, Epstein E et al: Mucous membrane grafting for severe palpebral vernal conjunctivitis. Ophthalmology 101:1879, 1983

40. Friedlander MH: Diseases affecting the eye and skin. p. 76. In: Allergy and Immunology of the Eye. Harper & Row, Hagerstown, MD, 1979

41. Foster CS, Rice BA, Dutt JE: Immunopathology of atopic keratoconjunctivitis. Ophthalmology 98:1190, 1991

42. Morgan SJ, Williams JH, Walls AF et al: Mast cell hyperplasia in atopic keratoconjunctivitis: an immunohistochemical study. Eye 5:729, 1991

43. Tuft SJ, Kemeny DM, Dart JKG et al: Clinical features of atopic keratoconjunctivitis. Ophthalmology 98:150, 1991

44. Huber-Spitzy V, Bohler-Sommeregger K, Arocker-Mettinger E, Grabner G: Ulcerative blepharitis in atopic patients—is Candida species the causative agent? Br J Ophthalmol 76:272, 1992

45. Korb DR, Greiner JV, Finnemore VM, Allansmith MR: Biomicroscopy of papillae associated with wearing of soft contact lenses. Br J Ophthalmol 67:733, 1983

46. Meisler DM, Krachmer JH, Goeken JA: An immunopathologic study of giant papillary conjunctivitis associated with an ocular prosthesis. Am J Ophthalmol 92:368, 1981

47. Allansmith MR, Korb DR, Greiner JV et al: Giant papillary conjunctivitis in contact lens wearers. Am J Ophthalmol 83:697, 1977

48. Allansmith MR: Giant papillary conjunctivitis. J Am Optom Assoc, suppl. 61:S42, 1990

49. Mackie IA, Wright P: Giant papillary conjunctivitis—an iatrogenic disease resembling vernal conjunctivitis. p. 524. In Pepys J, Edwards AM (eds): The Mast Cell: Its Role in Health and Disease. Pitman Medical, London, 1979

50. Ballow M, Maenza R, Yamase H, Donshik PC: An animal model for contact lens-induced giant papillary conjunctivitis. Invest Ophthalmol Vis Sci 28:39, 1987

51. Ehlers WH, Donshik PC, Gillies C et al: The induction of an inflammatory reaction (similar to giant papillary conjunctivitis) by chemotactic factors derived from conjunctival cells. Invest Ophthalmol Vis Sci, suppl. 31:S241, 1990

52. Hann LE, Cornell-Bell AH, Marten-Ellis C, Allansmith MR: Conjunctival basophil hypersensitivity lesions in guinea pigs: analysis of upper tarsal epithelium. Invest Ophthalmol 27:1255, 1986

53. Greiner JV: Papillary conjunctivitis induced by an epithelialized corneal foreign body. Ophthalmologica 196:82, 1988

54. Mandell RB: Contact Lens Practice: Basic and Advanced. Charles C Thomas, Springfield, IL, 1965

55. Molinari JF: Giant papillary conjunctivitis management in hydrogel contact lens wearers. J Br Con Lens Assoc 3:94, 1982

56. Meisler DM, Berzins UJ, Krachmer JH, Stock EL: Cromolyn: treatment of giant papillary conjunctivitis. Arch Ophthalmol 10:1608, 1982

57. Smolin G, O'Conner GR: Ocular Immunology. Lea & Febiger, Philadelphia, 1981

58. Donshik PC, Ballow M, Luistro A et al: Treatment of contact lens-induced giant papillary conjunctivitis. CLAO J 10:346, 1984

59. Spring TF: Reactions to hydrophilic lenses. Med J Aust 1:449, 1974

60. Douglas JP, Lowder CY, Lazorik R, Meisler DM: Giant papillary conjunctivitis associated with rigid gas permeable contact lenses. CLAO J 14:143, 1988

61. Mackie IA, Wright P: Giant papillary conjunctivitis (secondary vernal) in association with contact lens wear. Trans Ophthal Soc UK 98:6, 1978

62. Hatinen A, Terasverta M, Fraki JE: Contact allergy to components in topical ophthalmological preparations. Acta Ophthalmol 63:424, 1985

63. Eiermann HJ, Larsen W, Maibach HI et al: Prospective study of cosmetic reactions: 1977–1980. J Am Acad Dermatol 6:909, 1982

64. Sendele DP: Chemical hypersensitivity reactions. Int Ophthalmol Clin 26:25, 1982

17 Substance Abuse

JOHN L. BAKER

INTRODUCTION

Drug abuse refers to the use of illegal substances as well as the inappropriate and usually excessive use of licit substances. Despite programs directed at preventing drug use and treating drug abusers, drug abuse continues to be an urgent social problem and significant national health crisis.[1] Current discussions about health care costs and management include containing the spread of acquired immunodeficiency syndrome (AIDS) and hepatitis, both of which can in part be attributed to drug abuse.

Many factors contribute to drug abuse. Curiosity, peer pressure, escape from everyday problems, feelings of alienation from society, and rejection of the establishment are frequently noted reasons. The psychological characteristics of abusers and drug availability are also important considerations.[1]

The cardiac, pulmonary, vascular, and cerebral systems are all susceptible to the direct toxic effects, allergic reactions, idiosyncratic responses, and side effects caused by drugs. Accelerated ventricular rhythm and pulmonary hypertension are complications seen in drug abusers that contribute to fatalities.[2,3] In cases of overdose, home remedies such as intravenous injection of milk or mayonnaise can contribute to mortality and morbidity in addicts.[4]

The manifestations of drug abuse, are not limited to their direct pharmacologic actions. Other manifestations result from infectious or embolic sources. Drug abusers often show a disregard for aseptic technique. Sharing injection paraphernalia and diluting drug materials in vehicles ranging from tap water to urine can cause a direct infusion of organisms into the bloodstream or subcutaneous tissue.[2-4]

Abused drugs can be inhaled, ingested, smoked, injected into the soft tissue, or injected directly into a vein. Subcutaneous and intravenous injections pose the most serious health risk to the drug abuser.

Drug abusers can be a difficult population to study. Their medical histories are often unreliable and can vary with each questioner.[4] Drug abusers will often attempt to conceal or minimize their history of abuse.

The ocular effects of drug abuse can be helpful in the identification of drug abusers. Common symptoms such as blurred vision, headaches, and eye pain may be indications of drug abuse and should be investigated thoroughly. Table 17-1 outlines the ocular effects of commonly abused drugs.[1,2] Other more serious consequences, such as emboli and infection, can contribute to significant visual loss.

Drugs and their contaminants can have a profound effect on a patient's health and visual status. It is imperative that the eye care provider recognize the ocular manifestations of drug abuse as early as possible so that appropriate counseling and medical evaluation can be initiated.

Table 17-1. Ocular Effects of Commonly Abused Drugs

Drug	Effects
Opiates Morphine Codeine Heroin Meperidine (Demerol) Methadone (Dolophine) Propoxyphene (Darvon) Pentazocine (Talwin) Fentanyl (Sublimaze) Butorphanol (Stadol) Nalbuphine (Nubain)	Pupil changes (extreme miosis) Decrease intraocular pressure Ptosis Nystagmus Diplopia Blurred vision Stevens-Johnson syndrome Increased accommodation
Marijuana	Visual and auditory hallucinations Diplopia Accommodation impairment Transient visual disturbance Photophobia Nystagmus Blepharospasm Lid and conjunctival congestion Dyschromatopsia Ciliary injection Reduced intraocular pressure
Stimulants Amphetamines Methylphenidate (Ritalin) Phenmetrazine (Preludin) Cocaine	Mydriasis with decreased pupil reaction Decreased accommodation and convergence Visual hallucinations Blue tinge to vision Posterior subcapsular cataracts Decreased vision Microaneurysms
Depressants Barbituates Nonbarbituate sedative-hypnotics Methaqualone (Qualude) Chloral hydrate Glutethimide (Doriden) Ethchlorvynol (Placidyl) Paraldehyde Benzodiazepines Antianxiety agents Diazepam (Valium) Chlordiazepoxide (Librium) Oxazepam (Serax) Flurazepam (Dalmane) Lorazepam (Ativan)	Irregularities of binocular coordination Loss of optokinetic response Pursuits replaced by low-amplitude saccades Nystagmus Optic atrophy Weakened convergence Ptosis Diplopia Dyschromatopsia Visual hallucinations Retinal vasoconstriction Bilateral retinal hemorrhage Conjunctival hemorrhage Nystagmus Blurred vision Nerve palsies Visual hallucinations
Hallucinogens LSD Mescaline Psylocibin Psilocin Phencyclidine (PCP) Dimethyltrytamine Diethyltrytamine 2,5-dimethoxy-4-methyl-amephetamine (DOM) 3,4-Methylene-dioxy-amphetamine (MDA) 3,4-Methylene-dioxy-methamphetamine (MDMA) 5-Methoxy-MDA (MMDA, ecstacy)	Vivid and bizarre hallucinations Ptosis Decreased corneal reflex Lack of spontaneous eye movements Papilledema Retinal hemorrhage Optic neuropathy Mydriasis Decreased accommodation Blurred vision
Inhalants Nitrous oxide (laughing gas) Organic compounds Industrial solvents Degreasers Aerosol propellants	Hyperemia Nystagmus Lacrimation Retinal hemorrhages Papilledema Optic atrophy

CASE REPORT

A 45-year-old man presented for a general eye examination because he had broken his reading-only glasses. The patient stated that his vision was good at distance without a correction. He began wearing reading glasses at his last eye examination 4 years ago. The ocular history was unremarkable. The patient denied previous eye problems and stated that other than his visit to the eye doctor 4 years ago, he had never had his eyes examined.

The patient also denied having any medical problems, although he was not currently under a physician's care. His last visit to a medical doctor was approximately 10 years ago. The patient appeared poorly nourished. He stated he was 5'11'' tall and weighed 145 pounds. He admitted his diet was "not good," that he drank a six-pack of beer every day, and smoked at least two packs of cigarettes a day. He denied previous treatment for alcohol and/or drug abuse.

Entering unaided visual acuity was 20/25^{-2} OU at distance and 20/40 at near. Pupil testing was normal, with round, reactive pupils in each eye and no afferent pupillary defect. Confrontation visual field testing was normal for each eye. There was no evidence of strabismus by unilateral cover test, but the patient lacked stereopsis with Randot testing and did not appreciate gross forms. Color vision testing was also reduced in each eye with Ishihara plates. The patient denied previous awareness of a color vision deficit and was able to identify objects in the examination room correctly by color.

A refraction revealed a minimal distance correction of pl $^-$0.50 × 090 OD and −0.25 −0.25 × 085 OS with no improvement in vision. A tentative add of +1.25 gave the patient 20/25 vision in each eye at near.

While this near prescription was being trial framed, the color vision and stereopsis were rechecked, but there was no improvement. D-15 color testing revealed random errors in each eye. Amsler grid testing at this time was also normal with no reported scotomas or metamophopsia.

Slit lamp examination was normal. Mild blepharitis was present in each eye, but the lids, cornea, conjunctiva, iris, and anterior chamber appeared healthy. Intraocular pressure by Goldmann applanation tonometry wa 16 mmHg OU. The blood pressure measured on the right arm while the patient was seated was 170/100 mmHg. More significant was the presence of scarring in a tracklike pattern in the antecubital fossa. The blood pressure was also checked on the left arm, with a result of 166/98 mmHg. Scarring was also present in the antecubital fossa of the left arm.

A dilated pupil examination revealed a clear lens in each eye. The peripheral retina was normal in each eye, with no evidence of neovascularization. The optic nerves of each eye were obliquely inserted with a temporal choroidal crescent. No evidence of optic nerve neovascularization was seen, but pallor of the temporal aspect of the optic nerve was questionably noted.

More striking was the appearance of small, glistening particles scattered in the posterior pole of each eye (Figs. 17-1 and 17-2 and Plates 17-1 and 17-2). No evidence of hemorrhage or exudate was seen.

On repeated questioning, the patient did admit to intravenous drug abuse starting when he was 19 and continuing for approximately 15 years. The patient stated he had been "clean" since that time, following incarceration and drug rehabilitation. Attempts to question this patient further about amount and frequency of drug abuse were unsuccessful.

The results of the eye examination were explained to the patient. A spectacle correction for reading-only glasses was provided to the patient at his request. The differential diagnosis for the cause of the decreased vision was toxic/nutritional amblyopia versus macular ischemia due to intravenous drug abuse. The patient was scheduled for a visual field test and fluorescein angiogram to determine the cause of the vision loss.

The patient was also advised to see a physician regarding his elevated blood pressure. The patient was advised of the possible systemic complications associated with intravenous drug abuse, particularly the pulmonary complications. The patient denied difficulty breathing and declined to schedule a medical appointment at our facility, stating he would consult his own physician.

The patient did not return for his scheduled follow-up appointments, and attempts to contact him were unsuccessful because the phone number and address he supplied us were inaccurate.

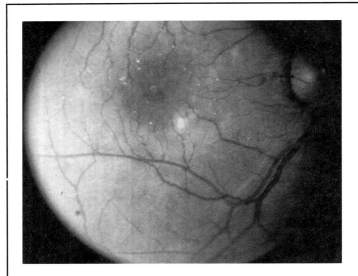

Fig. 17-1. Right eye. Note the small, refractile particles in the perimacular area. (See also Plate 17-1).

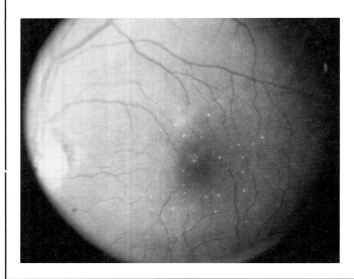

Fig. 17-2. Left eye. Note the talc particles trapped by the small arterioles in the perimacular area. (See also Plate 17-2).

SIGNS AND SYMPTOMS

Talc retinopathy results from the repeated intravenous injection of drugs intended for oral use (Fig. 17-2 and Plate 17-2). Talc retinopathy also results from the injection of illicit substances that have been diluted or "cut" with inert fillers. Crushed tablets are diluted with water to prepare a suspension suitable for injection. The suspension is often boiled and then passed through a crude filter. Typical materials include cigarette filters, cotton fibers, or gauze. The filtered material is then injected intravenously, subcutaneously, or intramuscularly.[5] The drug abuser experiences a subjective high or rush accompanied by a "talc flash" at the time of injection.[6] *Talc flash* refers to the phenomenon of perceived light flashes seconds after intravenous injection.[7] This effect can be heightened by injecting the suspension without passing it through a filter.[8]

The tablets generally contain inert fillers such as cornstarch and talc. Other fillers include lactose, sucrose, polyethylene glycol, tragacanth, and magnesium stearate.[9] Talc (hydrous magnesium silicate) has a crystalling structure and appears whitish to light green.[10]

Commonly injected substances include methadone

hydrochloride, methylphenidate hydrochloride (Ritalin), "blue velvet" (paregoric and tripelennamine hydrochloride), meperidine hydrochloride, oxycodone, opium, pentazocine, pentazocine (Talwin), and barbiturates.[9,11–13] (Multidrug abuse is common among drug abusers.[5])

The drug suspension gains access to the venous system through intravenous injection. The venous system returns the drug-contaminated blood to the auricle of the right side of the heart. After passing to the right ventricle, the blood is pumped via the pulmonary arteries to the lung. The vasculature of the lungs is composed of fine blood vessel networks with decreasing capillary lumen size. These fine capillaries allow arterialization (oxygenation) of the blood. The oxygenated blood is then returned to the left auricle of the heart via the pulmonary veins. After passing to the left ventricle, the blood is transported throughout the body by the systemic circulation. Complications of drug abuse, however, affect the lung more frequently than any other organ.[6]

The lumen size of the smallest pulmonary capillaries is known to be approximately 7 μm.[6] The suppliers of talc indicate that approximately 50 percent of talc particles are larger than 5 μm and approximately 25 percent are larger than 10 μm.[14] Particles of talc greater than 7 μm will become trapped in the lumen of the pulmonary capillaries. Initially, the systemic circulation is protected from larger talc emboli by the pulmonary vasculature. These small capillaries trap the larger particles and act as a filter.[15]

With repeated injection, the particles that lodge in the lung induce endothelial proliferation within the blood vessels and granuloma formation within the lungs. Talc is known to be capable of causing granulomatous lesions in tissue and was first described in tissue of postoperative patients in 1933.[16] This has been demonstrated by biopsy and autopsy studies.[6,17]

The granuloma formation causes further occlusion of larger arteries within the lung. These changes develop after chronic, long-term drug abuse. Interstitial fibrosis is the ultimate result, which causes diminished diffusion capacity, and is associated with lung stiffening in the advanced stages.[17] As a result of this obstruction, pulmonary vascular perfusion decreases, and resistance to perfusion increases. This results in angiothrombotic pulmonary hypertension.[13]

The major consequence of pulmonary hypertension is an increase in the work required by the right ventricle of the heart to pump blood through the pulmonary circulation. This increased work load can lead to cor pulmonale, a hypertrophy or failure of the right side of the heart. Cor pulmonale predisposes those affected to syncope (transient loss of consciousness), precordial pain (pain over the anterior surface of the body overlying the heart and lower thorax), and sudden death. Cardiac catheterization has demonstrated pulmonary hypertension caused by talc in drug abusers.[18]

The changes that develop in the lung are compounded by chronic drug use. As pulmonary hypertension increases, collateral blood vessels develop within the lung.[6]

The collateral circulation does not act as a satisfactory filter to drug fillers. Drug-contaminated blood bypasses the pulmonary circulation and gains access to the left side of the heart and thus the systemic circulation. With access to the systemic circulation, talc embolization occurs to many other organs, including the eye.[19] Other systems affected by talc emboli include the spleen, kidney, liver, bone marrow, skin, and lymph nodes.[9]

The ocular manifestations of intravenous drug abuse are noted in Table 17-2.[10–12,14,15,20]

Retinal deposits, known as *talc retinopathy*, are the most common ocular findings. The deposits are an embolic phenomenon caused by drugs and their contaminants. These deposits usually appear as tiny, glistening particles scattered throughout the fundus but concentrated in the macular region.[11]

In 1972 Atlee[11] was the first to describe particles scattered throughout the fundi in 17 known drug addicts.[11] The amount of particles was greater in addicts who had injected the greatest amount of drugs intra-

Table 17-2. Ocular Manifestations of Intravenous Drug Abuse

Retinal deposits
Macular ischemia
Peripheral retinal neovascularization
Optic disc neovascularization
Vitreous hemorrhage
Tractional retinal detachment

venously. His examination of these patients also described venous engorgement, blotch hemorrhages, and cotton-wool patches. Because the particles appeared to be in a linear arrangement, he suggested they were contained within smaller retinal blood vessels.

Following the death of one of his patients, Atlee[11] examined a microscopic stained section using polarized light, which revealed numerous birefringent particles in the capillaries of the nerve fiber and inner nuclear layers of the retina. He noted that these particles were characteristic of talc, which had been previously described in other organ systems. Vessel examination revealed talc in the capillaries, small arterioles, venules, and even choriocapillaris. Atlee found no evidence of granuloma formation.

Murphy et al.,[10] in 1978, reported 17 addicts who presented with the characteristic small, white, glistening dots concentrated most heavily in the macular area.

In 1979, Friberg et al.[14] presented a case report of a patient with decreased vision and central scotomas secondary to macular ischemia. Fluorescein angiography demonstrated absence of perifoveal capillaries, arteriolar attenuation, and tortuosity of small venules.

Friberg et al.[14] introduced the idea that the accumulation of talc in the retinal microvaculature resulted in direct occlusion of the retinal capillaries. They believed that the talc itself, or endothelial proliferation induced by the talc, led to the vaso-occlusive changes demonstrated by fluorescein angiography. Cerebral angiography in drug addicts had previously revealed small artery occlusive disease as the most common angiographic finding.[4]

Friberg et al.[14] believed that the acute stages of capillary occlusion led to the retinal hemorrhages and cotton-wool spots seen in some drug addicts.

Kresca et al.,[12] also in 1979, were the first to report peripheral retinal neovascularization and vitreous hemorrhage in a drug addict exhibiting characteristic talc retinopathy. Kresca et al.[12] suggest that although the posterior pole was more susceptible to the retinopathy because of the denser capillary net and greater blood flow in that area, blood flow had been reduced to a more critical level in the retinal periphery. They also suggest that the changes that developed secondary to vaso-occlusion disease resulting in peripheral neovascularization between areas of perfused posterior retina and nonperfused anterior retina could be a model for other vaso-occlusive diseases such as proliferative sickle cell retinopathy.

In 1979 in a case report, Brucker[20] corroborated the presence of peripheral retinal neovascularization with associated tractional retinal detachment and vitreous hemorrhage in a drug addict with talc retinopathy. His report also was important because he noted for the first time the presence of a fibrovascular membrane involving the optic nerve.

Schatz and Drake[6] in 1979 reported on 12 patients with talc particles located in the inner layers of the retina. Larger particles were noted in the retinal vessels, but smaller ones could be seen only when ophthalmoscopic photographs were correlated with well-resolved fluorescein angiograms. These authors also noted that, although vascular occlusion with capillary nonperfusion was not a common complication, it could occur and result in irreversible visual loss.

Schatz and Drake[6] also noted that talc particles probably caused retinal capillary endothelial damage that could result in capillary leakage seen on fluorescein angiography. This complication seemed to be greater when combined with systemic hypertension.

Tse and Ober[5] in 1980 reported their findings of 28 intravenous drug abusers. Their report was significant because it was the first to demonstrate all the peripheral vascular changes that are also seen in proliferative sickle cell retinopathy. These changes are noted in Table 17-3.

Tse and Ober[5] further supported the idea that the talc particles, when combined with endothelial proliferation and further embolization, lead to lumen occlusion.

Obstruction of blood vessels leads to sluggish blood flow and retinal ischemia, which causes neovascular

Table 17-3. Proliferative Peripheral Stages in Sickle Cell Retinopathy

Peripheral arteriolar occlusion
Peripheral arteriolar-venular anastomosis
Neovascular and fibrous proliferation
Vitreous hemorrhage
Retinal detachment

proliferation as seen in other vaso-occlusive disease. The fragile neovascular vessels are prone to breakage with resultant vitreous hemorrhage. Ultimately, vitreoretinal traction results in retinal detachment.

Tse and Ober[5] also note that the duration of drug abuse and cumulative number of tablets injected influenced the number of talc particles detected in the fundus and the severity of the retinopathy. Although lack of filtering contributed to the severity of the retinopathy, it did not significantly affect visual acuity. The authors point out that preservation of central vision is the rule rather than the exception, despite evidence of compromised macular perfusion.

DIFFERENTIAL DIAGNOSIS

The differential diagnosis for talc retinopathy is noted in Table 17-4.[6,10,14]

Gunn's Dots

Gunn's dots are tiny white or glistening colorless dots located at the level of the internal limiting membrane. They are concentrated most heavily in the posterior pole and are believed to be reflections arising from small elevations or depressions of the retinal surface. Similar to other retinal reflections, Gunn's dots become less conspicuous with age and may be absent by the third or fourth decade.[21] The amount of fundus pigmentation and higher refractive errors may limit their visibility. Gunn's dots may be confused with talc particles because they generally occur in the same age group.[10] Gunn's dots, however, will vary in size and appearance depending on the positioning of the examiner's light source.

Multiple Cholesterol Emboli

Multiple cholesterol emboli may resemble the mild form of talc retinopathy when only a few talc particles are present.[10] Associated with carotid vascular disease, Hollenhorst's plaques tend to be greater in size (10 to 250 μm[22]) because they do not have to pass through the respiratory circulation to gain access to the eye. Although cholesterol emboli often appear yellow-white and highly reflective like talc, they generally occur in older patients with other evidence of atherosclerotic disease, which usually allows them to be distinguished from talc. In addition, the distribution of talc in the retina tends to be symmetric between the two eyes compared to the bilateral and multiple distribution of cholesterol emboli.

Nephropathic Cystinosis

Nephropathic cystinosis is an autosomal recessive condition that is characterized by deposition of cystine in ocular and nonocular tissues. The diagnosis of this condition is usually established at a young age (1 or 2 years) because of continued vomiting that leads to dehydration.[23] Systemic complications include renal transplantation by 9 to 10 years of age in approximately 50 percent of those affected.[24] Ocular signs include crystal deposits in the corneal stroma, conjunctiva, iris, and anterior lens surface. The corneal deposits may lead to symptoms of light sensitivity secondary to epithelium breakdown.[25]

Retinal changes include pigment mottling at the level of the retinal pigment epithelium that may lead to pigment clumping and areas of depigmentation.[23] In addition crystal deposits within the retina may also be noted.[25] These crystals have been described as refractile and are believed to represent cystine crystals either in the choroid or pigment epithelium.[10]

Talc retinopathy is not usually confused with nephropathic cystinosis, because those affected with this condition manifest numerous systemic and ocular features not characteristic of talc retinopathy. The location of the crystals at the level of the pigment epithelium also helps distinguish them from the more superficial talc crystals.

Flecked Retina Syndrome

The flecked retina syndrome is a group of disorders that includes fundus albipunctatus, fundus flavimaculatus, and drusen.[26] Fundus albipunctatus is a stationary disorder characterized by yellow-white dots in the fundus and an abnormally slow rate of dark adaptation.[27] The presence of a congenital night blindness helps differentiate this condition from talc

Table 17-4. Differential Diagnosis for Talc Retinopathy

Gunn's dots
Multiple cholesterol emboli—Hollenhorst's plaques
Nephropathic cystinosis
Flecked retina syndrome
Oxalate crystals from methoxy-flurane anesthesia
Crystalline retinopathy
Tamoxifen retinopathy

retinopathy. Clinically, the retinal lesions in fundus albipunctatus appear to be at the level of the pigment epithelium.[28]

Fundus flavimaculatus is a condition characterized by yellow-white flecks in the retina of the posterior pole along with maculopathy. Visual symptoms develop in childhood, and vision rapidly deteriorates to 20/200 before stabilizing.[29] Most of these patients (90 percent) demonstrate a dark choroid on fluorescein angiography. The term *dark choroid* describes the absence of background fluorescence during dye transit that is normally seen during fluorescein angiography.[30]

Fundus flavimaculatus can usually be distinguished from talc retinopathy because of the onset of visual symptoms at a young age. The ill-defined yellowish spots or dots seen with fundus flavimaculatus, which are ophthalmoscopically visible before maculopathy,[29] also occur at the level of the retinal pigment epithelium.[31]

Drusen may occur in several ophthalmoscopically different forms. Hard (nodular) drusen have a yellowish-white color and are pinpoint size. They have a hyaline structure and represent a localized disorder of the retinal pigment epithelium.[32] Soft (granular) drusen are larger than hard drusen and have indistinct edges and tend to be confluent. This change represents a serous detachment at the level of Bruch's membrane along with the retinal pigment epithelium.[32] Calcified (glistening) drusen represent a dystrophic change of the previously described drusen.[32] This change has the greatest similarity to talc retinopathy because of its glistening ophthalmoscopic appearance. Because drusen changes occur at the level of the retinal pigment epithelium, this condition should be easy to differentiate from talc retinopathy.[10]

Oxalate Crystal Deposition

Calcium oxalate crystals are a rare finding in the retina. The crystals appear as a rectangular yellow-white deposit in the middle and inner layers of the retina distributed most commonly along retinal arteries.[33] Deposition occurs most commonly as part of hereditary hyperoxaluria. This is a rare autosomal recessive condition that causes an error in glycoxylate metabolism leading to widespread calcium oxylate crystal deposition in diverse tissues, including the eye.[34] Symptoms associated with this crystal deposition

usually develop in early childhood and early adulthood and are related to kidney failure.

Retinopathy can also develop secondary to prolonged methoxyflurane abuse.[33] Ingestion of oxalate or its precursors (ethylene-glycol antifreeze, rhubarb) can also lead to this retinopathy.[35]

Talc emboli are usually smaller than oxalate crystals and are trapped in the capillary or precapillary arterioles. The calcium oxalate crystals are larger and are seen preferentially along the larger retinal arteries. The significant medical history in most of these individuals also helps establish the cause of the oxalate crystals.

Crystalline Retinopathy

Various hereditary crystalline retinopathies may resemble talc retinopathy. The disorders are varied but result in a striking appearance of crystal deposition in the fundus. These crystals are hypothesized to be secondary to a metabolic disorder at the level of the pigment epithelium photoreceptor complex.[36] This location helps distinguish these conditions from talc retinopathy.

Tamoxifen Retinopathy

Recently, tamoxifen has been noted to cause refractile intraretinal opacities in the nerve fiber and inner plexiform layers.[37] This medication is a nonsteroidal antiestrogenic agent used in the treatment of postmastectomy patients[38] and patients with metastatic breast carcinoma.[37] This significant medical history easily helps distinguish this condition from talc retinopathy.

The location and size of talc crystals, within the inner retinal layers associated with retinal capillaries helps identify this condition in most cases. A careful medical history and fundus examination can rule out many of the other conditions in the differential diagnosis. If the patient admits to intravenous drug abuse or if evidence of intravenous drug abuse is observed, the diagnosis is often easily established.

OCULAR EXAMINATION

The diagnosis of talc retinopathy can usually be established by slit lamp indirect ophthalmoscopy or fundus examination with a Goldmann or Hruby lens. The ocular examination of a suspected drug abuser is de-

Table 17-5. Ocular Examination

Dilated fundus examination with slit lamp indirect ophthalmoscopy or fundus lens (Goldmann or Hruby)
Fluorescein angiography
Visual field (Optional)

scribed in Table 17-5. The presence of small talc particles deposited most heavily in the superficial retinal layers of the posterior pole helps establish this diagnosis.

In a patient with suspected talc retinopathy, fluorescein angiography can also be useful in the evaluation.[5,6,14] Fluorescein angiography may reveal absence of perifoveal capillaries and arteriolar attenuation with tortuosity of small venules.[14] Subtle microvascular changes and leakage as well as microaneurysms may become apparent at the level of the pigment epithelium.[6] Choriocapillaris occlusion and capillary occlusion may also be visible with fluorescein angiography.[5,6]

Visual field testing is usually normal except in the rare circumstance of decreased vision secondary to macular ischemia. In these cases a central scotoma may be present.[14]

Color vision, pattern-shift visual-evoked responses, dark adaptation,[14] as well as photopic and scotopic electroretinograms (ERGs)[19] are also usually normal. A focal ERG may be abnormal in patients with macular ischemia and decreased vision.[14]

Vitreous fluorophotometry may show evidence of breakdown of the blood–retinal barrier.[19]

Table 17-6. Differential Diagnosis of Peripheral Retinal Neovascularization

Diabetes
Branch retinal vein occlusion
Carotic insufficiency
Sickle cell hemoglobinopathy
Hemoglobin C trait
Eale's disease
Sarcoidosis
Macroglobulinemia
Polycythemia
Leukemia
Uveitis
Periphlebitis
Retinopathy of prematurity
Incontinentia pigmenti

Capillary nonperfusion, as a result of capillary closure by obstruction with talc particles, becomes visible by fluorescein angiography. This rare but serious complication can lead to peripheral neovascularization. This in turn can result in the serious visual complications of preretinal and vitreous hemorrhages, as well as retinal detachment.

The differential diagnosis of peripheral retinal neovascularization is extensive and is noted in Table 17-6.[5,6,12,20]

SYSTEMIC EVALUATION

Mortality rates for drug abusers are considerably greater than expected for their age. Acute reaction to dosage and overdosage accounts for the highest percentage of fatalities in drug abusers. Overdose (acute intravenous narcotism) causes death as a result of the sudden collapse of the pulmonary system and pulmonary edema.[39]

Diseases that are unusual in the general population may occur with increased frequency among addicts.[40] Hepatitis and AIDS are well-known systemic complications of intravenous drug abuse. Other complications are noted in Table 17-7.[3,29,41,42]

The initial venous entry site in drug abuse is often the antecubital fossa.[3] Repeated injections leads to scarring of these veins. Veins of the back of the hand or lower extremities often become the next sites for repeated injections. As a last resort, the parenteral drug abuser will use "skin popping" when subcutaneous veins are no longer accessible.[3]

When drug abuse is suspected and the patient admits drug abuse, the case history should explore the following[5]:

Table 17-7. Systemic Complications of Intravenous Drug Abuse

Acquired immunodeficiency syndrome
Hepatitis
Septicemia
Bacterial and fungal endocarditis
Tetanus
Tuberculosis
Skin abscesses
Thrombophlebitis
Pulmonary hypertension
Cor pulmonale

1. Duration of abuse
2. Average number of tablets per injection
3. Frequency of injection
4. Method of injection

The most serious ocular and systemic complications are associated with the chronic abuser.

If drug abuse is suspected, but the patient denies such use, examination of the skin in the areas where injection occurs most commonly can prove helpful. Hyperpigmentation or cutaneous "railroad track" scars due to repeated puncture of skin overlying accessible veins in the antecubital fossa of the forearm are a hallmark of drug abuse.[3,40] Obtaining a blood pressure measurement gives the doctor an excellent opportunity to examine this important area in a nonthreatening manner. Patients may use elaborate tattoos to disguise injection sites.[3,40]

Skin popping, the technique of subcutaneous injection, often results in bacterial or chemical skin abscesses. These abscesses may leave two types of characteristic lesions[40]:

1. Round, macular hyperpigmented lesions with poorly defined borders
2. Round or oval depressions with sharp borders that have a "punched-out" appearance; overlying these lesions, the epithelium is intact but appears atrophic, shiny, and/or depigmented

Once systemic drug abuse is confirmed by the patient or suspected by the ocular and/or physical findings,

Table 17-8. Medical Evaluation

General testing
    General physical examination with blood pressure
    Chest radiograph
    Complete blood count with differential
    Urinalysis
Recommended testing
    Venereal Disease Research Laboratory test
    Erythrocyte sedimentation rate
    Liver scan
    Electrocardiogram
    Pulmonary function tests
    Blood urea nitrogen
    Creatinine
    Electrolyte
Additional testing when retinal neovascularization is present
    2-Hour postprandial blood glucose
    Hemoglobinelectrophoresis
    Purified protein derivative
    Angiotensin-converting enzyme

the patient should be advised to seek medical consultation for a general physical examination.[5] This is particularly true when the patient has complaints consistent with dyspnea.

Because the lung is a common site of damage, pulmonary radiographs are usually recommended.[5,9,14,43] Radiographs may demonstrate reticulonodular infiltration with associated cardiomegaly.[5] Pulmonary function studies may demonstrate ventilatory disturbance of a restrictive type secondary to the granulomatosis infiltration resulting in lung fibrosis.[5]

The medical evaluation of an intravenous drug abuser is outlined in Table 17-8.[5,12,14,20,43]

REFERENCES

1. McLane N, Carroll D: Ocular manifestations of drug abuse. Sur Ophthalmol 30:298, 1986
2. Urey J: Some ocular manifestations of systemic drug abuse. J Am Optom Assoc 62:832, 1991
3. Michaelson J: Nonocular manifestations of parenteral drug abuse. Sur Ophthalmol 30:314, 1986
4. Rumbaugh CL, Bergeron RT, Fong HCH: Cerebral angiographic changes in the drug abuse patient. Radiology 101:335, 1971
5. Tse DT, Ober RR: Talc retinopathy. Am J Ophthalmol 90:624, 1980
6. Schatz H, Drake M: Self-injected retinal emboli. Ophthalmology 86:468, 1979
7. Michelson JB, Whitcher JP, Wilson S, O'Connor GR: Possible foreign body granuloma of the retina associated with intravenous cocaine addiction. Am J Ophthalmol 87:278, 1979
8. Siepser SB, Magargal LE, Augsburger JJ: Acute bilateral microembolization in a heroin addict. Ann Ophthalmol 13:699, 1981
9. Hopkins B: Pulmonary angiothrombotic granulomatosis in drug offenders. JAMA 221:909, 1974
10. Murphy SB, Jackson WB, Pare JAP: Talc retinopathy. Can J Ophthalmol 13:152, 1978
11. Atlee WE: Talc and cornstarch emboli in eyes of drug abusers. JAMA 219:49, 1972.
12. Kresca LJ, Goldberg MF, Jampol LM: Talc emboli and retinal neovascularization in a drug abuser. Am J Ophthalmol 87:334, 1979
13. Lee J, Sapira JD: Retinal and cerebral microembolization of talc in a drug abuser. Am J Med Sci 265:75, 1973
14. Friberg TR, Gragoudas ES, Rogan CDJ: Talc emboli and macular ischemia in intravenous drug abuser. Arch Ophthalmol 97:1089, 1979
15. Johnston EH, Goldbaum LR, Whelton RL: Investigation of sudden deaths in addicts. Med Ann DC 38:375, 1969
16. Wendt VE, Puro HE, Shapiro J et al: Angiothrombotic pulmonary hypertension in addicts: "blue velvet" addiction. JAMA 188:755, 1964
17. Douglas FG, Kafilmout KJ, Patt NL: Foreign particle embolism in drug addicts: respiratory pathophysiology. Ann Intern Med 75:865, 1971
18. Robertson CH, Reynolds RC, Wilson JE: Pulmonary hypertension and foreign body granulomas in intravenous drug abusers. Am J Med 61:657, 1976

19. Jampol LM, Setogawa T, Rednam KRV, Tso MOM: Talc retinopathy in primates. Arch Ophthalmol 99:1273, 1981
20. Brucker AJ: Disk and peripheral retinal neovascularization secondary to talc and cornstarch emboli. Am J Ophthalmol 88:864, 1979
21. Ballantyne AJ, Michaellson IC: Textbook of the fundus of the eye. E & S Livingstone, Edinburgh, 1970
22. Hollenhorst RW: Vascular status of patients who have cholesterol emboli in the retina. Am J Ophthalmol 61:1159, 1966
23. Richler M: Ocular manifestations of nephropathic cystinosis. Arch Ophthalmol 109:358, 1991
24. Kaiser-Kupfer M: Ocular manifestations of metabolic disorders. Curr Opin Ophthalmol 3:221, 1992
25. Kaiser-Kupfer M: Long-term ocular manifestations in nephropathic cystinosis. Arch Ophthalmol 104:706, 1986
26. Krill AE, Klien BA: Flecked retina syndrome. Arch Ophthalmol 74:496, 1965
27. Miyake Y, Shiroyama N, Sugita S et al: Fundus albipunctatus associated with cone dystrophy. Br J Ophthalmol 76:375, 1992
28. Marmor MF: Long-term follow-up of the physiologic abnormalities and fundus changes in fundus albipunctatus. Ophthalmology 97:380, 1990
29. Lambert SR: Degenerative retinal diseases in childhood. Semin Ophthalmol 6:219, 1991
30. Vliss AE: Dark choroid in posterior retinal dystrophies. Ophthalmology 94:1423, 1987
31. McDonnell P: Fundus flavimaculatus without maculopathy. Ophthalmology 93:116, 1986
32. Green W: Pathologic features of senile macular degeneration. Ophthalmology 92:615, 1986
33. Wells CG, Johnson RJ, Qingli L et al: Retinal oxalosis. Arch Ophthalmol 107:1638, 1989
34. Small KW, Letson R, Scheinman J: Ocular findings in primary hyperoxaluria. Arch Ophthalmol 108:89, 1990
35. Novak MA, Roth AS, Levine MR: Calcium oxalate retinopathy associated with methoxyflurane abuse. Retina 8:230, 1988
36. Grizzard WS, Deutman AF, Jijhuis F, Aan DeKerk A: Crystalline retinopathy. Am J Ophthalmol 86:81, 1978
37. Chang T, Gunder JR, Ventresca MR: Low-dose tamoxifen retinopathy. Can J Ophthalmol 27:148, 1992
38. Gerner EW: Ocular toxicity of tamoxifen. Ann Ophthalmol 21:420, 1989
39. Cherubin CE: Medical sequelae of narcotic addiction. Ann Intern Med 76:23, 1967
40. Sapira JD: The narcotic addict as a medical patient. Am J Med 45:555, 1968
41. Hopkins GB, Taylor DG: Pulmonary talc granulomatosis. Am Rev Respir Dis 101:101, 1970
42. Louria DB, Hensle T, Rose J: Major medical complications of heroin addiction. Ann Intern Med 67:1, 1967
43. Bluth LL, Hanscom TA: Retinal detachment and vitreous hemorrhage due to talc emboli. JAMA 246:980, 1981

18 Sexually Transmitted Disease

G. RICHARD BENNETT

INTRODUCTION

Interest in the study of sexually transmitted diseases (STDs) and their ocular manifestations has renewed for a variety of reasons. An alarming increase in STDs has occurred spite of the recent explosion in research, clinical diagnosis, and treatment. A resurgence of syphilis and gonorrhea is of great concern to those clinicians who examine patients at risk of these diseases. The pandemic of acquired immunodeficiency syndrome (AIDS) has brought other sexually transmitted diseases to the attention of the medical community because of the increasing frequency with which such diseases as gonorrhea and syphilis are found in AIDS patients and in patients positive for the human immunodeficiency virus (HIV). The optometrist must therefore consider these diseases in the AIDS era and perform appropriate serologic testing for syphilis on all AIDS patients with ocular inflammation.[1]

STDs have significant ocular manifestations and are critically important as a possible cause of a variety of ocular conditions. Ocular manifestations of STD may include such diverse conditions as corneal ulceration, conjunctivitis, nerve palsies, uveitis, inflammatory retinal disease, lid lesions, and secondary glaucoma. Once the causative agent is identified, it is often possible to treat the pathogen responsible for the secondary ocular disease. The optometrist must consider other STDs once a positive result is obtained because of the possibility that the patient may have multiple infections, especially if the patient is immunocompromised.

CASE REPORT

A 36-year-old white man presented with a chief complaint of reduced vision in the right eye, pain, and photophobia for approximately 14 days. The patient had returned to a substance abuse center, having voluntarily discontinuing treatment there for several weeks. During his hiatus from the substance abuse center, no medical care had been available. His medical history included intravenous substance abuse, several instances of trauma, and treatment for gonococcal urethral infection.

A physical examination revealed an entering visual acuity of hand motion in the right eye and 20/20 in the left. Neither multiple pinhole nor subjective refraction improved visual acuity. Pupil testing showed a classic Argyll Robertson pupil with miosis and light-near dissociation. Slit lamp biomicroscopy showed a hazy, edematous cornea, 2+ cell and flare, and posterior synechiae in the right eye. The left eye was normal in appearance. Intraocular pressure, as measured by Goldmann applannation tonometry, revealed pressures of 32 mmHg OD and 18 mmHg OS. A dilated fundus examination showed a nonrhegmatogenous retinal detachment confirmed by B-scan ultrasonography and demonstrating choroidal effusion. A Venereal Disease Research Laboratory (VDRL) test was positive at a titer of 1:18, as was a fluorescent treponemal antibody absorption (FTA-ABS) test. Informed con-

---

sent was obtained and, and HIV enzyme-linked immunosorbent assay (ELISA) was performed, which was positive and confirmed by Western blot.

The patient was treated with 2.4 million U of benzathine penicillin G initially. The anterior uveitis and elevated intraocular pressures were initially treated with topical prednisolone and scopolaminne and timolol maleate ophthalmic solutions, respectively. Unfortunately, the patient was lost to follow-up when he left the substance abuse center with no address.

EPIDEMIOLOGY

The epidemiology of STDs changed during the past several years. STDs are a recognized worldwide problem, not localized to a geographic region. STDs respect no class, race, or socioeconomic group and must be considered as a possible cause when ocular disease of unknown origin is present. The development of resistant organisms has made treatment more difficult and has aided the resurgence of these diseases because the infected individuals may continue to be sexually active. Finally, a significant factor in the worldwide spread of STDs is the large number of asymptomatic carriers who continue to spread the disease while exhibiting no symptoms for an extended period. These considerations make the study of STDs important and relevant to the optometrist. The purpose of this chapter is to review the more common STDs, their ocular manifestations, and appropriate management. Chapter 19 covers the ocular manifestations of AIDS. For a more encyclopedic discussion of STDs, the reader should consider Insler's excellent text *AIDS and Other Sexually Transmitted Diseases and the Eye*.[2]

ACQUIRED SYPHILIS

Fracastorius of Verona (1485 to 1553), physician, poet, physicist, geologist, and astrologist, is thought to have contributed the name *syphilis* to that disease known at the time as the French disease, Neapolitan disease, or big pox.[3] Syphilis was observed all over Europe after the unsuccessful siege of Naples in 1495 and remains a worldwide problem today. Ophthalmic manifestations of acquired syphilis were first described during this period and provide early clinical descriptions of eyelid lesions, uveitis, keratitis, and conjunctivitis. Clinical cases of syphilis increased dramatically, and as many as 5 to 10 percent of Americans at one time had syphilis, according to surveys published in the 1880s. In recent years, reported cases of syphilis peaked in the early 1940s, but the disease remains an important cause of ophthalmic disease. A recent study reports a 66 percent increase in the disease between 1981 and 1989.[4]

Microbiology

The causative organism of syphilis is the spirochete *Treponema pallidum*, a spiral bacteria about 10 to 13 μm in length. This spirochete is a facultative anaerobic organism and can persist in the host in spite of an intact immune system. Although viable spirochetes remain active in the host during secondary and tertiary stages of the disease, the host is resistant to reinfection during this period. This adaptable organism can incorporate fatty acids from host cells. Fluorescent-antibody dark-field testing easily demonstrates spirochetes.

Transmission

The most common mode of transmission is sexual or other direct contact. Young, sexually active individuals are at highest risk of contacting the disease, and substance abuse is often linked today with increased risk of infection. It was reported around the turn of the century that examining physicians were at risk from infected patients, and a significant number contracted ocular primary syphilitic infections in this manner.[5] Although infection through nonsexual contact and fomites is certainly possible, sexual contact remains the primary mode of transmission of this disease.

Clinical Stages

The first presenting sign of syphilis is a painless skin chancre with associated local lymphadenopathy appearing at the site of infection. The chancre may be located on the external genitalia, anus, mouth, eyelid, or conjunctiva. The exposed individual has a high rate of contracting syphilis from an infected individual, with a conversion of between 33 and 50 percent. This infected chancre appears following approximately a 3-week incubation period. This clinical stage of the disease is known as *primary syphilis* and may be so subtle as to allow the infection to go undetected.

Secondary syphilis is a secondary stage of bacteremia with disseminated mucocutaneous lesions and generalized lymphadenopathy. This hematogenous dissemination of the disease generally presents about 6 weeks after the appearance of the primary chancre. This stage of syphilis is characterized by a variety of signs and symptoms, including generalized malaise, fever, sore throat, disseminated maculopapular skin rash (hence, the name "pox"), joint pain, and headache. A variety of ocular findings are observed at this stage (see the section, *Ocular Manifestations*). An important concept is the multiorgan involvement of this stage and the wide range of potential involvement.

In individuals with an intact immune system, a period of latency occurs without proper treatment. This latent period is characterized by the disappearance of the symptoms and clinical signs of the diseases as the patient's immune system suppresses the disseminated syphilis. At this point, the individual usually is asymptomatic, but serologic testing will be positive.

Tertiary syphilis develops many years after the onset of untreated or undertreated syphilis in about 33 percent of cases. The classic lesions of tertiary syphilis are gummas, focal granulomatous-like necrotic lesions that are a result of localized obliterative endarteritis. Syphilis has been called the "great imitator" because of the complex variety of signs and symptoms that can accompany the disease. Gummas can involve virtually any target organ, including the eye and adnexa. Major areas of tertiary involvement include neurosyphilis and cardiovascular syphilis as a result of localized endarteritis. Neurosyphilis may present as meningitis, and up to 10 percent of untreated patients will develop central nervous system involvement. This is clinically determined by lumbar puncture and examination of the cerebrospinal fluid. The light-near dissociation of syphilis (Argyll Robertson pupil) is caused by focal obliterative changes in the rostral midbrain. These obliterative changes, when found in the posterior roots and columns of the spinal cord, produce the paresthesias, ataxia, impotence, and loss of bladder control found in tabes dorsalis. Cardiovascular syphilis may also present in a variety of ways, including coronary artery stenosis, aortic aneurysm, and temporal arteritis.

Congenital syphilis classically manifests as Hutchin-

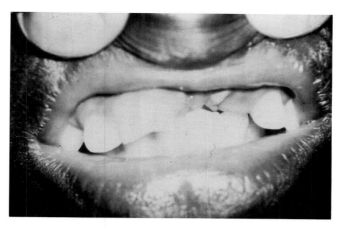

Fig. 18-1. Malformed "notched" teeth in Hutchinson's triad. (Photograph by Ms. Jane Stein.) (See also Plate 18-1).

son's triad of interstitial keratitis, deafness, and malformed "notched" teeth (Fig. 18-1 and Plate 18-1). Congenital syphilis is the result of transplacental transmission of the spirochete, generally after the fourth month of pregnancy in a mother with untreated primary, secondary, or latent syphilis. In addition to Hutchinson's triad, a variety of manifestations of congenital syphilis are noted, including rhinitis, hepatosphlenomegaly, osteochondritis, bony abnormalities, as well as ocular abnormalities (Fig. 18-2 and Plate 18-2).

Diagnostic Tests

Laboratory testing for syphilis includes both serologic testing as well as direct examination of scrapings of mucocutaneous lesions by dark-field or phase-contrast microscopy. Obviously, mucous patches or skin lesions must be present for scrapings, and this limits the usefulness of microscopic examination in many patients.

Serologic testing includes both quantitative nonspecific tests and tests for specific treponemal antibody. Nonspecific tests include the VDRL test and are generally used to monitor the effectiveness of antibiotic treatment. As the patient is treated, the reactive results decline and are an indication of therapeutic efficacy. Two specific tests for syphilis are the FTA-ABS test and the microhemagglutination assay for antibodies to *T. pallidum* (MHA-TO). As with any serologic test, the optometrist must consider relative sensitivity and specificity of these tests. Table 18-1 suggests clini-

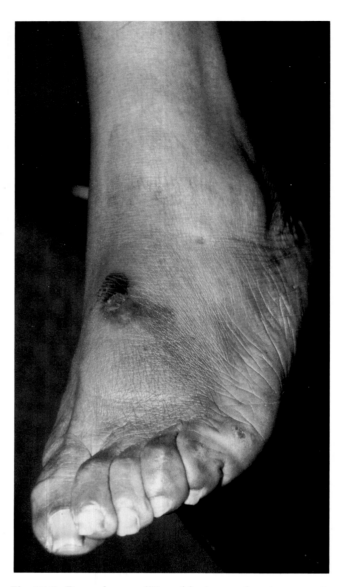

Fig. 18-2. Bony abnormalities of foot secondary to congenital syphilis. (Photograph by Ms. Jane Stein.) (See also Plate 18-2).

Table 18-1. Clinical Indications for Serologic Tests for Syphilis

Any potential ocular manifestation of syphilis in a patient with another STD
Argyll Robertson pupil or unexplained pupillary abnormalities
Keratitis or keratouveitis of unknown origin
Recurrent uveitis of unknown origin
Idiopathic subluxated lenses
Scleritis, chorioretinal inflammation of unknown origin
Optic atrophy or papillitis of unknown origin

cal indications for performing serologic tests for syphilis for the optometrist.

Ocular Manifestations

Primary syphilis may present with ocular findings of conjunctival or eyelid chancre. Primary syphilis in newborn babies may present in this manner after contamination from the birth canal during delivery.

Ocular manifestations of secondary syphilis present in a variety of ways; all can involve virtually any ocular tissue. The eyelids may be involved in the generalized skin rash of secondary syphilis and is often associated with alopecia of the lashes and eyebrows. Conjunctivitis and blepharitis may also be found with the generalized rash. Orbital inflammation and orbital periostitis have been reported during this phase of the disease. Episcleritis is generally found during secondary syphilis, whereas scleritis is more commonly found late in the disease.

Anterior uveitis is a common manifestation of secondary syphilis and may be the only clinical indication of recurrent secondary syphilis. The incidence of uveitis associated with secondary syphilis was believed to be extremely high before effective treatment for the disease. There are many reports in the modern literature of secondary syphilitic uveitis presenting as a single clinical entity or in conjunction with other clinical signs such as altitudinal field loss, frontal balding, and palmar skin lesions.[6] Iris roseolae may precede the uveitis. These transient reddish spots or tufts may correspond to localized areas of infection. Less commonly found are iris papules associated with secondary syphilis. The papules are transient and may be missed.[7] Dacryocystitis and dacryoadenitis have also been reported.

Glaucoma is found in secondary syphilis and may be associated with uveitis, neovascularization of the anterior chamber angle, hypertrophy of Descemet's membrane, or to multiple intraepithelial cysts. These secondary glaucomas may be rather refractory to treatment. Optic neuritis, chorioretinitis, and neuroretinitis have all been described during secondary syphilis and frequently are associated with meningitis. Retinal findings of retinal pigment epithelial proliferation, narrowed retinal blood vessels, and chorioretinal atrophy can be confused with retinitis pigmentosa. The "salt and pepper" fundus appearance of syphilis generally has many areas of chorioretinal atrophy, unlike retinitis pigmentosa. Neuroretinitis associated with secondary syphilis presents as a collection of waxy macular exudates, superficial "flame" hemorrhages, cotton-wool spots, and sheathed arterioles. The nerve may be swollen and the retina takes on a grayish, thickened appearance.

Ciliochoroidal effusion may be associated with secondary syphilis and can cause significant secondary ocular complications. Ciliochoroidal effusion may cause nonrhegmatogenous retinal detachment in patients with secondary syphilis. These detachments are difficult to treat and may recur.[8] Another significant complication of ciliochoroidal effusion is acute angle closure glaucoma. I reported a case of bilateral angle closure glaucoma in a patient with syphilis and AIDS.[9]

Hutchinson[10] made many observations relative to the ocular manifestations of syphilis, and his term "interstitial keratitis" describes the stromal keratitis secondary to syphilis. Stromal keratitis may be caused by acquired syphilis but is generally the result of congenital syphilis. Interstitial keratitis generally appears from infancy to the early 20s and probably represents a hypersensitivity reaction to the spirochete. In congenital syphilis, treatment of the mother in the first trimester or the infant before the age of 3 months can prevent stromal keratitis. Later treatment does not have a beneficial effect on the course of the interstitial keratitis.

The clinical course of syphilitic keratitis is most often associated with a concurrent uveitis and perilimbal episcleritis. From an initial "ground-glass" hazy appearance to the cornea, corneal neovascularization begins to give a "salmon-patch" appearance to the cornea. This stage of intense corneal inflammation is usually bilateral (80 percent of congenital cases) and persists for months. After spontaneously resolving, the inflammation results in the characteristic corneal scarring, thinning, and alteration of Descemet's membrane. Stromal "ghost vessels" persist indefinitely and may be patent to plasma flow but not erythrocytes. Although antibiotic therapy during this stage of inflammation is not useful, aggressive topical therapy with cycloplegics and steroids may reduce sequelae.

The ocular manifestations of tertiary syphilis are characterized by gummas resulting from localized endarteritis. These gummas may be found in a variety of ocular structures and may be misdiagnosed. A gumma of the upper eyelid from tertiary syphilis may resemble a chalazion. The iris and ciliary body are relatively common sites for the gummas associated with tertiary disease. Iris gummas may lead to sectoral iris atrophy but usually are small. By contrast, a ciliary body gumma may present as a large mass in the anterior chamber angle. Gummas of the choroid and retina are associated with neovascularization. The retina may take on an atrophic appearance in tertiary syphilis.

Neurosyphilis is a common sequellae in tertiary syphilis and has a varied presentation. Common ocular manifestations include cranial nerve palsies, extraocular muscle involvement, ptosis, and optic atrophy. The previously described Argyll Robertson pupil with miosis and light-near dissociation remains a valuable clinical sign of neurosyphilis. Visual fields are often abnormal in tertiary syphilis but difficult to characterize because of the many potential sites of involvement, including the retina, optic nerve, optic tract and chiasm, lateral geniculate body, and visual radiation abnormalities. Visual field manifestations may be as severe as total cortical blindness.

Therapy

The most critical element in the effective treatment of a patient with syphilis is accurate and early diagnosis. The signs and symptoms of syphilis can be confusing and may lead experienced clinicians to a mistaken diagnosis. Because even an intact immune system will not eliminate the spirochete, effective antibiotic therapy must be administered. Benzathine penicillin G (2.4 million U IM) remains highly effective in the treatment of syphilis. Alternative therapy in cases of penicillin allergies or resistant organisms includes ceftriaxone, tetracycline, and erythromycin. It is important to consider related STDs because of the high rate of multiple infections, especially in immunocompromised patients.

INCLUSION CONJUNCTIVITIS (CHLAMYDIA)

Chlamydia is thought to be the most common sexually transmitted infection in the developed world, with 3 to 4 million Americans infected per year. The ocular manifestation of genital chlamydial infection is inclusion conjunctivitis and is found in about 1 percent of these cases. The conjunctivitis associated with genital chlamydia may be found most commonly in patients aged 15 to 40 years old and represents a significant percentage of cases of conjunctivitis those age groups.[11] Concomitant gonococcal infection is common in patients with genital chlamydial infection and supports the growing evidence that individuals infected with one STD should be carefully screened for other related STDs.

Neonatal inclusion conjunctivitis continues to be a significant public health problem, especially because the common incubation period of 5 to 12 days after birth generally means the infant already has been discharged from the hospital. One study suggests that between 7 and 12 percent of women were infected with chlamydia just before delivery.[12]

Microbiology

The causative organism of inclusion conjunctivitis is *Chlamydia trachomatis,* sereotypes D through K. *Chlamydia trachomatis* sereotypes A, B, Ba, and C cause trachoma. These organisms are obligate intracellular parasites and replicate by binary fission. Once thought to resemble large viruses, chlamydial organisms contain both RNA and DNA and thus more closely resemble higher order bacteria. The chlamydiae cannot synthesize *adenosine triphosphate* and need a host cell for replication. Chlamydial organisms replicate during a 48-hour growth cycle, during which infectious elementary bodies attach to host cells, reorganize into reticulate bodies, and finally are released as new elementary bodies following cell rupture. The release of these infectious elementary bodies and the subsequent infection of other epithelial cells probably account for the characteristic acute inflammatory response. In the eye, conjunctival epithelial cells become the host cells for the organism to maintain their growth cycle.

Transmission

Direct exposure to infected genital tract secretions is by far the most common mode of chlamydial transmission. As in other STDs, asymptomatic sexual partners may serve as an important reservoir for infection. Inclusion conjunctivitis may result from direct exposure to infected genital tract secretions, hand-to-eye transmission, or even hand-to-eye-to-hand infection. Because other organisms can cause acute conjunctivitis, the early descriptions of "swimming pool" conjunctivitis may be inaccurate. Adenovirus may be the

culprit in many of these reported cases. In an experimentally induced infection in human volunteers, the incubation period of this disease was found to be 2 to 19 days.[13] Neonatal cases involve an exposure to the organism during vaginal delivery through an infected cervix, which results in an approximately 50 percent rate of inclusion conjunctivitis. These babies are also at high risk of associated chlamydial pneumonia.

Clinical Features

The associated presentation of chlamydia in adults is characterized by a nonspecific urethritis in men and cervicitis, acute urethral syndrome, and pelvic inflammatory disease in women. Unfortunately, scarring and resultant infertility may occur in women long before symptoms of chlamydial disease occur. Chlamydia may also be associated with salpingitis, perihepatitis, and otitis media. Many infected individuals may be asymptomatic and unknowing carriers of the infection.

Diagnostic Tests

All diagnostic testing for suspected chlamydial infection should be done with the understanding that gonococcal infections and syphilis must also be ruled out. Conjunctival scrapings may be examined under the microscope to detect evidence of chlamydial infection. The scrapings are generally obtained from the lower palpebral conjunctiva and stained with Giemsa. Chlamydial inclusions often present as fine blue-purple granules clustered around the nucleus. Only about one-half the patients with chlamydial disease will have a positive Giemsa examination, and fluorescent antibody studies and culture techniques are more useful clinically. The fluorescent antibody studies are based on the binding of antibodies to the chlamydial inclusion body or the surface antigen of the exposed organisms. Because of the expense of many of these tests, adult inclusion conjunctivitis generally is treated with a clinical trial of systemic antibodies and testing is done only when a clear diagnosis is not evident.

Ocular Manifestations

Neonates classically present with an acute inclusion conjunctivitis between 5 and 12 days after birth. The condition is marked by purulent discharge, lid edema, and papillary formation and may be associated with pseudomembrane formation with the sequellae of conjunctival and corneal scarring. This does not usually occur in adult disease. Because of the possible confusion of inclusion conjunctivitis with gonococcal conjunctivitis or staphylococcal, streptococcal, or pneumococcal conjunctivitis, laboratory testing is frequently ordered to differentiate these neonatal eye infections.

Adult inclusion conjunctivitis often presents as a chronic, follicular conjunctivitis in contrast to the papillary response of the neonate. The disease may have an acute or subacute onset with symptoms of pain, photophobia, redness, and lid swelling. A mucopurulent discharge is present, and the conjunctivitis may be unilateral or asymmetric. If the untreated inclusion conjunctivitis does not resolve spontaneously, the presenting signs and symptoms may last for months. Slit lamp biomicroscopy usually reveals marked foliculosis with involvement of the palpebral conjunctiva, the superior and inferior fornices, around the limbus, caruncle, and on the plica. Superficial punctate keratitis often develops about 14 days after the onset of the conjunctivitis, and peripheral and central subepithelial infiltrates are common. More serious corneal complications may occur in untreated disease and include persistent infiltrates with vision loss, vascularization of the cornea, and corneal pannus, especially superiorly in the corena. Preauricular lymphadenopathy commonly is found in conjunction with the inclusion conjunctivitis. An anterior uveitis may accompany the conjunctivitis and keratitis, especially in individuals with associated collagen vascular disease.

Differential Diagnosis

As in the neonatal form of the disease, multiple conditions are easily confused with adult inclusion conjunctivitis. Trachoma is probably the most serious of the masquerading conditions and is a potentially blinding condition. Trachoma has been found in certain geographic areas and is associated with severe lid scarring and corneal pannus. Misuse of topical ophthalmic solutions, chronic application of topical solutions (glaucoma patients), toxic reactions to eye drops, and contact lens-related solutions, and the normal folliculosis of young individuals have all been confused with chlamydial inclusion conjunctivitis. Table 18-2 shows a partial list of clinical entities easily confused with inclusion conjunctivitis.

A careful history can often make the differential diag-

Table 18-2. Conditions Often Confused With Inclusion Conjunctivitis

Adenovirus conjunctivitis and keratitis
Folliculosis of young individuals (normal)
Herpes simplex keratitis
Molluscum contagiosum
Toxic reactions
    Chronic eye-drop use
    Contact lenses
    Contact lens solutions
Trachoma

nosis of chlamydial inclusion conjunctivitis much easier. When diagnostic evaluation and clinical evidence are insufficient to make a definitive diagnosis, laboratory evaluation is necessary.

Treatment

Fortunately, the effective treatment of chlamydial inclusion conjunctivitis is relatively straightforward after accurate diagnosis. The goal of treatment is systemic antibiotic therapy to eliminate the chlamydial infection, which halts the ocular and systemic problems associated with the disease. In neonates, oral erythromycin is usually given for 14 days. In adult inclusion conjunctivitis, both systemic tetracycline and doxycycline may be given for 3 weeks to eradicate the chlamydial infection. Failure of systemic treatment may be due to a variety of factors, including noncompliance with mediation and failure to treat infected sexual partners. Topical erythromycin ointment at night is not necessary with proper systemic treatment but may help alleviate symptoms until the systemic antibiotics become effective. Chlamydial infection must be suspected in cases of follicular conjunctivitis and ruled out, especially in individuals likely to be infected.[14]

HERPES SIMPLEX VIRUS

Herpes simplex is another sexually transmitted disease with a long history, first described by Herodotus almost 2,000 years ago.[15] In 1920, Professors Doerr and Vochting[16] described herpetic central nervous system symptoms following corneal inoculation, which led to the explanation of recurrent herpetic disease secondary to latent virus in sensory neurons. Herpes simplex virus (HSV) has traditionally been classified as type I, commonly associated with herpes simplex keratitis, and type II, genital herpes. Current evidence suggests that type I and type II may infect either area, and neither is restricted to "above the belt" or "below the belt." In the past 20 years, the incidence of sexually transmitted HSV infection has increased 10-fold and it is currently the second most common STD in North America.

Microbiology

The agent of infection in HSV is a double-stranded DNA virus in the *Herpetoviridae* family. Close cousins include cytomegalovirus, Epstein-Barr virus, and varicella-zoster virus, which is the causative agent of chickenpox and shingles. HSV replicates within the cell nucleus and may remain dormant for intervals between active episodes of infection. During these latent periods, the virus remains within sensory neurons and is noninfectious. The actual site of the latent virus depends on the location of the primary infection. Once reactivated by a "trigger" factor, the virus travels to the peripheral site by axonal flow and replicates with active shedding of the virus and/or formation of a herpetic lesion. A variety of mechanisms may serve as the "triggor" factor to reactivate the latent virus and includes such diverse entities as fever, trauma, sunburn, stress, ultraviolet light, menstruation, surgery, sexual intercourse, and immunosuppression. Conventional assays are not useful in detecting latent HSV.

Transmission

The virus is transmitted by direct contact with an infectious individual or, more rarely, via formites. Neonatal herpes is transmitted from the infected mother to the newborn at delivery through the birth canal or by infection spreading to the fetus after the membrane ruptures. Rarely, a contaminated fetal monitor may be the source of the infection. The adult genital form of the disease is transmitted via direct sexual contact with an infected partner who is actively shedding virus at the time. The virus may be found in body secretions or in the epithelial lesions during the active episodes of the disease. Although a very high rate of transmission is likely during periods of active shedding from lesions, virus may be recovered even in the secretions of asymptomatic individuals.[17] Ocular herpes simplex may be transmitted in the same manner. Direct contact with body secretions or genital lesions of an infected individual, indirect transmission via hands or contaminated fomites such as a moist towel, or autoinoculation of a patient with genital infection (usually from contaminated hands) all transmit the virus to the eye.

Clinical Features

Normally, symptoms appear in adult primary genital HSV infection 2 to 12 days after sexual contact with an infected partner. The newly infected individual may be virtually asymptomatic or show extensive paresthesia and burning of the genital area, aching and generalized malaise, fever, and painful vesicular skin lesions. As with other STDs, patients with HSV are more at risk of other STDs and should be screened for them. After the initial crusting of skin lesions and resolution of symptoms, a latency period will occur with an almost 80 percent chance of reactivation during the first 6 months after the first episode of genital herpes. The great variation in presentation of the genital disease may be due in part to the patient's prior exposure to nongenital herpes at some point. Recurrent disease is likely to be less symptomatic than the initial presentation. HSV type II may cause more prolonged and symptomatic disease than type I.

Ocular Manifestations

Primary ocular HSV infection is often a disease of childhood with HSV type I as the causative agent. HSV type II also can cause primary ocular infection, often with a more severe and prolonged clinical course. Only extensive testing by culture and tissue analysis can differentiate between type I and II herpetic infection; because the two strains are treated identically, this is rarely done. Signs and symptoms of primary ocular HSV infection secondary to genital disease may include a follicular conjunctivitis, blepharitis, keratitis, subepithelial infiltrates, photophobia, foreign body sensation, tearing, and blurred vision appearing 1 to 2 weeks after inoculation. The primary ocular infection may present as vesicular eruptions of the lid or skin around the eyes. Following resolution of the primary episode, the virus retreats via retrograde axonal flow and remains latent in the trigeminal, ciliary, and superior cervical ganglia. The recurrent bouts of ocular HSV infection most often present as an epithelial keratitis.

Recurrent adult ocular HSV infection of the cornea often presents as a superficial punctate or stellate keratitis, which increases in size and later forms white plaques of opaque epithelial cells. Grayson[18] describes a "palisading" of epithelial cells at the periph-

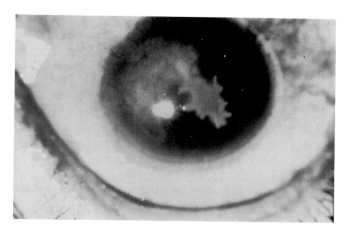

Fig. 18-3. Herpetic corneal ulcer. (Courtesy of Dr. Andrew Gurwood.) (See also Plate 18-3.)

ery of each plaque. The characteristic dendrites are formed by the enlargement and development of these plaques. The dendritic ulcer stains with both sodium fluorescein and rose bengal and may occur at the primary site of infection or elsewhere. With recurrent disease, the presence of keratic precipitates directly behind the lesion may be noted, and decreased corneal sensation is common. Inappropriate treatment with topical steroids can significantly worsen the course and prognosis of the disease (Fig. 18-3 and Plate 18-3). The dendrites may develop into geographic and ameboid ulcers and spread into the stroma. With stromal keratitis, a concurrent anterior uveitis usually is present and may involve significant corneal scarring and corneal vascularization. Tropic ulcers (postinfectious herpetic erosions) may damage the basement membrane, possibly with a neurotrophic component.

Herpetic keratitis—especially if a delay in diagnosis coupled with inappropriate topical steroid treatment has allowed progression—may result in stromal keratitis with stromal abscess. Differential diagnosis may be difficult, and cultures must be used to rule out secondary infection. Interstitial keratitis mimicking syphilis may even occur, with decreased visual acuity and dense vessels observed in the corneal stroma. A concurrent uveitis is not unusual.

Therapy

Oral acylovir remains the most effective treatment of nonocular HSV and is effective in reducing the severity of symptoms and the duration of virus shedding.

In a recent study, daily suppressive acyclovir was found to be efficacious and well tolerated in normal adults with frequently recurring genital herpes simplex infection.[19] Annual Papanicolaou smears are recommended for women with a history of genital HSV infection because of the associated risk of reproductive tract malignancies.

One of the first antiviral agents used against ocular HSV infection was idoxuridine. Idoxuridine acts by competitively inhibiting the uptake of thymidine into the DNA molecule; thus causing a faulty DNA chain and inhibiting virus synthesis. Unfortunately, the drug also affects corneal epithelial metabolism and is a relatively toxic drug with poor corneal penetration. Adenine arabinoside has been found to be less toxic than idoxuridine and has been used in cases of idoxuridine failure. Adenine arabinoside acts as an inhibitor of DNA polymerase and prevents the lengthening of the DNA chain. The drug has been associated with toxic side effects and must be used with this understanding. Trifluorothymidine has shown superior penetration to both idoxuridine and adenine arabinoside and is also more efficacious against HSV, especially ulcers previously treated with topical steroids. Acyclovir ointment is now the therapy of choice and is easily used with oral acyclovir in cases of severe disease or systemic involvement. It is important to remember that associated conditions must also be treated appropriately. For instance, topical cycloplegic agents may be used to treat concurrent bouts of uveitis, and topical antibiotics may be used to treat an associated bacterial infection.

GONOCOCCAL INFECTIONS

In ophthalmia neonatorum, hyperacute conjunctivitis secondary to *Neisseria gonorrhoeae* must be ruled out. Just before the turn of the century, almost 10 percent of newborns suffered from gonococcal ophthalmia with gonococcal keratitis. Following the use of the Crede's prophylaxis of using 2-percent silver nitrate drops, the incidence of gonococcal ophthalmia dramatically decreased. Older children and adults acquire gonococcal infectious by direct or indirect contact. Sexual contact is the normal route of transmission, but other contact with infected individuals (including ophthalmic examination) has been reported. Systemically, gonococcal infections are associated with acute infectious disease of the urethra, cervix, and rectum.

Microbiology

The causative organism of gonococcal infections in *N. gonorrhea*, a gram-negative diplococcus that may invade an intact mucosal surface. These intracellular kidney-shaped cocci may be distorted after antibiotic exposure, may not decolorize well, and may be difficult to evaluate because of poor staining.[18]

Transmission

Transmission is generally by sexual contact and other direct or indirect contact with an infected individual. In ophthalmia neonatorum, the risk of transmission from an infected mother to her infant is likely less than 2 percent with Crede's prophylaxis.[20] By contrast, it is estimated that sexual intercourse with an infected man carries a risk of greater than 50 percent. Many individuals have no signs or symptoms of the disease and may remain asymptomatic carriers.

Ocular Manifestations

This highly infectious disease has a dramatic hyperacute ocular presentation of marked hyperemia, copious purulent discharge, with subconjunctival hemorrhage, chemosis, and pseudomembrane formation. It can cause infiltration and ulceration of an intact cornea, a rare microbiologic entity. The conjunctivitis has an incubation period of about 2 to 7 days. A ring abscess may develop from a confluent series of peripheral ulcers and may lead to perforation of the cornea.

Treatment

Traditionally, penicillin and tetracycline have been the first-line therapy in gonococcal conjunctivitis and keratitis. Unfortunately, resistant strains of gonococcus have been observed, and thus therapy recommendations have been changed.[21] Currently, intravenous ceftriaxone is the systemic drug of choice in the treatment of adult and neonatal gonococcal ophthalmia.[22] In adults, a several-week course of oral doxycycline or erythromycin may be added to the ceftriaxone. Topical treatment consists of bacitracin or erythromycin at frequent intervals.

SUMMARY

There has been an explosion in the clinical investigation and research of STDs. The prevalence of these diseases and their ocular manifestations are staggering. In one study, 27 percent of jailed women were found to be positive for chlamydial cervical infection.[14] Obviously, patients found to be positive for one STD should carefully be evaluated for associated sexually transmitted infections, especially HIV infection. Richert et al.[23] described nearly 1 million sexually transmitted infections discovered in STD clinics in 1990. The optometrist must be aware of the sometimes difficult differential diagnosis and be prepared to evaluate the patient for associated STDs.

REFERENCES

1. Schultz S, Araneta MRG, Joseph SC: Neurosyphilis and HIV infection. N Engl J Med 317:1474, 1987
2. Insler MS (ed): AIDS and Other Sexually Transmitted Diseases and the Eye. Grune & Stratton, Orlando, FL, 1987
3. Ackernecht EH. A Short History of Medicine. Ronald Press, New York, 1968
4. Rolfs RT, Nakashima AK: Epidemiology of Primary and Secondary Syphilis in the U.S., 1981–1989. JAMA 264:1432, 1990
5. Fournier A: Prophylaxie de al Syphilis. J. Reuff, Paris, 1903
6. Belin MW, Baltch AL, Hay PB: Secondary syphilitic uveitis. Am J Ophthalmol 92:2, 1981
7. Schwartz LK, O'Connor GR: Secondary syphilis with iris papules. Am J Ophthalmol 90:3, 1980
8. DeLuise VP, Clark SW, Smith JL, Collart P: Syphilitic retinal detachment and uveal effusion. Am J Ophthalmol 94:757, 1982
9. Bennett GR, Kay M, Muchnick B: Bilateral angle-closure glaucoma secondary to the acquired immune deficiency syndrome (AIDS). Paper presented to the American Academy of Optometry, Toronto, Canada, December 1986
10. Hutchinson J: A Clinical Memoir on Certain Diseases of the Eye and Ear: Consequent on Inherited Syphilis. John Churchill, London, 1863
11. Ronnerstam R, Persson K, Hansson H et al: Prevalence of chlamydial eye infection in patients attending an eye clinic, a VD clinic, and in healthy persons. Br J Ophthalmol 69:35, 1985
12. Alexander ER, Harrison RH: Role of chlamydia trachomatis in perinatal infection. Rev Infect Dis 5:713, 1983
13. Dawson C, Wood TR, Rose L et al: Experimental inclusion conjunctivitis in man: III. Keratitis and other complications. Arch Ophthalmol 78:341, 1967
14. Holmes MD, Safyer SM, Bickell NA et al: Chlamydial cervical infection in jailed women. Am J Public Health 83:551, 1993
15. Mettler C: History of Medicine. Blakiston, Philadelphia, 1947
16. Doerr R, Vochting K: Etudes sur le virus de l'herpes febrile. Rev Gen Ophthalmol (Paris) 34:409, 1920
17. Deardorff SL, Deture FA, Drylie DM et al: Association between herpes hominis type II and the male genitourinary tract. J Urol 112:126, 1974
18. Grayson M: Diseases of the cornea. CV Mosby, St. Louis, 1979
19. Kaplowitz LG, Baker D, Gelb L: Prolonged continuous acyclovir treatment of normal adults with frequency recurring genital herpes simplex infection. JAMA 265:747, 1991
20. Rein MF: Epidemiology of gonococcal infections. p. 12. In Roberts RB (ed): The gonococcus. John Wiley & Sons, New York, 1977
21. Schwarcz SK, Zenilman JM, Schnell D: National surveillance of antimicrobial resistance in *Neisseria gonorrhoeae*. JAMA 264:1413, 1990
22. Parker JS: An update on treatment of gonococcal ophthalmia. Arch Ophthalmol 109:613, 1991
23. Richert CA, Peterman TA, Zaid AA et al: A method for identifying persons at high risk for sexually transmitted infections: opportunity for targeting intervention. Am J Public Health 83:520, 1993

19 Acquired Immunodeficiency Syndrome

CONNIE L. CHRONISTER

INTRODUCTION

As the number of cases of acquired immunodeficiency syndrome (AIDS) increases in the 1990s, eye care practitioners will be faced with the examination and management of these unique and clinically challenging patients. This chapter discusses the ocular mani-festations in patients with human immunodeficiency virus (HIV) and AIDS. The course of HIV infection can be plotted according to the patient's immunologic state and many of the ocular manifestations. Eye care practitioners may be an integral part of the initial diagnosis of HIV infection by discovering its ocular sequelae.

CASE REPORT

A 27-year-old black woman presented with a history of crack cocaine drug abuse. She admitted occasional prostitution activities to support her cocaine habit. She presented with a chief complaint of ocular burning, grittiness, and mild foreign body irritation of 3 months' duration. She also complained of occasional floating spots in both eyes, which had occurred for many years. She had been diagnosed with HIV 7 years before this examination. She denied any history of ocular opportunistic infections or carcinomas. She had no history of opportunistic systemic infections but had been feeling "run down," with symptoms of swollen glands, mild malaise, recurrent fevers, and other flu-like symptoms. She claimed to be in "good health," and her last CD4$^+$ T-helper cell count was 210 cells/mm^3. She took five 100-mg tablets of AZT (zidovudine) per day. The patient also reported a history of genital chlamydial infection before her diagnosis of HIV infection. She denied any other systemic conditions or the presence of any drug allergies.

Ocular examination revealed a best corrected visual acuity of 20/20 OU. Her ocular motilities were smooth and intact, and her pupil responses were equal, round, and reactive with a negative afferent pupillary defect. Her confrontation fields were full in both eyes. Slit lamp examination revealed a reduced tear meniscus that contained debris, mild corneal epithelial stippling, and a reduced tear break-up time of 7 seconds OD and 8 seconds OS (Fig. 19-1 and Plate 19-1). Her intraocular pressure was normal, with Goldmann applanation tonometry readings of 15 mmHg OD and 16 mmHg OS. A dilated fundus evaluation revealed a normal optic nerve with C/D (cup to disc) ratios of 0.3 × 0.3 OU. Cotton-wool spots (CWSs) as well as blot and dot hemorrhages were noted in the macular region in both eyes (Fig. 19-2 and Plate 19-2).

The patient was considered to be HIV infected and not to have full-blown AIDS. To be diagnosed with AIDS, a patient must have either an opportunistic in-

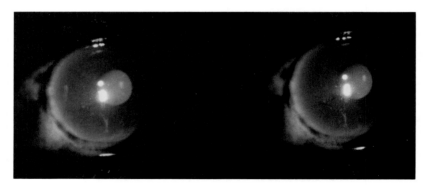

Fig. 19-1. The patient from the case report: a premenopausal woman infected with HIV. She presented with a reduced break-up time, debris in the tear film, and a reduced tear meniscus. She had symptomatology of dry eye secondary to HIV infection. (Photograph courtesy of Jane Stein). (See also Plate 19-1.)

fection or a CD4$^+$ T-helper cell count of less than 200 cells/mm^3. It is the CD4$^+$ T-helper cells (a subpopulation of lymphocytes) that are primarily infected and destroyed by HIV. The level of CD4$^+$ T-helper cells is often referred to as the "CD4 count." The average CD4$^+$ count in a normal healthy adult is 1,000/mm^3. Her ocular irritation was secondary to a dry eye condition that can occur in HIV-infected patients. This was treated with artificial tear supplements to be used at least four times per day. The presence of cotton-wool patches is a classic ocular presentation of HIV infection and should be monitored every 3 to 6 months.

Over the next year, the patient's condition quickly deteriorated. I examined her every 3 months to moni-

tor for any ocular opportunistic infections and advised her to return immediately if she noted any visual changes. Nine months after her initial visit, she returned for her third follow-up visit. Until this visit, her dry-eye condition was controlled with the artificial tears and her cotton-wool patches had not increased significantly. This visit, she reported a drastic decrease in her CD4$^+$ T-helper cell count. She also stated that she had recently been hospitalized for *Pneumocystis carinii* pneumonia. She was not as coherent and as reliable a historian as she had been in the past, and it was difficult to ascertain what medications she was taking and what her exact CD4$^+$ count was on her last check-up. All she knew was that it was much lower than it had been in the past. She seemed to be experiencing AIDS dementia.

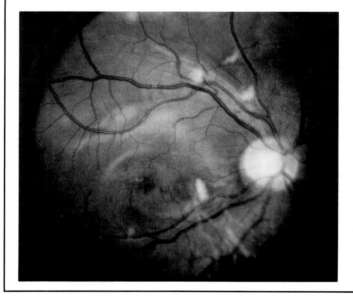

Fig. 19-2. Cotton-wool spots and retinal microvascular changes. (Photograph courtesy of Jane Stein.) (See also Plate 19-2.)

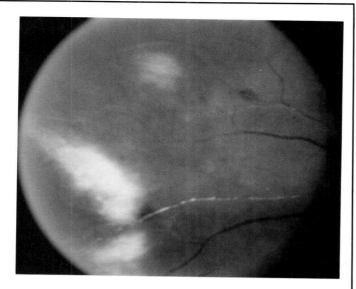

Fig. 19-3. Early cytomegalovirus exhibited in the superior nasal quadrant of the retina. (Photograph courtesy of Jane Stein.) (See also Plate 19-3.)

Fortunately, her best corrected acuity had remained at 20/20 OU, and her external signs and symptoms remained unchanged except for a questionable inferior temporal defect on confrontation testing of the left eye. She had a red vascularized elevation on her left upper lid that appeared to be early Kaposi sarcoma. Dilated fundus examination revealed extensive microvascular changes with numerous CWS and hemorrhages in both eyes. The superior nasal quadrant in the left eye contained a patch of retinal necrosis, hemorrhaging, and vascular sheathing approximately 4 disc diameters in size. A sharp demarcation line between affected and unaffected retina was noted (Fig. 19-3 and Plate 19-3). The vitreous contained numerous inflammatory cells and debris, and a few cells could be seen in the anterior chamber.

The left eye had developed cytomegalovirus (CMV) retinitis, and the patient was immediately referred to a retinal specialist for treatment with either ganciclovir or foscarnet. She was initially treated with ganciclovir, and the CMV was controlled for several weeks. Unfortunately, her CD4 count had become dangerously low (10 cells/mm^3) due to the concurrent use of ganciclovir and AZT. Both ganciclovir and AZT cause bone marrow suppression and usually cannot be used together. The patient needed to continue AZT to control the HIV infection. Foscarnet was then used instead of ganciclovir, because its side effects do not include bone marrow suppression and it can be taken with AZT. The retinal specialist continued to care for the patient, and she maintained some vision until her death 8 months after the diagnosis of CMV infection. Her Kaposi sarcoma remained small and the elevation did not interfere with lid function, so it was simply monitored.

Discussion: This patient exhibited some of the more common ocular manifestations of HIV infection and AIDS. Following is a more detailed discussion of the examination and management of an HIV-infected patient.

EXAMINATION

History

HIV has attacked mainly white men age 25 to 45 years (Centers for Disease Control [CDC] informational hotline, personal communication, 1993) (Fig. 19-4). Recently, the number of women infected with HIV has increased dramatically (CDC informational hotline, personal communication, 1993). Today, especially in urban settings, many women are contracting AIDS. Many of these women are either intravenous drug abusers or drug abusers who resort to prostitution to support their habits. Many women also are contracting HIV from heterosexual activities with HIV-infected men. Even though homosexual or bisexual men continue to be the overwhelmingly majority of those who become HIV infected, practitioners must be aware of other high-risk groups and transmission categories for HIV infection (Fig. 19-5). High-risk behaviors can often be elicited in the history if it is tactfully and care-

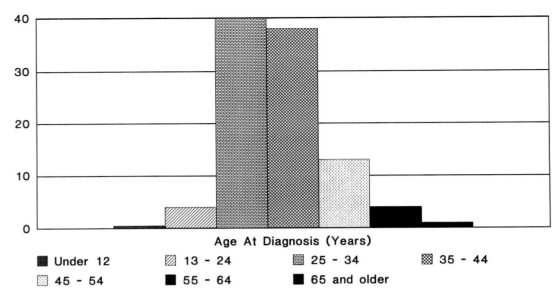

Fig. 19-4. Age categories of AIDS patients (expressed as a percentage of total AIDS cases). (Data from Centers for Disease Control.[76])

fully taken, and this information can alert the practitioner to possible HIV-infected patients (Table 19-1).

AIDS initially was mainly a disease of white homosexual or bisexual men. The disease now crosses all sexual, racial and socioeconomic barriers (Fig. 19-6). The stereotypical AIDS patient is a thing of the past. An estimated 5 to 10 million people are infected with HIV worldwide, and 1 million are infected in the United States (CDC, personal communication, 1993).

The general systemic manifestations of HIV infection

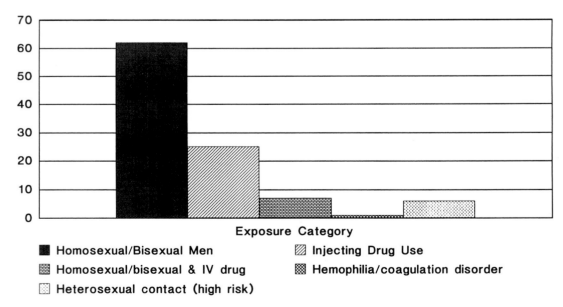

Fig. 19-5. Transmission (exposure) categories for HIV infection (expressed as a percentage of total AIDS cases). (Data from Centers for Disease Control.[76])

Table 19-1. High-Risk Groups for HIV Infection

Sexually active homosexual men
Intravenous drug abusers
Hemophiliacs or persons with coagulation disorders
Heterosexual persons who have sexual intercourse with persons
   at risk
Recipients of blood transfusions, blood components, or tissue
Children of mothers with or at risk of HIV infection

can help to alert a practitioner that a patient is infected. Five to twenty percent of patients will experience a mild flu-like illness 4 to 12 weeks after becoming infected with HIV.[1] Active primary infection occurs during seroconversion and is not diagnostic because it is so similar to the common flu. It usually lasts only 2 weeks. The virus then becomes latent in the host's system for a variable amount of time. The average latency is approximately 10 years.[1] During this period, most patients are not aware of their HIV infection but can transmit the disease. Latency is referred to as the chronic asymptomatic infection stage. After latency, the virus causes persistent generalized lymphadenopathy and the patient experiences enlarged lymph nodes. Progression of the infection leads to active disease; the patient experiences weight loss, persistent fever, night sweats, skin rashes, fatigue, and oral thrush. Not until the patient contracts an opportunistic infection or shows severe immunodeficiency (CD4$^+$ cell count less than 200 cells/mm^3) is full-blown AIDS is diagnosed (CDC, personal communication).

By knowing the different stages of the disease, the eye care practitioner can ask patients specific questions about their general systemic health, such as the following:

Have you been very fatigued lately?
Have you experienced recurrent fever or night sweats?
Have you had any recurring oral infections or sores?
Have you had any skin rashes?
Have you lost weight or had appetite loss?
Have you had recurrent diarrhea?

Certainly, yes to any of these questions is not fully diagnostic but could aid in determining whether the patient is experiencing symptoms caused by HIV infection.

When looking for full-blown AIDS the patient can be asked:

Have you ever been tested for HIV infection?
Have you had pneumonia, and what was the cause of your
   lung infection?
Have you had any recurrent infections?
What medications have you been taking?
Have you ever had your CD4$^+$ T-cell count taken?
If so, what was your latest CD4$^+$ T-cell count?

These questions may seem basic, but many diagnosed AIDS patients may be reluctant to state whether they are infected; the eye care practitioner can find out about the infection indirectly. Furthermore, many full-blown AIDS patients experience dementia and simply forget to give pertinent information or are poor

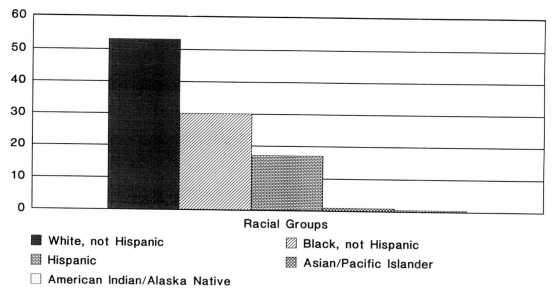

■ White, not Hispanic   ▨ Black, not Hispanic
▦ Hispanic   ▩ Asian/Pacific Islander
☐ American Indian/Alaska Native

Fig. 19-6. Percentages of racial groups infected with AIDS. (Data from the Centers for Disease Control.)

Table 19-2. CD4 Count and HIV Infection

Stage of HIV Infection	CD4 Count Range (cells/mm³)
Initial illness (active retroviral syndrome)	1,000–500
Asymptomatic carrier (latency)	750–500
Early symptomatic (non-life-threatening infections, chronic symptoms)	500–100
Late symptomatic (life threatening infections, carcinomas and severe symptoms)	200–50
Advanced HIV infection (severe infections, high risk of death)	50–0

(Adapted from DeVita et al.,[1] with permission.)

historians. The preceding lists are a starting point and are not inclusive.

The CD4⁺ T-helper lymphocyte count is a valuable marker for the course of HIV infection because it is the CD4⁺ T-helper cells that are mainly infected and depleted by HIV infection. The lower the CD4⁺ T-helper cell count, the more advanced the HIV disease. Therefore, the lower the CD4⁺ T-helper cell count, the more immunosuppressed the patient, and the more likely the patient has had or will develop life-threatening opportunistic infections (Table 19-2).

When examining HIV-infected patients, the eye care practitioner should always ask for their most recent CD4⁺ T-helper cell count. If the number is less than 200 cells/mm³, they have full-blown AIDS; as this number decreases, the patient should be examined more frequently for monitoring of opportunistic ocular infections[1,2] (CDC, personal communication).

The medications commonly taken by HIV-infected patients are for either HIV itself or the opportunistic infections. The three medications approved by the Food and Drug Administration (FDA) commonly used to treat HIV infection are AZT (zidovudine, Retrovir), ddI (dideoxycytosine), or ddC (Zalcitabine, HIVID). All inhibit the replicative cycle of HIV. None are fully effective in eradicating HIV. They simply improve longevity and quality of life. The common opportunistic infections seen in HIV patients and their treatments are listed in Table 19-3.[2]

OCULAR MANIFESTATIONS

Microvascular Changes

The most common ocular manifestation of HIV infection are cotton-wool patches and retinal microvascular changes. Studies have reported that CWSs have

Table 19-3. Major Systemic Opportunistic Infections and Neoplasms

Major Pathogen	Major Diseases	Common Treatments (Not All Inclusive)
Viral Infections		
Cytomegalovirus	Retinitis, colitis	Ganciclovir, foscarnet
Herpes Simplex	Mucocutaneous ulcer	Acyclovir, foscarnet
Herpes Zoster	Vesiculobullous eruptions	Acyclovir
Protozoal Infections		
Pneumocystis carinii	Pneumonia	Trimethoprim, sulfamethoxazole, pentamidine, primaquine, dapsone, bactrim
Toxoplasma gondii	Central nervous system lesion, chorioretinitis	Pyrimethamine, sulfadiazine, clindamycin
Cryptosporidum muri	Diarrhea, cholecystis	None
Fungal Infections		
Candida albicans	Oral thrush, gastrointestinal tract Endophthalmitis	Ketoconazole, fluconazole, amphotericin B Amphotericin B
Cryptococcus neoformans	Meningitis, endophthalmitis, optic neuritis	Amophotericin B, fluconazole
Bacterial Infections		
Mycobacterium tuberculosis	Pneumonia	Isoniazide, pyridoxine, rifampin, pyrazinamide, ethambutol
Streptococcus pneumoniae	Pneumonia	
Haemophilus influenzae	Pneumonia	
Mycobacterium avium intracellulare	Gastrointestinal tract	
Neoplasms		
Kaposi sarcoma	Vascularized tumors	Systemic chemotherapy, immune response modifiers, excision, cryotherapy, radiotherapy

Table 19-4. Common Causes
of Cotton-Wool Spots

Diabetes mellitus
Systemic hypertension
Collagen vascular diseases
AIDS (HIV infection)
Leukemia
Severe anemia
Retinal vein obstruction

been found in 45 to 100 percent of AIDS patients.[3-7] CWSs are areas of ischemia that occur from blockade of axoplasmic flow, swollen interrupted axons, and edema in the nerve fiber layer of retina. Table 19-4 lists the common causes of CWS. The optometrist should consider the list of differentials for the causes of CWS before concluding that a patient may be HIV infected. Cotton-wool patches in HIV-infected patients resolve in 4 to 6 weeks. This resolution was noted in the patient in the case report, but as old ones resolved, new ones were forming, along with retinal hemorrhages. Retinal hemorrhages have been seen in 8 to 40 percent of HIV-infected patients.[8,9] Microaneurysms and ischemic macular edema have been observed in HIV-infected patients.[8-11] The microvascular changes seen in HIV-infected patients are often likened to the appearance of early diabetic retinopathy (Fig. 19-2).

To effectively monitor the progression of retinal microvascular changes, an understanding of the cause of microvascular disease in HIV-infected patients is helpful. The pathogenesis remains under question, but several studies have addressed this question.[5-12] Ultrastructural retinal vascular changes that have been observed include loss and degeneration of pericytes, swollen endothelial cells, thickened basal lamina, and narrowed capillary lumina.[6] Causes of these ultrastructural changes remain to be determined but have been hypothesized. HIV has been isolated in the endothelial cells that line retinal blood vessels.[12] Therefore, HIV may directly infect the retinal capillaries and cause microvascular disease.[12] HIV infection causes an increase in the amount of circulating immune complexes, and these may deposit in the walls of capillaries and cause capillary occlusion.[8] Other studies have examined altered viscosity of blood and altered blood flow in HIV-infected patients.[11] If the blood viscosity increases, retinal ischemia may result.[11]

Regardless of the cause, the presence of CWSs in an HIV-infected patient is a significant prognostic sign.[5] Patients who exhibited CWSs were more immunocompromised and had lower CD4+ T-helper cell counts than those with clear retinas.[5,7,10] The patient in the case report was immunocompromised on the initial visit with a CD4+ T-helper cell count of 210 cells/mm[3] and mild symptomatology. CWSs are rarely found in HIV-infected patients who have minimal to no signs of HIV infection. By contrast, CWSs have been found in 31 percent of AIDS-related complex patients (patients with flu-like symptoms and lymphadenopathy), and these patients were more likely to more quickly develop full-blown AIDS than AIDS-related complex patients without CWSs.[10] Again, the patient in the case report proved this to be true: she developed full-blown AIDS within a relatively short period of exhibiting CWSs. The presence of CWSs indicates a compromised blood–retina barrier and compromised capillaries.[13] This patient developed CMV shortly after exhibiting cotton-wool patches and retinal microvascular changes. Opportunistic infections such as CMV may more easily infect the retina through viremic seeding. In other words, the compromised retinal arcades and capillaries allow infection to more easily reach the retina. Follow-up should be done every 6 months unless the patient exhibits a decline in the CD4+ T-helper cell count. Then follow-up should be done every 3 months or more frequently if necessary. Routine retinal photography is also helpful in the follow-up of these patients.

Conjunctiva of HIV-infected patients have also exhibited microvascular changes.[11] Observations of alterations in blood flow of arterioles and venules of capillaries have included granular appearance of blood column, aggregation of red blood cells, decreased rate of blood flow, capillary dilation, microaneurysms, short vessel segments of irregular caliber, and isolated vessel fragments.[11] These changes have been most apparent on inferior, perilimbal, bulbar conjunctiva and have been reported in 75 percent of HIV-infected patients.[11] Most likely, the cause of the conjunctival vessel changes is the same as the cause of retinal CWSs.[11]

Opportunistic Ocular Infections

CMV retinitis is the most common ocular opportunistic infection seen in AIDS patients and was the first ocular opportunistic infection exhibited in the case report. CMV retinitis is the second most common ocular manifestation of HIV infection and is seen in 15 to 40 percent of AIDS patients.[4,14] After contracting CMV, patients are most likely very immunocompromised.[14] The patient in the case report contracted CMV very late in the course of her HIV infection. CMV usually occurs when a patient has a very depleted CD4+ count. It affects central vision only when visually important structures such as the macula or optic nerve are infected with CMV. Fortunately, this patient had peripheral retinal involvement and was treated before the infection reached the macula or optic nerve, sparing her vision. Her peripheral field loss was the result of the CMV infection.

CMV retinitis has a characteristic appearance (Fig. 19-3). Many optometrists have referred to CMV retinitis as the "pizza fundus" or "cottage cheese and ketchup fundus."[15] Active CMV infection causes granular white patches along the retinal vessels[15] (Fig. 19-7 and Plate 19-4). The inflammation often follows the vascular arcades, and necrotic foci coalesce to form large patches of retinal necrosis with extensive edema, hemorrhaging, and exudate.[15] The infection spreads like a brush fire to invade the entire retina within 3 to 6 months.[16] Untreated infection can lead to retinal detachment and blindness.

Two FDA-approved drugs are used to treat CMV—ganciclovir and foscarnet. These drugs treat ocular as well as other systemic infections caused by CMV. Ganciclovir and foscarnet inhibit the replication of CMV. They are intravenous medications that require hospitalization for the initial induction doses. An outpatient maintenance dose is needed to prevent reactivation of infection. Using ganciclovir, improvement of the retinitis is seen in 81 percent of treated patients with complete remission in 61 percent of treated patients.[17] Because of ganciclovir's relatively good success rate, it was the drug initially used in the case report. Intravitreal injection of ganciclovir has been done experimentally with varying results and was not attempted in the reported case.[18]

The adverse effects of ganciclovir treatment include bone marrow suppression or neutropenia and long-term breakthrough progression of retinitis in 35 percent of treated patients.[19] Because AZT also causes neutropenia, great care must be taken in the administration of AZT with ganciclovir. Often, a decision must be made by both the patient and practitioner whether to administer ganciclovir to preserve vision or continue AZT therapy to control HIV infection. Because CMV patients are usually severely immunocompromised, the median survival rate of AIDS patients treated with ganciclovir is 8 months.[20]

Foscarnet, an alternative drug to ganciclovir, was FDA approved in the fall of 1991. Foscarnet does not suppress the bone marrow nor cause the side effects of AZT and ganciclovir. Therefore, both AZT and foscarnet can be used simultaneously to treat CMV retinopathy and HIV infection.[20] It does not appear to be quite as effective against CMV as ganciclovir. Response to therapy was good in 47 of treated patients.[21] Side effects of foscarnet include renal toxicity as well as anemia.[21]

Many other drugs are used experimentally for the treatment of CMV retinitis. Recently AZT was used in conjunction with acyclovir in an AIDS patient infected with herpes stomatitis and CMV.[22] This treatment regimen successfully controlled the retinal lesions for 28 months.[22] With the patient in the case report, only FDA-approved drugs were used. To enroll a patient in a clinical trial or to obtain information call the AIDS clinical trial hotline (1-800-TRIALS-A).

Early diagnosis of CMV retinitis is essential to initiate early treatment and to allow patients the option of participating in a clinical trial. As AIDS patients become more immunocompromised, they should be monitored every 3 months.

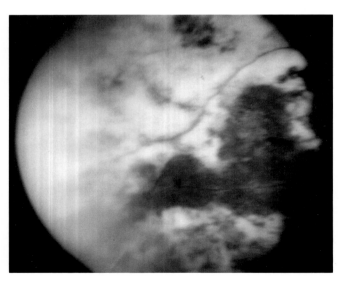

Fig. 19-7. Advanced CMV. Note the white granular retinal necrosis, exudate, and hemorrhaging that are characteristic of CMV retinitis. (Photograph courtesy of Jane Stein.) (See also Plate 19-4.)

Dry Eye

Dry eye in HIV-infected women has been reported, but most of literature discusses this condition in men.[23–25] Dry eye in a premenopausal woman is rare unless the patient has concurrent collagen vascular or autoimmune disease affecting the lacrimal gland. Dry eye is rare in healthy young men but has commonly been reported in HIV-infected men. One study reported keratoconjunctivitis sicca in 21 percent of HIV-infected men.[24] It is hypothesized that HIV-infected patients develop a sicca complex similar to that in Sjögren syndrome.[25] In HIV-infected patients, the lacrimal gland is rendered dysfunctional by the immune attack on the parenchyma of the gland. The disease process is not identical to Sjögren syndrome, but the two conditions have been compared.[25] Aggressive ocular lubrication is recommended for these patients.

Kaposi Sarcoma

Kaposi sarcoma is a slowly progressive, vascular malignancy seen in 24 percent of AIDS patients.[26] Although it tends to be most common in male homosexual HIV-infected patients, it can be seen in any HIV-infected patient. Ocular Kaposi sarcoma is a vascular malignancy commonly seen on the eyelids, caruncle, and conjunctiva (Fig. 19-8). Conjunctival lesions could easily initially be mistaken for a subconjunctival hemorrhage. Lack of regression of a red conjunctival lesion in an HIV patient should alert the practitioner to Kaposi sarcoma malignancy. Treatment of Kaposi sarcoma includes chemotherapy, immunotherapy, radiotherapy, cryotherapy, and excision.[26]

Viral Infections

Herpes Simplex

Herpes simplex keratitis has been reported in patients with AIDS. It is not clear whether the incidence of herpes simplex is greater in HIV-infected patients than in patients with normal immune systems. Herpes simplex keratitis in HIV-infected patients can be more difficult to manage than in immunocompetent patients. Herpes simplex keratitis in AIDS patients shows a predilection for peripheral cornea and limbus versus central cornea. The corneal lesions are unilateral and either dendritic or geographic (Fig. 19-9). Stromal involvement is rare. Herpes simplex also causes skin follicles, follicular conjunctivitis, and punctate keratitis. Recurrences are common with a prolonged clinical course.

Herpes simplex mucocutaneous ocular infection is usually managed initially with topical antivirals. In HIV-infected patients, topical antivirals are often effective for herpes simplex keratitis. The common antiviral agents used are vidarabine (Vira-A) ointment four times daily and trifluridine (Viroptic) solution every 2 hours.[27,28] Idoxuridine (IDU, Stoxil) ointment has been used in the past but is often not the current drug of choice. Acyclovir (Zivorax) ointment has been used experimentally for deeper corneal infections and skin lesions.[29] Occasionally, in immunocompromised HIV-infected patients, severe infections occur and require oral acyclovir in conjunction with topical antivirals.[30,31] Occasionally, acyclovir-resistant mucocutaneous herpes simplex infections occur in HIV-infected patients. Other antiviral agents such as vidarabine

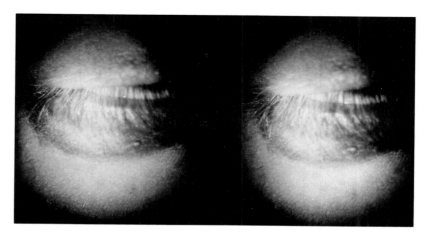

Fig. 19-8. Kaposi sarcoma on the lower lid. (Photograph courtesy of Jane Stein.) (See also Plate 19-5.)

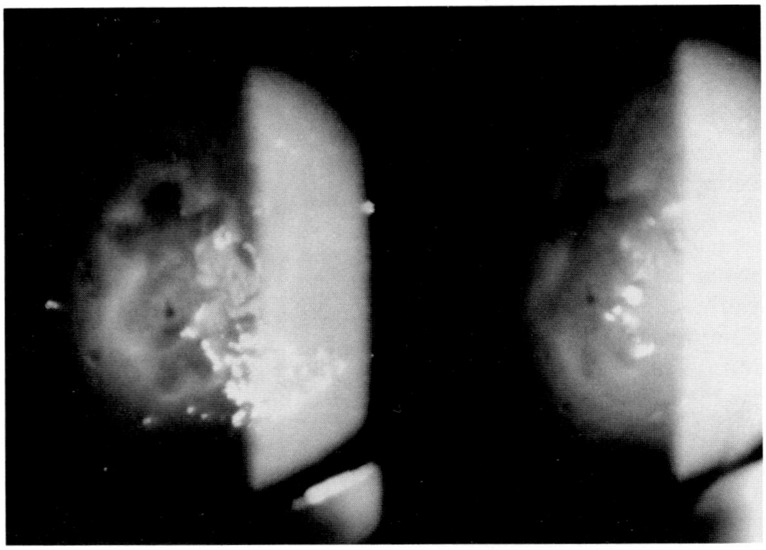

Fig. 19-9. Herpes simplex corneal dendrite. (Photograph courtesy of Jane Stein.) (See also Plate 19-6.)

and foscarnet have been used. Foscarnet had superior efficacy and less frequent toxicity than AZT.[32,33] Topical steroids should always be avoided in cases of active epithelial keratitis. Occasionally, however, if there is stromal inflammation only, steroids can be carefully used to control the stromal inflammation that results in response to viral antigens. The discretionary use of topical steroids in immunocompromised HIV-infected patients should only occur in conjunction with aggressive use of antivirals.

Although rare, herpes simplex retinitis can occur in AIDS patients. It is characterized by large confluent patches of retinal necrosis with retinal hemorrhage. Herpes simplex retinitis causes less hemorrhaging and less of a "cheesy appearance" than CMV retinitis. It spreads by continuous extension, causing an absolute field defect. Lesions resolve centrally, leaving mottled gray atrophy. Herpes simplex retinitis is treated with intravenous acyclovir.

Herpes Zoster

Herpes zoster ophthalmicus, commonly seen in elderly patients, can cause both anterior and posterior segment disease in HIV-infected patients. When herpes zoster infection is seen in patients younger than 40 years old, HIV infection or other causes of severe immunosuppression such as chemotherapy or organ transplantation should be suspected.[34] Herpes zoster ophthalmicus may be the first manifestation

of HIV infection and can have important prognostic implications for an HIV-infected patient. HIV-infected patients with herpes zoster infection are at increased risk of developing full-blown AIDS.

Herpes zoster ophthalmicus in AIDS or HIV-infected patients is characterized by a severe vesiculobullous rash along the distribution of the ophthalmic division of the trigeminal nerve. Along with the rash, an AIDS patient could develop conjunctivitis, keratitis, and uveitis. A recurrent dendriform keratitis that is due to herpes zoster can occur in HIV-infected patients due to the severe immunosuppression allowing active replication of the virus on the cornea. Chronic herpes zoster keratitis in HIV-infected patients can sometimes be confused with herpes simplex infection.

Also reported in HIV-infected patients has been a zoster retinitis that is rare yet visually devastating because it causes a severe necrosis that often leads to retinal detachment.[35,36] It is similar in appearance to CMV retinitis, but it can be differentiated from CMV by its lack of severe hemorrhaging.[35,37] Unlike CMV, it also tends to spare the retinal vessels and the vitreous. It is a rapidly progressive retinal necrosis characterized by outer retinal, multifocal lesions that can coalesce and cause retinal detachment.[35,37] The course of herpes zoster infection in AIDS patients can be chronic and require prolonged treatment with oral or intravenous acyclovir.[35,38] Unfortunately, herpes zoster retinal necrosis can be resistant to treatment with oral or intravenous acyclovir.[35]

Molluscum Contagiosum

Infection with molluscum contagiosum (pox virus) has been reported in AIDS patients.[39,40] Molluscum is a benign, common viral disease of the skin. It usually appears in children with normal immunity around the face or eyelids or in adults around the genitalia as a sexually transmitted disease. It usually comprises less than 20 lesions and is self-limiting with spontaneous resolution in 3 to 12 months.

In AIDS patients, molluscum has been characterized by a large number of lesions that do not resolve spontaneously.[39] The lesions tend to be larger and more confluent than in immunocompetent patients and involve the face and extremities.[40] Recurrences within 6 to 8 weeks are common after surgical removal or cryotherapy of the lesions.[39] The effectiveness of the treatment of molluscum contagiosum remains under question.

Protozoal Infections

Toxoplasmosis

In the "non-AIDS" population, toxoplasmosis is the most common cause of infectious retinitis.[41] Toxoplasmosis, in the immunocompromised host, is becoming a major cause of mortality and can cause life-threatening encephalitis, pneumonia, or myocarditis. In AIDS patients, central nervous system infection is the most common manifestation of toxoplasmosis.[41] Retinochoroiditis from toxoplasmosis occurs in 1 percent of AIDS patients and is the second most common form of retinal infection seen in AIDS patients.[41,42] Its appearance is similar to retinochoroiditis in "non-AIDS" patients, except new lesions often occur distant from old pre-existing toxoplasmic scars.[43] This suggests acquired infection rather than activation of latent infection. Unlike CMV retinitis, toxoplasmosis rarely causes retinal hemorrhaging (Fig. 19-10). This difference usually assists the optometrist in the differentiation of CMV from toxoplasmosis retinal infection.

Active toxoplasmosis infection in AIDS patients can be difficult to treat. Treatment usually includes pyrimethamine, clindamycin, and sulfadiazine.[43] Other ocular complications from toxoplasmosis include chronic iridocyclitis, cataract formation, secondary

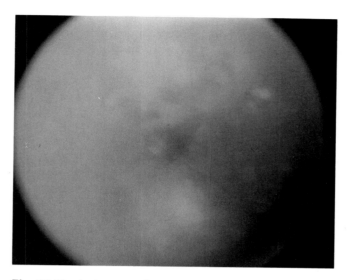

Fig. 19-10. Active toxoplasmosis adjacent to a scar due to toxoplasmosis. (Photograph courtesy of Jane Stein.) (See also Plate 19-7.)

glaucoma, band keratopathy, cystoid macular edema, retinal detachment, and optic atrophy.

Pneumocystis Carinii

Pneumocystis carinii pneumonia is the most common systemic opportunistic infection in AIDS patients, yet it rarely causes ocular infection. Pneumocystis infects the eye by causing unilateral or bilateral multifocal choroidal lesions that cluster in the posterior pole.[44] The choroidal lesions are round, yellow-white, flat, or slightly raised and can lead to serous detachments. The choroiditis is very difficult to treat. Intravenous pentamidine, methoprim, and sufamethoxazole have been used to control serous retinal detachment and progression of pneumocystis choroiditis.[44,45]

Bacterial Infections

Tuberculosis

Mycobacterium tuberculosis is becoming a more common cause of pneumonia in AIDS patients. HIV immunosuppression has caused a resurgence of this highly contagious infection. In addition to causing systemic infection, tuberculosis choroiditis has been reported in AIDS patients.[46] Tuberculosis choroiditis is characterized by hazy, granulomatous lesions with retinal phlebitis. Chronic iridocyclitis can also occur in ocular tuberculosis.

Unfortunately, tuberculosis has developed some resistant strains, and treatment can be extremely difficult.[47] Isonazide with pyridoxine, rifampin, pyrazinamide, and ethambutol have been used to treat tuberculosis but sometimes with limited success. Tuberculosis tends to occur in patients that are relatively less immunologically suppressed (CD4 counts of 350 mm cells/mm^3 or less) than other opportunistic infections such as CMV.[1] Patients with tuberculosis can easily transmit this very infectious organism via respiratory droplets. Therefore, when patients with tuberculosis are being examined, both the eye care practitioner and the patient should wear a mask.

Syphilis

An association exists between syphilis and HIV infection. Genital syphilitic ulcers may favor the acquisition of HIV infection; therefore, the prevalence of syphilis in HIV-infected individuals is higher. The natural course of syphilitic infection is accelerated when concurrent HIV infection exists. Syphilis is known as the great imitator and can be clinically present in many different ways. This is also true of HIV-infected syphilitic patients. They can develop uveitis, ocular nerve palsies, episcleritis, scleritis, neuroretinitis, and optic neuritis.[48–50] Treatment can be difficult in these patients. Although recurrence of infection is common in HIV-infected patients, intravenous penicillin is recommended for ocular syphilis.[49]

Other Bacterial Infections

Numerous bacterial ocular infections have been reported that affect both the anterior and posterior segments. Bacterial endogenous retinitis has been reported in AIDS patients, but it is very rare.[51] As with all ocular infections in HIV-infected patients, these rare bacterial infections can be difficult to treat[52,53] (Table 19-5).

Most HIV-infected patients who have developed corneal bacterial ulcers had pre-existing conditions such as exposure keratitis, herpes simplex, or contact lens wear.[52] Therefore, HIV infection itself probably does not predispose a patient to bacterial corneal ulcers. Infections that result after some insult to the cornea, however, may be particularly severe.[54] Contact lens wear in HIV-infected patients therefore should be discouraged.

Table 19-5. Examples of Bacterial Corneal Ulcers in HIV-Infected Patients[a]

Infecting Organism	Treatment	Outcome
Pseudomonas aeruginosa	Fortified topical cefazolin and gentamicin	Perforation
Staphylococcus aureus	Fortified topical gentamicin	Perforation
Staphylococcus epidermidis	Fortified topical cefazolin and gentamicin	Resolved
Capnocytophaga ochracea	Fortified topical gentamicin sulfate and cefazolin sodium switched to erythromycin ointment	Resolved

[a] All the patients had pre-existing corneal conditions.
(Adapted from Shuler, et al.,[52] with permission.)

Fungal Infections

Cryptococcus and candidal retinal lesions seen in AIDS patients are similar to those seen in other immunocompromised patients. Candidal endophthalmitis is very common in intravenous drug abusers. It initially presents as yellow-white, small, inner retinal colonies that spread into the vitreous. This produces vitreous seeding with puff balls and condensation of the posterior vitreous face.[55] The retinal lesions can be treated with systemic amphotericin or ketoconazole, with or without fluocystosine or rifampin. The vitreal lesions need to be treated with intravitreal and intravenous amphotericin with or without vitrectomy.

Cryptococcus tends to cause choroiditis, often with optic nerve involvement. Bilateral vision loss in AIDS patients with cryptococcus is often due to optic neuropathy with cryptococcal meningitis. Without treatment, cryptococcal meningitis is fatal. The ocular infection needs aggressive treatment with amphotericin B and flucytosine with maintenance doses of amphotericin B.[56]

Histoplasmosis is a rare fungal ocular pathogen seen in AIDS patients. Histoplasmosis yeasts have been identified in the retina, optic nerves, and uveal tract of AIDS patients.[54,57] As with cryptococcus, it is treated with amphotericin B or ketoconazole.

Many ocular opportunistic infections are seen in HIV-infected and AIDS patients. These infections are summarized in Table 19-6. Note that this list is not comprehensive because new opportunistic infections are constantly being reported. Most of the ocular op-

Table 19-6. Ocular Opportunistic Infections and Neoplasms

Infections	Ocular Infection	Clinical Appearance	Treatment	Additional Comments
Viral Infections				
Cytomegalovirus	Retinitis	"Pizza fundus" full-thickness retinal necrosis and hemorrhage	Ganciclovir (IV) Foscarnet (IV)	Most common ocular opportunistic infection (20–40%)
Herpes simplex	Anterior segment (skin vesicles, follicular conjunctivitis, dendritic ulcer)	Severe skin vesicles and corneal ulceration	Oral or IV Acyclovir	Severe form in AIDS patients
	Retinitis	Retinal necrosis (significant intra-retinal hemorrhage)	Vidarabine (Vira-A) Trifluorothymidine (Viroptic) Foscarnet (IV)	
Herpes Zoster	Anterior segment (conjunctivitis, keratitis, vesicular eruptions, uveitis, retinitis)	Severe skin vesicles and keratitis Retinal necrosis	Acyclovir (IV and PO)	Herpes Zoster in young patients indicates possible HIV infection (4% of AIDS patients)
Molluscum contagiosum (pox virus)	"Warts" on eyelids	Benign epithelial tumor	Direct cautery, cryodestruction, surgical removal	Severe form in AIDS patients; spread by direct or indirect contact
Protozoal				
Toxoplasmosis	Chorioretinitis	Full-thickness necrosis Minimal hemorrhage, marked vitritis	Pyrimethamine Sulfadiazine Clindamycin	20–30% AIDS patients (systemic infection) 1% chorioretinitis
Pneumocystis carinii	Choroiditis	Choroidal inflammation (serous detachment)	Pentamidine (IV) Methoprim (IV) Sufamethoxazole (IV)	Rarely causes eye infection
Bacterial				
Tuberculosis	Chorioretinitis	Mainly choroidal involvement (yellow-white choroidal nodule)	Rifampin, pyridoxine, isonazide, pyrazinamide, ethambutol	Rarely affects eye; common cause of pneumonia
Syphilis	Uveitis, extraocular muscle (EOM) palsies, episcleritis, scleritis, neuroretinitis, optic neuritis	Greater imitator (variable) neuroretinitis (retinal necrosis)	Penicillin (IV)	Variable presentation
Pseudomonas Staphylococcus Neisseria gonorrhoeae Capnocytophagia Chlamydia	Ulcer and conjunctivitis	Corneal infiltrate with excavation Red eye	Varies depending on causative agent	Always culture ulcers and conjunctivitis from HIV-infected patients
Fungal				
Cryptococcus neoformans Candida albicans Sporothrix schenckii Histoplasmosis	Chorioretinitis, endophthalmitis, keratitis	Endophthalmitis (small white fluffy infiltrates, spread to overlying vitreous, vitreal haze with white fluffy lesions, vitreal abscess)	Amphotericin B (IV) Flucytosine Ketoconazole	Fungal infections, although rare in general population, should not be overlooked in HIV-infected patients

portunistic infections seen in HIV-infected patients are similar in clinical presentation and appearance to those seen in other patients but are much more severe and more difficult to treat.

NEUROPHTHALMIC MANIFESTATIONS

The neurophthalmic manifestations of HIV infection are numerous, and many are due to the opportunistic ocular infections. If the retina becomes infected, HIV-infected patients may show extensive field loss. Optic nerve infection can result in vision loss as well as an afferent pupillary defect.[58,59] HIV infection can also cause nerve damage that can present as a facial paresis or extraocular muscle (EOM) paresis.[60,61] Lymphoma is the second most common malignancy associated with AIDS.[62] Primary central nervous system lymphoma and systemic lymphoma with central nervous system involvement can cause diplopia from oculomotor, trochlear, or abducens nerve involvement.[62] Primary eyelid non-Hodgkin's lymphoma has been reported in a patient with AIDS.[63] Orbital and ocular large cell lymphomas in HIV-infected patients are rare.[62] Any neurophthalmic abnormality should be carefully investigated in an HIV-infected patient.

OCULAR HIV INFECTIONS

HIV infects nervous tissue in other areas of the body, and the retina does not appear to have escaped. HIV has been isolated from retinal tissues, vitreous, and choroid.[13] HIV has been found in all the retinal layers, but it appears to primarily infect Müller cells, the support cells of the retina.[13] Some HIV-infected patients have exhibited reduced acuity without apparent cause.[64,65] Their retinas as well as ocular media appear clear. They have exhibited reduced color vision and contrast sensitivity.[65] These findings may be the result of HIV infecting Müller cells, which are necessary for proper retinal function. HIV may be the cause of CWSs through infection of retinal vascular endothelial cells. More research is needed to confirm the effects of the presence of HIV in the retina.

INFECTION CONTROL PROCEDURES

Every patient should be treated as potentially infectious. Many HIV-infected individuals are not aware of their infection but can transmit the virus. Hand washing before each patient care encounter is an ef-

Table 19-7. CDC Recommendations for Preventing Possible Transmission of HIV From Tears

1. Wash hands immediately after a procedure and between patients. Gloves are advised when there is a break in the integrity of the skin.
2. Instruments that come into direct contact with external surfaces of the eye should be wiped clean and disinfected by soaking 5–10 minutes in one of the following:
   a. Fresh solution of 3% hydrogen peroxide
   b. Fresh solution of 1:10 dilution of household bleach or sodium hypochlorite (updated in 1987 to 1:100)
   c. 70% Ethanol
   d. 70% Isopropyl alcohol
   These devices should be thoroughly rinsed in tap water and dried before reuse.
3. Contact lenses used in trial fitting should be disinfected in between fittings by one of the following regimens:
   a. Commercially available hydrogen peroxide disinfecting systems. (This is for PMMA, gas-permeable and soft contact lenses.)
   b. Standard heat disinfection system for soft lenses.
   Cold chemical disinfectants used in standard contact solutions have not yet been thoroughly tested for their activity against HIV.

(Adapted from Centers for Disease Control.[70])

fective hygienic procedure that prevents the transmission of many pathogens including HIV. Instruments can be cleaned with common household disinfectants such as Lysol or dilute household bleach (1:10 dilution). Instruments that contact the cornea, conjunctiva, or tears need to be properly disinfected because HIV has been isolated in all these ocular tissues or fluids.[66–68]

The CDC has published specific recommendations for the disinfection of Goldmann applanation tonometer tips and other eye-contact devices.[69,70] A 10-minute soak in one of the selected disinfectants is recommended (Table 19-7). An enzymatic contact lens vial can be easily modified to serve as receptacle for soaking tonometer tips.[71] Reports show that after repeated soaking in alcohol, Goldmann tonometer tips become severely damaged.[72,73] Therefore, although recommended by the CDC, it is not financially practical to soak tonometer tips in alcohol because they need to be replaced frequently. Although not recommended by the CDC, swabbing with 70 percent isopropyl alcohol swabs or 3 percent hydrogen peroxide has been shown to be effective in disinfecting the tips.[74] Alcohol should be allowed to air dry before applanating the cornea because it may cause a corneal chemical burn or "tattoo" (Fig. 19-11). Surgical instruments

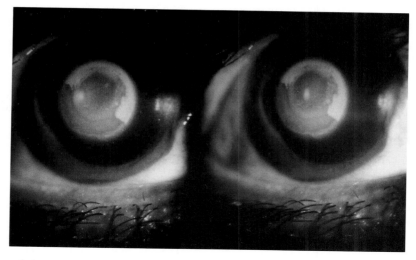

Fig. 19-11. Corneal chemical burn or "tattoo" secondary to a wet alcohol disinfected tonometer tip. (Photograph courtesy of Jane Stein.) (See also Plate 19-8.)

should be sterilized with autoclaving or ethylene oxide gas.

Contact lens fitting poses a potential mode of HIV transmission. HIV is inactivated by both heat and hydrogen peroxide contact lens disinfection systems.[70] The efficacy of other cold chemical contact lens disinfection systems has not been established and therefore cannot be currently recommended for the disinfection of trial-fitting lenses.

Latex gloves are usually not necessary for routine ocular evaluation. If the optometrist has a skin break and will contact infectious body fluids, gloving is recommended.[69] Eye protection, masking, and growing are required only when exposure to infectious bodily fluids that require universal precautions is certain.[75] To date, no evidence exists of proven transmission of HIV via contact with tears. The potential for transmission, however, remains; therefore, the infection protocols described must be adhered to.

CONCLUSIONS

HIV infection has been epidemic in the 1980s and 1990s, and no cure is in sight, although a great deal of research is being done to produce a vaccine. The transmission rates of HIV remain alarming, and HIV is infiltrating into many different segments of the population in both the United States and worldwide. Eye care practitioners must stay abreast of the new devel-

opments for the examination and management of the ocular manifestations of HIV infection.

REFERENCES

1. DeVita VT, Hellman S, Rosenberg SA: AIDS Etiology, Diagnosis, Treatment, and Prevention. p. 126. JB Lippincott, Philadelphia, 1992
2. Wormser GP: AIDS and Other Manifestations of HIV Infection. Raven Press, New York, 1992
3. Kestelyn P, dePerre PV, Rouvroy D et al: A prospective study of the ophthalmic findings in the acquired immune deficiency syndrome in Africa. Am J Ophthalmol 100:230, 1985
4. Holland GN, Pepose JS, Pettit TH et al: Acquired immune deficiency syndrome: ocular manifestations. Ophthalmology 90: 859, 1983
5. Freeman WR, Chen A, Henderly DE et al: Prevalence and significance of acquired immunodeficiency syndrome—related retinal microvasculopathy. Am J Ophthalmol 107:229, 1989
6. Newsome DA, Green WR, Miller ED et al: Microvascular aspects of acquired immune deficiency syndrome retinopathy. Am J Ophthalmol 98:590, 1984
7. Gabrieli CB, Angarano G, Moramarco A et al: Ocular manifestations in HIV-seropositive patients. Ann Ophthalmol 22:173, 1990
8. Pepose JS, Holland GN, Nestor MS et al: Acquired immune deficiency syndrome. Pathogenic mechanisms of ocular disease. Ophthalmology 92:472, 1985
9. Freemen WR, Lerner CW, Mines JA et al: A prospective study of the ophthalmic findings in the acquired immune deficiency syndrome. Am J Ophthalmol 97:133, 1984
10. Brezin A, Girard B, Rosenheim M et al: Cotton wool spots and AIDS related complex. Int Ophthalmol 14:37, 1990
11. Engstrom RE, Holland GN, Hardy WD, Meiselman HJ: Hemorheologic abnormalities in patients with human immunodeficiency virus infection and ophthalmic microvasculopathy. Am J Ophthalmol 109:153, 1990
12. Pomerantz RJ, Kuritzkes DR, DE LA Mont SM et al: Infection of the retina by human immunodeficiency virus type I. N Engl J Med 317:1643, 1987

13. Cellini M, Baldi A: Vitreous fluorophotometric recordings in HIV infection. Int Ophthalmol 15:37, 1991
14. Henderly DE, Freeman WR, Smith RE et al: Cytomegalovirus retinitis as the initial manifestation of the acquired immune deficiency syndrome. Am J Ophthalmol 103:316, 1987
15. Hennis HL, Scott AA, Apple DJ: Cytomegalovirus retinitis. Surv Ophthalmol 34:193, 1989
16. Gross JG, Bozzette SA, Mathews WC et al: Longitudinal study of cytomegalovirus retinitis in acquired immune deficiency syndrome. Ophthalmology 97:681, 1990
17. Jabs DA, Enger C, Bartlett JG: Cytomegalovirus retinitis and acquired immunodeficiency syndrome. Arch Ophthalmol 107: 75, 1989
18. Henry K, Cantrill H, Fletcher C et al: Use of intravitreal ganciclovir (dihydroxy propoxymethyl guanine) for cytomegalovirus retinitis in a patient with AIDS. Am J Ophthalmol 103:17, 1987
19. Weisenthal RW, Sinclair SH, Frank I, Rubin DH: Long-term outpatient treatment of CMV retinitis with ganciclovir in AIDS patients. Br J Ophthalmol 73:996, 1989
20. Jacobson MA, Drew WL, Feinberg J et al: Foscarnet therapy for ganciclovir-resistant cytomegalovirus retinitis in patients with AIDS. J Infect Dis 163:1348, 1991
21. Fanning MM, Read SE, Benson M et al: Foscarnet therapy of cytomegalovirus retinitis in AIDS. J Acquire Immune Defic Syndr 3:472, 1990
22. Carter JE, Shuster AR: Zidovudine and cytomegalovirus retinitis. Ann Ophthalmol 24:186, 1992
23. Chronister CL: Dry eye in an HIV-infected female. Clin Eye Vis Care 4:61, 1992
24. Lucca JA, Farris RL, Bielory L, Caputo AR: Keratoconjunctivitis sicca in male patients infected with human immunodeficiency virus type 1. Ophthalmology 97:1008, 1990
25. Couderc LJ, D'Agay MF, Danon F et al: Sicca complex and infection with human immunodeficiency virus. Arch Intern Med 147:898, 1987
26. Everetti A, Wong KL: Ophthalmic manifestations in AIDS. In Fujikawa LS (ed): AIDS and the Eye. Ophthalmol Clin North Am 1:53, 1988
27. Eggleston M: Therapy of ocular herpes simplex infections. Infect Control 8:294, 1987
28. Menage MJ, de Clercq E, van Lierde A et al: Antiviral drug sensitivity in ocular herpes simplex virus infection. Br J Ophthalmol 74:532, 1990
29. Grant ED: Acyclovir (Zovirax) ophthalmic ointment: a review of clinical tolerance. Curr Eye Res 6:231, 1987
30. Schwab IR: Oral acyclovir in the management of herpes simplex ocular infections. Ophthalmology 95:423, 1988
31. Young TL, Robin JB, Holland GN et al: Herpes simplex keratitis in patients with acquired immune deficiency syndrome. Ophthalmology 96:1476, 1989
32. Safrin S, Crumpacker C, Chatis P et al: A controlled trial comparing foscarnet with vidarabine for acyclovir resistant mucocutaneous herpes simplex in the acquired immunodeficiency syndrome. N Engl J Med 325:551, 1991
33. Chatis PA, Miller CH, Schrager LE, Crumpacker CS: Successful treatment with foscarnet of an acyclovir resistant mucocutaneous infection with herpes simplex virus in a patient with acquired immunodeficiency syndrome. N Engl J Med 320:297, 1989
34. Sandor EV, Millman A, Croxson TS, Mildvan D: Herpes zoster ophthalmicus in patients at risk for the acquired immune deficiency syndrome (AIDS). Am J Ophthalmol 101:153, 1986
35. Forster DJ, Dugel PU, Frangieh GT et al: Rapidly progressive outer retinal necrosis in the acquired immunodeficiency syndrome. Am J Ophthalmol 110:341, 1990
36. Margolis TP, Lowder CY, Holland GN et al: Varicella-zoster virus retinitis in patients with the acquired immunodeficiency syndrome. Am J Ophthalmol 112:119, 1991
37. Chess J, Marcus DM: Zoster-related bilateral acute retinal necrosis syndrome as presenting sign in AIDS. Ann Ophthalmol 20:431, 1988
38. Schuman JS, Orellana J, Friedman AH, Teich SA: Acquired immunodeficiency syndrome (AIDS). Sur Ophthalmol 31:384, 1987
39. Kohn SR: Molluscum contagiosum in patients with acquired immunodeficiency syndrome (letter). Arch Ophthalmol 105: 458, 1987
40. Robinson MR, Udell IJ, Garber PF et al: Molluscum contagiosum of the eyelids in patients with acquired immune deficiency syndrome. Ophthalmology 99:1745, 1992
41. Jabs DA: Ocular toxoplasmosis. Int Ophthalmol Clin 30:264, 1990
42. de Smet MD, Nussenbatt RB: Ocular manifestations of AIDS. JAMA 266:3019, 1991
43. Gagliuso DJ, Teich SA, Friedman AH, Orellana J: Ocular toxoplasmosis in AIDS patients. Trans Am Ophthalmol Soc 88:63, 1990
44. Foster RE, Lowder CY, Meisler DM et al: Presumed *Pneumocystis carinii* choroiditis. Ophthalmology 98:1360, 1991
45. Dugel PU, Rao NA, Forster DJ et al: *Pneumocystis carinii* choroiditis after long term aerosolized pentamidine therapy. Am J Ophthalmol 110:113, 1991
46. Blodi BA, Johnson MW, McLeish WM, Gass JDM: Presumed tuberculosis in a human immunodeficiency virus infected host (letter). Am J Ophthalmol 108:605, 1989
47. Edlin BR, Tokars JI, Grieco MH et al: An outbreak of multidrug-resistant tuberculosis among hospitalized patients with the acquired immunodeficiency syndrome. N Engl J Med 326:1514, 1992
48. Becerra LI, Ksiazek SM, Savino PJ et al: Syphilitic uveitis in human immunodeficiency virus infected and noninfected patients. Ophthalmology 96:1727, 1989
49. McLeish WM, Pulido JS, Holland S et al: The ocular manifestations of syphilis in the human immunodeficiency virus type 1-infected host. Ophthalmology 97:196, 1990
50. Levy JH, Liss RA, Maguire AM: Neurosyphilis and ocular syphilis in patients with concurrent human immunodeficiency virus infection. Retina 9:175, 1989
51. Davis JL, Nussenblatt RB, Bachman DM et al: Endogenous bacterial retinitis in AIDS. Am J Ophthalmol 107:613, 1989
52. Shuler JD, Engstrom RE, Holland GN: External ocular disease and anterior segment disorders associated with AIDS. Int Ophthalmol Clin 29:98, 1989
53. Nanda M, Pflugfelder SC, Holland S: Fulminant pseudomonal keratitis and scleritis in human immunodeficiency virus-infected patients. Arch Ophthalmol 109:503, 1991
54. Schuman JS, Friedman AH: Retinal manifestations of the acquired immune deficiency syndrome (AIDS): cytomegalovirus, candida albicans, cryptococcus, toxoplasmosis, and pneumocystis carinii. Trans Ophthalmol Soc UK 103:177, 1983
55. Golnik KC, Newman SA, Wispelway B: Cryptococcal optic neuropathy in acquired immune deficiency syndrome. J Clin Neuro Ophthalmol 11:96, 1991
56. Macher A, Rodrigues MM, Kaplan W et al: Disseminated bilateral chorioretinitis due to Histoplasma capsulatum in a patient with acquired immunodeficiency syndrome. Ophthalmology 92:1159, 1985
57. Specht CS, Mitchell KT, Bauman AE, Gupta M: Ocular histoplasmosis with retinitis in a patient with acquired immunodeficiency syndrome. Ophthalmology 98:1356, 1991
58. Lipson BK, Freeman WR, Beniz J et al: Optic neuropathy associated with cryptococcal arachnoiditis in AIDS patients. Am J Ophthalmol 107:523, 1989
59. Winward KE, Hamed LM, Glaser JS: The spectrum of optic nerve disease in human immunodeficiency virus infection. Am J Ophthalmol 107:373, 1989

60. Belec L, Georges AJ, Vuillecard E et al: Peripheral facial paralysis indicating HIV infection. Lancet 1:1421, 1988
61. Hamed LM, Schatz NJ, Galetta SL: Brainstem ocular motility defects and AIDS. Am J Ophthalmol 106:437, 1988
62. Friedman DI: Neuro-ophthalmic considerations. Ophthalmol Clin North Am 4:449, 1991
63. Goldberg SH, Fieo AG, Wolz DE: Primary eyelid non-hodgkins lymphoma in a patient with acquired immunodeficiency syndrome (letter). Am J Ophthalmol 113:216, 1992
64. Brodie SE, Friedman AH: Retinal dysfunction as an initial ophthalmic sign in AIDS. Br J Ophthalmol 74:49, 1990
65. Quiceno JI Capparelli E, Sadun SA et al: Visual dysfunction without retinitis in patients with acquired immunodeficiency syndrome. Am J Ophthalmol 113:8, 1992
66. Fujikawa LS, Salahuddin SZ, Ablashi D et al: HTLV III in the tears of AIDS patients. Ophthalmology 93:1479, 1986
67. Fujikawa LS, Salahuddin SZ, Ablashi D et al: Human T-cell leukemia/lymphotropic virus type III in the conjunctival epithelium of a patient with AIDS. Am J Ophthalmol 100:507, 1985
68. Salahuddin SZ, Palestine AG, Heck E et al: Isolation of the human T-cell Leukemia/lymphotropic virus type II from the cornea. Am J Ophthalmol 101:149, 1986
69. Centers for Disease Control: Recommendations for prevention of HIV transmission in health care settings. MMWR, suppl. 36(2):1s, 1987
70. Centers for Disease Control: Recommendations for preventing possible transmission of human T-lymphotropic virus III/lymphadenopathy-associated virus from tears. MMWR 34:533, 1985
71. Chronister CL, Dell WM, Ellis R: A simple guard against the AIDS virus. Rev Optom 126:75, 1989
72. Chronister CL, Russo P: Effects of disinfecting solutions on tonometer tips. Optom Vis Sci 67:818, 1990
73. Lingel NJ, Coffey B: Effects of disinfecting solutions recommended by the Centers for Disease Control on Goldmann tonometer biprisms. J Am Optom Assoc 63:43, 1992
74. Pepose JS, Linette G, MacRae S: Disinfection of Goldmann tonometers against human immunodeficiency virus type I. Arch Ophthalmol 107:983, 1989
75. Centers for Disease Control: Update: universal precautions for prevention of transmission of human immunodeficiency virus, hepatitis B virus and other blood-borne pathogens in health care settings. MMWR 37:377, 1988
76. Centers for Disease Control and Prevention: AIDS (HIV) Surveillance Report. February 1993. U.S. AIDS Cases Reported through December 1992.

20 Bacterial Disease

MARCUS G. PICCOLO

INTRODUCTION

The manifestation of bacterial disease in the human body is significantly varied. It consists of bacterial infections to any part of the body. The infectious process may be the result of virulent pathogens, surgery, trauma, or a compromised host. Normally, the immune system is well adapted to controlling transient inoculations of bacteria. This normal defense mechanism is mediated through direct cellular engulfment by phagocytic cells or the activities of immunoglobulins or antitoxins produced by the immune system. If however, the patient is compromised by a dysfunctional immune system or the presence of other predisposing diseases such as diabetes or if the inoculum is more than the immune system can control, the patient will manifest an active infection. Although predisposing factors may favor one site for an infection over another, virtually any tissue or organ system is susceptible to bacterial infection.

When infection is present in the body, the eye may become involved in several ways: as a remote site of seeding by infectious emboli (metastatic endophthalmitis), by extension of infection from tissues adjacent to ocular or orbital structures (orbital cellulitis secondary to sinus infection), or as a secondary site of infection spread by vectors such as the hand (infection of at-risk ocular tissues during upper respiratory infections).

This chapter deals with the ramifications of ocular or periocular infections secondary to established bacterial infection at some site within the body other than the eye. The factors that cause the initial systemic infections are beyond the scope of this chapter. Two broad topics are discussed: metastatic endophthalmitis and the acute orbit.

METASTATIC ENDOPHTHALMITIS

Metastatic endophthalmitis is an infection of the eye that is the result of bacterial seeding from a distant locus of infection. The manifestation of metastatic endophthalmitis and the primary site of infection can be quite varied. What is constant about metastatic endophthalmitis is the necessity for blood or lymph-borne infective emboli to be present, resulting in bacteremia. Bacteremia may be clinically asymptomatic, or it may evolve rapidly to the syndrome of septic shock.[1] Systemic findings present in bacteremia may include fever, leukocytosis, and malaise. Although endophthalmitis may manifest at the same time or before systemic findings, the patient is frequently diagnosed as septic before the onset of the ophthalmic manifestation.[2] This suggests that many of the patients with metastatic endophthalmitis are hospitalized before ophthalmic involvement.

Although the primary site of infection could be anywhere in the body, some common primary conditions or sites include meningitis, endocarditis, urinary tract infection, gastrointestinal infection, skin or wound infections, pulmonary infections, septic arthritis, and bacteremia with no remote foci of infection.[2–4] The most common sites of systemic involvement for metastatic endophthalmitis are meningitis, endocarditis, and urinary tract infection.[4] This implies that whenever metastatic endophthalmitis is suspected, a complete physical examination is mandatory, preferably by a specialist in infectious disease.

Although metastatic endophthalmitis is considered a rare condition, several case reports are available in the literature.[2–6] The following is a synopsis of two of five cases reported by Greenwald et al.[2]

CASE REPORT #1

A 15-year-old girl was hospitalized with meningitis and bilateral endophthalmitis. She had been febrile and feeling ill for 3 days. Her systemic symptoms were typical of meningitis and included purpuric skin rash, stiff neck, headache, and mental confusion. Her ocular symptoms developed on the day of admission to the hospital and included decreased vision and redness. Her prior health was good, with the exception of esotropia and amblyopia of the left eye.

A clinical diagnosis of meningitis was made in the emergency room. Ophthalmic evaluation of the right eye revealed mild conjunctival injection, a clear cornea, a small temporally layered hypopyon, normal pupils, and a normal fundus. The left eye showed marked conjunctival infection, moderate haziness of the cornea and anterior chamber, a hypopyon lying primarily on the inferior and nasal iris, and immobility of the pupil. The left fundus could not be seen. Intraocular pressure by Schiotz tonometry was 17 mmHg OD and 24 mmHg OS. Anterior chamber paracentesis was performed on the left eye, and microscopic examination of gram-stained aqueous demonstrated polymorphonuclear leukocytes (PMNs) containing gram-negative diplococci. Cerebrospinal fluid (CSF) contained 9,500 white blood cells/mm^3 (95 percent PMNs). No bacteria were seen in gram-stained CSF. Cultures of blood, urine, CSF, and aqueous were negative, but countercurrent immunoelectrophoresis of urine was positive for meningococcus group C.

Treatment was begun immediately with intravenous penicillin G (3.0 million U every 6 hours). Topical 5 percent homatropine was administered to the left eye, and prednisolone phosphate 1 percent drops were added for both eyes after 2 days, but no topical or subconjunctival antibiotics were given. The appearance of the right eye returned to normal within 24 hours. The left eye gradually improved, beginning 2 days after admission. One week later, the only abnormalities were a small fibrin precipitate at the center of the anterior lens capsule and a discrete opacity in the nasal vitreous. The fundus was normal, and vision was 20/50. The patient made a complete recovery from the meningitis and was discharged after 2 weeks.

CASE REPORT #2

A 35-year-old man developed bilateral endophthalmitis while hospitalized for treatment of gram-negative sepsis. He had been well until several days before admission, when he developed fever associated with vomiting and mild abdominal pain. Systemic evaluation revealed a systolic heart murmur, hyperglycemia, a hepatic lesion on computed tomographic (CT) scan that was thought to represent an abscess and blood cultures positive for *Klebsiella pneumoniae*. Initial treatment included intravenous tobramycin and cefazolin (treatment was initiated before the recognition of ocular involvement); the organism had proved sensitive to both by laboratory report. On the third hospital day, the patient reported decreased vision in the right eye. Ophthalmic evaluation revealed mild conjunctival injection, a clear cornea, mild anterior chamber reaction, and heavy vitreous infiltration by inflammatory cells, which completely obscured the fundus. Vision was hand movements in the right eye. Examination of the left eye showed only a few retinal hemorrhages (some with pale centers). The vitreous was clear and vision was 20/25. Diagnostic aspiration of vitreous and injection of 400 μg of tobramycin plus 360 μg of dexamethasone into the vitreous cavity was performed on the right eye a few hours after the diagnosis of metastatic endophthalmitis was made. Culture of the aspirate was negative.

On the following day, the vision of the left eye dropped to finger counting. Examination findings of the left eye were similar to those in the right eye. Ultimately, the patient underwent core vitrectomy with injection of gentamicin and dexamethasone in the right eye and core vitrectomy with injection of gentamicin in the left eye. At the time of surgery, titers of the vitreous concentrations of the systemically administered drugs were assessed. Systemically administered drugs were found to be at therapeutic levels within the vitreous. The retina, which was visible at the time of surgery, was reported to be hemorrhagic and necrotic. Despite all therapeutic efforts, vision fell to light perception bilaterally and did not improve. The vitreous cleared gradually to reveal opaque white retina in both eyes. The patient recovered from his systemic sepsis after prolonged antibiotic treatment.

Classification

The preceding cases represent very different presentations and outcomes for metastatic endophthalmitis. Greenwald et al.[2] present a classification scheme that accounts for the various presentations of metastatic endophthalmitis. Their classification includes categories such as focal (anterior or posterior), anterior diffuse, posterior diffuse, and panophthalmitis. Their classification scheme is summarized in Table 20-1. A description of each of the elements within their classification follows.

Focal

Focal manifestation of metastatic endophthalmitis is the mildest form of the disease. It typically takes the appearance of whitish plaques or nodules in the iris, ciliary body, choroid, or retina. Anterior segment lesions are typically less than 3 mm in size, while posterior segment lesions are from 1 to 10 disc diameters in size. The lesions are associated with moderate-to-marked cellular reaction in the aqueous or the vitreous; however, external ocular manifestation is typically mild. Posterior focal disease may cause un-

deraction of the extraocular muscle closest to the lesion. Because of the focalization of the infection, it is likely that the inoculum is small and well contained by body defenses. This form of the disease has an excellent prognosis for full recovery with little loss of function of the affected tissues.

Anterior Diffuse

Anterior diffuse metastatic endophthalmitis typically manifests with severe generalized inflammation of the anterior segment and moderate-to-severe inflammation of the conjunctiva, mild-to-moderate edema of the conjunctiva and eyelids, but limited or no involvement of the posterior segment. Corneal edema, hypopyon, fibrous clots, and elevated intraocular pressure are the rule. Visualization of the posterior segment may be difficult or impossible because of the severity of the anterior segment reaction. In cases in which the posterior segment cannot be observed, ultrasound is suggested. Anterior chamber cultures and smears are typically positive. Vitreous cultures may become positive if the disease advances without treatment.

Table 20-1. Clinical Classification of Metastatic Bacterial Endophthalmitis

	Anterior Focal	Posterior Focal	Anterior Diffuse	Posterior Diffuse	Panophthalmitis
Orbit/EOMs	Normal	No proptosis; ± limited motility	Normal	No proptosis; ± limited motility	Proptosis; poor motility
Lids	Normal or mild edema	Normal of mild edema/ptosis	Mild–moderate edema	Mild–moderate edema/ptosis	Marked edema/ptosis
Conjunctiva	Mild–moderate reaction	Normal or mild reaction	Moderate–marked reaction	Mild–marked reaction	Marked reaction
Cornea	Mild–moderate haze	Clear ± precipitates	Moderate–marked haze	Clear to mild haze ± precipitates	Moderate–marked haze
Anterior chamber	Moderate–marked reaction ± hypopyon	Mild–moderate reaction ± hypopyon	Marked reaction + hypopyon	Mild–marked reaction ± hypopyon	Marked reaction + hypopyon
Iris/pupil	Microabscess; poor movement; ± late synechiae	Normal or mildly limited movement; no synechiae	Poorly seen; no movement; ± late synechiae	Mild–markedly limited movement; ± late synechiae	Poorly seen; no movement
Viteous	Poorly seen; ± anterior opacity – posterior echoes	Moderate–marked cells; moderate haze	Poorly seen; ± anterior opacities – posterior echoes	Marked cells; totally opaque + posterior echoes	Poorly seen; totally opaque + posterior echoes
Fundus (when seen)	Normal	Discrete lesion; normal areas	Normal	White retina; ± emboli	Necrotic retina pathologically
Tension	Normal–high	Low–normal	Typically high	Low–high	Typically high
Prognosis	Excellent	Good	Good	Poor	Very poor

(From Greenwald et al.,[2] with permission.)

Anterior diffuse metastatic endophthalmitis is likely the result of extensive bacterial seeding to the anterior segment. Some combination of the lens–iris barrier, the forward flow of aqueous, the presence of a fibrin clot, or synechia likely may prevent or slow the posterior spread of infection in the eye. Case 1 is an example of this type of presentation.

This form of the disease typically has a good prognosis and rarely results in blindness if recognized and managed early. Potential sequelae are persistent corneal edema, synechia formation, glaucoma, or cataract.

Posterior Diffuse

Posterior diffuse metastatic endophthalmitis manifests as intense inflammation of the vitreous such that the retina is unobservable. Case 2 is an example of this manifestation of the disease. The prognosis is extremely poor, and recovery of useful vision is very unlikely. The anterior segment and external ocular structures may manifest mild-to-severe inflammation. Cultures of the aqueous may be negative; however, pretreatment aspirations of vitreous should be positive for the offending pathogen (the vitreous aspirate in Case 2 was probably negative because treatment was in progress at the time the sample was taken). Posterior diffuse disease is likely the result of occlusion of the central retinal artery with a septic embolus. The initial embolus likely breaks apart and proceeds downstream, further seeding sites within the posterior segment. In addition to the infectious process, ischemia is likely a cause of tissue damage. The end result is a totally destroyed retina with little or no chance of visual recovery. The evolution of the disease is very swift, often causing irreversible damage before disease recognition.

Panophthalmitis

Metastatic panophthalmitis results in inflammation of the eye and orbit, most likely as the result of primary seeding of the orbit with subsequent seeding of the globe. Marked lid edema, proptosis, and limitations of eye movements are common. The media is typically opaque, and the intraocular pressure is generally very high. Cultures of either aqueous or vitreous are likely to be positive. Other forms of metastatic endophthalmitis are likely to progress to panophthalmitis if left untreated. Blindness is the undoubted result of this manifestation of the disease. Phthisis or enucleation are very likely.

Clinical Presentation

Cases 1 and 2 represent very different presentations of metastatic endophthalmitis, with very different outcomes. Both cases had bilateral involvement, although only about 25 percent of reported cases of metastatic endophthalmitis are bilateral.[2] Certain organisms such as meningococcus, Escherichia coli and Klebsiella spp. tend to cause a higher percentage of bilateral cases.[2] Although any organism could cause a bacteremia resulting in metastatic endophthalmitis, certain organisms tend to be more likely pathogens. Gram-positive organisms such as streptococcus spp. and Staphylococcus aureus are commonly involved. These organisms tend to cause primary infections involving skin wounds or meningitis.[2] Another gram-positive organism that tends to be associated with metastatic endophthalmitis is Bacillus cereus. Unlike other organisms, when B. cereus is involved, a primary focus of infection is rarely found; however, cultures of blood and urine are likely to be positive. A strong association exists between B. cereus and intravenous injection. Therefore, this organism should be suspected whenever the patient is an intravenous drug abuser. Gram-negative organisms such as Neisseria meningitidis and Haemophilis influenzae are commonly associated with meningitis and metastatic endophthalmitis. Enteric gram-negative bacteria including E. coli, Klebsiella, Serratia, and Pseudomonas are not uncommon causes of metastatic endophthalmitis. These organisms usually are associated with infections of the gastrointestinal tract or the urinary tract.[2]

Perhaps one of the largest influences on prognosis is delay in diagnosis with inappropriate initial treatment. Several reported cases in the literature suggest that the initial diagnosis was conjunctivitis, acute glaucoma, or noninfectious uveitis.[2] The overall condition of the patient must be assessed and considered when making the initial diagnosis so that appropriate therapy may be instituted.

Treatment

Treatment for metastatic endophthalmitis is controversial. The typical treatment for primary endophthalmitis includes possible vitrectomy and intravitreal as well as periocular administration of appropriate antibiotics.[7] The use of systemic antibiotics alone is thought to be inadequate due to the blood–ocular barrier and the likelihood that adequate intraocular titers of systemically administered drugs would be too low.[3] Greenwald et al.[2] suggest that the pathophysiology of metastatic endophthalmitis differs significantly from primary endophthalmitis in that the pathogen enters the ocular tissues through the vasculature and as a result impedes the blood–ocular barrier. This results in enhancement of the ocular titers of systemically applied drugs, which is not seen in conditions where the blood–ocular barrier is intact. Greenwald et al.[2] therefore advocate the primary use of appropriate intravenous antibiotics as a first line treatment rather than intravitreal injections. Case 2 illustrates the adequate titers of systemically administered antibiotics within the vitreous before the application of local antibiotics. Also, cultures of external ocular tissues tend not to correlate with the offending pathogen cultured from intraocular cultures or blood cultures. The use of topical antibiotics therefore is not advocated. Topical steroids and cycloplegics may be of benefit, however, as illustrated in Case 1. Although the method of drug delivery, the quickness of diagnosis, and the appropriateness of the specific drug is important, the prognosis is most likely determined by the classification of the presentation. The range of outcomes varies from complete visual recovery to enucleation or phthisis.

THE ACUTE ORBIT

The acute orbit consists of any one of an array of presentations, including preseptal cellulitis, subperiosteal abscess, orbital cellulitis, orbital abscess, and finally cavernous sinus thrombosis. The cause of the acute orbit is varied. The specific presentation is influenced by the cause. In most cases, the acute orbit is the result of bacterial inoculation from purulent infections of the skin of the face or eyelids, sinuses, trauma, or surgery.[8] Many other less common causes have also been reported, including infections spreading from the teeth, otogenous infections spread via the venous sinuses, extradural and cerebral abscess, and syringing or probing of the lacrimal sac.[9] Infectious diseases such as typhoid, tuberculosis, syphilis, subacute bacterial endocarditis, and others may present as an acute orbit.[9] Although fungus infection has been implicated in some presentations (especially associated with diabetes or immunosuppression), bacterial involvement is the rule.[8] Many patients who present with preseptal or orbital cellulitis give a history of recent upper respiratory infection or sinusitis.[9] This is especially common in children younger than age 6, and in these children the most likely cause is *H. influenzae*.[8] The great majority of reported cases of acute orbit occurs in patients younger than 20 years of age.

Following is a synopsis of two of three cases reported by Noel et al.[10]

CASE REPORT #3

Four days before hospital admission, a 13-year-old boy complained of frontal headache and pain and discomfort around the right eye. On the fourth day of symptoms, the parents noted redness and swelling of the lids. The patient experienced diplopia on attempted upgaze.

Clinical findings were visual acuity of 20/20 OU, marked swelling of the lids delimited by the septum, limitation of elevation, and 4 mm of proptosis. Oral temperature was 37.8°C, and the leukocyte count was elevated. Two blood cultures were done, both of which showed no growth.

Treatment was initiated with intravenous cloxacillin and chloramphenicol, but the fever and proptosis persisted. The ocular motility became limited on abduction as well as on elevation despite 48 hours of antibiotic therapy. A CT scan showed right frontal and ethmoid sinusitis, as well as inferolateral displacement of the globe and displacement of the medial rectus. Radiologic evaluation was unable to determine whether a frank abscess existed or only inflammation of the tissues.

Because of the deteriorating clinical condition despite 48 hours of intravenous antibiotic, an external ethmoidectomy was performed. Purulent material was found and drained from the sinus; however, no pus was localized between the bone and the periorbitum. The frontal sinus was also drained. The aspirate was positive for β-hemolytic streptococcus, which was sensitive to penicillin, ampicillin, and chloramphenicol.

After a 5-day postoperative period maintaining intravenous drugs, the patient was switched to a 14-day course of oral ampicillin therapy. Two weeks after surgery, the proptosis had resolved and the ocular motility returned to normal.

CASE REPORT #4

Three days before hospital admission of a 3½-year-old girl, nasal discharge developed. One day before admission, the parents noted mild swelling of the left lower lid, which rapidly increased. Clinically, at the time of admission, the upper and lower lids were markedly swollen and erythematous. No sign of proptosis or chemosis was present. Axillary temperature was 37.5°C, and the leukocyte count was elevated.

Treatment was initiated with intravenous cefuroxime. On the following day, proptosis was evident, and abduction as well as adduction became limited. Intravenous clindamycin was added to the therapy. Forty-eight hours after admission, the child began to show improvement. She was afebrile, the swelling decreased, and the extraocular motility improved. Blood cultures taken on admission were positive for *Streptococcus pneumoniae*, which was sensitive to ampicillin, chloramphenicol, penicillin, and clindamycin. The cefuroxime and clindamycin were replaced with intravenous penicillin G. Over the next 24 hours, lid swelling, proptosis, and limitation of motility reappeared.

A CT scan revealed anterolateral displacement of the globe by a soft tissue mass adjacent to the left ethmoid sinus.

Because of the patient's worsening condition and CT findings, drainage of the left frontal, maxillary, and ethmoidal sinus was done. The periorbita was elevated with a collection of purulent material beneath it.

Postoperative therapy was accomplished with cefuroxime and clindamycin intravenously for 10 days, at the conclusion of which a 5-day course of oral amoxicillin/clavulanate was given. Two months after surgery, the visual acuity, lids, and motility were all normal.

Classification

Moloney et al.[9] present a classification scheme of the acute orbit that is based on an earlier classification by Chandler et al.[11] and Smith and Spencer.[12] The following is a description based on the classification of Moloney et al.[9]

Stage 1: Preseptal Cellulitis

Preseptal cellulitis is an inflammation of the periocular structures anterior to the orbital septum. The clinical presentation includes edema of one or both eyelids, warmth, tenderness of the eyelids, chemosis, and closure of the palpebral fissure. The condition may be unilateral or bilateral. Typically, the globe is uninvolved.

Stage 2: Subperiosteal Abscess

A subperiosteal abscess is a collection of pus between the bony orbit and the periosteum that lines the orbit (periorbita). Clinically, marked preseptal cellulitis and chemosis are observed. Asymmetric proptosis is usually present, with the displacement away from the site of the abscess. Limitation of ocular mobility may be present with diplopia in some fields of gaze. Marked tenderness of the area between the bony orbital margin and the globe in the area near the abscess may be present. Pus may extend anteriorly into the lids and may break through the skin forming a fistula. Visual acuity may be compromised.

Stage 3: Orbital Cellulitis

Orbital cellulitis is an inflammation within the retrobulbar tissues, within the orbit, enclosed by the periorbita. Clinically, marked preseptal cellulitis and chemosis are noted. Axial proptosis is present as well as asymmetric displacement if subperiosteal abscess is manifest. Other findings may include pain in the eye, ocular pain on attempted eye movement, ocular tenderness, limited mobility of the globe due to orbital congestion and edema, external ophthalmoplegia, internal ophthalmoplegia (depending on the severity of the presentation), decreased visual acuity, or blindness. In addition, other orbital structures may be involved, resulting in anesthesia of the V1 and V2 branches of the trigeminal nerve, as well as, hyperesthesia of the nasociliary branch. The intraocular pressure may be elevated.

Stage 4: Orbital Abscess

Orbital abscess represents an organization of pus within the orbit confined by the periorbita. In addition to the findings in orbital cellulitis, afferent pupillary defects may be present. Internal findings may include venous congestion and disc edema. Pus may spread forward into the lid or conjunctiva and break through to the surface.

Stage 5: Cavernous Sinus Thrombosis

Cavernous sinus thrombosis is an inflammation of the cavernous sinus. The nerves running through the sinus may be affected. Clinically, the signs are initially unilateral, but progress to being bilateral. The clinical findings may include proptosis and palsies of cranial nerves III, IV, and VI, which result in decreased ocular motility. Meningitis or meningeal irritation may be present. Dilation of the episcleral veins is a characteristic finding. Ocular motility may remain affected even after successful treatment.

This classification does not necessarily represent a progression of events. Each of the stages may present independently depending on the specific cause.

Etiology

As previously stated, the acute orbit can arise from many sources. The causes can be broadly classified as endogenous or exogenous. Exogenous sources of infection that cause the acute orbit include surgery, trauma, and infections of the skin of the middle third of the face. The pathogens involved are typically those that are found as normal inhabitants of the skin and include *S. aureus, S. pyogenes,* and other staphlococcal and streptococcal spp.[8] Chronic infections of the skin around the lids and eyes, such as impetigo, are certainly risk factors for preseptal cellulitis, and potentially for orbital cellulitis. The valveless anatomy of the venous system in this area of the face enhances the blood-borne inoculation of tissues deep to the primary infection.

Endogenous causes of the acute orbit center around spread of infection from infected sinuses or upper respiratory infection (URI). The most likely pathogens are those that normally inhabit the nasopharynx and sinuses. Examples of two of the most common potential pathogens are *H. influenzae* and *S. pneumoniae. H. influenzae* is a nonsuppurative pathogen, commonly associated with URI in children younger than 6 years of age. The method of inoculation of the orbit is usually via blood or lymph channels.[8] In addition, URI is often associated with concurrent or subsequent sinus infection. The typical pathogens in sinus infections are staphylococci and streptococci species and *H. in-*

fluenzae. Of those patients presenting with acute orbit, may have histories of chronic recurring sinusitis or asthma.[9] Although blood cultures are frequently negative, it is still recommended that they be taken to help identify potential pathogens.[13] Although anaerobic pathogens are possible, their involvement is rare, especially in children.

The spread of infection from the sinuses is most common from the ethmoidal sinus through the medial thin bony wall of the orbit (lamina papyraccea). The spread may be through natural foramina within the bone, dehiscences, or venous channels.[8] Although, this manner of spread is commonly associated with the formation of subperiosteal abscess, the formation of subperiosteal abscess is not absolute, and orbital cellulitis may develop without abscess. Other sinuses may also contribute to direct seeding of the orbit, including the frontal, maxillary, and sphenoid sinuses.[8,9,14] Infections of the sphenoid sinus, in addition to potentially causing an acute orbit, have a greater likelihood of causing meningitis and sepsis due to the deep location of the sinus.[14] The spread of infection, once it is established in the orbit, is usually anteriorly. Abscess within the orbit may rupture on the conjunctiva, whereas subperiosteal abscess is more likely to rupture onto the medial skin of the lids.[9] Although the spread of infection is usually anterior, the potential posterior spread could be devastating, causing cavernous sinus thrombosis. Cavernous sinus thrombosis has a tendency to cause greater neurologic deficits such as internal and external ophthalmoplegia, blindness, and hyperesthesia and hypoesthesia of the trigeminal nerve as well as the potential for meningitis and death.[15] An important diagnostic clue for the manifestation of cavernous sinus thrombosis is the initial presentation of unilateral signs that quickly progress to bilateral signs.

Management

The strategy for management of the acute orbit includes early identification and diagnosis, laboratory analysis of blood, nasal discharge or any presenting purulent material, immediate empiric antibiotic therapy, radiographic evaluation, including CT scans, and potential surgical exploration of the orbit with drainage of the sinuses or any found abscess. The choice of antibiotic is aimed at the most likely potential pathogens. In general, β-lactam drugs, including penicillin, ampicillin, cloxacillin, nafcillin, as well as other antibiotics such as clindamycin, vancomycin, chloramphenicol, and others are commonly used. First- and second-generation cephalosporins are also frequently preferred by some physicians. Samad and Riding[13] suggest that the use of cefuroxime (a second-generation cephalosporin) as compared with cloxacillin resulted in the necessity of fewer surgical outcomes. The authors admit, however, that those patients placed on cloxacillin may have had more advanced disease, which may have influenced a higher number of surgical outcomes. The initial means of drug delivery should be intravenous followed by a course of oral antibiotics.

If clinical improvement is not noted within 24 to 48 hours, a CT scan is recommended to help in the identification and localization of subperiosteal abscess. This information may help to guide the surgeon during an exploration of the orbit for purposes of decompression and drainage. In addition, the imaging will help identify involved sinuses, which may also require drainage. In both of the presented cases, orbital exploration and drainage of the sinuses was necessary to remove the primary focus of infection. In one case (Case 4) a subperiosteal abscess was identified and drained. Although frank abscess can be controlled with antibiotic therapy alone, the drainage of the abscess hastens the recovery and eliminates the pressure, which may cause serious ocular problems such as loss of vision secondary to optic nerve compression or stretching, proptosis, and other neurologic manifestations. In some cases, even though vision is lost during the acute episode of the presentation, it returns after decompression of the orbit and resolution of the infection.

In addition to the management of the orbit, attention must be paid to the globe. The proptosis has the potential to cause secondary problems associated with exposure. Exposure keratitis, corneal necrosis, and perforation could result from excess exposure of the cornea. Efforts must be made to maintain corneal integrity and health in addition to addressing the primary problem.

The patient presenting with the acute orbit usually requires close supervision and observation within a hospital setting. Although exogenous sources of infection can cause an acute orbit, bacterial infections of the respiratory tract and sinuses are very common primary sources of infection. Prompt diagnosis and therapy are key in decreasing the ocular morbidity associated with this presentation.

CONCLUSION

Both metastatic endophthalmitis and the acute orbit are serious vision-threatening diseases that are often treated with systemic antibiotics and surgical intervention. As optometrists begin to move into the hospital setting, they will be called on more frequently to consult on ophthalmic presentations of ill patients. Both of the diseases discussed require early recognition and prompt and aggressive therapy to decrease serious sequelae. It is of prime importance that optometrists are well able to recognize these ocular manifestations of systemic disease and participate within the health-care delivery system.

REFERENCES

1. Fishman MC, Hoffman AR, Klausner RD, Thaler MS: Medicine. 3rd Ed. JB Lippincott, Philadelphia, 1991
2. Greenwald MJ, Wohl LG, Sell CH: Metastatic bacterial endophthalmitis: a contemporary reappraisal. Surv Ophthalmol 31: 81, 1986
3. Quirk JA, Beaman MH, Blake M: Community-acquired pseudomonas pneumonia in a normal host complicated by metastatic panophthalmitis and cutaneous pustules. Aust NZ J Med 20:254, 1990
4. Hornblass A, To K, Coden DJ, Ahn-Lee S: Endogenous orbital cellulitis and endogenous endophthalmitis in subacute bacterial endocarditis. Am J Ophthalmol 108:196, 1989
5. Wang F, Wang L, Liu Y et al: Successful treatment of metastatic endophthalmitis. Ophthalmologica 198:124, 1989
6. Cordido M, Fernandez-Vigo J, Cordido F, Rey AD: Bilateral metastatic endophthalmitis in diabetics. Acta Ophthalmologica 69:266, 1991
7. Wilson FM: Basic and Clinical Science Course. Section 9. Intraocular Inflammation and Uveitis. American Academy of Ophthalmology, San Francisco, 1992
8. Jones DB, Steinkuller PG: Strategies for the initial management of acute preseptal and orbital cellulitis. Trans Am Ophthalmol Soc 86:94, 1988
9. Moloney JR, Badham NJ, McRae A: The acute orbit, preseptal cellulitis, subperiosteal abscess and orbital cellulitis due to sinusitis. J Laryngol Otol, suppl. 12:1, 1987
10. Noel LP, Clarke WN, Macdonald N: Clinical management of orbital cellulitis in children. Can J Ophthalmol 25:11, 1990
11. Chandler JR, Langenbrunner DJ, Stevens ER: The pathogenesis of orbital complications in acute sinusitis. Laryngoscope 80: 1414, 1970
12. Smith AF, Spencer JF: Orbital complications resulting from lesions of the sinuses. Ann Otol Rhinol Laryngol 57:5, 1948
13. Samad I, Riding K: Orbital complications of ethmoiditis: B.C. Children's Hospital experience, 1982–89. J Otolaryngol 20:6, 1991
14. Oktedalen O, Lilleas F: Septic complications to sphenoidal sinus infection. Scand J Infect Dis 24:353, 1992
15. DiNubile MJ: Septic thrombosis of the cavernous sinuses. Arch Neurol 45:567, 1988

Index

Note: Page numbers followed by f indicate figures; those followed by t indicate tables.